D1386467

$16/50
618 RIV

MANUAL OF
CLINICAL PROBLEMS IN
OBSTETRICS AND
GYNECOLOGY

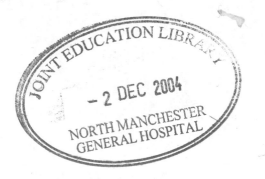

JOINT EDUCATION LIBRARY

– 2 DEC 2004

NORTH MANCHESTER
GENERAL HOSPITAL

G

FIFTH EDI

EDITED BY
MICHEL E. RIVLIN, M.D.
Associate Professor
Department of Obstetrics and Gyn
University of Mississippi Medical Cent
Jackson, Mississippi

RICK W. MARTIN, M.D.
Associate Professor
Department of Obstetrics and Gynecology
University of Mississippi Medical Center
Jackson, Mississippi

FOREWORD BY
WINFRED L. WISER, M.D.
Chairman emeritus, and Professor
Department of Obstetrics and Gynecology
University of Mississippi Medical Center
Jackson, Mississippi

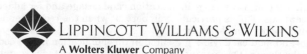 LIPPINCOTT WILLIAMS & WILKINS
A **Wolters Kluwer** Company
Philadelphia · Baltimore · New York · London
Buenos Aires · Hong Kong · Sydney · Tokyo

NCOTT

rt of it may be
, or utilized by any
ermission from the
al articles and reviews.
uals as part of their official
ed by the above-mentioned

Publication Data

obstetrics and gynecology / edited by
Martin ; foreword by Winfred L. Wiser. —

ographical references and index.
17-2201-2 (alk. paper)
gnancy—Complications.   2. Gynecology.   I. Rivlin, Michel
II. Martin, Rick W.
DNLM: 1. Obstetrics Handbooks.   2. Gynecology Handbooks.
3. Labor Complications Handbooks.   4. Pregnancy Complications
Handbooks. WQ 39 M294 1999]
RG571.M28   1999
618—dc21
DNLM/DLC   99-25744
for Library of Congress   CIP

Care has been taken to confirm the accuracy of the information presented and to describe generally accepted practices. However, the authors, editors, and publisher are not responsible for errors or omissions or for any consequences from application of the information in this book and make no warranty, expressed or implied, with respect to the currency, completeness, or accuracy of the contents of the publication. Application of this information in a particular situation remains the professional responsibility of the practitioner.

The authors, editors, and publisher have exerted every effort to ensure that drug selection and dosage set forth in this text are in accordance with current recommendations and practice at the time of publication. However, in view of ongoing research, changes in government regulations, and the constant flow of information relating to drug therapy and drug reactions, the reader is urged to check the package insert for each drug for any change in indications and dosage and for added warnings and precautions. This is particularly important when the recommended agent is a new or infrequently employed drug.

Some drugs and medical devices presented in this publication have Food and Drug Administration (FDA) clearance for limited use in restricted research settings. It is the responsibility of the health care provider to ascertain the FDA status of each drug or device planned for use in their clinical practice.

10   9   8   7   6   5   4   3   2   1

For Sarah, Katy, Janice, Joel, and David

CONTENTS

Contributing Authors xv
Foreword by *Winfred L. Wiser* xix
Preface xxi

OBSTETRICS

I. HEMORRHAGE IN PREGNANCY

1. Abortion 5
   Brian K. Rinehart

2. Ectopic Pregnancy... 10
   Randall S. Hines

3. Gestational Trophoblastic Disease 13
   Michel E. Rivlin

4. Placenta Previa 18
   Kenneth G. Perry Jr.

5. Abruptio Placentae 21
   Kenneth G. Perry Jr.

II. HYPERTENSION IN PREGNANCY

6. Essential Hypertension 29
   Garland D. Anderson

7. Pregnancy-Induced Hypertension 33
   Garland D. Anderson

8. Eclampsia.. 39
   Garland D. Anderson

III. INFECTIONS IN PREGNANCY

9. Viral Infections During Pregnancy..................................... 47
   Everett F. Magann

10. Urinary Tract Infection in Pregnancy.................................. 51
    Mendley A. Wulfsohn

11. Venereal Diseases in Pregnancy 55
    Mark H. Einstein

IV.   PREEXISTING DISEASES IN PREGNANCY

12.   Pulmonary Disease in Pregnancy 65
       James A. Bofill

13.   Cardiovascular Disease in Pregnancy 71
       Everett F. Magann

14.   Diabetes Mellitus Associated with Pregnancy 74
       Rick W. Martin

15.   Thyroid Disease in Pregnancy 78
       Brian K. Rinehart

V.   MORE HIGH-RISK PREGNANCIES

16.   Pregnancy in the Adolescent 85
       Sister Clarice Carroll

17.   Advanced Maternal Age and Management of the Grand
       Multipara. 91
       Michel E. Rivlin

18.   Multifetal Gestations 95
       William E. Roberts

19.   Rh Isoimmunization 101
       Kenneth G. Perry Jr.

20.   Postterm Pregnancy 105
       James Nello Martin Jr.

21.   Anemias and Hemoglobinopathies in Pregnancy 108
       Dom A. Terrone

22.   Preterm Labor 113
       Everett F. Magann

23.   Premature Ruptured Membranes 117
       Brian K. Rinehart

24.   Fetal Demise 122
       Garland D. Anderson

25.   Surgery and Trauma in Pregnancy 126
       Michel E. Rivlin

26.   Hyperemesis Gravidarum 130
       Sister Clarice Carroll

27.   Intrauterine Growth Restriction 134
      Dom A. Terrone

VI.   FETAL MALPOSITIONS

28.   Breech Presentation 143
      James A. Bofill

29.   Nonbreech Abnormal Presentations, Positions, and Lies 146
      Michel E. Rivlin

30.   Hydramnios and Oligohydramnios 149
      Richard L. Rosemond

VII.   LABOR AND DELIVERY

31.   Analgesia and Anesthesia for Labor and Delivery 157
      *L. Wayne Hess, Randall C. Floyd, Robert F. Fraser II,
      and Susan E. Winkelmann*

32.   Forceps and Vacuum Extraction 160
      Richard L. Rosemond and Rudolph P. Fedrizzi

33.   Cesarean Birth 163
      Steven A. Culbert

34.   Failure to Progress in Labor................................... 168
      Michel E. Rivlin

35.   Cephalopelvic Disproportion 171
      Baha M. Sibai, Farid Mattar, and Dorel Abramovici

36.   Fetal Distress in the Intrapartum Period 175
      Michel E. Rivlin

37.   Delivery of the Small and Large Infant 179
      Barbara B. Hogg and Debora F. Kimberlin

VIII.   PUERPERIUM

38.   Lactation and Lactation Suppression 185
      Harriette Hampton

39.   Postpartum Hemorrhage 189
      Baha M. Sibai, Farid Mattar, and Dorel Abramovici

40.   Puerperal Infections   194
       Marian H. Ascarelli

41.   Deep Vein Thrombosis and Pulmonary Embolism   199
       Baha M. Sibai

42.   Postpartum Depression   204
       Cheryl A. Glass and Joseph P. Bruner

IX.   ADVANCES IN OBSTETRICS

43.   Antepartum Diagnosis of Fetal Anomalies   211
       *L. Wayne Hess, Darla B. Hess, Randall C. Floyd, and
       Robert F. Fraser II*

44.   Genetic Counseling   214
       Joseph P. Bruner and Cheryl A. Glass

45.   Antepartum Assessment of Fetal Well-Being   223
       Christy Michelle Isler

46.   Laboratory Tests of Fetal Lung Maturity   226
       Neil S. Whitworth

GYNECOLOGY

X.   GENERAL GYNECOLOGY

47.   Uterine Fibroids   237
       Abraham Rubin

48.   Prolapse   241
       Michel E. Rivlin

49.   Stress Incontinence   246
       Mendley A. Wulfsohn

50.   Dysmenorrhea and Pelvic Pain   251
       Michel E. Rivlin

51.   Endometriosis   256
       Randall S. Hines

52.   Pediatric Gynecology   260
       Michel E. Rivlin

53.   Laparoscopy and Hysteroscopy   264
       Michel E. Rivlin

54.   Hysterectomy   270
       Michel E. Rivlin

XI. INFECTIOUS AND VENEREAL DISEASES

55. Gonorrhea 277
     Michel E. Rivlin

56. Syphilis.. 281
     Michel E. Rivlin

57. Genital Herpes.. 285
     Michel E. Rivlin

58. Chlamydia 289
     Michel E. Rivlin

59. Human Papillomavirus...................................... 292
     Michel E. Rivlin

60. Acquired Immunodeficiency Syndrome........................ 297
     Michel E. Rivlin

61. Vaginitis 303
     Abraham Rubin

62. Toxic Shock Syndrome 306
     Michel E. Rivlin

63. Pelvic Inflammatory Disease 310
     Michel E. Rivlin

64. Pelvic Abscess.. 314
     Michel E. Rivlin

65. Genital Tuberculosis 318
     Michel E. Rivlin

XII. CONTRACEPTION

66. Hormonal Contraception 325
     Michel E. Rivlin

67. Intrauterine Devices 330
     Michel E. Rivlin

68. Barrier and Chemical Contraceptives 333
     Marc Vatin

69. Female Sterilization 336
     Marc Vatin

XIII. INFERTILITY

70. Evaluation of the Infertile Couple 343
     John D. Isaacs Jr.

71. Treatment of Male-Associated Infertility 345
     John D. Isaacs Jr.

72. Treatment of Female-Associated Infertility 348
     John D. Isaacs Jr.

73. Anovulatory Infertility 351
     Bryan D. Cowan

XIV. HUMAN SEXUALITY

74. Adolescent Sexuality 359
     Michel E. Rivlin

75. Alterations in Sexuality with Aging, Drugs, and Disease 363
     Michel E. Rivlin

76. Inhibited Female Sexual Desire, Excitement, and Orgasm 367
     Michel E. Rivlin

77. Problems of Orgasmic Response in the Male....................... 370
     Michel E. Rivlin

78. Dyspareunia and Vaginismus 374
     Michel E. Rivlin

79. Rape, Incest, and Abuse 377
     Michel E. Rivlin

XV. GYNECOLOGIC ENDOCRINOLOGY

80. Amenorrhea 385
     Randall S. Hines

81. Hyperprolactinemia 388
     Cecil A. Long

82. Precocious Puberty 391
     Harriette Hampton

83. Hirsutism and Virilization 394
     Bryan D. Cowan

84. Dysfunctional Uterine Bleeding 399
    Bryan D. Cowan

85. Premenstrual Syndrome 402
    Michel E. Rivlin

86. Menopause 406
    Cecil A. Long

87. Gonadal Dysgenesis 410
    Randall S. Hines

88. Androgen Insensitivity and Disorders of Androgen Action 412
    Randall S. Hines

XVI.   GYNECOLOGIC ONCOLOGY

89. Non-neoplastic and Intraepithelial Neoplastic Vulval Conditions 419
    Michel E. Rivlin

90. Carcinoma of the Vulva 422
    Michel E. Rivlin

91. Cervical Intraepithelial Neoplasia 425
    Michel E. Rivlin

92. Carcinoma of the Cervix 429
    Michel E. Rivlin

93. Endometrial Hyperplasia 433
    Michel E. Rivlin

94. Endometrial Carcinoma 438
    Michel E. Rivlin

95. Uterine Sarcoma 441
    Michel E. Rivlin

96. Benign Ovarian Neoplasms 445
    Michel E. Rivlin

97. Ovarian Carcinoma 450
    Michel E. Rivlin

98. Surgery.. 454
    Michel E. Rivlin

99. Radiation Therapy 458
    Michel E. Rivlin

100.   Chemotherapy in Gynecologic Cancer 464
       Michel E. Rivlin

101.   Benign Breast Disorders 468
       Galen V. Poole

102.   Malignant Breast Disease 474
       Galen V. Poole

Subject Index.. 483

CONTRIBUTING AUTHORS

Dorel Abramovici, M.D.
Instructor, Department of Obstetrics and Gynecology, University of Tennessee, 853 Jefferson Avenue, Suite B102, Memphis, Tennessee 38103

Garland D. Anderson, M.D.
Professor and Chairman, Department of Obstetrics and Gynecology, University of Texas Medical School, 301 University Boulevard, Galveston, Texas 77555

Marian H. Ascarelli, M.D., F.A.C.O.G.
Perinatologist, Department of Pikes Peak Maternal-Fetal Medicine, Memorial Hospital, 1400 East Boulder Street, Colorado Springs, Colorado 80906

James A. Bofill, M.D.
Department of Obstetrics and Gynecology, Pitt County Memorial Hospital, Greenville, North Carolina; Department of Obstetrics and Gynecology, East Carolina University School of Medicine, 600 Moye Boulevard, Greenville, North Carolina 27858

Joseph P. Bruner, M.D.
Director of Fetal Diagnosis and Therapy, Department of Obstetrics and Gynecology, Vanderbilt University Medical Center, Nashville, Tennessee; Assistant Professor, Department of Obstetrics and Gynecology, Vanderbilt University School of Medicine, B-1100 Medical Center North, Nashville, Tennessee 37212

Sister Clarice Carroll, R.N., C.N.M., M.S.N.
Nurse Practitioner, Department of Obstetrics and Gynecology, University Medical Pavilion, Jackson, Mississippi; Assistant Professor, Department of Obstetrics and Gynecology, University of Mississippi Medical Center, 2500 North State Street, Jackson, Mississippi 39216

Bryan D. Cowan, M.D.
Professor and Director, Department of Obstetrics and Gynecology, University Hospitals and Clinics, University of Mississippi Medical Center, 2500 North State Street, Jackson, Mississippi 39216

Steven A. Culbert, M.D.
Resident, Department of Obstetrics and Gynecology, Saint Barnabas Medical Center, Old Short Hills Road, Livingston, New Jersey 07039

Mark H. Einstein, M.D.
Chief Resident, Department of Obstetrics and Gynecology, Saint Barnabas Medical Center, Old Short Hills Road, Livingston, New Jersey 07039

Rudolph P. Fedrizzi, M.D.
Chief, Department of Perinatal Medicine, Holy Cross Hospital, 1397 Weimer Road, Taos, New Mexico 87571

Randall C. Floyd, M.D.
Department of Obstetrics and Gynecology, University of Missouri, N609 Health Sciences Center, One Hospital Drive, Columbia, Missouri 65212

Robert F. Fraser II, M.D.
Assistant Professor, Department of Obstetrics and Gynecology, University of Missouri Health Sciences Center and University of Missouri School of Medicine, 301B McHaney Hall, Columbia, Missouri 65212

Cheryl A. Glass, R.N.C., M.S.N., W.H.N.P.
Nurse Practitioner, Department of Obstetrics and Gynecology, Vanderbilt University Medical Center, B-1100 Medical Center North, Nashville, Tennessee 37212

Harriette Hampton, M.D.
Faculty and Associate Professor, Department of Obstetrics and Gynecology, University of Mississippi Medical Center, 2500 North State Street, Jackson, Mississippi 39216

Darla B. Hess, M.D.
Director of Noninvasive Section, Co-Director of Fetal Laboratory Cardiology, Departments of Medicine and Obstetrics and Gynecology, Staffot Life Hospital, Health Sciences Center, Columbia, Missouri; Associate Professor, Departments of Medicine and Obstetrics and Gynecology, University of Missouri, 100 Hospital Drive, Columbia, Missouri 65212

L. Wayne Hess, M.D.
Professor and Chairman, Department of Obstetrics and Gynecology, University of Missouri Medical Center, N624 Health Sciences Center, One Hospital Drive, Columbia, Missouri 65212

Randall S. Hines, M.D.
Assistant Professor, Department of Obstetrics and Gynecology, University of Mississippi Medical Center, 2500 North State Street, Jackson, Mississippi 39216

Barbara B. Hogg, M.D.
Fellow and Instructor, Department of Obstetrics and Gynecology, University of Alabama, 618 South 20th Street, Birmingham, Alabama 35233

John D. Isaacs Jr., M.D., F.A.C.O.G
Assistant Professor, Department of Obstetrics and Gynecology, University of Mississippi, 2500 North State Street, Jackson, Mississippi 39216

Christy Michelle Isler, M.D.
Fellow, Maternal-Fetal Medicine, Department of Obstetrics and Gynecology, University of Mississippi Medical Center, 2500 North State Street, Jackson, Mississippi 39216

Debora F. Kimberlin, M.D.
Assistant Professor, Department of Obstetrics and Gynecology, University of Alabama, 618 South 20th Street, Birmingham, Alabama 35233

Cecil A. Long, M.D.
Department of Obstetrics and Gynecology, Brookwood Medical Center, 2006 Brookwood Medical Center Drive, Suite 508, Birmingham, Alabama 35209

Everett F. Magann, M.D.
Maternal-Fetal Medicine, Department of Obstetrics and Gynecology, University of Mississippi Medical Center; Associate Professor, Department of Obstetrics and Gynecology, University of Mississippi Medical School, 2500 North State Street, Jackson, Mississippi 39216

James Nello Martin Jr., M.D.
Director, Department of Obstetrics and Maternal-Fetal Medicine, University of Mississippi Medical Center; Professor, Department of Obstetrics and Gynecology, University of Mississippi Medical School, 2500 North State Street, Jackson, Mississippi 39216

Rick W. Martin, M.D.
Associate Professor, Department of Obstetrics and Gynecology, University of Mississippi Medical Center, 2500 North State Street, Jackson, Mississippi 39216

Farid Mattar, M.D.
Instructor, Department of Obstetrics and Gynecology, University of Tennessee, 853 Jefferson Avenue, Suite E102, Memphis, Tennessee 38103

Kenneth G. Perry Jr., M.D.
Director, Prenatal Diagnostic Center, Mississippi Baptist Medical Center, Jackson, Mississippi; Clinical Associate Professor, Department of Obstetrics and Gynecology, University of Mississippi Medical Center, 2500 North State Street, Jackson, Mississippi 39216

Galen V. Poole, M.D.
Director and Professor, Department of Surgery, University of Mississippi Medical Center, 2500 North State Street, Jackson, Mississippi 39216

Brian K. Rinehart, M.D.
Fellow, Maternal-Fetal Medicine, Department of Obstetrics and Gynecology, University of Mississippi Medical Center, 2500 North State Street, Jackson, Mississippi 39216

Michel E. Rivlin, M.D.
Associate Professor, Department of Obstetrics and Gynecology, University of Mississippi Medical Center, 2500 North State Street, Jackson, Mississippi 39216

William E. Roberts, M.D.
Professor, Department of Obstetrics and Gynecology, University of Mississippi Medical Center, 2500 North State Street, Jackson, Mississippi 39216

Richard L. Rosemond, M.D.
Director, Athens Maternal-Fetal Medicine, 1270 Prince Avenue, Suite 304, Athens, Georgia 30606

Abraham Rubin, M.D.
Associate Clinical Professor (Visiting), Department of Obstetrics and Gynecology, Michael Reese Hospital, 2900 South Ellis Street, Chicago, Illinois 60616

Baha M. Sibai, M.D.
Chief, Department of Obstetrics and Gynecology, Regional Medical Center of Memphis, Memphis, Tennessee; Professor, Department of Obstetrics and Gynecology, University of Tennessee, 853 Jefferson Avenue, Suite E102, Memphis, Tennessee 38103

Dom A. Terrone, M.D.
Fellow, Department of Obstetrics and Gynecology, University of Mississippi Medical Center and University of Mississippi Medical School, 2500 North State Street, Jackson, Mississippi 39216

Marc Vatin, M.D.
Clinical Assistant Professor, Department of Obstetrics and Gynecology, George Washington University, 901 23rd Street Northwest, Washington, D.C. 20037

Neil S. Whitworth, M.D.
Professor, Department of Obstetrics and Gynecology, University of Mississippi Medical Center, 2500 North State Street, Jackson, Mississippi 39216

Susan E. Winkelmann, M.D.
Assistant Professor, Department of Obstetrics and Gynecology, University of Missouri; University of Missouri Medical Center, N601 Health Sciences Center, One Hospital Drive, Columbia, Missouri 65212

Mendley A. Wulfsohn, M.D.
Clinical Assistant Professor, Department of Urology, Mount Sinai School of Medicine of the City University of New York, New York, New York; Attending Physician, Department of Urology, Adult and Pediatric Urology Center, P.A., 1100 Clifton Avenue, Clifton, New Jersey 07013

FOREWORD

This outstanding teaching volume is unique in its approach to providing in-depth information about major topics in a simple, readable fashion. The list of authors demonstrates a variety of qualified teachers and practitioners with the ability to provide crucial information in a succinct but forceful manner. The annotated references following each topic are invaluable to medical students and residents, as well as the busy practicing physician.

Michel E. Rivlin is a dedicated, highly competent teacher who constantly strives to uncover greater vehicles for learning. This volume demonstrates his interest in providing better patient care through an improved method of learning.

Winfred L. Wiser, M.D.
Chairman emeritus, and Professor
University of Mississippi Medical Center
Jackson, Mississippi

PREFACE

The objectives of this fifth edition have not changed from those of the previous editions. The first objective is to give the reader a summary of each topic. The second is to add detailed information and a focused bibliography. The third is to prepare the reader for board examinations, grand rounds, or equivalent presentations. The final objective is to provide the essential background for a clear understanding of the clinical management of obstetric and gynecologic patients.

The term "manual" suggests the liberal use of boldface print, subheadings, lists, and algorithms. The reader will not find these in this volume. It is our belief that the human mind retains information and learns best in response to straightforward, lucid storytelling, which was our goal in the presentation of the material. Certainly, the reader will readily see the skeleton behind the fleshed-in chapter separable from the individual components of the easily assimilable whole. Chapters consist of definition, epidemiology, etiology, pathogenesis, clinical features, diagnosis, therapy, and prognosis. We are satisfied that the material is equally suitable for students, residents, general physicians, and specialist physicians. In fact, health care providers responsible for the obstetric and gynecologic care of women will find the material beneficial.

We thank Dr. John C. Morrison for placing the facilities of his department at our disposal, the Vicksburg Hospital Medical Foundation for its continuing support, and Lippincott Williams & Wilkins for its publishing expertise. In addition, thanks to Dr. Winfred L. Wiser for providing the foreword, and to Gail Head, Vickie Moore, and Rochella Simpson for typing the manuscript.

OBSTETRICS

I. HEMORRHAGE IN PREGNANCY

1. ABORTION

Brian K. Rinehart

Abortion is defined as the termination of pregnancy prior to neonatal viability and may be either spontaneous or induced. Neonatal viability may be defined by a number of means, but gestational age of 24 weeks or fetal weight of 500 g is often used. Spontaneous abortion is more commonly referred to as a *miscarriage*. The term applies to gestations that spontaneously abort prior to 20 weeks' gestation. Elective or therapeutic abortion is the termination of pregnancy by medical intervention.

The incidence of spontaneous abortion in clinically recognized pregnancy is between 15% and 22%, and the incidence of unrecognized abortion may be as high as 40%–50%. Therefore, spontaneous abortion is a common occurrence in human reproduction. Spontaneous abortion usually occurs prior to 8 weeks' gestation, with only 3% of viable pregnancies being lost after 8 weeks. After 16 weeks' gestation, only 1% of viable pregnancies will abort. As maternal age increases, the incidence of spontaneous abortion increases and doubles between 20 and 40 years of age. Pregnancies that do abort have usually undergone fetal demise several weeks before the onset of clinical symptoms.

There are numerous etiologies that contribute to the rate of spontaneous abortion in humans. The most common of these is chromosomal aneuploidy. The incidence of chromosomal anomalies in fetuses that abort is approximately 50%, and the majority of these have autosomal trisomies (22%). The most common trisomy is of autosome 16 (7%). Monosomy X (45, X) (8%) is the single most common chromosomal anomaly found in abortuses. Other chromosomal abnormalities that contribute to the incidence of spontaneous abortion include triploidy (7%), Robertsonian and reciprocal translocations (5%), and chromosomal mosaicism (1%). Other contributing factors include medical diseases such as systemic lupus erythematosis, diabetes mellitus, and thyroid disease. Luteal phase defect remains controversial as a cause of recurrent abortion. Antiphospholipid antibody syndrome has also been implicated as a cause. Asherman's syndrome (intrauterine synechiae), uterine malformation, and incompetent cervix have all been shown to be associated with an increased risk of spontaneous abortion.

Habitual or recurrent abortion is defined as the occurrence of three or more spontaneous abortions without a live birth. The incidence of habitual abortion is 0.3%–0.4% for the general population. The incidence of a fourth spontaneous abortion occurring in these patients is only 25%–30%. Habitual aborters should undergo an evaluation which includes a complete history and physical, thyroid-stimulating hormone (TSH), mid-luteal phase serum progesterone measurement, evaluation for evidence of diabetes, and a hysterosalpingogram or hysterosonography to rule out Asherman's syndrome and uterine malformation. Patients should also be screened for evidence of anticardiolipin antibodies and lupus anticoagulant. Chromosomal analysis of the patient and her partner should be performed if the earlier tests are normal.

Spontaneous abortion may be classified by clinical presentation. Missed abortion is defined as intrauterine fetal demise prior to 20 weeks' gestation or 500 g fetal weight without clinical symptoms. The utility of this terminology is limited, since in most patients with spontaneous abortion fetal demise occurs several weeks before the onset of symptoms; therefore, all spontaneous abortions are missed abortions at some point in time. Inevitable abortion is the occurrence of vaginal bleeding and cervical dilation prior to embryonic or fetal demise. Incomplete abortion occurs when only a portion of the products of conception are spontaneously expelled.

Elective or therapeutic abortion is the intentional termination of pregnancy prior to fetal viability. Prior to 1973, abortion was illegal in the United States. Currently, approximately 1.6 million pregnancy terminations are performed annually in the United States. Ninety percent of all abortions are performed in the first trimester (the average gestational age being 8–9 weeks). Sixty percent of all abortions are provided to women younger than 25 years of age, and the highest rate of abortion (39%–50%) is among teenagers. Approximately 35% of patients undergoing termination of pregnancy have had a prior therapeutic abortion (70%, one prior abortion; 22%, two prior abortions; 8%, three or more prior abortions).

Induced abortion may be carried out by a number of medical or surgical means. Postcoital contraception has become more widely available in recent years, and the ingestion of approximately 100 µg of ethinyl estradiol in the form of a combined oral contraceptive within the first 72 hours after intercourse, with repetition of the dose in 12 hours, has been successful in interrupting pregnancy 75% of the time. Mifepristone (RU-486) is a progesterone receptor antagonist which can induce abortion in 85% of patients who ingest a single dose at up to 5 weeks' gestation. The addition of a prostaglandin E_1 (PGE$_1$) or a PGE$_2$ analogue will increase the efficacy of RU-486 to approximately 95%. RU-486 is currently unavailable in the United States. The combination of methotrexate and misoprostol has also been used in early first-trimester gestations. Misoprostol, a PGE analogue, can also be used as a single agent for medical induction of abortion in the first and second trimesters and has been used to cause expulsion of retained products of conception in incomplete abortion.

Common methods of medically inducing abortion in the second trimester include the use of vaginal PGE$_2$ suppositories and the intraamniotic injection of hypertonic saline, prostaglandin $F_{2\alpha}$, or a combination of urea and prostaglandin $F_{2\alpha}$. The efficacy of these methods can be increased by the addition of mechanical cervical dilators such as laminaria or other hygroscopic cervical dilators. High-dose pitocin protocols for the induction of second-trimester pregnancy termination have also been described. Hypernatremia may occur after intraamniotic hypertonic saline injection, and water intoxication is a rare complication of high-dose oxytocin.

Surgical pregnancy termination may be performed in the first or second trimester. Dilation and curettage involves the evacuation of the uterus by a combination of suction and sharp curettage, and may be performed between 8 and 12 weeks' gestation. Dilation and evacuation involves the use of any of a number of specialized forceps to disarticulate the fetus in addition to applying suction and sharp curettage. This may be performed after 12 weeks' gestation. Dilation and evacuation by an experienced practitioner is the safest means of second-trimester pregnancy termination.

Multiple pregnancy reduction is the termination of one or more gestations in a multifetal gestation. This procedure is performed by the injection of 2–3 mEq of KCl into the fetal thorax in order to reduce the risk of preterm delivery in higher-order multifetal gestations. The fetus injected is commonly the most accessible fetus, unless one or more of the fetuses has obvious anomalies. Risks of this procedure include bleeding, infection, and loss of the other fetuses.

Complications after pregnancy termination are relatively rare. The maternal mortality rate after elective abortion was 0.4 per 100,000 cases in 1987 as compared to 4.1 per 100,000 in 1972. This can be compared with the maternal mortality rate of 9 per 100,000 live births in 1995. As gestational age increases, and maternal age and parity increases, the risk of maternal mortality increases. The procedure-specific mortality rate for dilation and curettage is 0.5 per 100,000 cases, and the risk of maternal mortality increases by sixfold for dilation and evacuation, 13-fold for instillation methods, and 95-fold for hysterotomy/hysterectomy. Anesthesia complications were implicated in 29% of these deaths between 1983 and 1987, with pulmonary embolism, infection, and hemorrhage also contributing.

Complications of abortion can be divided into immediate and delayed types. The immediate complications include hemorrhage, uterine perforation, cervical laceration, hematometra, and vasovagal reaction. Hemorrhage requiring blood transfusion occurs more frequently with instillation methods of abortion when compared to dilation and curettage or dilation and evacuation. Uterine perforation occurs in 0.2–2.0 per 100 cases. The most common site of perforation is the uterine fundus and up to 90% of these may go undetected. When fundal perforation occurs and there is no evidence of bowel injury, the procedure may be completed under ultrasound guidance. Perforation of the uterus laterally is more likely to cause significant bleeding. Bleeding from cervical lacerations can often be controlled by suture ligature at three and nine o'clock to control bleeding from the cervical branch of the uterine artery.

Late complications of pregnancy termination include retained products of conception, infection, and continuation of pregnancy. Incomplete abortion often presents with vaginal bleeding and a soft, tender, globular uterus. Repeat dilation and curettage can be used to remove the remaining products of conception. Infection occurs in less than 1% of patients undergoing dilation and curettage, 1.5% of patients undergoing dilation and evacuation, and 5% of patients undergoing intraamniotic instillation of prostaglandins or hypertonic saline. Continuation of pregnancy is a rare complication and may be more likely in patients who have had an early first-trimester termination. Septic abortion may follow either spontaneous or therapeutic abortion. The mortality rate for these patients is between 0.4 and 0.6 per 100,000. Escherichia coli, Bacteroides fragilis, and the gram-positive cocci are commonly involved. The infection may progress from involving the products of conception to the uterus, the adnexa, and then to generalized sepsis. Treatment involves rapid evaluation with a complete blood count (CBC), urinalysis, and electrolyte panel, as well as coagulation panel, chest x-ray, and blood cultures in septic-appearing patients. Treatment includes fluid resuscitation, broad spectrum antibiotics (ampicillin, gentamycin, and clindamycin or an equivalent regimen), and evacuation of the uterus after achieving therapeutic serum levels of antibiotics. Uterine evacuation can usually be performed by dilation and curettage or dilation and evacuation, but hysterectomy will sometimes be necessary. Patients with septic abortion should be closely monitored for signs of renal failure, disseminated intravascular coagulation, septic shock, and adult respiratory distress syndrome.

Spontaneous abortion is a significant problem in human reproduction, and elective pregnancy termination continues to be a controversial topic in both medicine and society. The ability to successfully manage these entities and the associated complications remains important for any physician who cares for reproductive age women.

General
1. Edmonds DK, et al. Early embryonic mortality in women. *Fertil Steril* 1982; 38:447.
   Before 12 weeks of pregnancy, 61.9% of conceptuses will be lost. Most of these losses (91.7%) occur subclinically without the knowledge of the mother.
2. Rock JA, Zacur HA. The clinical management of repeated early pregnancy wastage. *Fertil Steril* 1983;39:12.
   A good review with an extensive bibliography.
3. Castadot RG. Pregnancy termination: techniques, risks, and complications and their management. *Fertil Steril* 1986;45:1.
   Review of the standard techniques with an excellent list of references.
4. Houwert-DeJong MH, et al. Habitual abortion: a review. *Eur J Obstet Gynecol Reprod Biol* 1989;30:39.
   This is an excellent review article on habitual abortion that discusses many of the classic as well as the new studies in the literature.
5. Ryan KJ. Abortion or motherhood, suicide and madness. *Am J Obstet Gynecol* 1992;166:1029.
   The author discusses the legal history of abortion in the United States and different ethical views on the subject.

Etiology
6. Chervenak FA, et al. When is termination of pregnancy during the third trimester morally justifiable? *N Engl J Med* 1984;310:501.
   This landmark article addresses the very difficult question of when termination of pregnancy can be carried out in the third trimester.
7. Stray-Pedersen B, Stray-Pedersen S. Etiologic factors and subsequent reproductive performance in 195 couples with a prior history of habitual abortion. *Am J Obstet Gynecol* 1984;148:140.
   Blighted ovum, chromosomal abnormalities, and uterine malformation are the most common causes of habitual abortion.
8. Coulam CB. Unexplained recurrent pregnancy loss: epilogue. *Clin Obstet Gynecol* 1986;29:999.

This summarizes the relative frequency of the established causes of this complex problem and suggests appropriate tests for its evaluation.

9. Mishell DR Jr. Recurrent abortion. *J Reprod Med* 1993;38:250.
   Most fetal causes of recurrent abortion consist of genetic or chromosomal abnormalities; most maternal causes are congenital or acquired uterine abnormalities.

10. Christian OB, Christian BS. Prospective study of anticardiolipin antibodies in immunized and untreated women with recurrent spontaneous abortions. *Fertil Steril* 1992;53:328.
    Anticardiolipin levels did not increase after the active immunization of women with recurrent spontaneous abortions. Prospectively, anticardiolipin-positive patients did not miscarry more often than did patients without this antibody.

11. Ecker JL, Laufer MR, Hill JA. Measurement of embryotoxic factors is predictive of pregnancy outcome in women with a history of recurrent abortion. *Obstet Gynecol* 1993;81:84.
    In early pregnancy, the production of embryotoxic factors predicts a subsequent spontaneous abortion; absence of these factors predicts a viable pregnancy.

12. McIntyre JA, et al. Clinical, immunologic, and genetic definitions of primary and secondary recurrent spontaneous abortions. *Fertil Steril* 1984;42:849.
    This elegant paper proposes that maternal antipaternal immunity can be related to spontaneous abortion and thus supports the use of immunotherapy to prevent pregnancy losses in certain abortion-prone women.

13. Sider D, et al. Cytogenetic studies in couples with recurrent pregnancy loss. *South Med J* 1988;81:1521.
    The lymphocyte karyotype from 232 couples with habitual abortion was studied. There was no significant difference in the incidence of chromosomal abnormalities between those having two losses and those having three or more. Because abnormalities were present in 6%, the authors recommend that this test be considered after two losses.

14. Clark SL. Bleeding during early pregnancy. *Female Patient* 1989;14:71.
    This offers an excellent clinical approach to bleeding during early pregnancy. Abortion was most common, but other important entities were included in the differential diagnosis.

Diagnosis

15. Castle D, Bernstein P. Cytogenetic analysis of 688 couples experiencing multiple spontaneous abortions. *Am J Med Genet* 1988;29:549.
    This discusses the significance of balanced translocations, inversions, sex chromosome aneuploidies, and mosaicisms in the cause of multiple abortions.

16. Scott JP, et al. Immunologic aspects of recurrent abortion and fetal death. *Obstet Gynecol* 1987;70:645.
    Mechanisms that prevent rejection of the conceptus and maternal immunologic aberrations that may cause repeated abortions are reviewed.

17. MacKenzie WE, et al. Spontaneous abortion rate in ultrasonographically viable pregnancies. *Obstet Gynecol* 1988;71:81.
    Spontaneous abortion at less than 10 weeks' gestation was up to three times higher than that at greater than 10 weeks' gestation; this may have implications when deciding on the timing of first-trimester diagnostic procedures.

18. Chervenak FA, et al. The need for routine sonography prior to late abortion. *NY State J Med* 1985;31:4.
    The need for an ultrasound study to document fetal age prior to abortion is recommended.

Treatment

19. Dicker D, et al. Spontaneous abortion in patients with insulin-dependent diabetes mellitus: the effect of preconceptional diabetic control. *Am J Obstet Gynecol* 1988;158:1161.
    The authors confirm the evidence accumulated in the recent literature that metabolic control around the time of conception and in the early weeks of pregnancy

may be the determining factor favoring abortion, above the rate in the normal population, in women with insulin-dependent diabetes mellitus.
20. Fuchs AR, et al. Prostaglandin $F_{2\alpha}$, oxytocin, and uterine activation in hypertonic saline-induced abortion. *Am J Obstet Gynecol* 1984;150:27.
   This discusses the possible mechanism of action of hypertonic saline in the induction of abortion.
21. Romero R, et al. Sonographic monitoring to guide the performance of postabortal uterine curettage. *Am J Obstet Gynecol* 1985;151:51.
   The information in this article is of particular value in the management of postabortal endometritis with retained products of conception.
22. Methods of mid-trimester abortion. *ACOG Tech Bull* no. 109, October 1987.
   Despite reductions in the percentage of mid-trimester abortions, each year in the United States more than 100,000 women obtain legal abortions at 13 menstrual weeks or more. Techniques, morbidity and mortality, and recommendations are presented.
23. Cameron IT, Baird DT. Early pregnancy termination: a comparison between vacuum aspiration and medical abortion using prostaglandin (16,16 dimethyl-trans-Δ_2-PGE$_1$ methyl ester) or the antiprogestogen RU-486. *Br J Obstet Gynaecol* 1988; 95:271.
   Compares the efficacy of these medical techniques with vacuum aspiration.
24. Ulmann A, et al. Medical termination of early pregnancy with mifepristone (RU-486) followed by a prostaglandin analogue. *Acta Obstet Gynecol* 1992;71:278.
   This study conducted in 16,369 women is the largest to date and shows that the administration of RU-486 followed by a prostaglandin analogue provides an efficient and safe medical alternative to surgical intervention for early pregnancy termination, provided that the recommended protocol is adequately followed and the contraindications to prostaglandins are respected.
25. El-Refaey H, et al. Medical management of missed abortion and an embryonic pregnancy. *BMJ* 1992;305:1399.
   The article shows that these conditions can be managed medically up to 13 weeks' gestation without the need to resort to surgery or anesthesia.
26. Henshaw RC, et al. Medical management of miscarriage: non-surgical uterine evacuation of incomplete and inevitable spontaneous abortion. *BMJ* 1993; 306:894.
   The use of antigestagens and prostaglandins may replace operative evacuation, in the treatment of miscarriage, thus freeing up surgical resources for other means.
27. Johnson N. Intracervical tents: usage and mode of action. *Obstet Gynecol Surv* 1989;44:410.
   A comprehensive review of the use of these adjuncts to cervical dilatation.
28. Jacot FRM, et al. A five-year experience with second-trimester induced abortions: no increase in complication rate as compared to the first trimester. *Am J Obstet Gynecol* 1993;168:633.
   For suction curettage at less than 15 weeks, the complication rate was 5.1% versus 2.9% with dilatation and evacuation at 15–20 weeks.
29. Jain JK, Mishell DR. How clinical studies rate abortion induction with misoprostol. *Contemp Obstet Gynecol* 1997;42(9):57.
   A good summary of medically induced abortion.
30. Winkler CL, et al. Mid-second trimester labor induction: concentrated oxytocin compared with prostaglandin E_2 vaginal suppositories. *Obstet Gynecol* 1991; 77:297.
   A retrospective comparison of PGE$_2$ suppositories with high-dose oxytocin.
31. Owen J, et al. Midtrimester pregnancy termination: a randomized trial of prostaglandin E_2 versus concentrated oxytocin. *Am J Obstet Gynecol* 1992; 167:1112.
   A randomized trial comparing PGE$_2$ suppositories with high-dose oxytocin.
32. Ho P, et al. Vaginal misoprostol compared with oral misoprostol in termination of second-trimester pregnancy. *Obstet Gynecol* 1997;90:735.
   A randomized controlled trial which demonstrates that vaginal misoprostol is more effective than oral misoprostol in induction of labor in the second trimester.

33. Chung T, et al. A medical approach to management of spontaneous abortion using misoprostol. Extending misoprostol treatment to a maximum of 48 hours can further improve evacuation of retained products of conception in spontaneous abortion. *Acta Obstet Gynecol Scand* 1997;76:248.
    Misoprostol can be successfully used to manage spontaneous abortion.
34. Zinaman MJ, et al. Estimates of human fertility and pregnancy loss. *Fertil Steril* 1996;65:503.
    A prospective observational study to determine clinical and subclinical spontaneous abortion rates in a normal population.
35. Evans MI, et al. International, collaborative experience of 1789 patients having multifetal pregnancy reduction: a plateauing of risks and outcomes. *J Soc Gynecol Invest* 1996;3:23.
    A review of an international database of experience with multifetal pregnancy reduction.
36. Bradley LD, Andrews BJ. Saline infusion sonography for endometrial evaluation. *Female Patient* 1998;23:12.
    A good review of the uses and techniques of hysterosonography.

Complications
37. Berkowitz RL, et al. Selective reduction of multifetal pregnancies in the first trimester. *N Engl J Med* 1988;318:1043.
    Discusses the practical techniques and ethical dilemmas involved in this procedure.
38. Boulot P, et al. Multifetal pregnancy reduction: a consecutive series of 61 cases. *Br J Obstet Gynaecol* 1993;100:63.
    Selective termination reduces but does not prevent early preterm labor. The procedure is of value in pregnancies with more than three fetuses and should be considered carefully for triplet pregnancies.
39. Grimes DA, Cates W Jr, Selik RM. Fetal septic abortion in the United States. *Obstet Gynecol* 1981;57:739.
    Fetal septic abortion remains an important national health problem. Reducing the patient's reliance on hazardous illegal abortions is an important means of eliminating septic abortion deaths.
40. Fackow EC, Astiz ME. Pathophysiology and treatment of septic shock. *JAMA* 1991;266:548.
    Septic abortion persists as a cause of septic shock. Newer therapeutic modalities, including immunologic interventions and pharmacologic therapies, are described. Excellent review with extensive bibliography.

2. ECTOPIC PREGNANCY

Randall S. Hines

A pregnancy in which the fertilized ovum implants on any tissue other than the endometrium is considered an ectopic pregnancy (EP). Approximately 95% of the cases of EP occur in the fallopian tube, with the majority in the ampullary (81%), infundibular, isthmic, and cornual (interstitial) segments in descending frequency. Nonoviductal EP occurs in the abdominal cavity, ovaries, or cervix, between the layers of the broad ligament (intraligamentous), or in a congenital rudimentary uterine horn. The coexistence of both an intrauterine and extrauterine gestation (heterotopic pregnancy) is extremely rare, but occurs in assisted reproductive technologies in one per 100 pregnancies. From 1970 to 1989, in the United States, EP comprised 2% of all pregnancies and led to 13% of all pregnancy-related deaths.

The destruction of the normal tubal anatomy remains the major cause of EP and is the explanation in about 50% of the cases. The histologic changes associated with pelvic inflammatory disease (PID) are found in about half of the tubes removed for EP. There is a sevenfold increase in the EP rate following documented salpingitis. Previous operation for an EP, previous tubal ligation, and conservative tubal procedures for the treatment of infertility are also important risk factors. Probably related to PID are other important risk indicators, such as age and ethnicity (i.e., a threefold increased incidence in women older than 35 years of age versus those younger than 35 and a 60% higher risk in black or Hispanic women than in white women). Although the use of oral contraceptives reduces the risk of EP by about 90%, the use of an intrauterine device (IUD) may increase the risk of EP, in that, when pregnancy does occur (<2%), about 4%–17% will be an EP. The greatest risk occurs during the first year after removal of the IUD and when the device has been in place for more than 2 years. Similarly, although less than 3% of women become pregnant after tubal sterilization, 15%–50% of these pregnancies are ectopic. Salpingitis isthmica nodosa, the microscopic presence of tubal epithelium in the oviductal wall, generally in the proximal portion, also predisposes to EP.

The other occurrences of EP are probably a result of hormonal imbalance, aberrations in tubal motility, and abnormalities in the embryo, including transmigration to the opposite tube and genetic abnormalities. Hormonal factors that have been implicated include an increased incidence of EP with the use of the progesterone mini-pill, postcoital estrogens, and the progesterone-containing IUD. Congenital tubal anomalies secondary to intrauterine diethylstilbestrol exposure are associated with a fivefold increased risk of EP. Women undergoing in vitro fertilization and ovulation induction are also at increased risk (5%), although this risk is probably related to associated tubal disease. Approximately 60% of the fetuses of EPs are malformed, and 30% have grossly abnormal chromosomal patterns. Previously induced abortion does not seem to be a risk factor for the occurrence of EP.

As with an intrauterine pregnancy (IUP), tubal gestation does not reside within the lumen but within the tubal wall. The trophoblast also invades vessel walls, so that the usual vasoconstrictive response to hemorrhage cannot occur. Embryonic death and tubal abortion are the most common outcomes of EP. Hemorrhage is frequently self-limiting, and, in some cases, a pelvic hematocele forms, composed of bowel, omentum, and dense adhesions. This is referred to as *chronic EP*.

Rarely, secondary implantation on another pelvic structure results in an abdominal pregnancy. Abdominal pregnancy resulting from primary implantation is even less common than that after secondary implantation. Cervical pregnancy occurs when the placenta attaches below the peritoneal reflection and the uterine vessels. Ovarian pregnancy is diagnosed when Spiegelberg's criteria are met: the tube is intact, ovarian tissue is present in the sac wall, and the sac is in the normal position of the ovary. Rudimentary horn pregnancy results from nidation in the atretic horn of a bicornuate uterus.

About 70% of those patients who are not diagnosed early present with the classic triad of symptoms, consisting of amenorrhea, abdominal pain, and abnormal vaginal bleeding. Symptoms of pregnancy are uncommon, whereas dizziness, shoulder pain, and syncope occur only when blood loss is heavy. Irregular bleeding stems from sloughing of the decidua, occasionally as a decidual cast. Pain is most often experienced in the pelvis or abdomen, and usually occurs at approximately 4–6 weeks' gestation. Rupture with intraperitoneal bleeding generally occurs at 6–10 weeks. Abdominal and pelvic tenderness is the most consistent sign. In only half of the cases can an adnexal mass be palpated. The uterus is enlarged in about 30% of the cases, but rarely beyond 8 weeks' gestation size. Cul-de-sac fullness, orthostatic hypotension, and other evidence of intraperitoneal bleeding may be present. The most common misdiagnoses include PID, abortion, a ruptured corpus luteum cyst, appendicitis, adnexal torsion, endometriosis, dysfunctional uterine bleeding, and gastroenteritis. Leukocytosis is found in one third of the cases of EP, and temperature elevations above 38°C are found in approximately 20%.

Another group of patients present earlier in the natural course of the disease, and this group is growing more common, such that, in some centers, more than 80% of the patients are now diagnosed before tubal rupture. This diagnostic advance has primarily followed upon the availability of quantitative assays of human chorionic gonadotropin (hCG). During the first 40 days of pregnancy, the hCG titer doubles approximately every 2 days. Failure to do so is strong evidence of abnormal gestation, either ectopic or intrauterine. The additional performance of vaginal ultrasonography greatly enhances the information supplied by the hCG reading, generally to exclude EP by demonstrating an intrauterine gestational sac (5–6 weeks), fetal pole, yolk sac, or fetal heartbeat (6–7 weeks). The level of hCG at which the sac becomes visible is referred to as the *discriminatory zone*, and many centers have reported this to range from 2,000 to 3,000 mIU/ml. (For abdominal ultrasound, this level is generally about 6,500 mIU/ml.) Caution must be exercised in applying these values because of the difference in assays. The quantitation of hCG may be reported using one of two reference standards. It is vital that the standard used be stated. The levels just given are quoted from the International Reference Preparation (IRP; 1 ng hCG = 10 mIU); the other standard is the Second International Reference Standard (Second IS; 1 ng hCG = 5 mIU). Sonography identifies a tubal gestational sac in less than one fourth of the EP cases; however, a solid adnexal mass or fluid in the cul-de-sac are highly important findings.

Uterine curettage may be helpful when the patient does not desire pregnancy and may reveal chorionic villi. The presence of decidual changes or the Arias-Stella reaction in the absence of villi is highly suggestive of EP. Culdocentesis has been used in the past to detect intraperitoneal blood via aspiration from the cul-de-sac. This test is used less frequently today. Laparoscopy is used in confusing cases, and false-positive and false-negative findings occur in 2%–5% of the laparoscopies.

Treatment of the hemodynamically unstable patient includes volume resuscitation with the administration of crystalloid and type-specific blood as needed, together with early operation. EP remains a medical emergency. Salpingectomy is the traditional treatment for large EPs or those associated with significant hemorrhage. In recent years, the use of more conservative surgical procedures has become the standard for clinically stable patients. The procedures include linear salpingostomy and segmental resection. Each may be performed via a laparoscope or by laparotomy. Linear salpingostomy is done primarily for ampullary ectopics and is typically performed by incising the tube over the pregnancy and removing the ectopic. Closure of the tube is not required. Segmental resection and later anastamosis may be performed for patients with isthmic ectopics. The laparoscopic approach is favored for all stable patients.

Several nonsurgical methods are now used in the treatment of small unruptured tubal gestations. These methods include expectant management while awaiting spontaneous regression, and may have merit in those patients with persistent low hCG levels after a conservative tubal surgical procedure for EP. Another technique is the use of chemotherapy (primarily methotrexate), which is effective in the treatment of trophoblastic disease. Methotrexate has major side effects including neutropenia and stomatitis.

To summarize the results of the various surgical and medical therapies, the following numbers have been taken from a 1997 review of the literature. The rate of IUP following linear salpingostomy is 61% with a recurrent EP rate of 15%. (Laparoscopy and laparotomy yield equivalent rates with laparoscopy requiring less hospitalization.) For patients who have the tube removed, the IUP rate is 38% and the recurrent EP rate is 10%. For patients treated with single-dose methotrexate, 84% did not require further treatment, the IUP rate was 54%, and the recurrent EP rate was 8%.

The key to proper treatment of EP is early evaluation in pregnant patients with bleeding or pain. With early intervention, medical and surgical options can be discussed, and the possibility of future pregnancy remains high.

General
1. Alexander JM, et al. Treatment of the small unruptured ectopic pregnancy: a cost analysis of methotrexate versus laparoscopy. *Obstet Gynecol* 1996;88:123.
   Initial methotrexate is a cost-effective alternative to laparoscopic salpingostomy in the treatment of the small unruptured ectopic pregnancy.
2. Tal J, et al. Heterotopic pregnancy after ovulation induction and assisted reproductive technologies: a literature review from 1971 to 1993. *Fertil Steril* 1996;66:1.
   With early diagnosis and skillful treatment, the outcome of the intrauterine pregnancy is favorable and its survival rate should increase in the future.

3. Mantzavinos T, Kanakas N, Zourlas PA. Heterotopic pregnancies in an in vitro fertilization program. *Clin Exp Obstet Gynecol* 1996;23:205.
A review of the impact of assisted reproductive technology on ectopic pregnancy.
4. Ewen S. Ectopic pregnancy. Adnexal masses. *Infertil Reprod Med Clin North Am* 1995;6:615.
An updated review of ectopic pregnancy.
5. Yao M, Tulandi T. Current status of surgical and nonsurgical management of ectopic pregnancy. *Fertil Steril* 1997;67:421.
Compiled statistics on treatment of ectopic pregnancy.
6. Goldner TE, et al. Surveillance for ectopic pregnancy—United States, 1970–1989. *MMWR CDC Surveill Summ* 1993;42(SS-6):73.
A review of the statistics of ectopic pregnancy in the United States.

---

3. GESTATIONAL TROPHOBLASTIC DISEASE

Michel E. Rivlin

Gestational trophoblastic neoplasms arise from fetal tissue in the mother and are composed of both syncytiotrophoblast and cytotrophoblast. Trophoblastic tissue produces human chorionic gonadotropin (hCG), and the amount produced correlates with the amount of tissue present. Gestational trophoblastic disease (GTD) includes hydatidiform mole, invasive mole, choriocarcinoma, and placental site trophoblastic tumor. The latter three are also referred to as gestational trophoblastic tumors (GTTs). Classification is further based on high-risk and low-risk factors, and whether the disease is metastatic or nonmetastatic. A complete hydatidiform mole occurs in one of 1,500 pregnancies in the United States. The incidence may be higher elsewhere, especially in the Far East, although these differences may be due to reporting problems. Choriocarcinoma occurs in 2%–5% of the patients with GTD; after a hydatidiform mole in half of these cases, term pregnancy in one fourth, and abortion or ectopic pregnancy in the remainder. The risk of molar pregnancy is greater in adolescents and in women over 40, but most patients are aged 25–29.

Molar pregnancy consists of two separate entities, partial and complete mole. They differ in chromosomal pattern, histopathologic characteristics, and clinical presentation. The complete mole has a 46XX karyotype in 90% of cases. The molar chromosomes are of paternal origin. In general, a haploid (23X) sperm fertilizes an ovum and then duplicates its own chromosomes; the maternal chromosomes are absent or inactivated. The remainder are 46XY, apparently resulting from the fertilization of an empty ovum by two separate sperm. Partial moles have a triploid karyotype (69 XXY or 69XYY), after the fertilization of a normal ovum by two sperm, in two-thirds of instances; the remainder have a diploid karyotype (46XX or 46XY). Diffuse swelling, absent villus vasculature, and trophoblastic hyperplasia characterize the chorionic villi in the setting of complete moles with no identifiable embryonic or fetal tissues. Partial moles exhibit focal swelling of the villi with focal trophoblastic hyperplasia, marked scalloping of the villi, and identifiable embryonic or fetal tissue. The fetuses identified with partial moles generally have the stigmata of triploidy, such as hydrocephalus, syndactyly, and growth retardation. If the fetus is normal, a twin pregnancy with a complete mole should be considered. About 25% of hydatidiform moles are partial, as shown by histologic review. Complete moles give rise to persistent GTT in about 15%–25% of cases. In contrast, a postmolar tumor develops in only 4%–9% of the patients with partial moles. Completing the spectrum of GTD is the uncommon placental-site trophoblastic tumor. This tumor is composed almost entirely of intermediate trophoblast, and, unlike the usual GTD, there is little necrosis or hemorrhage. Human chorionic gonadotropin is produced as in all forms of GTD, but at much lower levels, and the major secretion is human placental lactogen. Furthermore, unlike the other forms of GTD, the response to chemotherapy is poor, so that, when this rare diagnosis is made, hysterectomy is usually indicated because there is a definite risk of malignancy.

Vaginal bleeding is the most frequent early sign of an abnormal gestation. Anemia, hyperemesis, abdominal pain, and, rarely, the passage of grapelike vesicles are less common signs. In the setting of complete moles, one half of the patients present with a uterus 4 weeks or more larger than their dates in terms of gestational weeks. Bilateral theca-lutein ovarian cysts are present in 15%–25%. Less frequently, clinical pregnancy-induced hypertension (10%–15%) or hyperthyroidism may be seen. Patients with partial moles do not usually have these clinical features. The differential diagnosis includes ectopic pregnancy and abortion. The diagnosis is made by very high levels of hCG, the demonstration of multiple echoes that display a "honeycomb" pattern on ultrasound images, or, occasionally, histologic examination of the aborted products of conception.

Initial management consists of suction curettage performed under general anesthesia, along with uterine stimulation by oxytocin. Although usually a safe procedure, complications include hemorrhage, infection, perforation, and acute respiratory failure secondary to pulmonary trophoblastic embolization. In the setting of nonmetastatic tumors and in older women who have completed having their families, a hysterectomy decreases the risk of choriocarcinoma and the need for further therapy. With primary hysterectomy, there is only a 3% chance that further treatment will be needed, which is well under the usual 15% expected incidence rate of the need for subsequent therapy. As a result, up to one third of molar pregnancies are managed by primary hysterectomy. Routine prophylactic chemotherapy has not been shown to clearly reduce the overall risk and is not generally advocated. Follow-up consists of weekly beta-hCG titers until negative for three consecutive determinations; thereafter, this should be done every 3 months for 1 year. Because an elevation of hCG level owing to a new pregnancy would complicate follow-up, oral contraceptives should be prescribed and careful counseling is essential. Generally, patients should not conceive for at least 1 year. The risk of persistent disease is less than 0.5% if the beta-hCG determination is negative for 3 months, and one in 500 if negative for 6 months after molar evacuation. The risk of another mole in a future pregnancy is one in 60, and if two moles have occurred, it is one in six.

The probability of persistent GTD can be estimated by assessing epidemiologic risk factors, including second molar pregnancy, older age, large uterus (over 16-week size), the presence of theca-lutein cysts, or a combination of these. The diagnosis is usually made when the beta-hCG level plateaus or rises over a 2-week period, as indicated by three serial levels. Sometimes curettage may reveal the presence of a lesion consistent with choriocarcinoma or very high levels of beta-hCG may persist after curettage, a finding associated with a high risk of uterine perforation. The workup for persistent GTD includes chest x-ray studies, abdominal and head computed tomography (CT) scan for metastatic lesions, and a pelvic sonogram to rule out the existence of a normal pregnancy. In the event of bleeding or suspicion that evacuation has been incomplete, a repeat suction curettage may be considered, although there is a real risk of perforation.

Nonmetastatic GTD (confined to the uterus) is usually treated on an outpatient basis using single-agent chemotherapy consisting of either methotrexate or dactinomycin. The methotrexate course may include folinic acid rescue. Moderate nausea or vomiting occurs in 80% of patients, but severe toxicity is rare. Dactinomycin produces some alopecia, and pigmentation problems may occur. Although both are known mutagens and teratogens, there does not seem to be an increased frequency of malformations in offspring of treated patients. Once hCG has returned to normal, two or three courses should then be given to obtain a relapse rate well under 5%. If first-line therapy is unsuccessful, another first-line drug may be used, although many would then use multiple drug regimens of middle-risk toxicity such as vincristine, cyclophosphamide, or etoposide, in various combinations. Current remission rates for nonmetastatic GTD approach 100%, and fertility can be preserved in most cases. Nonmetastatic GTD is practically synonymous with postmolar trophoblastic disease seen after molar evacuation.

Low-risk metastatic GTD is a diagnosis based on the absence of high-risk criteria. Specifically, these criteria comprise liver or brain metastases, prior failed chemotherapy, an interval of more than four months from the antecedent pregnancy to treatment, pretreatment serum hCG level greater than 40,000 mIU/ml, an antecedent term pregnancy, or a histologic diagnosis of choriocarcinoma or placental-site trophoblastic tumor. Most patients with high-risk GTD have choriocarcinoma. Up to one third of the patients have no gynecologic symptoms; the rest have uterine disease with vaginal bleeding or discharge. If vaginal lesions are present, biopsy is contraindicated because of the possibility of hemorrhage. Extrapelvic masses include pulmonary (75%), cerebral, and hepatic metastases, which cause dyspnea, hemoptysis, respiratory embarrassment, severe headaches, nausea, vomiting, and neurologic symptoms. Visceral metastases may cause hemorrhage intraperitoneally or into the bowel. Magnetic resonance imaging (MRI) and ultrasound scans are important diagnostic aids. The keystone of management is the beta-hCG assay with the vital proviso that, even when hCG is no longer detected, 10^4 to 10^5 viable cells may still be present. Various prognostic staging-scoring systems are available to aid in the identification of patients at risk for treatment failure, in the hope that prompt treatment with more effective regimens may improve survival.

The management of high-risk disease entails the aggressive use of multiagent chemotherapy. The emphasis is placed on alternating non–cross-resistant drug regimens given frequently to prevent the emergence of drug-resistant clones of cells. For instance, one regimen alternates etoposide, dactinomycin, and methotrexate/folinic acid with vincristine and cyclophosphamide. From the beginning of therapy, drugs must be administered according to their most effective schedules, with nothing held in reserve for future use. Drug effects are predictable and not idiosyncratic. During treatment courses, daily blood counts and chemistries are determined. Therapy is suspended for white cell counts under 3,000, platelets under 100,000, or significant changes in renal or hepatic function. Generally, 5-day courses are given every 7–10 days for several cycles. Consideration is given to altering drug therapy if hCG levels plateau or rise, or if the metastases increase in size or number. A plateau is defined as no change in the titer in three separate assays performed over 15 days. Surgical treatment may consist of a hysterectomy, thoracotomy, or craniotomy to remove well-localized disease. Radiotherapy should be used only for the management of nonresectable disease because the responses are usually incomplete. The therapy for high-risk disease should be left to experts. Occasionally, a high-risk patient has been treated with single-agent therapy, making subsequent multiagent therapy more toxic and chances for response poor.

Complete remission is an hCG titer that remains in the normal range for 3 consecutive weeks. Cure is considered achieved if the patient is disease free for 5 years. Shadows on chest x-ray studies representing nonviable pulmonary metastases may persist for 6 months or more. Cerebral abnormalities on CT scan also persist for long periods; thus, while serial hCG titers remain normal, these changes can be disregarded. Drug resistance lies at the heart of therapeutic failure, and no active drug should remain in reserve. Early diagnosis and treatment carried out at major centers prevents low-risk patients from becoming high-risk patients.

Reviews
1. Society of Gynecologic Oncologists Clinical Practice Guidelines. Practice guidelines: gestational trophoblastic disease. *Oncology (Huntingt)* 1998;12:455.
   Although the risk for GTT after a partial molar pregnancy is of the order of one in 200, compared with one in 12 after a complete molar pregnancy, these patients still require gonadotropin follow-up to ensure that complete remission has taken place.
2. Hammond CB, Evans AC. Gestational trophoblastic disease. *Curr Ther Endocrinol Metab* 1997;6:603.
   The trend toward earlier diagnosis provides a problem for the pathologist because of the similarity that exists between the morphology of the early complete and partial mole.

3. Berkowitz RS, Goldstein DP. Recent advances in gestational trophoblastic disease. *Curr Opin Obstet Gynecol* 1998;10:61.
   Patients with persistent disease after a partial molar pregnancy usually have nonmetastatic tumors.

Etiology
4. Parrazzini F, et al. Dietary factors and risk of trophoblastic disease. *Am J Obstet Gynecol* 1988;158:93.
   The role of dietary factors has been studied repeatedly in the context of GTD because of the differences in incidence related to race and socioeconomic status. The etiology, however, remains largely unknown.
5. Fisher RA, Newlands ES. Gestational trophoblastic disease. Molecular and genetic studies. *J Reprod Med* 1998;43:87.
   Various kinds of abnormal fertilization cause different molar syndromes. Because all the chromosomes in complete moles are paternal, they are complete allografts (transplants). The expression of human leukocyte antigens by molar tissue is similar to that of the normal first-trimester placenta.
6. Di Cintio E, et al. The epidemiology of gestational trophoblastic disease. *Gen Diagn Pathol* 1997;143:103.
   Reports of a very high incidence of GTD in Asia, Africa, and South Central America may have been exaggerated due primarily to selection bias in the patients studied at university hospitals.

Diagnosis
7. Rotmensch J, Rosenshein NB, Block BS. Comparison of human chorionic gonadotropin regression in molar pregnancies and post-molar nonmetastatic gestational trophoblastic neoplasia. *Gynecol Oncol* 1988;29:82.
   Once chemotherapy is started for postmolar nonmetastatic GTD, the disappearance of hCG is the same as that of spontaneously regressing postevacuation moles. The regression curves can therefore identify those at high risk for failure of primary therapy.
8. Kohorn EI, McCarthy SM, Taylor KJ. Nonmetastatic gestational trophoblastic neoplasia. Role of ultrasonography and magnetic resonance imaging. *J Reprod Med* 1998;43:14.
   Imaging techniques are not decisive in nonmetastatic disease; with metastases, they play an integral role in diagnosis, staging, and management.
9. Fox H. Differential diagnosis of hydatidiform moles. *Gen Diagn Pathol* 1997; 143:117.
   Serial sonography in conjunction with serial hCG evaluation may occasionally be indicated, either early in the first trimester or when there is a live fetus with a focus of molar tissue in the placenta.
10. Smith ET, et al. Renal metastases of malignant gestational trophoblastic disease: the use of intravenous urography in staging. *Gynecol Oncol* 1985;20:317.
    Renal metastases are documented in up to 48% of fatal cases of choriocarcinoma. In this study, intravenous urography was a poor technique for staging, and CT scan is recommended in its place.

Complications
11. Kumar J, Ilancheran A, Ratnam SS. Pulmonary metastases in gestational trophoblastic disease. A review of 97 cases. *Br J Obstet Gynaecol* 1988;95:70.
    Beta-hCG titers should always be obtained from women with unexplained urinary, gastrointestinal, or pulmonary bleeding as well as from those with central nervous system tumors or atypical pelvic malignancies.
12. Newman RB, Eddy GL. Association of eclampsia and hydatidiform mole: case report and review of the literature. *Obstet Gynecol Surv* 1988;43:185.
    Recommends the liberal use of prophylactic antiseizure medication when treating GTD with hypertension, neurologic complaints, or other evidence of pregnancy-induced hypertension.

13. Kelly MP, et al. Respiratory failure due to choriocarcinoma: a study of 103 dyspneic patients. *Gynecol Oncol* 1990;38:149.
    The cause of respiratory insufficiency in GTD is probably multifactorial, including trophoblastic embolization, toxemia, hyperthyroidism, and vigorous transfusion therapy.
14. Goodwin TM, Hershman TM. Hyperthyroidism due to inappropriate production of human chorionic gonadotropin. *Clin Obstet Gynecol* 1997;40:32.
    Clinical hyperthyroidism occurs in a small number of patients with trophoblastic neoplasia.
15. Crawford RA, et al. Gestational trophoblastic disease with liver metastases: the Charing Cross experience. *Br J Obstet Gynecol* 1997;104:105.
    The incidence of hepatic involvement ranges from 5% to 20% of the cases of high-risk metastatic GTT. The best chemotherapeutic regimen is still undetermined.
16. Schechter NR, et al. Prognosis of patients treated with whole-brain radiation therapy for metastatic gestational trophoblastic disease. *Gynecol Oncol* 1998; 68:183.
    The combination of chemotherapy and brain radiation may cure 50%–80% of patients with brain metastases.

Treatment
17. Fisher PM, Hancock BW. Gestational trophoblastic diseases and their treatment. *Cancer Treat Rev* 1998;43:69.
    The GTDs are the prototype human tumors used in investigating the pharmacokinetics of chemotherapy because of their sensitivity to the drugs and the presence of an ideal tumor marker (hCG) that accurately reflects the tumor burden.
18. Homesley HD. Single-agent therapy for nonmetastatic and low-risk gestational trophoblastic disease. *J Reprod Med* 1998;43:69.
    Although methotrexate and actinomycin-D appear to be equally effective, the optimal single-agent has not yet been identified.
19. Bower M, et al. EMA/CO for high-risk gestational trophoblastic tumors: results from a cohort of 272 patients. *J Clin Oncol* 1997;15:2636.
    EMA/CO (etoposide, methotrexate, actinomycin-D, cyclophosphamide, vincristine) appears superior to the combination of methotrexate, actinomycin, and cyclophosphamide in the treatment of patients with prognostic scores of 8 or higher. Cisplatin is also active, and many oncologists include this agent in treating high-risk patients.
20. Newlands ES, et al. Management of resistant gestational trophoblastic tumors. *J Reprod Med* 1998;43:111.
    Salvage therapy options include surgery, the addition of platinum, and high-dose chemotherapy with autologous bone marrow transplantation.
21. Newlands ES, et al. Management of placental site trophoblastic tumors. *J Reprod Med* 1998;43:53.
    Because of the relatively poor response to chemotherapy and the inability to predict the biologic behavior of this tumor, prompt hysterectomy is recommended.
22. Soper JT, Hammond CB. Role of surgical therapy and radiotherapy in gestational trophoblastic disease. *J Reprod Med* 1987;32:663.
    The coordination of chronic aggressive multiagent chemotherapy, irradiation, and surgical intervention may be necessary in patients with GTD. Up to 25% of the deaths are due to the toxic complications of therapy in patients with resistant disease.

Prognosis
23. Berkowitz RS, et al. Gestational trophoblastic disease. Subsequent pregnancy outcome, including repeat molar pregnancy. *J Reprod Med* 1998;43:81.
    These patients can expect a normal reproductive outcome in the future if successfully treated with chemotherapy alone.
24. Wenzel L, et al. The psychological, social, and sexual consequences of gestational trophoblastic disease. *Gynecol Oncol* 1992;46:74.
    Significant levels of anxiety, anger, fatigue, confusion, sexual problems, and pregnancy concerns persist for a protracted period.

25. Goldstein DP, et al. Revised FIGO staging system for gestational trophoblastic tumors. Recommendations regarding therapy. *J Reprod Med* 1998;43:37.
    The three available prognostic classification systems are the FIGO staging system, the National Institutes of Health prognosis classification, and the World Health Organization scoring system.
26. Cole LA. hCG, its free subunits and its metabolites. Roles in pregnancy and trophoblastic disease. *J Reprod Med* 1998;43:3.
    Mean levels of free beta-hCG are 3.5-fold higher in the presence of a benign partial mole versus that in normal pregnancy, 11-fold higher in the presence of benign complete mole, and 30-fold higher in patients with choriocarcinoma.

4. PLACENTA PREVIA

Kenneth G. Perry Jr.

Placenta previa is defined as the abnormal implantation of the placenta in the lower uterine segment over the internal cervical os and accounts for approximately 20% of all cases of antepartum hemorrhage. Placenta previa is classified according to the degree of placental encroachment on the cervical os. A total placenta previa completely covers the internal os, and may be central, anterior, or posterior. In the case of a partial placenta previa, the placenta covers part of the internal os, while a marginal placenta previa just reaches the edge of the internal os. In a low-lying placenta, the placental edge is within 5 cm of the cervix but does not reach the internal os. In the second trimester, a complete previa is found in approximately 5% of all pregnancies, with more than 90% of them resolving by the time of delivery. The overall incidence of placenta previa is one in 200 deliveries at term. Because all forms of placenta previa have the potential for leading to severe antepartum hemorrhage and maternal and perinatal morbidity, management is based on the clinical presentation and not the classification.

Factors that have been associated with implantation in the lower uterine segment and placenta previa include advanced maternal age, increased parity, multiple gestations, prior uterine operation, spontaneous and induced abortions, smoking and cocaine use, and a previous placenta previa. The risk of recurrence for placenta previa may be as high as 10%–15%.

The risk of abnormal placental attachment (accreta, increta, or percreta) increases when placentation occurs in the lower uterine segment. This is especially true when a placenta previa is diagnosed in a patient who has undergone a previous cesarean section. The risk of a placenta accreta is approximately 5% in cases of previa without prior uterine surgery. This risk increases to 25% after one cesarean delivery and further increases to approximately 50% after two cesarean births.

The most common clinical manifestation of placenta previa is substantial bright red vaginal bleeding occurring in the third trimester, particularly at 28–34 weeks' gestation. This is the time prior to parturition when the lower uterine segment thins and disruption of a portion of the implantation site can occur. As many as 20% of these patients present with uterine contractions, while approximately 10% present with uterine irritability suggestive of placental abruption. The mean gestational age at the time of the first bleeding episode is 30 weeks, with 25% of the patients presenting before 30 weeks. Physical examination reveals a soft, nontender uterus, and the fetus may be unengaged in an abnormal lie, either transverse or breech. The differential diagnosis includes abruption, vasa previa, genital tract trauma, excessive show, cervical lesions, cervicitis, nongenital bleeding (rectum or bladder), and blood dyscrasias. However, one third to one half of the cases of third-trimester bleeding may remain unexplained.

Placenta previa is almost exclusively diagnosed on the basis of ultrasound findings, and a pelvic examination is contraindicated until the diagnosis of previa is excluded.

Transabdominal ultrasound is very accurate in the detection of placental location. Even so, a false-positive rate of 10% has been reported, usually attributed to an overdistended bladder or an anterior placenta. A false-negative rate of 7% has also been noted and may result from a posterior or lateral placental location that is obscured by the fetal head. Translabial ultrasonography is also useful for locating the placenta and appears to be more accurate than transabdominal sonography. In contrast, transvaginal ultrasound performed by experienced operators can confirm the diagnosis of placenta previa in almost 100% of the patients.

Clinically, the diagnosis of placenta previa can be made by palpation of the placenta through the cervix during a procedure known as a double setup. Though rarely indicated today, the use of the double setup assumes delivery is indicated, adequate blood replacement is available, and the patient is in the operating room prepared for cesarean delivery with a complete operating team in attendance. A speculum examination is performed initially, followed by a digital examination. If placental tissue is palpated, then cesarean section is performed immediately. The only indication for a double setup is when the ultrasound finding is inconclusive, the patient's condition is stable, the patient appears to be in active labor, and vaginal delivery is a consideration.

Management of the pregnancy complicated by placenta previa depends on (1) the gestational age of the fetus, (2) the maternal and fetal condition, and (3) the extent of vaginal bleeding. As with any cause of substantial antepartum hemorrhage, the mother's condition should be stabilized, external fetal monitoring begun, blood studies obtained, and blood products made available. If the vaginal bleeding persists or significant fetal distress is noted, then immediate cesarean section is indicated. If bleeding ceases and the fetus is immature (<36 weeks), then expectant management is appropriate, with modified bed rest until significant bleeding occurs or fetal lung maturity is documented by amniocentesis. The maternal hematocrit should be maintained at 30% or greater by the administration of supplemental iron or blood transfusions, or both. In those cases complicated by uterine contractions in which abruption has been excluded, tocolysis in the form of magnesium sulfate therapy may be utilized. In addition, steroids to accelerate fetal lung maturity should be administered in the gravida remote from term. Rh-negative patients are at risk for isoimmunization resulting from a fetal-maternal transfusion, and should be given Rh_0 (D) immune globulin (RhoGAM). Serial ultrasound examinations performed at 3-week intervals and weekly fetal assessments in the form of a nonstress test or biophysical profile are useful. An ultrasound examination can document normal fetal growth and show placental migration, should it occur.

If delivery becomes necessary, cesarean section is the method of choice, with the type of uterine incision depending on placental location. In general, the placenta should be avoided during delivery, thus mandating a low-segment vertical or classic incision. In the setting of a posterior placenta and a well-developed lower uterine segment, a low-segment transverse cesarean incision may be chosen with minimal attendant risk of additional blood loss. Irrespective of the uterine incision, the administration of prophylactic antibiotics is indicated.

The outcome for both mother and fetus in the setting of placenta previa is generally favorable. The maternal mortality rate is less than one per 1,000 and is most often a complication of infection or severe hemorrhage associated with placenta accreta, uterine atony, or the placenta previa itself. Preterm delivery poses the greatest risk to the fetus; however, other perinatal complications include growth retardation, anemia, asphyxia, and acute blood loss. Because of these various complications, the clinical management of placenta previa requires a team approach, with close cooperation among the obstetric, neonatal, and anesthesia personnel.

General
1. Benedetti TJ. Obstetric hemorrhage. In: Gabbe SG, Niebyl JR, Simpson JL, eds. *Obstetrics: normal and problem pregnancies,* 3rd ed. New York: Churchill Livingstone, 1996.
   A well-done overview of the clinical aspects of obstetric hemorrhage and specifically placenta previa.

2. Cunningham FG, et al., eds. *Obstetrical hemorrhage. Williams obstetrics*, 20th ed. Norwalk, CT: Appleton & Lange, 1997.
   A time-honored classic in the management of placenta previa.
3. Gallagher P, et al. Potential placenta previa: definition, frequency, and significance. *Am J Radiol* 1987;149:1013.
   A 5% incidence of second-trimester placenta previa is reported; complete forms of previa usually persist until the end of gestation versus infrequent persistence of the marginal or partial "potential placenta previa" forms.

Etiology
4. Rose GL, Chapman MG. Aetiological factors in placenta praevia—a case-controlled study. *Br J Obstet Gynaecol* 1986;93:586.
   Previous cesarean delivery, uterine curettage, and spontaneous abortion followed by uterine curettage are important etiologic factors in placenta previa.
5. Miller DA, Chollet JA, Goodwin TM. Clinical risk factors for placenta previa-placenta accreta. *Am J Obstet Gynecol* 1997;177:210.
   In women with placenta previa, advanced maternal age and prior cesarean section are independent risk factors for placenta accreta.
6. Macones GA, et al. The association between maternal cocaine use and placenta previa. *Am J Obstet Gynecol* 1997;177:1097.
   Cocaine use, prior cesarean section, previous elective abortion, and parity are associated with placenta previa.
7. Clark SL, Koonings PP, Phelan JP. Placenta previa/accreta and prior cesarean section. *Obstet Gynecol* 1985;66:89.
   Strikingly high incidence rates (25%, 50%, and 67%) of placenta accreta are to be expected when prior low-segment transverse cesarean section (1, 2, or 3, respectively) is coupled with placenta previa in the present gestation.
8. Newton ER, Barss V, Cetrulo CL. The epidemiology and clinical history of asymptomatic midtrimester placenta previa. *Am J Obstet Gynecol* 1984;148:743.
   An etiologic and epidemiologic analysis of asymptomatic placenta previa between 20 and 30 weeks' gestation as a high-risk pregnancy marker transcending considerations of bleeding alone.
9. Ananth CV, Smulian JC, Vintzileos AM. The association of placenta previa with history of cesarean delivery and abortion: a meta-analysis. *Am J Obstet Gynecol* 1997;177:1071.
   Evidence is given in this meta-analysis for the strong association between previous cesarean section, spontaneous or induced abortion and subsequent placenta previa. This risk increases with the number of cesarean deliveries.
10. Andres RL. The association of cigarette smoking with placenta previa and abruptio placentae. *Semin Perinatol* 1996;20:154.
    A review of the published literature regarding cigarette smoking and placenta previa.

Diagnosis
11. Kuhlman RS, Warsof S. Ultrasound of the placenta. *Clin Obstet Gynecol* 1996; 39:519.
    An excellent overview of ultrasound utilization for placental location.
12. Timor-Tritsch IE, Yunis RA. Confirming the safety of transvaginal sonography in patients suspected of placenta previa. *Obstet Gynecol* 1993;81:742.
    Confirms the safety of transvaginal ultrasound in the diagnosis and management of placenta previa.
13. Tan NH, et al. The role of transvaginal sonography in the diagnosis of placenta praevia. *Aust NZ J Obstet Gynaecol* 1995;35:42.
    Transvaginal sonography is more accurate than transabdominal sonography for the diagnosis of placenta previa, thus avoiding misdiagnosis and unnecessary hospitalization.
14. Dawson WB, et al. Translabial ultrasonography and placenta previa: does measurement of the os-placenta distance predict outcome? *J Ultrasound Med* 1996; 15:441.
    Translabial ultrasonography can be a useful adjunct for the diagnosis of placenta previa.

Treatment
15. Sauer M, Parsons M, Sampson M. Placenta previa: an analysis of three years' experience. *Am J Perinatol* 1985;2:39.
    A thorough retrospective analysis of one referral center's recent clinical experience (1981–1984) with central placenta previa management utilizing modern diagnostic and therapeutic modalities.
16. Silver R. Placenta previa: aggressive expectant management. *Am J Obstet Gynecol* 1984;150:15.
    Another excellent series with 4.2% perinatal mortality.
17. Gorodeski IG, Bahari CM. The effect of placenta previa localization upon maternal and fetal-neonatal outcome. *J Perinat Med* 1984;15:169.
    A well-presented institutional series of 165 gravidas from Israel, which found no association between type of placenta previa and character / timing of hemorrhage; a wealth of maternal and perinatal data highlights this article.
18. Chervenak FA, et al. Role of attempted vaginal delivery in the management of placenta previa. *Obstet Gynecol* 1984;64:798.
    The authors suggest that the double-setup finding of partial placenta previa near term can be managed by attempted vaginal delivery if blood loss is minimal during the examination and ensuing trial of labor.
19. Besinger RE, et al. The effect of tocolytic use in the management of symptomatic placenta previa. *Am J Obstet Gynecol* 1995;172:1770.
    This retrospective analysis suggests that tocolytic intervention in cases of symptomatic preterm previa can be associated with a significant prolongation of the pregnancy.
20. Wing DA, Paul RH, Millar LK. Management of the symptomatic placenta previa: a randomized, controlled trial of inpatient versus outpatient expectant management. *Am J Obstet Gynecol* 1996;175:806.
    This randomized study suggests that outpatient management of patients with symptomatic previa is an acceptable alternative in a select group of patients.

Complications
21. McShane PM, Heyl PS, Epstein MF. Maternal and perinatal morbidity resulting from placenta previa. *Obstet Gynecol* 1985;65:176.
    In cases of placenta previa, there is a significant correlation with need for neonatal transfusion, neonatal anemia, and the amount of intrapartum blood loss; respiratory distress syndrome in the neonate was the major cause of death.
22. Breen JL, et al. Placenta accreta, increta, and percreta. *Obstet Gynecol* 1977;49:43.
    An excellent clinical series of 40 patients with related placental complication.
23. Druzin ML. Packing of lower uterine segment for control of postcesarean bleeding in instances of placenta previa. *Surg Gynecol Obstet* 1989;169:543.
    A proposal is made for packing the lower uterine segment in cases of hemorrhage following cesarean section.

---

5. ABRUPTIO PLACENTAE

Kenneth G. Perry Jr.

Abruptio placentae (placental abruption) is the premature separation of a normally implanted placenta from its attachment to the uterus prior to the delivery of the fetus. It is characterized by the triad of (1) vaginal bleeding, (2) uterine hypertonus, and (3) fetal distress. Abruption occurs in approximately one in 120 deliveries and is responsible for 15% of the third trimester stillbirths. Severe abruptions are associated with an overall perinatal mortality in the range of 25%–35%.

The precise etiology of placental abruption is unknown; however, several associated factors have been noted. Maternal hypertension, whether chronic or pregnancy induced, is the most frequent condition found in abruptions and may be seen in as many as 50% of the cases. Rapid decompression of an overdistended uterus has also been implicated as in cases of multiple gestations following the delivery of the first twin or in hydramnios after rupture of the membranes. Other factors associated with placental abruption include maternal trauma, cocaine abuse, smoking, severe fetal growth restriction, prolonged rupture of membranes, chorioamniotis, and advanced maternal age. A prior history of an abruption is a significant risk factor with a reported risk of recurrence ranging from 5% to 17%. Unfortunately, there are no biochemical or biophysical tests predictive of abruption in subsequent pregnancies.

Hemorrhage into the decidual basalis with formation of a decidual hematoma is thought to initiate placental separation. Anomalies of the spiral arterioles as well as arteriolar weakness may be involved as the underlying pathologic mechanism. This separation of the decidua from the basal plate predisposes to further hemorrhage and dissection of the membranes from the uterine wall resulting in destruction and loss of placental function. If placental destruction is significant, then fetal distress and ultimately fetal death will occur. If blood dissects toward the cervix, then escape of blood into the vagina results in external hemorrhage. On the other hand, if dissection of blood is away from the cervix, the hemorrhage is said to be concealed, occurring in 10%–20% of the cases of abruption. This condition may only be discovered following delivery when examination of the placenta reveals a circumscribed depression on the maternal surface filled with a blood clot. In addition, blood may infiltrate the myometrium resulting in a Couvelaire uterus.

Placental abruptions can be classified according to the clinical and laboratory findings. Grade I or mild abruptions occur in 40% of the cases and are characterized by slight vaginal bleeding associated with mild uterine activity in the absence of maternal hypotension or fetal distress. Forty-five percent of abruptions are grade II and exhibit moderate uterine bleeding and uterine contractions without evidence of maternal shock or fetal distress. Coagulopathy, if present, is only mild. Severe abruptions, grade III, found in 15% of the cases, demonstrate severe uterine bleeding that results in maternal shock, coagulopathy and fetal death.

Clinically, the diagnosis of placental abruption should be suspected in any patient who presents with vaginal bleeding, uterine hyperactivity, and fetal distress. Even so, the signs and symptoms of placental abruption vary considerably. Approximately 80% of patients will present with vaginal bleeding, and more than 50% will have uterine contractions. Two-thirds of patients with clinically significant abruptions will complain of back pain and/or have uterine tenderness. In the absence of vaginal bleeding, uterine tone and tenderness may be more pronounced indicating a concealed abruption. Placenta previa as well as other causes of third trimester hemorrhage should be excluded. A degenerating leiomyomata, ovarian torsion, appendicitis, or any acute abdominal emergency must also be considered in the differential diagnosis.

Even though abruption is a clinical diagnosis, ultrasound may be useful, especially to rule out placenta previa as the cause of third trimester hemorrhage. The ultrasound diagnosis of placental abruption can be made with certainty in only a minority of the cases because the characteristic retroplacental hematoma is identified less than 5% of the time. Since false-positive as well as false-negative results are a problem, a negative ultrasound should not be used to exclude abruptio placenta.

Abruption is the most common cause of acute disseminated intravascular coagulopathy (DIC) in pregnancy. As many as 20% of gravidas with moderate to severe abruptions will have clotting defects. Activation of the clotting cascade is probably a result of release of thrombogenic material into the maternal circulation from the retroplacental clot. This results in an increase in fibrin-split products, hypofibrinogenemia, and prolonged coagulation with or without thrombocytopenia. Clinical manifestations of acute DIC include epistaxis, hematuria, oozing from puncture sites, purpura, and petechiae. Management of the patient with DIC includes delivery of the infant and supportive therapy in the form of volume replacement, transfusion of specific blood products, and the maintenance of cardiopulmonary integrity. Fortunately, postpartum hemorrhage is not usually a problem and oxytocin for uterine atony is usually effective.

Prompt and aggressive treatment of the patient with abruptio placentae is aimed at avoiding the complications of (1) hemorrhagic shock, (2) DIC, and (3) ischemia necrosis of vital organs (i.e., acute tubular necrosis resulting in renal failure). Vigorous blood and volume replacement with packed red blood cells and crystalloid is the initial therapy. Supplemental oxygen is indicated to decrease tissue hypoxia. A Foley catheter should be placed to monitor urine output and central monitoring should be implemented as needed. Continuous electronic fetal monitoring is useful in assessing fetal well-being. Initial laboratory studies include a complete blood count, creatinine, blood urea nitrogen, fibrin-split products, fibrinogen, prothrombin time, and a partial thromboplastin time. These tests need to be repeated every 4–6 hours until delivery and thereafter as indicated. The patient should be typed and cross-matched for 4 units of packed red blood cells. If DIC is evident then delivery of the infant is always appropriate and blood, fluid volume, and clotting factors (fresh frozen plasma or cryoprecipitate) are replaced while proceeding toward delivery. Timing and mode of delivery depend on fetal status and maternal condition as well as severity of the abruption. In general, a term pregnancy complicated by a mild abruption in the absence of fetal distress may be delivered vaginally. Amniotomy and the use of oxytocin can facilitate delivery. If, however, the fetus is immature and the abruption is mild, expectant management and the use of tocolytics in the form of magnesium sulfate are advocated by some authorities. Such conservative management protocols mandate close maternal and fetal monitoring as rapid deterioration can occur unexpectedly. On the other hand, fetal distress in a viable fetus mandates immediate delivery by cesarean section if vaginal delivery is not imminent. If a fetal demise complicates the abruption and the maternal condition is stable, then vaginal delivery should be attempted.

General
1. Cunningham FG, et al., eds. *Obstetrical hemorrhage. Williams obstetrics*, 20th ed. Norwalk, CT: Appleton & Lange, 1997.
   A premier review strengthened by decades of first-hand study and clinical observation.
2. Rasmussen S, et al. The occurrence of placental abruption in Norway 1967–1991. *Acta Obstet Gynecol Scand* 1996;75:222.
   This population-based cohort study reviews 14 years' experience in Norway with an incidence of 6.6 placental abruptions per 1,000 births.
3. Blumenfeld M, Gabbe SG. Placental abruption. In: Sciarra JJ, ed. *Gynecology and obstetrics. Vol. 2.* Philadelphia: Lippincott, 1991.
   An excellent overview of placental abruption.
4. Rasmussen S, et al. Perinatal mortality and case fatality after placental abruption in Norway 1967–1991. *Acta Obstet Gynecol Scand* 1996;75:229.
   This cohort study demonstrates the strong association between placental abruption and perinatal mortality.
5. Kramer MS, et al. Etiologic determinants of abruptio placentae. *Obstet Gynecol* 1997;89:221.
   Severe fetal growth restriction, prolonged rupture of membranes, chorioamnionitis, hypertension, cigarette smoking, and advanced maternal age are associated with placental abruption.
6. Ananth CV, Savitz DA, Williams MA. Placental abruption and its association with hypertension and prolonged rupture of membranes: a methodologic review and meta-analysis. *Obstet Gynecol* 1996;88:309.
   A meta-analysis of published studies on placental abruption that examines incidence, recurrence, and association with hypertensive disorders and rupture of membranes.
7. Higgins SD, Garite TJ. Late abruptio placenta in trauma patients: implications for monitoring. *Obstet Gynecol* 1984;63:10S.
   The importance of continuous fetal monitoring for 48 hours following severe maternal trauma is emphasized.

8. Kettel LM, Branch DW, Scott JR. Occult placental abruption after maternal hemorrhage. *Obstet Gynecol* 1988;71:449.
   Maternal trauma-induced occult placental abruption (no vaginal bleeding or uterine pain) can occur and be detectable only by continuous long-term fetal monitoring.
9. Landy HJ, Hinson J. Placental abruption associated with cocaine use: case report. *Reprod Toxicol* 1988;1:203.
   Substance abuse, particularly with cocaine, in the third-trimester appears to be associated with a significant risk of placental abruption.
10. Holmgren PA, Olofsson JI. Preterm premature rupture of membranes and the associated risk for placental abruption. Inverse correlation to gestational length. *Acta Obstet Gynecol Scand* 1997;76:743.
    Clinicians are made aware of the risk of abruption in patients with premature rupture of membranes, especially when rupture of membranes occurs in the second trimester with a history of bleeding.
11. Ananth CV, et al. Influence of hypertensive disorders and cigarette smoking on placental abruption and uterine bleeding during pregnancy. *Br J Obstet Gynaecol* 1997;104:572.
    The combined effects of hypertension and smoking had a greater influence on the risk of abruption than would have been expected based on individual effects.
12. Rasmussen S, Irgens LM, Dalaker K. The effect on the likelihood of further pregnancy of placental abruption and the rate of its recurrence. *Br J Obstet Gynaecol* 1997;104:1292.
    This cohort study cites a 4.4% risk of recurrence after a single abruption and a 19.2% risk following two.

Diagnosis
13. Nyberg DA, et al. Placental abruption and placental hemorrhage: correlation of sonographic findings with fetal outcome. *Radiology* 1987;164:357.
    Excellent review of the various sonographic findings attendant with placental abruption and how these correlate with perinatal outcome.
14. Sauerbrei EE, Pham DH. Placental abruption and subchorionic hemorrhage in the first half of pregnancy: U.S. appearance and clinical outcome. *Radiology* 1986;160:109.
    Sonographic features of placental abruption and factors related to prognosis are discussed for gravidas between 10 and 20 weeks' gestation with vaginal bleeding.
15. Mintz MC, et al. Abruptio placentae: apparent thickening of the placenta caused by hyperechoic retroplacental clot. *J Ultrasound Med* 1986;5:411.
    Apparent thickening of the placenta may be the only sonographic sign of placental abruption.

Treatment
16. Hurd WW, et al. Selective management of abruptio placentae: a prospective study. *Obstet Gynecol* 1983;61:467.
    Evaluates the place of individualized management of placental abruption and emphasizes that vaginal delivery for the less than 1,500-g fetus can be achieved safely if safeguards are built in.
17. Sholl JS. Abruptio placentae: clinical management in nonacute cases. *Am J Obstet Gynecol* 1987;156:40.
    Frequent inpatient fetal heart rate monitoring, tocolysis if indicated, and timely cesarean delivery are indicated for the nonacute preterm placental abruption.
18. Heinonen PK, Kajan M, Saarikoski S. Cardiotocographic findings in abruptio placentae. *Eur J Obstet Gynecol Reprod Biol* 1986;23:75.
    Tocographic monitor tracings associated with placental abruption are discussed as a diagnostic aid and a management tool.
19. Grimes DA, Steele AO, Hatcher RA. Rh immunoglobulin use with placenta previa and abruptio placentae. *South Med J* 1983;76:743.
    Six of 25 Rh-negative gravidas with obstetric hemorrhage from abruptio placentae or placenta previa required more than 300 μg of Rh immune globulin.

Complications
20. Clark SL, et al., eds. *Disseminated intravascular coagulation. Critical care obstetrics.* Malden: Blackwell Science, 1997.

   Placental abruption is the most common obstetric cause of acute DIC; the goals of therapy, a simple management protocol, critical laboratory tests, and important considerations are well detailed in this superbly done treatise.
21. Knab DR. Abruptio placentae: an assessment of the time and method of delivery. *Obstet Gynecol* 1978;52:625.

   Analysis of 338 cases of abruptio placentae indicated that 75% of fetal deaths occurred more than 90 minutes after admission to the hospital, and almost 70% of all perinatal mortality occurred in infants who were delivered more than 2 hours after the time of diagnosis.
22. Harris BA Jr, Gore H, Flowers CE Jr. Peripheral placental separation: a possible relationship to premature labor. *Obstet Gynecol* 1985;66:774.

   A clinicopathologic investigation that suggests that peripheral placental separation ("marginal rupture") may play a role in some cases of preterm labor.
23. Neilson EC, Varner MW, Scott JR. The outcome of pregnancies complicated by bleeding during the second trimester. *Surg Gynecol Obstet* 1991;173:371.

   Perinatal mortality is high among pregnancies complicated by second trimester hemorrhage and especially those attributed to placental abruption. The mortality rate decreased in those gestations maintained into the third trimester.

II. HYPERTENSION IN PREGNANCY

6. ESSENTIAL HYPERTENSION

Garland D. Anderson

Hypertension is one of the most common medical complications of pregnancy, with reported incidence from 5% to 10%. One third to one half of these women have essential hypertension. There is a significant increase in the rate of stillbirths, pregnancy-induced hypertension (PIH), and small for gestational age (SGA) infants in women with a mean arterial pressure greater than 90 mm Hg during the second trimester. The overall perinatal mortality rate associated with hypertensive diseases of pregnancy ranges from 8% to 15%. The majority of the increase in perinatal mortality occurs in those women who develop superimposed PIH. Women with mild to moderate hypertension who are managed without antihypertensive medication and without superimposed PIH have outcomes similar to the general obstetric population.

Differentiating chronic essential hypertension complicating pregnancy from PIH can be very difficult. All pregnant women experience a decrease in blood pressure during the second trimester because the placenta is a low-resistance system parallel to the mother's circulation. Women with mild to moderate chronic hypertension may therefore be considered to have normal blood pressure readings if seen for the first time during midpregnancy. In late pregnancy, however, when the blood pressure rises to prepregnancy levels, the hypertension may then be erroneously attributed to PIH. Superimposed PIH occurs when PIH develops in addition to existing chronic hypertension.

The diagnosis of preexisting hypertension is confirmed only if present before pregnancy or before the 20th week of gestation. Essential hypertension may be diagnosed retrospectively when chronic hypertension is present at the postpartum visit. Other clues that favor the diagnosis of chronic preexisting hypertension include (1) hypertension associated with chronic diseases such as diabetes mellitus, renal disease, or collagen vascular disease; (2) abnormal optic fundi (e.g., hemorrhages or exudates); and (3) abnormal renal function test results (e.g., blood urea nitrogen level of >20 mg/dL or plasma creatinine level of >1 mg/dL).

Other chronic causes of elevated blood pressure must be considered. Vascular abnormalities (e.g., renal vascular disease and coarctation of the aorta), endocrinopathies (e.g., diabetes mellitus, pheochromocytoma, and hyperaldosteronism), and renal disease (e.g., glomerulonephritis, pyelonephritis, collagen vascular disease with renal involvement, and polycystic disease) should be included in the differential diagnosis. A flank bruit is suggestive of renovascular hypertension, whereas coarctation of the aorta can be detected by comparing arterial pressures in the upper and lower extremities.

The greatest risk associated with chronic essential hypertension during pregnancy is the increased occurrence of superimposed PIH. A diastolic pressure of ≥95 mm Hg has been associated with increased risk of fetal death. However, it is the development of superimposed PIH that jeopardizes the mother's life. Three common signs of superimposed PIH are accelerating hypertension, new onset or worsening of preexisting proteinuria, and worsening nondependent edema. The sudden onset of headaches, visual disturbances, tremulousness, or epigastric pain may suggest impending convulsion or eclampsia. The incidence of abruptio placenta is increased in women with chronic hypertension, with a reported incidence rate that ranges from less than 1% to upwards of 10% if superimposed PIH occurs. In a retrospective review of 265 cases of abruptio placentae, the incidence rate in the total obstetric population was 1.17%, compared with 10% in women with chronic hypertension.

Early documentation of gestational age is extremely important in the management of pregnant women with hypertension. A common fetal risk is intrauterine growth restriction or being SGA. Correlation of uterine size with menstrual dates, documentation of the first fetal heart tones heard by fetoscope, and baseline ultrasound are important. Fetal growth should be evaluated by serial ultrasonography. Growth restriction in the fetus is common in patients with chronic hypertension. Serial measurements that show increases in fundal height, progressive increases in estimated fetal weight, and appropriate increments in maternal weight are also good indications of fetal growth.

Plasma volume is reduced in pregnant women with chronic hypertension compared to that in normotensive gravidas. In addition, failure of the plasma volume to expand is associated with intrauterine growth retardation and intrauterine fetal demise.

Initial evaluation of pregnant women with essential hypertension should include careful examination of the optic fundi, renal evaluation by assessment of a 24-hour urine specimen for protein and creatinine clearance, and a chest x-ray study and/or electrocardiogram if the hypertension has been long-standing or if there is any question of heart disease. There is a high mortality rate in pregnant women with undiagnosed pheochromocytoma. Therefore, should symptoms warrant, a urine metanephrine test may be useful in the evaluation of women with severe hypertension.

Preconception counseling for women with chronic hypertension is ideal. A patient with chronic hypertension and a history of severe PIH or eclampsia has at least a 50% chance of recurrent PIH, whereas the normotensive patient with a past history of severe PIH or eclampsia has a one-in-four chance of recurrence. Unfortunately, the next episode may be more severe than the prior one and occur at an earlier stage of pregnancy.

The management of a pregnancy complicated by essential hypertension is controversial. Limitation of physical activity may be helpful once the disease process (superimposed PIH) is well established; however, it has no role in prevention of PIH. If superimposed PIH occurs, other routine household duties, shopping, and exercise should be curtailed. Dietary counseling should include discussion of sodium consumption. Excess sodium may exacerbate hypertension; however, its restriction may decrease placental perfusion. An appropriate diet includes 2–6 g of table salt per day, although this is truly not a low-salt diet. Many women with mild to moderate hypertension may not require medication during the first half of gestation.

An unresolved question in management is whether there is autoregulation of uterine blood flow in humans. If there is no autoregulation, placental perfusion will vary directly with maternal arterial pressure; in this case, a reduction in blood pressure might be detrimental to the fetus. On the other hand, if there is autoregulation, a reduction in blood pressure to normal would pose no problem. European obstetricians have been more aggressive in their treatment of women with chronic hypertension by attempting to maintain diastolic blood pressure under 90–100 mm Hg, but obstetricians in the United States usually do not institute therapy until the diastolic blood pressure exceeds 100 mm Hg because of fetal perfusion considerations.

Most authorities discontinue diuretic therapy in women once pregnancy is diagnosed. Initiation of diuretic therapy is contraindicated in pregnancy, except in the rare patient with pulmonary edema or congestive heart failure. Diuretics acutely reduce placental blood flow (as measured by the placental clearance of dehydroisoandrosterone sulfate). Women with chronic hypertension who receive diuretics during pregnancy have lower blood volumes than do hypertensive women who do not receive diuretics. When diuretic use is discontinued, there is then an increase in the plasma volume. Evidence also suggests that the long-term use of diuretics leads to reduced birth weight in the infants of such mothers. Electrolyte disturbances, fetal thrombocytopenia, and neonatal jaundice are also consequences of diuretic therapy.

If diuretics are relatively contraindicated, two management questions frequently arise: (1) What is the antihypertensive agent of choice, and (2) what course is proper for the pregnant woman who is already on an established antihypertensive regimen? Methyldopa (Aldomet) has traditionally been the preferred oral medication for treatment of hypertension in pregnancy. The customary initial dose is 750 mg/day (250 mg three times a day). This may be increased to a total of 2 g daily. If higher doses are required, a second agent should be added. A currently popular agent for management of acute life-threatening hypertension in pregnancy and maintenance therapy for chronic disease is labetalol, a combined alpha/beta blocker. The initial dose is 100–200 mg, two to three times daily; the maximum dose is 1,200 mg/day. Calcium channel blockers are other popular agents for management of hypertension during pregnancy.

Nifedipine has been studied extensively in its short-acting form for use during pregnancy. The initial dose is 20mg/day in divided doses up to a maximum of 120 mg/day. The only clearly contraindicated agents are angiotensin converting enzyme–inhibitors (ACE-I). These may cause fetal renal failure and fetal death. Diastolic pressures below 90–100 mm Hg are not desirable because of possible decreased placental perfusion. Medications should be prescribed when diastolic pressure exceeds 100–110 mm Hg and systolic blood pressure exceeds 160–180 mm Hg.

Antepartum fetal surveillance should be performed including nonstress test, biophysical profile, or contraction stress test performed at least weekly beginning at 34 weeks. In women with severe hypertension, a history of stillbirths, or a suspicion of an SGA fetus, these tests should be initiated at 28–32 weeks.

When superimposed PIH occurs, convulsions should be prevented by using magnesium sulfate. Any severe hypertension (systolic pressure of >160 mm Hg, diastolic pressure of >110 mm Hg) should be controlled with the intravenous administration of hydralazine or labetalol. Once superimposed PIH is diagnosed, delivery is the only cure. Induction of labor with oxytocin is recommended, unless an obstetric indication necessitates cesarean birth. The timing of delivery is a crucial question in all high-risk pregnancies. This decision is easy when the fetus is mature and the cervix is favorable for induction. Women with mild hypertension should be delivered by 40 weeks. When there is evidence of superimposed PIH or when severe intrauterine growth retardation is suspected, it is necessary to deliver the infant, even if preterm. Fetal survival after 32 weeks' gestation is excellent.

General
1. Walker JJ, Gant NF. *Hypertension in pregnancy*. London: Chapman and Hall Medical, 1980.
   A book reviewing both the basic science aspects and clinical management. Includes a critical analysis of major diagnostic and therapeutic questions on this subject.
2. Roberts JM, Perloff DL. Hypertension and the obstetrician-gynecologist. *Am J Obstet Gynecol* 1977;127:316.
   Concise review of hypertension problems in the female patient.
3. Rubin C. Hypertension in pregnancy. *J Hypertens Suppl* 1987;5:84.
   General article that summarizes current practice principles in the management of hypertension in pregnancy.
4. Witlin AG, Sibai BM. Hypertension in pregnancy: current concepts of preeclampsia. *Annu Rev Med* 1997;48:115.
   Overall review of hypertension and preeclampsia during gestation. Summarizes recent efforts involving prediction and prevention of preeclampsia using calcium and aspirin.
5. Working Group on High Blood Pressure in Pregnancy. National High Blood Pressure Education Program Working Group report on high blood pressure in pregnancy. *Am J Obstet Gynecol* 1990;163:1689.
   An overview of the current management of hypertension in pregnancy.
6. American College of Obstetricians and Gynecologists. Hypertension in pregnancy. *ACOG Tech Bull* no. 219, 1996.
   Provides definitions and standard of care management for hypertension in pregnancy.

Etiology
7. Lindheimer MD, Katz AI. Hypertension in pregnancy: advances and controversies. *Clin Nephrol* 1991;36:4.
   The advances made and remaining controversies regarding hypertension in pregnancy are discussed.
8. Marx JL. Natriuretic hormone linked to hypertension. *Science* 1981;212:1255.
   The author proposes that excess salt in the diet may produce hypertension by causing the release of a natriuretic hormone into the bloodstream. The effect of this mechanism is outlined.

9. Page EW, Christianson R. The impact of mean arterial pressure in the middle trimester upon the outcome of pregnancy. *Am J Obstet Gynecol* 1976;125:740. *Presents a simple formula for calculating the mean arterial pressure and demonstrates that perinatal mortality increases as the mean arterial pressure increases.*
10. Hunyor SN. Vascular, volume, and cardiac response to normal and hypertensive pregnancy. *Hypertension* 1984;6:196. *Hypertension during pregnancy may blunt the normal increase in plasma volume.*
11. de Boer K, et al. Enhanced thrombin generation in normal and hypertensive pregnancy. *Am J Obstet Gynecol* 1989;160:95. *The authors studied 79 women who were normotensive compared to 24 who were hypertensive. In the former, there was an increase in the plasma thrombin antithrombin III levels and a decrease in the protein S levels, whereas in the hypertensive patients, there was a reduction in the antithrombin III and protein C levels. The authors conclude that there is evidence for a prethrombotic state in normal pregnancy that is accentuated in those with hypertension.*
12. White WB, et al. Average daily blood pressure, not office blood pressure, determines cardiac function in patients with hypertension. *JAMA* 1989;261:873. *In this study, 720 patients underwent ambulatory blood pressure monitoring, and, when their readings at home were compared to those in the office, it was found that a significant portion were hypertensive only while visiting the physician.*

Diagnosis
13. Sibai BM, Anderson GD. Clues from blood volume changes in hypertensive pregnancies. *Contemp Obstet Gynecol* 1983;21:241. *Plasma volume determinations are useful in identifying babies at risk for intrauterine growth retardation and intrauterine fetal demise.*
14. Nicholas WC, et al. Does blood pressure cuff size make a difference in blood pressure readings? *J Miss State Med Assoc* 1985;26:31. *A large error in blood pressure measurement can result from using an inappropriate cuff size.*
15. Moutquin JM, et al. A prospective study of blood pressure in pregnancy. *Am J Obstet Gynecol* 1985;151:191. *In 1,000 patients, the sensitivity of simple but exact blood pressure assessment in predicting preeclampsia 9–12 weeks before clinical signs developed was evident.*
16. Thompson JA, et al. Echocardiographic left ventricular mass to differentiate chronic hypertension from preeclampsia during pregnancy. *Am J Obstet Gynecol* 1986;155:994. *Describes results that indicate increased left ventricular size in chronic hypertensive women.*
17. Villar MA, Sibai BM. Clinical significance of elevated mean arterial blood pressure in second trimester and threshold increase in systolic or diastolic blood pressure during third trimester. *Am J Obstet Gynecol* 1989;160:419. *The authors studied (longitudinally) 700 normotensive gravidas in an effort to predict preeclampsia. Neither a mean arterial pressure in the second trimester greater than 90 mm Hg nor a threshold increase in the systolic/diastolic blood pressure during the third trimester was predictive.*
18. Sibai BM. Diagnosis and management of chronic hypertension in pregnancy. *Obstet Gynecol* 1991;78:451. *The author reviews the diagnosis and management of hypertension in pregnancy and evaluates several treatment trials.*

Treatment
19. Lieb SM, et al. Nitroprusside-induced hemodynamic alterations in normotensive and hypertensive pregnant sheep. *Am J Obstet Gynecol* 1981;139:925. *The treatment of severe hypertension with sodium nitroprusside was studied in pregnant ewes. This agent was shown to reduce hypertension; the reduction in blood pressure was shown to increase uterine blood flow.*
20. Berkowitz RL. Anti-hypertensive drugs in the pregnant patient. *Obstet Gynecol Surv* 1980;35:191.

A comprehensive and up-to-date review of all ramifications of antihypertensive therapy during pregnancy.

21. Redman CW. Fetal outcome in trial of antihypertensive treatment in pregnancy. *Lancet* 1976;2:753.
    Often-quoted paper defending use of methyldopa during pregnancy.
22. Dudley DK. Minibolus diazoxide in the management of severe hypertension in pregnancy. *Am J Obstet Gynecol* 1985;151:196.
    Small dosages of intravenous diazoxide used in 34 patients with severe hypertension produced excellent results compared to those observed for conventional hydralazine therapy.
23. Mirro R, Milley JR, Holzman IR. The effects of sodium nitroprusside on blood flow and oxygen delivery to the organs of the hypoxemic newborn lamb. *Pediatr Res* 1985;19:15.
    The use of nitroprusside, which is normally a vasodilator, can decrease oxygen delivery to vital organs in the fetus and neonate during hypoxia.
24. Black HR. Fixed-dose combination therapy for hypertension. *Drug Ther* 1989; 19:80.
    The authors detail multiple combinations of antihypertensives formulated by a joint committee on the detection, evaluation, and treatment of high blood pressure. This is a must read for those who treat such patients.
25. Knott C. The treatment of hypertension in pregnancy—clinical pharmacokinetic considerations. *Clin Pharmacokinet* 1991;21:233.
    The author discusses the pharmacokinetic considerations with regard to different drugs used to treat hypertension in pregnancy.

Complications
26. Sibai BM, Abdella TN, Anderson GD. Pregnancy outcome in 211 patients with mild chronic hypertension. *Obstet Gynecol* 1983;61:571.
    Presents data on pregnancy outcome in women with mild hypertension.
27. Abdella TN, et al. Relationship of hypertensive disease to abruptio placenta. *Obstet Gynecol* 1984;63:365.
    A retrospective review of abruptio placenta in women with hypertension.
28. Mabie WC, Pernoll ML, Biswas MK. Chronic hypertension in pregnancy. *Obstet Gynecol* 1986;67:197.
    This report describes the outcome of 69 pregnancies in women with chronic hypertension.
29. Witlin AG, Friedman SA, Sibai BM. The effect of magnesium sulfate therapy on the duration of labor in women with mild preeclampsia at term: a randomized, double-blind, placebo-controlled trial. *Am J Obstet Gynecol* 1997;176:623.
    This report uses a placebo control to magnesium sulfate therapy to demonstrate no clinical effect of magnesium sulfate on labor.
30. Witlin AG, Sibai BM. Magnesium sulfate therapy in preeclampsia and eclampsia. *Obstet Gynecol* 1998;92:883.
    This provides a thorough review of the historical background and rationales for magnesium sulfate therapy in women with eclampsia and preeclampsia.

---

7. PREGNANCY-INDUCED HYPERTENSION

Garland D. Anderson

Hypertension unique to pregnancy is best termed *pregnancy-induced hypertension* (PIH). PIH is synonymous with preeclampsia-eclampsia (eclampsia being an extension of the preeclamptic process) and replaces the older term *toxemia*. Although the cause is unknown, there are many theories; none of these hypotheses, however, fully explains the disease entity. It is likely that the cause of PIH will be found to be multifactorial. Socioeconomic factors, nutritional deficiencies, and slow disseminated intravascular coagulation (DIC) have been postulated as etiologic agents, but may actually be only associated factors. Recent immunologic explanations are intriguing but not proven. There is a familial tendency observed for preeclampsia. In one large follow-up study of eclamptic women, preeclampsia occurred in 27% of the first pregnancies of sisters of eclamptic women. In 14% of the women who had severe PIH, severe preeclampsia developed in the second pregnancy. Any theory of PIH must explain the following observations: (1) PIH is principally a disease of primigravid women; (2) it is unique to humans; (3) it is associated with a large amount of trophoblasts; (4) there is coordination with chronic vascular disease; (5) there is a genetic predisposition; and (6) a viable fetus is not always present.

In a recent large prospective multicenter study of nulliparous women, only four characteristics predicted the development of preeclampsia (in order of importance): (1) systolic blood pressure at first prenatal visit, (2) obesity, (3) prior abortion or miscarriage, and (4) cigarette smoking. The higher the systolic blood pressure at the first prenatal visit, the higher the incidence of preeclampsia. Likewise, the more obese the women were at the start of pregnancy, the higher the incidence of preeclampsia. A prior abortion or miscarriage and cigarette smoking reduce the incidence of preeclampsia. Low-dose aspirin and calcium have both been felt to reduce the incidence of preeclampsia. However, large prospective studies have failed to demonstrate that low-dose aspirin or calcium supplementation prevents preeclampsia.

In terms of the basic physiology involved, hypertension is a consequence of either cardiac output or peripheral vascular resistance. Cardiac output remains normal during pregnancy; therefore, PIH results from increased peripheral vascular resistance. This vascular resistance is caused by the generalized vasospasm so characteristic of hypertension. Early in normal pregnancy, the mother's arteries become more refractory to the effects of pressor agents such as angiotensin II. The cause of this normal increase in vascular refractoriness is not known, but prostaglandins play a role. Many weeks before the onset of clinically detectable PIH, there is a loss of refractoriness to infused angiotensin. The results of angiotensin infusions can actually predict which normotensive patients are destined to acquire PIH. After the loss of vascular refractoriness to angiotensin but before the onset of clinical hypertension, there is a decrease in placental perfusion (as measured by the clearance of dehydroisoandrosterone sulfate). It is now understood that PIH is a chronic disease process and that hypertension occurs relatively late in its course. By the time elevated blood pressure is detected, the disease is well established.

The diagnosis of PIH is determined by the presence of hypertension in conjunction with proteinuria, edema, or both, after the 20th week of pregnancy. It is primarily a disease of the first pregnancy, and it occurs with higher frequency in younger (adolescent) and older (older than 35) primigravidas. The diagnosis of PIH in the multigravid woman is often incorrect and should be made only after ruling out cardiovascular and renal disease. Hypertension is defined as a blood pressure reading of greater than 140/90 mm Hg. Two blood pressure readings taken at least 6 h apart are required for determining this. Proteinuria is a more important diagnostic criterion than nondependent edema, but both normally occur later than hypertension. Significant proteinuria is defined as a protein level of 500 mg/dL or more per 24 hours, which approximates a 2+ urinary protein level. Edema is such a common occurrence that it is often not helpful for diagnosis. Nondependent edema is significant, but as many as eight in 10 normotensive women exhibit dependent edema.

Many authorities differentiate between mild and severe PIH. Mild disease consists of minimal to moderate elevations in blood pressure (systolic, <160 mm Hg; diastolic, <100 mm Hg), nondependent edema, and a proteinuria of less than 2 g in 24 hours. When one or more of the following occur, PIH is classified as severe: blood pressure greater than 160/110 mm Hg, proteinuria greater than 5 g in 24 hours, oliguria (<400 ml in 24 hours), visual blurring or scotomata, and pulmonary edema or cyanosis.

The diagnosis of PIH usually mandates hospitalization, but ambulatory treatment in questionable or mild cases with frequent follow-up also has a place in treating PIH.

Management must then be individualized according to the maturity of the fetus and the severity of PIH. If PIH arises at 37 or more weeks' gestation, little can be gained from procrastination. Even in the presence of mild PIH, oxytocin induction is indicated, particularly if the cervix is favorable. Severe PIH, even if associated with a premature fetus, demands intervention. There are also distinct warnings that eclampsia is imminent; these consist of accelerating hypertension, headache, visual blurring, scotomata, epigastric or upper quadrant abdominal pain, and tremulousness. The prompt administration of magnesium sulfate to prevent convulsions is needed when these signs are present.

Conservative management is appropriate only when the fetus is premature and the hypertension is not severe. The patient is allowed a regular hospital diet and light ambulation. Vital signs should be checked four times daily while she is awake. Weight is checked daily, and the urine protein level is checked frequently. Creatinine clearance is determined weekly, and serial sonography is performed every 3 weeks. The mother may be asked to record fetal movements, although nonstress tests, contraction stress tests, biophysical profiles, Doppler blood flow studies, or a combination of these assessment tests is usually conducted weekly or twice weekly in those who are managed conservatively. Biochemical monitoring consisting of the measurement of estriol, human placental lactogen, and pregnancy-specific protein levels is not usually helpful.

Once the patient is hospitalized, a spontaneous diuresis can be expected within the first 24 hours. This diuresis is reflected by a decrease in weight and an improvement in blood pressure, in addition to a large urinary output. If the patient becomes normotensive, it must be decided whether to continue hospitalization until delivery. For the woman who is unwilling or unable to accept hospitalization, home bed rest with daily blood pressure monitoring is the next best therapy. Whenever severe preeclampsia occurs, management is straightforward and consists of the prevention of convulsions with magnesium sulfate ($MgSO_4$), control of hypertension with intermittent hydralazine therapy, and delivery.

At least two large prospective randomized studies have demonstrated that $MgSO_4$ is the drug of choice for prevention of seizures and treatment of seizures in preeclampsia and eclampsia. Magnesium sulfate ($MgSO_4 \bullet 7H_2O$ USP) is a safe and efficient agent to prevent convulsions and can be given by the intramuscular or intravenous route. The standard intravenous dose used for many years was a 4-g loading dose (20%) delivered over 5–10 minutes followed by 1 g/hour (10 g of $MgSO_4 \bullet 7H_2O$ USP added to 1,000 ml of 5% dextrose in lactated Ringer's solution given at 100 ml/hour). Because of the low serum magnesium levels achieved at these dosages, the recommended regimen is now a 6-g loading dose delivered over 15–20 minutes followed by a maintenance dose of 2 g/hour. The intravenous method requires the use of continuous-infusion pumps, available personnel for infusion monitoring, the documentation of adequate renal function, and preferably the ability to determine serum magnesium levels on a rapid basis. The initial intramuscular dose is 10 g (50%), given after the intravenous loading dose and followed by 5 g given intramuscularly every 4 hours. Each 5 g of $MgSO_4$ consists of 10 ml of a 50% solution that is given in the upper outer quadrant of the buttock through a 3-inch (7.5-cm), 20-gauge needle. One milliliter of 2% lidocaine can be added to each dose for analgesia.

Maintenance of $MgSO_4$ may be continued without serial measurements of the serum magnesium level if the following criteria are met: (1) patellar reflex is present, (2) respirations are normal, and (3) urine output is at least 100 ml every 4 hours. Before any treatment, the normal serum magnesium level is 1.5 to 2 mEq/L, whereas the therapeutic maintenance range is 4 to 7 mEq/L. The earliest sign of magnesium toxicity is loss of the patellar reflex; this occurs at 7–10 mEq/L. Respiratory depression begins at 10–15 mEq/L and cardiac arrest at 30 mEq/L. Calcium gluconate is the antidote to $MgSO_4$ toxicity, and the dose is 1 g (10 ml of a 10% solution) given slowly over 3 minutes. Mechanical respiratory support may be necessary in these cases. An interesting subgroup of women with preeclampsia may present with the HELLP syndrome (hemolysis, elevated liver enzyme levels, and a low platelet count). Other coagulation tests such as the prothrombin time, the fibrinogen level, and partial thromboplastic time are normal. In some women who present with the HELLP syndrome, the diagnosis of PIH is delayed, or they may be diagnosed as having hypertension and started on antihypertensive therapy. Women who have the HELLP syndrome should be stabilized with $MgSO_4$ treatment and undergo prompt delivery. Antihypertensive medication is reserved for patients with a diastolic pressure greater than 110 mm Hg, and hydralazine is the drug of choice in this setting. It can be given by intermittent intravenous bolus infusion (5–10 mg); the preferred method is in 5-mg increments. It can also be given by continuous infusion (180 mg in 500 ml of 5% dextrose in water). To prevent hypotension, the continuous infusion should be discontinued when diastolic blood pressures enter the range of 90–100 mm Hg. Because of vasospasm, the patient with PIH has a contracted blood volume. This knowledge is important in management because volume contraction prohibits either volume expansion or depletion. Injudicious fluid therapy may then precipitate overload and pulmonary edema. In contrast, salt restriction or the use of diuretics may cause decreased placental perfusion. As a consequence of the diminished blood volume, the patient with PIH cannot withstand the same degree of blood loss at delivery that a normal woman can. A sudden reduction in blood pressure at delivery is usually the result of a profound blood loss.

Invasive hemodynamic monitoring has proved helpful in the management of a subset of patients with severe PIH and additional complications such as pulmonary edema, oliguria unresponsive to fluid challenge, sepsis, and the clinical need for blood transfusion or massive volume replacement. The pulmonary artery catheter is the technology of choice, owing to the limited and erroneous information that a central venous pressure may reveal in a patient with PIH. Severe PIH and its sequela, eclampsia, are largely preventable. The key to prevention is astute management. Patient education, close monitoring, and attention to subtle detail can reduce the morbidity, mortality, and expense associated with this disease.

General
1. Cunningham FG, et al. Hypertensive disorders in pregnancy. In: *Williams obstetrics,* 19th ed. Norwalk, CT: Appleton & Lange, 1993.
   A complete review of PIH.
2. Soutter WP. The haemodynamic pathophysiology of preeclampsia. *South Afr Med J* 1980;58:351.
   Reviews the hemodynamic characteristics of PIH. The overall role of therapeutic management is discussed.

Etiology
3. Yamaguchi M, Mori N. 6-Keto prostaglandin $F_{1\alpha}$, thromboxane B_2, and 13,14-dihydro-15-keto prostaglandin F concentrations of normotensive and preeclamptic patients during pregnancy, delivery, and the postpartum period. *Am J Obstet Gynecol* 1985;151:121.
   This elegant article giving details on the metabolites of prostaglandins demonstrates that prostacyclin plays an important role in the etiology of preeclampsia.
4. Page EW. On the pathogenesis of preeclampsia and eclampsia. *Br J Obstet Gynaecol* 1972;79:883.
   A complete work regarding the pathogenesis of preeclampsia and eclampsia. This work promotes McKay's theory regarding DIC.
5. Jouppila P, et al. Failure of exogenous prostacyclin to change placental and fetal blood flow in preeclampsia. *Am J Obstet Gynecol* 1985;151:661.
   Prostaglandins, specifically a deficiency in prostacyclin, are thought to be intimately involved with the development of preeclampsia. In this study, prostacyclin was given to 10 women with the disease, but no change in placental or umbilical blood flow occurred.
6. Zlatnik FK, Burmeister LF. Dietary protein and preeclampsia. *Am J Obstet Gynecol* 1983;147:345.
   The relationship of protein intake to the incidence of preeclampsia is examined.

7. Alderman BW, Sperling RS, Daling JR. An epidemiological study of the immuno-genetic etiology of preeclampsia. *BMJ* 1986;292:372.
   Presents a population-based study evaluating the incidence of PIH compared to race dissimilarities of the father and mother.
8. Benedetto C, et al. Reduced serum inhibition of platelet-activating factor activity in preeclampsia. *Am J Obstet Gynecol* 1989;160:100.
   The authors carefully studied women with preeclampsia, looking specifically at the inhibition of platelet-activating factor activity. They found this in most of the preeclamptics and consider that it might contribute to the hemostatic defect noted in these patients.
9. Arngrimsson R, et al. Genetic and familial predisposition to eclampsia and preeclampsia in a defined population. *Br J Obstet Gynaecol* 1990;97:762.
   The authors discuss the role of genetic and familial predisposition in the develop-ment of eclampsia and preeclampsia.
10. Zuspan FP. New concepts in the understanding of hypertensive disorders of pregnancy: an overview. *Clin Perinatol* 1991;18:653.
   The authors present the new concept regarding the pathophysiology of preeclampsia.

Diagnosis
11. Phelan JP, Yurth DA. Severe preeclampsia. I. Peripartum hemodynamic moni-toring. *Am J Obstet Gynecol* 1982;144:17.
   The cardiovascular changes that occur in the setting of severe preeclampsia are described for women who underwent Swan-Ganz monitoring during labor.
12. Chesley LC. Diagnosis of preeclampsia. *Obstet Gynecol* 1985;65:423.
   The diagnosis of mild preeclampsia may be wrong in more than half of the cases, although the clinical management appears to be correct for those women suspected of having the disorder.
13. Hays PM, Cruikshank DP, Dunn LJ. Plasma volume determination in normal and preeclamptic pregnancies. *Am J Obstet Gynecol* 1985;151:958.
   Plasma volume determination using the Evans blue technique was performed in nor-mal and preeclamptic patients. Those who were preeclamptic had a smaller plasma volume expansion, and their offspring were more likely to be growth retarded.
14. Sibai BM, et al. Effect of magnesium sulfate on electroencephalographic findings in preeclampsia-eclampsia. *Obstet Gynecol* 1984;64:261.
   Abnormal electroencephalographic recordings are common in patients with severe preeclampsia and are not altered by $MgSO_4$ treatment.
15. Romero R, et al. Clinical significance, prevalence, and natural history of throm-bocytopenia in pregnancy-induced hypertension. *Am J Perinatol* 1989;6:32.
   The authors of this study found that thrombocytopenia was encountered in 11.6% of the patients with PIH and, when present, it was correlated with a higher incidence of preterm delivery and intrauterine growth retardation. The lowest platelet count usu-ally appeared 48 hours after delivery, and recovery likewise took 2 additional days.

Treatment
16. Berkowitz RL. Antihypertensive drugs in the pregnant patient. *Obstet Gynecol Surv* 1980;35:191.
   Comprehensive, recent review of all the ramifications of antihypertensive therapy during pregnancy.
17. Sibai BM, et al. Reassessment of intravenous $MgSO_4$ therapy in preeclampsia-eclampsia. *Obstet Gynecol* 1981;57:199.
   The authors indicate that the standard dosage of $MgSO_4$ may be insufficient for many patients; they recommend adjusting the intravenous dosage of $MgSO_4$ for each patient.
18. Sibai BM, Graham JM, McCubbin JH. A comparison of intravenous and intra-muscular magnesium sulfate regimens in preeclampsia. *Am J Obstet Gynecol* 1984;150:728.

Intravenously and intramuscularly administered MgSO₄ was used in patients
with severe preeclampsia. At 1 g/hour given intravenously, the circulating level
was significantly lower than that associated with the intramuscular regimen.

19. Mabie WC, et al. A comparative trial of labetalol and hydralazine in the acute management of severe hypertension complicating pregnancy. *Obstet Gynecol* 1987;70:328.
    Study describes the use of labetalol in the treatment of a hypertensive crisis, com-
    pared to hydralazine treatment. Supports the contention that labetalol may be a
    safe and effective alternative.
20. Schwartz ML, Brenner W. Severe preeclampsia with persistent postpartum hemolysis and thrombocytopenia treated by plasmapheresis. *Obstet Gynecol* 1985;65:53S.
    Plasmapheresis was used to treat a patient with severe PIH, with good results.
21. Clark SL, et al. Severe preeclampsia with persistent oliguria. Management of hemodynamic subsets. *Am J Obstet Gynecol* 1986;154:490.
    Based on results of the study, the authors advise treatment based on hemodynamic
    variables evaluated by means of pulmonary artery catheterization.
22. Clark SL, Cotton DB. Clinical indications for pulmonary artery catheterization in the patient with severe preeclampsia. *Am J Obstet Gynecol* 1988;158:453.
    The authors review their own past experience with invasive hemodynamic moni-
    toring in PIH patients, and recommend its use in those women who are unre-
    sponsive to antihypertensives, develop pulmonary edema, or have persistent olig-
    uria and in some patients requiring conduction anesthesia.
23. Ramanathan J. Anesthetic considerations in preeclampsia. *Clin Perinatol* 1991; 18:875.
    The author discusses the special factors that should be considered before giving
    anesthesia to the woman with preeclampsia.
24. Witlin AG, Friedman SA, Sibai BM. The effect of magnesium sulfate therapy on the duration of labor in women with mild preeclampsia at term: a randomized, double-blind, placebo-controlled trial. *Am J Obstet Gynecol* 1997;176:623.
    Found that magnesium sulfate did not affect any component of labor but did
    necessitate a higher dose of oxytocin.
25. Sibai BM, et al. Risk factors for preeclampsia in healthy nulliparous women: a prospective multicenter study. *Am J Obstet Gynecol* 1995;72:642.
    This study found that prepregnancy weight, blood pressure, cigarette smoking,
    and prior abortions were the major factors that determined when a primipara
    developed preeclampsia.
26. Carroli G, et al. Calcium supplementation during pregnancy: a systematic review of randomized controlled trials. *Br J Obstet Gynaecol* 1994;101:753.
    This study is a review of the calcium supplement clinical trials.
27. Barton JR, Stanziano GJ, Sibai BM. Monitored outpatient management of mild gestational hypertension remote from term. *Am J Obstet Gynecol* 1994; 170:765.
    Reports the outcome of a group of preeclamptic women managed on an ambula-
    tory basis.
28. Sibai BM, Ramanathan J. The case for magnesium sulfate in preeclampsia-eclampsia. *Int J Obstet Anesth* 1992;1:167.
    Outlines why magnesium sulfate is the drug of choice to prevent or treat
    preeclampsia.
29. Lucas MJ, Leveno KJ, Cunningham FG. A comparison of magnesium sulfate with phenytoin for the prevention of eclampsia. *N Engl J Med* 1995;333:201.
    Large randomized study that demonstrated that magnesium sulphate is superior to
    phenytoin for the prevention of eclampsia.
30. The Eclampsia Trial Collaborative Group: Which anticonvulsant for women with eclampsia: evidence from the Collaborative Eclampsia Trial. *Lancet* 1995; 345:1455.
    Large multicenter study that demonstrates that MgSO₄ is the best way to prevent
    or control eclamptic seizures.

8. ECLAMPSIA

Garland D. Anderson

Eclampsia is the extension of pregnancy-induced hypertension (PIH) to the point of convulsion, coma, or both. Eclampsia is associated with an increased risk for both mother and newborn. Maternal mortality varies between 0% and 14%. Maternal morbidity is also increased because of complications that may affect multiple organ systems. Pulmonary complications include pulmonary edema and aspiration pneumonia. Abruptio placentae and disseminated intravascular coagulopathy are often complications. Intracerebral hemorrhage is the major cause of death. Other complications include acute renal tubular necrosis and ruptured liver, transient cortical blindness, and retinal detachment. The reported perinatal mortality is between 10% and 28%. Most of the perinatal mortality is due to prematurity, severe fetal growth retardation, and an increased incidence of abruptio placentae. Approximately 75% of eclampsia occurs antepartum and 25% occurs postpartum. Almost all cases (95%) of antepartum eclampsia occur during the third trimester. The remaining cases occur before 28 weeks' gestation. Eclampsia has rarely been reported to occur before 20 weeks' gestation. Most postpartum eclampsia occurs in the first 24 h postpartum. Some cases occur after 48 h postpartum and have been reported as late as 23 days postpartum. Fortunately, eclampsia is a largely preventable illness. The following are considered warnings that convulsion is imminent: acceleration of hypertension, epigastric right upper quadrant abdominal pain, visual blurring or scotomata, headache, and tremulousness. The presence of any of these signs demands the prompt administration of magnesium sulfate (MgSO₄). However, approximately 20% of the women in whom eclampsia develops have only mildly elevated blood pressure (80-90 mm Hg diastolic), often without proteinuria or edema. For this reason, all patients in labor who meet the blood pressure criterion of PIH should receive MgSO₄ therapy.

The cause of eclamptic convulsions is unknown. Both cerebral vasospasm and cerebral edema are incriminated but unproved as etiologic agents. One half of the cases of convulsions occur before labor, one fourth during labor, and most of the remainder within 48 h postpartum. Occasionally, eclampsia arises before 20 weeks' gestation and often 48 h postpartum. Eclampsia appearing more than 48 h postpartum is relatively common, and now represents 10% of the total cases of eclampsia. The seizures are grand mal in character, and typically, there is no antecedent aura. Tongue biting, urinary and fecal incontinence, injury from falls, and occasionally fractures are observed, as are transient apnea and cyanosis.

Care during the actual convulsion consists of gentle constraint and maintenance of an airway, then the administration of oxygen as soon as the convulsion ceases. A chest x-ray study is obtained to rule out aspiration. Blood is drawn for a complete blood count, liver profile, and serum electrolyte measurements, and an indwelling catheter is placed in the bladder for the measurement of hourly urine output. A stage of agitation is common after the postictal patient regains partial consciousness. A quiet room with subdued light and the presence of a family member are helpful. The management of eclampsia is straightforward. The convulsions are treated, blood pressure is controlled, and delivery is accomplished as soon as possible after stabilization of the mother's condition. Timing of delivery does not depend on the maturity of the fetus.

The agent of choice for the treatment of convulsions is MgSO₄. The following regimen has proved efficacious: 6 g of MgSO₄ in 20% solution given intravenously over 5–10 minutes, followed by a continuous maintenance infusion of 2 g/hour if there is no sign of maternal respiratory depression. If the patient has a recurrent seizure, another bolus of 2–4 g of MgSO₄ can be given over 3–5 minutes. We no longer use the maintenance dose of 1 g/h of MgSO₄, because this does not achieve therapeutic levels. Occasionally the maintenance dose has to be increased to greater than 2 g/hour if the urinary output is high. Another regimen frequently used is 4 g of MgSO₄ given intravenously over 4 minutes, followed immediately by 5 g (50%) given intramuscularly in each buttock and an intramuscular injection of 5 g every 4 hours. This 14-g loading dose can be given safely to any patient who has not already received $MgSO_4$. Another convulsion within 20 minutes or more after the initial dose is treated with additional intravenously administered (10%) $MgSO_4$ (with 2 g delivered slowly intravenously if the patient weighs less than 55 kg, or 4 g if the patient weighs more than 55 kg). The routine use of intravenous diazepam (Valium) or phenytoin sodium (Dilantin) in addition to the $MgSO_4$ should be avoided. These combinations may lead to aspiration, respiratory distress, or cardiac arrest. Only rarely does the patient continue to convulse after the second intravenous bolus of $MgSO_4$. In the rare instances, intravenous sodium amobarbital (Amytal), titrated as needed, may be helpful.

$MgSO_4$ causes a peripheral neuromuscular blockage through interference with acetylcholine release and action. This is clinically important if succinylcholine is used, because less of the muscle relaxant is then required for cesarean delivery or other surgical procedures. The synergism between $MgSO_4$ and succinylcholine explains the cases of prolonged muscle paralysis that arise postoperatively. Vasodilatation and a central cerebral sedative effect are also noted as actions of $MgSO_4$. Before any therapy, the normal serum magnesium level is 1.5–2.0 mEq/L. After a loading dose of 4 g, given intravenously, and the maintenance infusion of 1 g of $MgSO_4$ per hour, serum magnesium levels range from 2.2–4.1 mEq/L within 2 hours. The levels return to normal within 6 hours if no further magnesium is given. A maintenance dose of 5 g, given intramuscularly every 4 hours, results in a therapeutic range of between 4 and 7 mEq/L. Even with a 4-g loading dose of $MgSO_4$ and 1 g of $MgSO_4$ per hour, it may take 6–8 hours to achieve therapeutic levels. We now recommend a 6-g intravenous loading dose of $MgSO_4$, followed by a maintenance dose of 2 g/hour, to more rapidly arrive at a reasonable level.

Because the kidneys excrete magnesium, renal disease or oliguria requires a reduction in the dose or cessation of $MgSO_4$ treatment. The earliest sign of magnesium toxicity is loss of the patellar reflex, occurring at 7–10 mEq/L. Respirations are depressed at 10–15 mEq/L and cardiac arrest occurs at about 30 mEq/L. A maintenance regimen of $MgSO_4$ (delivered either by the intramuscular or intravenous route) should not be administered without obtaining serial serum magnesium levels, unless the following criteria are confirmed: (1) the patellar reflex is present (2) respirations are normal, and (3) urine output is at least 100 ml every 4 hours. The intramuscular regimen consists of 5 g given every 4 hours up to 24 hours postpartum, whereas the intravenous maintenance is 2 g/hour up to 24 hours postpartum. Calcium gluconate is the antidote to $MgSO_4$. In case of respiratory depression, the dose is 1 g (10 ml of a 10% calcium gluconate solution) administered intravenously over 3 minutes. Mechanical respiratory support may be necessary if respiratory depression develops.

The blood pressure may be normal immediately after a convulsion, although the hypertension usually resumes. If the patient remains normotensive or if the convulsion occurs more than 48 hours postpartum, causes of convulsions other than eclampsia should be considered, although eclampsia can occur more than 48 hours postpartum. Other causes include epilepsy, a cerebrovascular accident, central nervous system tumor, electrolyte disturbances, and hypoglycemia.

Intravenously administered hydralazine is the drug of choice to control the hypertension associated with eclampsia. Its use is reserved for a blood pressure of 170/110 mm Hg or greater. Hydralazine is given by intravenous bolus in 5- to 10-mg increments every 15–20 minutes. Blood pressure is measured every 5 minutes initially and every 15 minutes after becoming stable. The goal of therapy is to maintain the diastolic blood pressure between 90 and 100 mm Hg. If the diastolic blood pressure drops below 90 mm Hg, the injections should be discontinued. One may begin with 5 mg and increase (if necessary) in 5-mg increments until the diastolic pressure is 90–100 mm Hg. Rarely, hypotensive episodes may occur. Because hydralazine has a relatively long half-life, care must be taken to avoid hypotension.

The definitive cure of eclampsia is delivery, although it is best to wait until the mother's condition is stable on $MgSO_4$ therapy before proceeding to effect delivery. This is usually accomplished 4–8 hours after the last convulsion. Even if the cervix is unfavorable for induction, oxytocin stimulation may be successful. The fetus should be carefully monitored during labor. Many fetuses of eclamptic women have intrauterine growth retardation. They may have little placental reserve and may not tolerate labor. The incidence of placental abruption is also greatly increased in the setting of eclampsia, and this may lead to sudden fetal distress. The exception is the woman at less than 32 weeks' gestation, particularly if she has a long uneffaced cervix. In this type of woman, one usually opts for cesarean delivery. The eclamptic patient, like the one with severe PIH, has a contracted blood volume. Hemoconcentration is a consistent finding. Puerperal hemorrhage, even of a magnitude tolerated by the normal pregnant patient, can lead to the dangerous underperfusion of vital organs in eclamptic women. A sudden reduction in blood pressure at the time of delivery or immediately postpartum is usually the consequence of excessive blood loss. Because of their contracted blood volume, women with eclampsia should be typed and crossmatched for blood.

Eclampsia occurring more than 48 hours postpartum has one characteristic different than antepartum eclampsia or eclampsia occurring within 48 hours postpartum. In almost all cases of so-called late postpartum eclampsia, there is an immediate diuresis following the convulsion. When the catheter is inserted in the bladder, 400–500 ml of urine may be obtained. Urine output of 100–300 ml for the next several hours frequently occurs.

Most of the women who develop late postpartum eclampsia have severe headaches or visual disturbance before the onset of their convulsion. Approximately 50% of these women had been diagnosed as having preeclampsia before convulsion. Any woman with a history of convulsion more than 48 hours postpartum who is hypertensive and has proteinuria or edema should be considered eclamptic. If there are localizing findings on the neurologic examination or the patients do not improve rapidly following control of their blood pressure and seizures, they should have a full array of neurodiagnostic tests looking for other causes of the seizures.

The patient may frequently inquire about the risk of recurrent severe PIH or eclampsia. Women who have eclampsia are at increased risk for preeclampsia as well as abruptio placentae in future pregnancies. The young primigravida who has experienced this disease has a much more favorable prognosis than the older multigravida with chronic hypertension and superimposed preeclampsia-eclampsia. There is a one-in-four chance of recurrent PIH if the patient is normotensive. In the setting of chronic hypertension, the recurrence risk is even higher. The earlier in gestation that eclampsia occurs, the higher the incidence of preeclampsia-eclampsia in future pregnancies. The risk of chronic hypertension was also higher on long-term follow-up in the women who developed eclampsia earlier in gestation.

General
1. Villar MA, Sibai BM. Eclampsia. *Obstet Gynecol Clin North Am* 1968;15:355.
   An excellent and thorough review of the diagnosis, treatment, and management of eclampsia.
2. Zuspan FP. Toxemia of pregnancy. In: Sciarra JJ, McElin TW, eds. *Gynecology and obstetrics. Vol. 2.* Hagerstown, MD: Harper & Row, 1985.
   A 20-page review of all aspects of PIH, with excellent references.
3. Mendlowitz M. Toxemia of pregnancy and eclampsia. *Obstet Gynecol Surv* 1980;35:327.
   An in-depth review regarding the basic science aspects of the preeclampsia-eclampsia syndrome, with 70 references.
4. Wright JP. Anesthetic consideration in preeclampsia/eclampsia. *Anesth Analg* 1983;62:590.
   A review of the anesthetic considerations in women with eclampsia, with 116 references.
5. Bergsjo P. Familiar and remote clinical problems: remedies in 1922. *Acta Obstet Gynecol Scand* 1992;71:166.
   Historical account of the management and outcome of eclampsia in 1922.
6. Lopez-Llera MM. Main clinical types and subtypes of eclampsia. *Am J Obstet Gynecol* 1992;166:4.
   Describes the vast experience of a hospital in Mexico treating eclampsia and reports a high maternal mortality.

7. Sibai BM, Sarinoglu C, Mercer BM. Eclampsia. VII. Pregnancy outcome after eclampsia and long-term prognosis. *Am J Obstet Gynecol* 1992;166:1757.
    This article describes the long-term follow-up and prognosis in a large number of women who had eclampsia.

Etiology

8. Porapakkham S. An epidemiologic study of eclampsia. *Obstet Gynecol* 1979;54:26.
    The epidemiologic characteristics in 298 cases of eclampsia were studied. Inadequate antenatal care was a major factor in maternal and perinatal mortality.
9. Hankins GDV, et al. Longitudinal evaluation of hemodynamic changes in eclampsia. *Am J Obstet Gynecol* 1984;150:506.
    Extracellular and extravascular fluid mobilization occurs long after delivery in patients with eclampsia. Fluid management is particularly important in these patients.
10. Pitkin RM. Calcium metabolism in pregnancy and the perinatal period: a review. *Am J Obstet Gynecol* 1985;151:99.
    Calcium homeostasis may be related to toxemia. This fine review containing 135 references dealing with calcium metabolism may help demonstrate this relationship.
11. Romero R, et al. Toxemia: new concepts in an old disease. *Semin Perinatol* 1988; 12:302.
    Offers a very good diagrammatic depiction of what we know about the cause of toxemia, or PIH, with particular reference to eclampsia. It also contains 291 references.

Diagnosis

12. Sibai BM, et al. The late postpartum eclampsia controversy. *Obstet Gynecol* 1980; 55:74.
    Purportedly, eclampsia does not occur before the twentieth week and after a few days postpartum. This study deals with women who were diagnosed as eclamptic by exclusion, although the seizures occurred much later than is commonly acceptable for such a diagnosis.
13. Dahmus MA, Barton JR, Sibai BM. Cerebral imaging in eclampsia: magnetic resonance imaging versus computed tomography. *Am J Obstet Gynecol* 1992; 167:935.
    This article focuses on the value of magnetic resonance imaging versus computed tomography in the evaluation of the eclamptic patient.
14. Lubarsky SL, et al. Late postpartum eclampsia revisited. *Obstet Gynecol* 1994; 83:502.
    Describes the prior clinical course, workup, and outcome of 54 women who developed eclampsia ≥48 hours postpartum.
15. Pritchard JA, et al. The Parkland Memorial Hospital protocol for treatment of eclampsia: evaluation of 245 cases. *Am J Obstet Gynecol* 1984;148:951.
    A classic presentation of a successful management protocol prepared by author with extensive experience.
16. Sibai BM, et al. Reassessment of intravenous $MgSO_4$ therapy in preeclampsia eclampsia. *Obstet Gynecol* 1981;57:1991.
    This reference offers evidence that the current methods of $MgSO_4$ management in the treatment of eclampsia may not be adequate.
17. Zuspan FP, Zuspan KJ. Strategies for controlling eclampsia. *Contemp Obstet Gynecol* 1981;18:135.
    An in-depth review of the therapeutic choices for treating eclampsia, with a detailed section on the delivery of the eclamptic patient.
18. Little BC, et al. Treatment of hypertension in pregnancy by relaxation and biofeedback. *Lancet* 1984;1:865.
    Biofeedback is used during pregnancy to lower blood pressure. Postpartum, this may prove helpful in eclamptic patients with high blood pressure.
19. Tondriaux A, et al. Hemodynamic effects of magnesium sulfate in eclampsia. *Clin Exp Hypertens* 1983;B2:405.

The hemodynamic effects of MgSO$_4$ are decreased venous compliance, decreased preload, and reduced cardiac output.

20. Sibai BM, et al. Eclampsia treatment and referral. *South Med J* 1982;75:267.
    Guidelines for the treatment and stabilization of patients for subsequent referral to a tertiary care center are offered.
21. Koontz WL, Reid KH. The effect of pretreatment with magnesium sulfate on the initiation of seizure foci in anesthetized cats. *Am J Obstet Gynecol* 1989;160:508.
    The effects of parental magnesium sulfate before the initiation of seizure foci in anesthetized cats were studied, and no significant difference in terms of benefit was found between the experimental group and the control groups not so treated. The mechanism of magnesium sulfate's therapeutic effect remains unknown.

Complications
22. Richards AM, et al. Active management of the unconscious eclamptic patient. *Br J Obstet Gynecol* 1986;93:554.
    Discusses management of the woman who remains unconscious following eclamptic seizures.
23. Lucas MJ, Leveno KJ, Cunningham FG. A comparison of magnesium sulfate with phenytoin for the prevention of eclampsia. *N Engl J Med* 1995;333:201.
    Large randomized study that demonstrated that magnesium sulfate is superior to phenytoin for the prevention of eclampsia.
24. Eclampsia Trial Collaborative Group. Which anticonvulsant for women with eclampsia: evidence from the Collaborative Eclampsia Trial. *Lancet* 1995; 345:1455.
    Large multicenter study that demonstrates that MgSO$_4$ is the best way to prevent or control eclamptic seizures.
25. Sibai BM, Anderson GD, McCubbin JH. Eclampsia. II. Clinical significance of laboratory findings. *Obstet Gynecol* 1982;59:153.
    Describes the significance of the laboratory findings in women with eclampsia.
26. Sibai BM, et al. Eclampsia. III. Neonatal outcome, growth, and development. *Am J Obstet Gynecol* 1983;146:307.
    The short-term follow-up in children whose mothers had eclampsia is detailed.
27. Mansa KJ, et al. Hepatic hemorrhage without rupture in preeclampsia. *N Engl J Med* 1985;312:424.
    Hepatic swelling with subsequent rupture is a dreadful complication of preeclampsia-eclampsia. This case report graphically describes such a case.
28. Hill WC, Gill PJ, Katz M. Maternal paralytic ileus as a complication of magnesium sulfate tocolysis. *Am J Perinatol* 1985;2:47.
    The use of MgSO$_4$ for tocolysis or for the treatment of toxemia can result in paralytic ileus if too much of the medication is used, as demonstrated by this case report.
29. Montan S, Ingemarsson I. Intrapartum fetal heart rate patterns in pregnancies complicated by hypertension. *Am J Obstet Gynecol* 1989;160:283.
    Hypertensive pregnancies, particularly eclampsia, accounted for more than one-fifth of all ominous intrapartum fetal heart rate tracings. A high index of suspicion for fetal distress should be kept in mind when eclampsia is diagnosed.
30. Cunningham FG, Fernandez CO, Hernandez C. Blindness associated with preeclampsia and eclampsia. *Am J Obstet Gynecol* 1995;172:1291.
    Describes the course in 15 women with severe preeclampsia or eclampsia who temporarily developed cortical blindness.
31. Witlin AG, et al. Cerebrovascular pathology complicating pregnancy—beyond eclampsia. *Am J Obstet Gynecol* 1997;176:1139.
    Describes the presentation and course of a group of women who present with cerebrovascular disorders that may be confused with eclampsia.
32. Barton JR, Sibai BM. Cerebral pathology in eclampsia. *Clin Perinatol* 1991; 18:891.
    Describes the cerebral pathophysiology, diagnosis, and treatment of cerebral complications involving eclampsia.

III. INFECTIONS IN PREGNANCY

9. VIRAL INFECTIONS DURING PREGNANCY

Everett F. Magann

Approximately 5% of all pregnancies are complicated by viral infections. The predominant viral infections in pregnancy which affect the mother and/or fetus include rubella, hepatitis, cytomegalovirus, herpes, human immunodeficiency virus and parvovirus (B-19). Other infections including enteroviruses and rhinoviruses do occur during pregnancy but have not been associated with birth defects and/or fetal morbidity. Overall viral infections generally cause minimal maternal morbidity but the fetal effects range from developmental delay and mental retardation to structural abnormalities and fetal death in utero.

A primary rubella infection is communicable for 1 week before and 4 days after appearance of the rash. The rash normally lasts for 3 days. Prodromal symptoms include fever, headaches, malaise, and pharyngitis prior to the rash. The risk of congenital infection is related to the gestational age of the mother at the time of the infection. An infection in the first 4 weeks of pregnancy has a risk of 50%, a risk of 25% during weeks 4–8, a 10% risk during weeks 8–12, and <1% risk after week 12. The fetal effects include cataracts, retinopathy, microcephaly, cardiac defects, intrauterine growth restriction, and hearing loss. The most common cardiac defect observed is patent ductus arteriosus, but the most specific is pulmonic stenosis. The diagnosis of a rubella infection is made by complement fixation, hemagglutination inhibition, and cord blood IgM after 22 weeks. Breast-feeding is not contraindicated in women with a primary rubella infection during pregnancy. Immune globulin does not protect against congenital rubella. The rubella vaccine is a live attenuated vaccine and does cause detectable antibodies in 95% of cases. On theoretical grounds women should not receive this vaccine during pregnancy or within 3 months of conception; however, to date no birth defects have been reported in women receiving this vaccine during or just prior to conception.

Acute viral hepatitis is one of the most common and acute viral infections encountered in pregnancy. There are five distinct types of viral hepatitis: types A, B, C, D, and E. The two types that have clinical implications in pregnancy are types B and C. The maternal symptoms associated with an acute infection of hepatitis include malaise, fatigue, anorexia, nausea, right upper quadrant pain, and jaundice. Hepatitis B is a small DNA virus that accounts for 40%–45% of all cases of hepatitis. Acute infections occur in 1–2 per 1,000 pregnancies and chronic infections are present in 5–15 per 1,000 pregnancies. Eighty-five percent to 90% of all women who become infected with hepatitis B will have a complete recovery with the remaining 10%–15% becoming chronically infected. Those individuals who are chronically infected are at risk for the development of chronic and persistent hepatitis, cirrhosis, and ultimately death. Hepatitis B is transmitted by both parental and sexual contact. The virus has three major structural antigens: surface antigen (HB$_s$Ag), core antigen (HB$_c$Ag), and e antigen (HB$_e$Ag). The perinatal transmission of hepatitis B is 10%–20% if HB$_s$Ag is present and 90% with the presence of both the HB$_s$Ag and HB$_e$Ag. Chronic carriers can be identified by persistent levels of HB$_s$Ag.

Neonatal immunoprophylaxis is 85%–95% effective in preventing neonatal hepatitis B infection. All pregnant women should be screened for hepatitis B on their first prenatal visit. The CDC recommends universal immunoprophylaxis for all newborn infants. If the mother is seronegative the newborn receives the vaccine only. If the mother is seropositive, the newborn receives the vaccine and the immunoglobulin (HBIG). This treatment method is effective as 85%–95% of the perinatal transmission takes place at the time of delivery.

Hepatitis C, a single-stranded RNA virus, accounts for 10%–20% of all cases of hepatitis in the United States. The principal risk factors for hepatitis C are multiple blood transfusions and use of intravenous drugs. Ninety percent of posttransfusion hepatitis is hepatitis C. Heterosexual contact has also been shown to be a mechanism of transmission. The diagnosis of hepatitis C is a very specific IgG that turns positive within 6 months of an acute infection. The majority of patients with hepatitis C are asymptomatic with <25% becoming jaundiced. A chronic infection develops in up to 50%–80% of patients, with 20%–30% of these women developing cirrhosis (mean progression time is 19 years). Hepatocellular cancer is associated with hepatitis C infection; the exact prevalence remains unknown. There is a potential for transmission during pregnancy, delivery, and breast-feeding. The risk of transmission in PCR-positive women (indicates active viral replication in the liver) is 2%–20%. Interferon, 3 million units given 3 times a week for up to 6 months, has been suggested as therapy for hepatitis C, but a permanent response occurs in only 15%–20% of women.

Herpes simplex virus is a double-stranded DNA virus which is sexually transmitted. The primary infection of herpes may be asymptomatic or characterized by clusters of acutely painful ulcers on mucosal surfaces, and bilateral inguinal lymphadenopathy. The virus gains entry at the skin surface through direct contact with a person who is shedding the virus and persists in sensory nerve root ganglia from which it can subsequently establish recurrent infections. The risk of neonatal infection after a primary outbreak is up to 50% if the primary infection occurs within 4 weeks of a vaginal delivery. First-episode herpes infection in pregnancy is also associated with an increased risk of intrauterine growth restriction and premature labor. With recurrent genital herpes infections, the risk of transmission from the mother to the fetus is 1%–4% and is dependent on the presence of active lesions at the time of delivery. Recurrent infection is preceded in up to 40% of cases by a prodrome (pain or itching sensation at the skin site where the outbreak is about to occur). Transplacental transmission is thought to occur only with a primary infection acquired during pregnancy and the rate of transmission is thought to be very rare. The gold standard for diagnosis is isolation of the virus by tissue culture. The Jzanck smear and pap smear are rarely used for diagnosis because of low sensitivity, and newer techniques with antigens have not gained widespread acceptance, also because of low sensitivities. The rate of spontaneous abortions is probably increased with primary infections but not with recurrent infections. Congenital infections are manifest as cutaneous scarring, hydrocephalus, chorioamnionitis, and hepatosplenomegaly. An infection acquired during delivery is characterized by skin lesions, pneumonitis, neurologic sequel, and ophthalmologic sequel, and those infants surviving have significant morbidity including seizures. In women with a history of genital herpes infection, an examination of the perineum, vulva, vagina, and cervix is performed upon presentation in labor. If no lesions were detected upon admission to labor and delivery, then vaginal delivery is permitted. Delivery should only be abdominal if lesions are present to prevent fetal exposure through an infected birth canal. Cesarean delivery is not completely protective, as 20%–30% of babies who develop neonatal HSV infections have been delivered abdominally. Acyclovir therapy is available and may be most useful in primary infections and recurrent infections but its influence on pregnancy outcome is currently unknown. Studies using acyclovir in both primary and recurrent infections are continuing. No studies to date demonstrate that acyclovir is a teratogen or harmful when administered during pregnancy.

Varicella is a DNA virus that is characterized by a primary infection, chickenpox, and a recurrent infection that remains dormant in the dorsal root ganglia for many years becoming reactivated years later as herpes zoster (shingles). The onset of the disease is in the early spring, and it is highly infectious, resulting in up to 95% of women becoming seropositive prior to their childbearing years. Clinically, varicella is spread by aerosol droplet. The incubation period is 10–21 days, and it can be infective 1–2 days prior to the appearance of the skin lesions and until all the lesions have become crusted over. The incidence of varicella infection in pregnancy is 0.1–0.5 per 1,000 pregnancies. In women who do not recall having varicella in childhood, only 8% will be seronegative. The fetal abnormalities associated with varicella infection in pregnancy are cutaneous scars (cicatricial skin lesions of the extremities), intrauterine growth restriction, cortical atrophy, limb hypoplasia, eye abnormalities (cataracts, chorioretinitis, microphthalmia, Horner's syndrome) neurologic abnormalities (hydrocephalus, cortical atrophy, mental retardation) and limb abnormalities (hypoplasia, abnormal or absent digits). The risk of developing varicella syndrome with first trimester exposure is 2.2%. A targeted ultrasound appears to be the best method to determine the presence and severity of the infection. Varicella may be complicated by pneumonia in 10%–15% of adults, and the current treatment is with intravenous acyclovir 10–15 mg/kg three times per day for 7 days. Neonatal mortality is 10%–30% in neonates who develop the disease 5 days prior to birth or 2 days following birth, and is usually secondary to encephalitis. If immunity is uncertain and exposure has occurred then the patient's immune status should be determined. Susceptible patients should be given varicella immune globulin (VZIG). The usual dose is one vial per 10 kg of maternal weight up to five vials. VZIG does not decrease the rate of infection, but does decrease the complication rate. Acyclovir should be considered if chickenpox is diagnosed during pregnancy. Acyclovir has not been associated with any congenital abnormalities. Varivax is a live attenuated virus which has been recently approved for use. It is administered as 0.5 ml in two doses with the second dose 4–8 weeks later, and pregnancy should be avoided for 3 months. The risk of congenital infection in women who received the vaccine just prior to or during early pregnancy is uncertain and currently under investigation. No congenital abnormalities have been reported with varicella zoster (shingles) in pregnancy.

Cytomegalovirus (CMV) is a double-stranded DNA herpesvirus and is the most common intrauterine infection affecting 30,000–40,000 U.S. newborns each year with 9,000 of these children having permanent serious sequelae. CMV is species-specific with no known non-human vector for transmission in nature. Infection results from personal contact with an individual who is shedding the virus. The virus is shed in many body fluids, including saliva, urine, semen, breast milk, and cervical secretions. Day-care workers are at increased risk (11%) of seroconversion during pregnancy. Nurses working in intensive care units and with renal dialysis patients do not appear to be at increased risk of seroconversion. The fetal effects include microcephaly, hydrocephaly, periventricular calcifications, blindness, deafness, chorioretinitis, microphthalmia, hepatosplenomegaly, mental retardation, and fetal death in utero. Those infants surviving the initial infection are at risk for significant developmental and neurologic dysfunction, including mental retardation, hearing loss (60%–70%), language and learning disabilities, motor abnormalities, and visual disturbances. The risk of an intrauterine infection with a primary disease during pregnancy is 30%–40% and the risk with recurrent disease in 0.2%–1%. CMV infection prior to pregnancy is a protective factor for the fetus. At the time of birth, 90% of affected infants are asymptomatic, but 10%–15% of these may have delayed effects including deafness and developmental delay. Ten percent of the affected neonates will be symptomatic at birth, with 20%–30% of those infants dying. The presence of an IgG antibody to CMV indicates an exposure to CMV in the past. The presence of IgM antibody to CMV in a woman who was previously negative to CMV indicates a recent infection. Fetal diagnosis is based on amniotic fluid cultures or PCR analysis of amniotic fluid.

HIV is the third leading cause of death of U.S. women 25–44 years of age and in some metropolitan areas is the leading cause of death. Currently, it is estimated that 7,000 births take place each year in the United States to HIV-infected women. More than 90% of all HIV infections in children worldwide and virtually all of the new cases in children are the result of perinatal transmission. The rate of perinatal transmissions is 13%–35%. HIV infection is caused by an RNA retrovirus. When the infection occurs, the virus becomes incorporated into the host genome. HIV remains dormant for a number of years and then becomes activated, leading to progressive deterioration of the immune system and susceptibility to opportunistic infections and neoplasms. All pregnant women should be offered HIV testing as part of their routine antenatal care. Perinatal transmission may occur antepartum, intrapartum, or postpartum. Transmission is increased by amniocentesis, the presence of other sexually transmitted disease (particularly those with ulcerations), preterm delivery, high viral load in the mother, premature rupture of membranes, and breast-feeding. The transmission rate has been decreased from 25.5% to 8.3% with the use of Zidovudine (AZT). AZT is given to HIV-infected women after the 14th week of pregnancy at a dose of 100 mg five times a day. Upon admission to labor and delivery, a 2 mg/kg loading dose is given followed by a continuous infusion of 1 mg/kg until delivery. The neonate is administered AZT syrup at 2 mg/kg every 6 hours for the first 6 weeks of life. Breast-feeding should be avoided because of an increased risk of HIV transmission from the infected mother to her newborn child by 10%–20%. Universal precautions should be used on all obstetric patients as if all of them were HIV positive. Higher seroconverison rates in health care workers is observed with visible blood contamination and deeper injuries. AZT used for postexposure prophylaxis does offer some protection.

Human parvovirus B19 is the only proven parvovirus which affects humans. Human parvovirus is also known as fifth disease or erythema infectious. This disease is often called the slapped cheek disease, because of the characteristic appearance of the hyperemic cheeks with spared nose and circumoral region observed in children. Its first appearance is within 14 days of exposure, followed by maculopapular rash of the trunk and extremities. In adults the disease is usually asymptomatic but may have fever (should not exceed 39°C), arthralgias (fingers, knees, and wrists) and arthritis. In patients with decreased erythroid precursors (sickle cell disease or thalassemia) nonimmune fetal hydrops and fetal death have been observed. This adverse outcome is because parvovirus replication is primarily in the erythroid precursors in the bone marrow and may induce an acute aplastic crisis. The diagnosis in the gravid woman is based on a positive IgM for B19 with a negative IgG indicating an acute infection within the past 7 days. A positive IgM and IgG for B19 is consistent with an infection in the past 7–120 days. PCR of amniotic fluid may be the best diagnostic test of an infected fetus. The affected fetus usually manifests nonimmune hydrops 4–6 weeks after maternal exposure. The rate of infection in pregnancies of <12 weeks is 19% and in pregnancies of >20 weeks is 6%. More recent studies have found the rate of spontaneous abortion, and neonatal and fetal death to be much lower and in a series of 52 IgM-positive for B19 women in pregnancy no pregnancy losses or fetal deaths were observed. The risk of maternal infection is highest if the source of exposure is the patient's own child. The risk of acquiring a parvovirus infection in pregnancy in susceptible women is 16.7%. If a pregnant woman has a documented infection, then she should be followed for signs of fetal hydrops with serial ultrasounds, as a fetal infection should be manifest within 3 months of the maternal infection. With very low rates of infection, the use of weekly ultrasounds to detect nonimmune hydrops has been questioned. However, some authors report a greater than 95% favorable fetal outcome without intrauterine transfusions in women followed prospectively in pregnancy with ultrasounds. If hydrops does develop, an intrauterine transfusion may be lifesaving. Parvoviruses have been associated with birth defects in animals but there is no correlation between B19 infections in pregnancy and birth defects.

Other viruses that are of neonatal importance are respiratory syncytial viruses and enteroviruses, which infrequently can cause infections in newborns but are not associated with complications in pregnancy or birth defects. Mumps has been associated with an increased risk of fetal loss in the first trimester, but not congenital anomalies. Measles in pregnancy increases the risk of prematurity and low birth weight infants, but not congenital anomalies.

General
1. Perinatal viral and parasitic infections. *ACOG Tech Bull* no. 177, February 1993.
   A review of cytomegalovirus, varicella, and human parvovirus.

Herpes
2. Brockehurst P. Genital herpes infection in pregnancy. *Fetal Matern Med Rev* 1997;9:163.
   A comprehensive review of current literature regarding genital herpes and genital herpes in pregnancy.

Hepatitis
3. Hepatitis in pregnancy. *ACOG Tech Bull* no. 174, November 1992.
   A review of hepatitis in pregnancy, diagnosis and treatment.
4. Snydman DR. Hepatitis in pregnancy. *N Engl J Med* 1985;313:1398.
   Etiology, epidemiology, and natural history of hepatitis in pregnancy.

HIV
5. Human immunodeficiency virus in pregnancy. *ACOG Tech Bull* no. 232, January 1997.
   A review of perinatal transmission, testing, counseling, and management during pregnancy is discussed.
6. Andrews EB, et al. Acyclovir in pregnancy registry: six year experience. *Obstet Gynecol* 1992;79:7.
   The results of the AIDS clinical trials group protocol 076 of asymptomatic women beyond the first trimester of pregnancy who had a CD4 count of >200/mm³.

Parvovirus B19
7. Harger JH, et al. Prospective evaluation of 618 pregnant women exposed to parvovirus B19: risks and symptoms. *Obstet Gynecol* 1998;91:413.
   Demographic and occupational information on 618 women exposed to parvovirus over a 6-year period and their risk of acquiring an infection and the risk of developing fetal hydrops.
8. Guidozzi F, Ballot D, Rothberg AD. Human B19 parvovirus infection in an obstetric population. *J Reprod Med* 1994;39:36.
   A prospective study of 64 IgM-positive women followed through pregnancy with ultrasound with a 95% favorable fetal outcome.

---

10. URINARY TRACT INFECTION IN PREGNANCY

Mendley A. Wulfsohn

Urinary tract infection (UTI) in pregnancy may be asymptomatic or symptomatic. To detect asymptomatic bacteriuria (ASB), which occurs in 4%–7% of pregnant women, a routine urine assessment, most often a urinalysis, and urine culture, should be performed at the first prenatal visit. A high incidence of ASB is associated with multiparity, sickle-cell trait, diabetes mellitus, high parity, and advancing age. It is also found more commonly in lower socioeconomic groups.

Symptomatic UTI most often reflects an exacerbation of preexisting ASB, facilitated by the changes that take place in the urinary tract during pregnancy. Patients who have an antenatal history of UTI and are found to have ASB in early pregnancy have a considerable chance of acquiring active UTI during pregnancy. In addition, women with a previous history of UTI have a 35%–50% chance of having ASB and may develop active UTI in late pregnancy. Therefore, despite initially negative urine culture results at the first visit, further cultures should be taken in this group of women at the beginning of the third trimester. Patients who have an initially positive culture result usually remain positive throughout pregnancy, unless they receive treatment, and acute pyelonephritis may develop in 20%–30% of them, compared to only 1% of the women with negative culture findings. It has been conclusively shown that progression to pyelonephritis can be effectively prevented in 97% of the cases by adequate antibiotic treatment of ASB.

Persistence or recurrence of infection despite adequate treatment suggests the presence of an underlying urologic disease, such as vesicoureteral reflux, obstructive uropathy, or urinary tract calculi. This is an indication for a postpartum urologic workup.

Symptomatic UTI may be confined to the bladder, and cause acute cystitis, or may be manifested as acute pyelonephritis. Acute bacterial cystitis complicates 0.3%–1.3% of pregnancies. The initial symptoms of cystitis consist of frequent urination, nocturia, urgency, and suprapubic discomfort. Hemorrhagic cystitis occasionally occurs. Cystitis must be distinguished from urethral syndrome (frequency-urgency syndrome), interstitial cystitis, and the physiologic frequency occurring during pregnancy. Patients with simple cystitis are usually afebrile, and the diagnosis rests on positive culture findings.

Acute pyelonephritis is a more serious complication during pregnancy. Ascending infection from the bladder is more likely to occur during gestation, accounting for the increased incidence of acute pyelonephritis during pregnancy. The usual presentation consists of acute flank pain and tenderness, more commonly on the right side. Irritative bladder symptoms as well as fever and chills are usually present because bacteremia is common. Pyelonephritis may be a dangerous illness in pregnancy, with a 3% incidence of septic shock and the attendant potential for maternal death. Respiratory insufficiency occurs in 2%–8% of patients. This may occur as a result of pulmonary edema or the development of adult respiratory distress syndrome. Renal dysfunction or anemia may occur. Pyelonephritis may also precipitate premature labor.

Urinary stasis is an important component of the pathophysiologic mechanism responsible for UTI in pregnancy. Hydronephrosis is found on the right side in 90% of pregnant women, compared to 60% on the left side. Ureteral dilatation begins during the seventh week and progresses until term. The dilated collecting system may hold up to 200 ml of urine, making it an ideal reservoir for UTI.

The cause of hydronephrosis and right-sided predominance has never been satisfactorily explained. Obstruction occurs at the level of the pelvic brim because hydronephrosis extends only to this level. The enlarged uterus may compress the ureter against the pelvic brim, and the ovarian veins, which dilate tremendously during late pregnancy, are also implicated. In addition, high progesterone levels may cause ureteral atonicity, as well as hypertrophy of the longitudinal muscle below the pelvic brim (Waldeyer's sheath). The right-sided predominance may stem from the fact that the right ureter crosses the pelvic brim at a sharper angle. In addition, the uterus more commonly lies toward the right, and a right-sided placenta is more common. After delivery, hydronephrosis gradually resolves and is usually completely resolved in all patients by the eighth week postpartum. Other factors that may be important in promoting UTI are the high position of the bladder as well as hypotonicity of the detrusor muscle. A decreased concentrating ability of the kidneys may cause the antibacterial activity of the urine to be diminished. The glycosuria and aminoaciduria of pregnancy provide an ideal culture medium for microorganisms.

When UTI does not respond to appropriate therapy, the presence of urinary calculi should be considered. The presence of a urea-splitting organism, particularly one of the Proteus species, and a persistently alkaline urine suggest calculus disease. The usual symptoms of severe renal colic may be absent during pregnancy, owing to the poor tone of the ureters. Although most calculi can be treated expectantly, an infected kidney that is obstructed by a ureteral calculus may require emergency decompression by the passage of a ureteral catheter or indwelling ureteral stent via a cystoscope or through a percutaneous nephrostomy. Rarely, endoscopic or operative removal of a ureteral calculus becomes necessary. The use of lithotripsy is contraindicated in pregnancy. Diagnosis of calculi during pregnancy may be difficult in view of the reluctance to perform x-ray studies, since radiation to the fetus has been associated with an increased risk of childhood malignancy. An excretory urogram (intravenous pyelogram), however, can be limited to a plain film and a 20-minute film, which is usually sufficient to arrive at a diagnosis. Ultrasonography is useful in detecting hydronephrosis. It can detect a stone in the kidney but usually not a ureteral calculus. Use of a transvaginal probe, however, improves the yield of ultrasound by identifying distal ureteral stones.

Acute pyelonephritis is associated with premature labor and delivery. Mild UTIs appear to have little effect on perinatal morbidity and mortality. There is evidence to suggest that labor may be triggered by phospholipase A, which can be produced by *Escherichia coli* and other gram-negative organisms. This in turn stimulates the production of prostaglandins E_2 and F_2, which initiates labor.

The diagnosis of UTI is based on the findings yielded by urine culture. A midstream clean-catch urine specimen should be obtained, and culture should be performed within 1 h. A dip culture medium is best used as an inexpensive screen for bacteriuria. Routine catheterization to obtain specimens should be avoided during pregnancy and labor, because there is a significant danger of this introducing infection. During pregnancy, catheterization carries a 4%–6% risk of producing symptomatic UTI, and some of these patients could eventually suffer chronic UTI and pyelonephritis. The suprapubic aspiration of urine is a safe and accurate method of collection, but is poorly accepted by both patients and physicians. Bacteriuria is considered significant if greater than 10^5 colonies of a single organism are present on culture. A colony count of 10_2 to 10_4 in an acutely symptomatic patient also signifies infection. On routine culture, a count of 10_4 to 10_5 colonies is equivocal, and the culture should be repeated; less than 10_4 is not significant. The presence of any bacteria after suprapubic aspiration or catheterization is an important finding. *E. coli* accounts for 86% of UTIs in pregnancy. Less commonly, *Proteus mirabilis*, Klebsiella species, Enterobacter species, staphylococcus saprophyticus, and group B beta-hemolytic streptococcus are found.

Pyuria alone is a poor indicator of UTI and indicates inflammation (infective or noninfective) in the urinary tract. Abacterial pyuria is commonly due to vaginal contamination or the use of antibiotics before culture is taken. The possibility of anaerobic or other fastidious organisms should not be overlooked. These include *Gardnerella vaginalis,* Lactobacilli, microaerophilic streptococci, and *Ureaplasma urealyticum.* Persistent abacterial pyuria may also be caused by tumors, ureteral calculi, analgesic abuse, and renal tuberculosis.

ASB in early pregnancy or simple cystitis should be treated with antibiotics for three to ten days. Preferred agents are ampicillin, nitrofurantoin, and cephalexin. Sulfa drugs are usually avoided in late pregnancy because they may produce jaundice in the infant. Tetracycline and quinolones should not be used during pregnancy. Nitrofurantoin should not be used if there is any suspicion of either the mother or the fetus having glucose-6-phosphate dehydrogenase deficiency. Careful follow-up is essential after treatment. Reculture of the urine should be done one week after cessation of the treatment and monthly thereafter. Recurrent infection may require repeated courses of low-dose antibiotic therapy throughout pregnancy (e.g., nitrofurantoin at bedtime). Failure to respond to the initial course of treatment necessitates a second course of appropriate antibiotic, based on sensitivity results. Further relapse of infection is highly suggestive of an underlying urologic abnormality, which requires evaluation postpartum.

Patients with acute pyelonephritis are usually toxic and dehydrated and may be in premature labor. They should be hospitalized, and treatment should consist of the administration of intravenous fluids and correction of electrolyte imbalances. Hemodynamic abnormalities and respiratory insufficiency must be aggressively managed. The intravenous administration of antibiotics is advisable. Ampicillin or a first-generation cephalosporin is the initial antibiotic of choice. As indicated by sensitivity results, antibiotics such as the second- or third-generation cephalosporins, Aztreonam, aminoglycosides, or extended spectrum penicillins (such as Piperacillin and Mezlocillin) may be required. If the infection does not respond to the appropriate antibiotics, obstructive uropathy and renal or perirenal abscess must be suspected. Renal sonography may be helpful in delineating these lesions. Occasionally, abscesses may form in a localized area of pyelonephritis, and these may require percutaneous or operative drainage. Termination of pregnancy to control UTI is rarely indicated.

In summary, UTI during pregnancy can usually be prevented by intense prenatal assessment and treatment. If it does occur, however, it should be treated promptly; otherwise, maternal and fetal compromise can occur. Comprehensive follow-up of patients with this problem is strongly recommended.

General
1. Patterson TF, Andriole VT. Bacteriuria in pregnancy. *Infect Dis Clin North Am* 1987;1:807.
   A general review of 76 references is offered on the etiology, pathogenesis, diagnosis, and management of UTI in pregnancy.
2. Farrar WE Jr. Infections of the urinary tract. *Med Clin North Am* 1983;67:187.
   Emphasizes the importance of screening for UTIs in early pregnancy and reviews subsequent management.

3. Dempsey C, et al. Characteristics of bacteriuria in a homogeneous maternal hospital population. *Eur J Obstet Gynecol Reprod Biol* 1992;44:89.
    A prospective study of more than 3,000 antenatal women revealed a 4.74% incidence of bacteriuria. Sixty-seven percent of these patients were asymptomatic or had a previous history of UTI. The mainstay of treatment was nitrofurantoin. There were no fetal or maternal complications.
4. Millar LK, Cox SM. Urinary tract infections complicating pregnancy. *Infect Dis Clin North Am* 1997;11:13.
    Comprehensive review of the etiology, pathogenesis, and treatment.

Etiology
5. Andriole VT, Patterson TF. Epidemiology, natural history, and management of urinary tract infections in pregnancy. *Med Clin North Am* 1991;76:359.
    ASB is the major risk factor for symptomatic UTI developing in pregnancy. Short-course therapy should be followed by repeat culture to document resolution of the bacteriuria.
6. Martinell J, Jodal U, Linin-Janson G. Pregnancies in women with and without renal scarring after urinary infections in childhood. *BMJ* 1990;300:840.
    Preexisting renal scarring and vesicoureteral reflux predispose to the occurrence of acute pyelonephritis in pregnancy.
7. Jones WA, Correa RJ, Ansell JS. Urolithiasis associated with pregnancy. *J Urol* 1979;122:335.
    There were 20 cases of calculi in 34,081 deliveries observed over a 12-year period.
8. Gilbert GL, et al. Bacteriuria due to ureaplasma and other fastidious organisms during pregnancy: prevalence and significance. *Pediatr Infect Dis* 1986;5:293.
    Ureaplasma urealyticum and Gardnerella vaginalis can be detected quite commonly in apparently healthy pregnant women. Women with Ureaplasma bacteriuria detected at the first antenatal visit are three times more likely to suffer preeclampsia.

Diagnosis
9. Chang PK, Hall MH. Antenatal prediction of urinary tract infection in pregnancy. *Br J Obstet Gynaecol* 1982;89:8.
    A combination of ASB and a history of UTIs signifies a considerable risk: such a woman is 10 times more likely to suffer active infection during pregnancy than a normal woman.
10. Pollock HM. Laboratory techniques for detection of urinary tract infection and assessment of value. *Am J Med* 1983;75:79.
    Review of laboratory methods for detecting bacteriuria and their importance. The findings of bacteria on uncentrifuged gram-stained smears correlates with the presence of significant bacteriuria. The possible presence of anaerobic organisms and Mycoplasma should not be overlooked.
11. Platt R. Quantitative definition of bacteriuria. *Am J Med* 1983;375:44.
    Existing data strongly support the threshold of 10^5 colonies per milliliter as the criterion for diagnosis of pyelonephritis and ASB.
12. Peake SL, Roxburgh HB, Langlois SLP. Ultrasonic assessment of hydronephrosis of pregnancy. *Radiology* 1983;146:167.
    Ultrasonography performed during the routine examination of pregnant women confirmed the high incidence of hydronephrosis.
13. North DH, et al. Correlation of urinary tract infection with urinary screening at the first antepartum visit. *J Miss State Med Assoc* 1990;31:331.
    A cost-effective outpatient assessment of ASB is presented. Single-dose antibiotic therapy was effective.
14. Stenqvist K, et al. Bacteriuria in pregnancy. Frequency and risk of acquisition. *Am J Epidemiol* 1989;129:372.
    The sixteenth gestational week is the optimal time for a single screening for bacteriuria in pregnancy.

15. Hagay Z, et al. Uriscreen, a rapid enzymatic urine screening test: useful predictor of significant bacteriuria in pregnancy. *Obstet Gynecol* 1996;87:410.
An attempt to cut costs in screening for ASB in pregnancy.

Treatment
16. Hankins GDV, Whalley PJ. Acute urinary tract infections in pregnancy. *Clin Obstet Gynecol* 1985;28:266.
Routine screening for ASB in pregnancy, followed by adequate therapy and urine culture surveillance, are important preventive measures. The considerable maternal morbidity associated with the development of acute pyelonephritis more than justifies the effort and expense necessary to implement screening methods.
17. Adelson MD, Graves WL, Osborne NG. Treatment of urinary infections in pregnancy using single versus 10-day dosing. *J Natl Med Assoc* 1992;84:73.
Single-dose therapy did not provide adequate cure or prevent reinfection.
18. Wing DA, et al. A randomized trial of three antibiotic regimens for the treatment of pyelonephritis in pregnancy. *Obstet Gynecol* 1998;92:249.
Ceftriaxone IM was as effective as IV ampicillin/gentamicin or cefazolin.
19. Duff P. Antibiotic selection in obstetric patients. *Infect Dis Clin North Am* 1997;11:1.
Pharmacology of the important antibiotics which can be used in pregnancy is reviewed together with dosage and costs.

Complications
20. Davison JM, Sprott MS, Selkon JR. The effect of covert bacteriuria on renal function in schoolgirls at 18 years and during pregnancy. *Lancet* 1984;2:651.
ASB treated by antibiotic coverage prevents clinical renal damage that is more evident in the pregnant than in the nonpregnant.
21. Hill JA, Devoe LK, Bryans CI. Frequency of asymptomatic bacteriuria in preeclampsia. *Obstet Gynecol* 1986;67:52.
A significant difference in the rate of ASB was found in patients with preeclampsia versus that in control subjects. In addition, preeclamptic patients with bacteriuria had substantially lower total serum protein and albumin levels.
22. Yasin SY, Doun SNB. Hemodialysis in pregnancy. *Obstet Gynecol Surv* 1988; 43:655.
Chronic UTIs during pregnancy may lead to renal disease severe enough to require hemodialysis. The authors have reviewed the literature in this exhaustive search and find that hemodialysis can be accomplished safely, if done properly.
23. Towers CV, et al. Pulmonary injury associated with antepartum pyelonephritis: can patients at risk be identified? *Am J Obstet Gynecol* 1996;164:974.
Rare before the second trimester, more likely to occur in the third trimester. This article emphasizes the importance of close monitoring for complications and of response to therapy.

11. VENEREAL DISEASES IN PREGNANCY

Mark H. Einstein

Venereal diseases are usually asymptomatic; few of the women who have signs seek medical advice because their symptoms are mild and transient. Furthermore, the clinical course of venereal disease may be even milder in pregnancy. The common venereal diseases contracted in pregnancy include trichomoniasis, gonorrhea, condyloma acuminatum, herpes, and syphilis.

Trichomonas vaginalis is transmitted by sexual intercourse, and women usually have more symptoms than men. The prevalence of *T. vaginalis* in pregnancy is 13% in an evaluation of nearly 14,000 gravid women. Risk factors include young age, history of gonococcal infection, use of tobacco, multiple sexual partners, poor education, and single marital status. Some report that there is an increase in preterm birth, preterm premature rupture of membranes, and intrauterine growth restriction with trichomonas, but this is not supported by all authors. The subjective symptoms include a profuse, frothy, foul-smelling vaginal discharge, accompanied by vulvar itching, dyspareunia, and dysuria. The wet smear, or the more sensitive *T. vaginalis* culture, is used to establish diagnosis. The most effective therapeutic agent is metronidazole (Flagyl), which may be administered in doses of either 250 mg orally three times a day for 7 days or 2 g orally in one dose. Metronidazole may be safely administered in the second and third trimester of pregnancy, but its use is contraindicated during the first trimester. Local measures, such as povidone-iodine (Betadine) sitz baths and sulfur creams, are advocated for relief in the first trimester but have low cure rates. Clotrimazole, in a 100-mg vaginal suppository inserted at bedtime for 7 days, may also provide symptomatic relief. Treatment of the sexual partner is strongly recommended, especially in the setting of recurrent cases. Lactating women may be treated with metronidazole, 2.0 g orally in a single dose, but should stop breast-feeding for 24 hours.

Gonorrhea is the most commonly reported venereal disease in the United States, with more than one million cases reported annually. The incidence rate of gonorrhea in the pregnant population is 0.5%–7%; 90% of these cases are asymptomatic. *Neisseria gonorrhoeae* is almost always spread by genital or oral contact. The gonococcus is most commonly found in the endocervix. From the cervix, the gonococcus may move into the endometrium, oviducts, and pelvic peritoneum. During pregnancy, the infection rarely ascends to the upper genital tract, although it can disseminate to other organs, such as the joints and skin, by hematogenous pathways. Untreated gonococcal infection in pregnancy has been associated with premature birth, low birth weight, preterm premature rupture of membranes, and chorioamnionitis. Patients with disseminated gonococcal infection usually initially exhibit a pyogenic arthritis accompanied by chills and fever. In uncomplicated cases, gonorrhea usually involves a transient dysuria, mild vaginal discharge, pharyngeal infection, or any combination of these symptoms.

The definitive diagnosis of gonorrhea is based on the results of culture on modified Thayer-Martin medium in an enriched (5%–10%) carbon dioxide atmosphere or using enzyme immunoassay or DNA probe. Gram's staining, even if the results are positive, may be an inaccurate method. Endocervical cultures yield the best results, although anorectal and pharyngeal sources for cultures should be considered. Both sexual partners should be examined and treated. Finally, a diagnostic test for concomitant syphilis is strongly recommended.

The recommended treatment for uncomplicated asymptomatic pregnant patients with gonorrhea consists of a single intramuscular administration of 250 mg of ceftriaxone or cefixime 400 mg orally. If chlamydial diagnostic testing is not available, empirical treatment for chlamydia should also be given. Because tetracyclines are contraindicated in pregnancy, this treatment should consist of azithromycin 1 gram orally in a single dose or erythromycin base 500 mg (or equivalent) taken orally four times a day for 7 days. Pregnant women who are allergic to beta-lactams should be treated with spectinomycin, 2 g intramuscularly, plus erythromycin. In pregnant patients hospitalized with severe infections, ceftriaxone, ceftizoxime, or cefotaxime may be given intravenously, or, if the infecting organism proves to be penicillin sensitive, parenteral penicillin may be used. Details of this therapy and of the treatment of neonates, infants, and children are beyond the scope of this chapter. A test of cure after the completion of antimicrobial therapy is not indicated because the effectiveness of recommended regimens is greater than 95%. Women with known recent exposure to gonorrhea should be treated as just described.

Condyloma acuminatum (venereal warts) represent a venereal disease caused by human papilloma virus (HPV) that is spread by sexual contact. It is estimated that 6%–60% of women are infected with HPV. The warts are most commonly found in the genital area during the years of maximal sexual activity. The Papanicolaou (Pap) test is not useful for diagnostic purposes because there are no specific cytologic findings involved. The initial lesion is usually a rough, cauliflower-like warty papilloma that appears in the perineal area. During pregnancy, the condyloma acuminatum may grow more rapidly and hinder vaginal delivery, making a cesarean delivery necessary in patients who have large, obstructing condylomata. The pregnant patient with condyloma acuminatum poses special problems because the usual treatment, topically administered podophyllin, should be avoided throughout pregnancy owing to its toxic properties. Aldara (Imiquimod) is a category B drug that can shrink lesions if used three times per week prior to sleeping and left on for 6–10 hours. Definitive therapy during pregnancy includes destructive methods of therapy (e.g., electrocautery, cryosurgery, or laser vaporization), combined with povidone-iodine douches and sitz baths. In the event of recurrent and persistent condyloma acuminatum, an autogenous vaccine has been used successfully.

Syphilis is primarily a sexually transmitted disease, and approximately 30% of the 25,000 annual cases occur in women. Additionally, there are 350 cases of congenital syphilis reported every year. During pregnancy, transplacental infection of the fetus may occur, resulting either in an asymptomatic newborn who later shows the stigmata of congenital syphilis or in fetal death. Syphilis is a chronic infectious process caused by the spirochete *Treponema pallidum*. Owing to its small size, it can be identified only by dark-field microscopy. Initial screening uses nontreponemal rapid plasma reagin (RPR) test or venereal disease research laboratory (VDRL) test. False-positive tests can occur in women with autoimmune disorders. Also, these tests are insensitive in the setting of very early or latent disease. A positive nontreponemal test can be confirmed with a treponema-specific test such as a fluorescent treponemal antibody absorption (FTA ABS) test or microhemagglutinin *T. pallidum* (MHA TP) test. Congenital syphilis can be confirmed by either a dark-field examination, if lesions are present, or by determining the immunoglobulin M (IgM)–FTA–ABS titer, which represents infant IgM antibodies produced as a result of active syphilitic infection.

After a 10- to 90-day incubation period, an indurated, nontender ulcer develops, known as a chancre. This primary lesion, accompanied by painless regional lymphadenopathy, usually appears on the external genitalia, in the vagina, or on the cervix. The chancre is followed by a bacteremic, or secondary stage if the disease is not treated. The clinical manifestations of secondary syphilis include skin rash, lesions on the palms and soles, mucous patches on mucosal surfaces and wartlike growths in the genital area (condyloma latum). In the absence of therapy, the clinical manifestations of tertiary syphilis occur some years after the initial infection, and include gummatous involvement of various organs as well as abnormalities in the cardiovascular and central nervous systems.

The effect of syphilis on the fetus depends on when the disease was contracted in relation to the time of gestation, and on the effectiveness of treatment. It has been shown that the placenta is permeable to the treponema organism throughout pregnancy. Clinical observation, however, has shown that, if a pregnant patient contracts syphilis during the first 16–18 weeks of gestation, it is less likely that the fetus will be affected. Nevertheless, untreated syphilis in pregnancy may result in early spontaneous abortion, nonimmune hydrops, premature labor, stillbirth, neonatal death, or congenital syphilis.

The treatment of incubating syphilis and syphilis of less than 1 year's duration includes benzathine penicillin G 2.4 million units total, half given intramuscularly in each buttock. For gravidas with syphilis of more than 1 year's duration or of unknown duration, the treatment of choice is also benzathine penicillin G 2.4 million units given intramuscularly weekly for 3 successive weeks for a total of 7.2 million units. Patients allergic to penicillin should undergo skin testing and desensitization, if necessary, done in collaboration with an expert. Erythromycin is somewhat effective in eradicating early maternal disease; however, it is poor at preventing and treating fetal infection. Finally, the treatment of syphilis with long-acting penicillin is not always effective in pregnant patients owing to the lower serum levels of antibiotics attained during pregnancy, versus those in the nonpregnant patient. Thus, the course of the pregnant patient should be monitored by the performance of monthly quantitative nontreponemal serologic tests, and the patient should be retreated if the titer rises. A fourfold decrease in titers should be seen within 3–4 months of treatment.

Chancroid, caused by *Haemophilus ducreyi*, is an acute and painful infection of the external genitalia and regional lymph nodes (bubo). It can be transmitted sexually. The diagnosis is made on the basis of findings yielded either by culturing material from the ulcers or bubo in a blood-containing medium or by biopsy of these lesions. Treatment with erythromycin 500 mg orally four times per day or ceftriaxone 250 mg once intramuscularly is recommended. Ciprofloxin 500 mg orally twice per day for 3 days may also be used. Azithromycin or a multiple-dose regimen is preferred in human immunodeficiency virus (HIV)–infected individuals.

Granuloma inguinale, caused by *Calymmatobacterium granulomatis* (also called *Donavania granulomatis*), a disease with a low incidence of infection, is spread by sexual intercourse. The initial lesion consists of a raised, painless papule that develops into central ulcerations accompanied by local, deep destruction of tissues and the formation of rectovaginal fistulas and pseudobuboes. The diagnosis is made by the finding of characteristic Donovan bodies in material aspirated from lymph nodes. Culture of *C. granulomatis* is also helpful. Tetracycline and erythromycin are effective agents in the treatment of early lesions, although only the latter can be used in pregnancy. Surgical intervention may be required for correction of advanced tissue destruction.

Lymphogranuloma venereum, caused by *Chlamydia trachomatis*, is a disease that is usually transmitted through sexual intercourse, and primarily affects the lymphatics and the lymph nodes (inguinal buboes). Common complications of the disease include rectovaginal fistulas, perirectal abscesses, and polypoid growths of the colon, with occasional malignant degeneration. The definitive diagnosis of lymphogranuloma venereum is made by a complement fixation test. Biopsy of the lesions, biochemical tests, and the Frei intradermal test (nonspecific) can also be used diagnostically. The recommended treatment in pregnancy consists of erythromycin 500 mg given orally four times per day for 21 days.

Molluscum contagiosum is a sexually transmitted viral (poxvirus group) cutaneous disease that involves the genital area. The diagnosis is based on the findings from microscopic examination of the lesion. Cryosurgery and electrocautery are utilized as methods of treatment.

C. trachomatis is the most prevalent sexually transmitted bacterial pathogen in the United States today. An estimated four million chlamydial infections occur annually. Because laboratory screening for this pathogen has become widely available, pregnant women who are at high risk for sexually transmitted disease should be routinely cultured in the third trimester. Treatment should be instituted in women with proven *C. trachomatis* infection or women whose sexual partners have nongonococcal urethritis or epididymitis. During pregnancy the suggested treatment is azithromycin 1 gram orally as a single dose or erythromycin base 500 mg orally four times per day for 7 days. When treatment fails, patients should be retreated, and male sexual partners should be treated with tetracycline or doxycycline.

Genital herpes infection is a viral disease that may appear acutely or chronically during pregnancy. The pregnancy registry has not shown an increased risk to developing fetuses from acyclovir. Doses of 200 mg orally five times daily for 7–10 days or 400 mg orally three times a day for 5–7 days may be considered. Alternatives, including valacyclovir and famciclovir, are considered category B pregnancy drugs but are approved only in nonpregnant patients. Because of the risk of neonatal transfer, frequent perineal inspection during pregnancy is important, as is notification of the pediatric personnel. Transmission of herpes virus to the fetus is prevented by cesarean delivery if a visible lesion is present or prodromal symptoms are present in a patient with known herpes infection.

The growing threat that HIV poses to reproductive-age women is of increasing concern. At the end of 1996, the cumulative number of diagnosed cases of acquired immunodeficiency syndrome (AIDS) in the United States was 581,429, with women accounting for 15% of this total and 20% of the new cases. HIV infection is now the leading cause of death in young women 25–44 years old in many U.S. states and cities. It is estimated that there are more than 7,000 HIV-infected infants born annually in the United States. Advanced disease states, low CD4 counts, and high viral loads have been associated with higher rates of perinatal transmission.

The first task in caring for a pregnant woman with HIV is to provide counseling that will allow an informed reproductive choice. HIV-positive women should be screened for other sexually transmitted infections, including syphilis, gonorrhea, chlamydia, and hepatitis B. Tuberculosis should also be excluded. Antibody titers of cytomegalovirus (CMV) and toxoplasma should be measured. Counseling concerning the risk of vertical transmission should be provided and the reproductive options outlined.

A multicenter trial of Zidovudine (AZT) in pregnancy was discontinued because of the remarkable drop observed in the rate of vertical transmission of HIV from 25.5% in the placebo group to 8.3% in the intervention arm. From then on, the standard use of AZT was rapidly formulated and widely used. AZT should be given 100 mg orally five times per day. During labor, intravenous administration of AZT should be given in a 1-hour loading dose of 2 mg/kg body weight followed by a continuous infusion of 1 mg/kg until delivery. Oral administration of AZT should be given to the newborn at a dose of 2 mg/kg every 6 hours for the first 6 weeks of life beginning 8–12 hours after birth. The primary adverse reaction of AZT is bone marrow suppression. The CD4 cell counts in patients with HIV infection should be monitored. Patients with low CD4 counts are at risk for acquiring opportunistic infections. If counts fall below 200/mm^3, prophylaxis against *Pneumocystis carinii pneumonia* should be instituted with Bactrim.

As the evolution of treatment and prophylaxis with drugs such as ddC, ddI, 3TC, d4T, and protease inhibitors continues it would be prudent to gain the assistance of an infectious disease specialist to ensure optimal care. Additionally, this will allow the patient an avenue for care after delivery.

There is no evidence that the mode of delivery alters the rate of HIV transmission. However, some measures, such as the avoidance of direct contact of the infected mother's vaginal secretions with the fetal blood (such as might occur during fetal scalp sampling or electronic scalp electrode application), and avoidance of rupturing membranes until necessary may diminish risk. Women in labor should be carefully assessed initially and periodically for any signs of chorioamnionitis and antibiotics initiated liberally when appropriate. Finally, there is little information regarding the postpartum management of HIV-infected women. Evidence suggests that HIV vertical transmission can occur during breast-feeding, and, therefore, HIV-infected patients should be advised not to breast-feed their infants.

General
1. Anastos K, Denenberg R, Solomon L. Human immunodeficiency virus infection in women. *Med Clin North Am* 1997;81:533.
   Comprehensive discussion on all aspects HIV disease in women.
2. Charles D. Syphilis. *Clin Obstet Gynecol* 1983;26:125.
   This comprehensive article details the diagnosis and treatment of syphilis during pregnancy.
3. Hoyt L. HIV infection in women and children. Special concerns in prevention and care. *Postgrad Med* 1997;102:165.
   General, easy-to-read article on HIV infection.
4. Human immunodeficiency virus infections. *ACOG Tech Bull* no. 169, June 1992.
   A concise review of the etiology, diagnosis, and vertical transmission of HIV in pregnancy—worth reading.
5. Jackson SL, Soper DE. Sexually transmitted diseases in pregnancy. *Obstet Gynecol Clin North Am* 1997;24:631.
   Well-organized, comprehensive discussion on STD diagnosis, screening, and treatment.
6. Martens KA. Sexually transmitted and genital tract infections during pregnancy. *Emerg Med Clin North Am* 1994;12:91.
   In-depth discussion of diagnosis, management, and potential obstetric consequences of selected STDs during pregnancy.

7. Ross SM. Sexually transmitted diseases in pregnancy. *Clin Obstet Gynecol* 1982; 9:565.
   A discussion of 12 venereal diseases and their impact on pregnancy.
8. Wendel PJ, Wendel GD Jr. Sexually transmitted diseases in pregnancy. *Semin Perinatol* 1993;17:443.
   Focuses mainly on treatment of STDs in pregnancy.

Etiology

9. Blanchard AC, Pastonek JG, Weeks T. Pelvic inflammatory disease including pregnancy. *South Med J* 1987;80:136.
   The authors report on three cases of acute gonococcal salpingitis that coexisted with pregnancy.
10. Hardy PH, et al. Prevalence of six sexually transmitted disease agents among pregnant inner-city adolescents and pregnancy outcome. *Lancet* 1984;2:333.
    This study demonstrated that T. vaginalis infection, either alone or in conjunction with C. trachomatis or Candida infection, was associated with small-for-gestation-age and low-birth-weight infants.
11. Holmes KK. The chlamydia. *JAMA* 1981;245:1718.
    This article considers chlamydia and how it affects pregnant and nonpregnant women. This is must reading for those interested in the chlamydia epidemic in the country.
12. Peckham C, Gibb D. Mother-to-child transmission of the human immunodeficiency virus. *N Engl J Med* 1995;333:298.
    Explanation of vertical transmission, natural history, and therapeutics of HIV disease. Great references.

Diagnosis

13. Brown ST, et al. Serological response to syphilis treatment. A new analysis of old data. *JAMA* 1985;253:1296.
    This article describes a curve for following the VDRL titer, which allows the clinician to identify early treatment failures and reinfections.
14. Stamm WE, et al. Diagnosis of chlamydia trachomatis infections by direct immuno-fluorescence staining of genital secretions. *Ann Intern Med* 1984;101:638.
    Direct immunofluorescence staining of genital secretions for chlamydia trachomatis in men, women, and pregnant women demonstrated high sensitivity and specificity and offers an alternative diagnostic approach to cell cultures.
15. Wendel GD Jr. Gestational and congenital syphilis. *Clin Perinatol* 1988;15:287.
    In this review, the author outlines the current status, epidemiology, and complications of syphilis. The presentation on maternal and neonatal syphilis is nicely organized.
16. Zbella EA, Deppe G, Elrad H. Gonococcal arthritis in pregnancy. *Obstet Gynecol Surv* 1984;39:81.
    A review of the clinical presentation, diagnostic criteria, and recommended treatment for women with gonococcal arthritis in pregnancy.

Treatment

17. Drugs for sexually transmitted diseases. *Med Lett Drugs Ther* 1995;37:117.
    Focuses specifically on treatment of STDs.
18. Minkoff H, Augenbraun M. Anti-retroviral therapy in pregnant women. *Am J Obstet Gynecol* 1997;176:478.
    Discussion of all anti-retroviral agents, animal studies, and a review of FDA use-in-pregnancy ratings.
19. Ryan GM Jr. Ambulatory management of venereal disease. In: Ryan GM Jr, ed. *Ambulatory care in obstetrics and gynecology.* New York: Grune & Stratton, 1980.
    The author describes the ambulatory management of gonorrhea and syphilis in both pregnant and nonpregnant patients.

Complications
20. Goldenberg RL, et al. Sexually transmitted diseases and adverse outcomes of pregnancy. *Clin Perinatol* 1997;24:23–41.
Comprehensive discussion on perinatal effects of STDs. Nice comparison tables.
21. Mascola L, et al. Congenital syphilis. Why is it still occurring? *JAMA* 1984; 252:1719.
A CDC epidemiological review of 50 cases of congenital syphilis. Improved prenatal care in high-risk populations and refined care efforts to control infectious syphilis would reduce this complication.
22. Nguyen D. Gonorrhea in pregnancy and in the newborn. *Am Fam Physician* 1984;29:185.
The prevalence of gonorrhea in pregnancy ranges from 0.2% to 15%. Maternal gonococcal infection is associated with ectopic pregnancy, premature birth, and ophthalmia neonatorum.
23. Solola AS, Ryan GM Jr, Ling FW. Gonorrhea during the intrapartum period. *Am J Obstet Gynecol* 1982;144:351.
A 1-month surveillance of 148 randomly selected women in labor detected 9.5% with a positive gonococcal culture. The authors recommend initial prenatal screening and repeat screening until term in high-risk populations.

IV. PREEXISTING DISEASES IN PREGNANCY

12. PULMONARY DISEASE IN PREGNANCY

James A. Bofill

It is important to remember that normal pregnancy engenders significant changes in cardiorespiratory physiology. These changes facilitate oxygen transfer from the mother to the fetus and carbon dioxide transfer from fetus to mother. Static lung volumes undergo predictable changes during pregnancy, and some of these changes are appreciable as early as 8 weeks' gestation. There is a 20% fall (about 400 ml) in functional residual capacity (FRC). As pregnancy approaches term there will be a small decrease (5%) in total lung capacity but vital capacity does not change appreciably. While static lung volumes may be decreased during pregnancy spirometry should not be significantly affected. The forced expiratory volume in one second, FEV_1, the most commonly measured parameter in pulmonary function testing, should not be significantly different in the pregnant patient. The hormonal milieu of pregnancy, most notably progesterone, will reliably stimulate respiratory drive. Total airway resistance is decreased during pregnancy, and chest wall compliance is also decreased. There are also important ventilatory changes during normal pregnancy. Minute ventilation increases by 40% and alveolar ventilation increases by about 50%, with both of these changes occurring in early gestation and becoming more pronounced as pregnancy advances. Tidal volume is increased by 40%, but there is no change in maternal respiratory rate. This hyperventilation is considered a progestational effect. Many pregnant women will complain of the sensation of dyspnea in early pregnancy. This is considered to arise from the patient's perception of the hyperventilation of pregnancy mentioned above.

Oxygen uptake and carbon dioxide production both increase in early normal pregnancy. Arterial blood gas analysis documents that this hyperventilation will decrease the $PaCO_2$ in normal pregnancy to 28–32 mm Hg. This decrease in maternal $PaCO_2$ allows for efficient transfer of CO_2 from fetus to mother. It is important to remember these normal changes when evaluating arterial blood gas data in pregnant women who are in the throes of an asthmatic exacerbation or in the setting of pneumonia. The decrease in maternal $PaCO_2$ is even more noticeable during labor, and this may induce a respiratory alkalosis. A respiratory alkalosis may impair uteroplacental blood flow, and epidural analgesia may minimize these changes.

Asthma will complicate 1%–3% of pregnancies. Asthmatic patients who present for antenatal care should be assessed for the clinical severity of their disease. Most commonly this is done by pulmonary function testing. Serial measurements of peak expiratory flow rate (PEFR), or peak flows, should be performed at each clinic visit and, if required, twice daily at home by the patient. A 10% decrease from the patient's baseline peak flow rate generally indicates a need for an increase in medication, while a 20% decrease frequently dictates that the patient present for medical evaluation and therapy. It is important to know which medications the patient uses, either intermittently or chronically, for her asthma. Likewise, it is important to know if the patient has required the use of glucocorticoids to control her bronchospasm in the past. A history of severe attacks which required hospitalization or intubation and mechanical ventilation may offer insight into the severity of the patient's condition.

Asthma is a disease of reversible airway obstruction and is characterized by inflammation of the airways and hyperresponsiveness of the bronchial tree. This bronchial hyperresponsiveness may arise secondary to drugs (e.g., aspirin), environmental pollutants (e.g., tobacco smoke), infections (e.g., viral or bacterial tracheobronchitis or pneumonia), allergens (e.g., pollens), exercise (e.g., cold-induced), psychosocial stress, or other poorly defined stimuli. The diagnosis of asthma is centered on the patient's history, the physical examination, and the response to bronchodilators. If there is a 15% improvement in the FEV_1 after treatment with an inhaled β-agonist, this is considered tacit evidence of reversible bronchoconstriction.

During an acute exacerbation of asthma there is air-trapping leading to alveolar overdistention and the patient is unable to easily exhale. Alveolar overdistention may lead to ventilation-perfusion deficits. This chain of events, if uninterrupted, may lead to hypoxemia and hypercarbia, which may require intubation and mechanical ventilation. During a severe attack the patient's systolic blood pressure may fall during forceful inhalation; this is termed the pulsus paradoxus. A chest x-ray is advisable to rule out an obvious pneumonia and to demonstrate the typically overexpanded lungs seen during a moderate or severe exacerbation. Noninvasive pulse oximetry, if available, is a reliable method to exclude hypoxemia. Blood gas analysis should bear in mind the expected changes seen in normal pregnancy. A $PaCO_2$ of 36–38 mm Hg may be normal in the nonpregnant individual but may be evidence of CO_2 retention in the pregnant patient. A thorough physical examination is important in the assessment of a symptomatic asthma patient who presents for care. Is the patient using the accessory muscles of respiration? Auscultation of the lungs may reveal inspiratory and expiratory wheezes if ventilation is not overly impaired. Bedside spirometry, using the FEV_1 or PEFR, may be measured before and after treatment with an inhaled β-agonist. The patient who remains hypoxic and who develops progressive hypercapnea or who becomes exhausted by the work of breathing will require intubation and mechanical ventilation. Liberal consultation with colleagues in internal medicine, emergency medicine, or pulmonology is prudent if a patient may require intubation.

Recent studies of pregnancy in asthmatic patients have revealed no significant difference in rates of preterm delivery, intrauterine growth restriction, or perinatal mortality when these patients are compared to women without asthma. Most studies agree that 10%–12% of patients may expect an exacerbation of their disease during labor. Patients who are delivered by cesarean may be at higher risk for a postpartum relapse of bronchospasm. The inhaled β-agonists are the most commonly used medications for asthma. The most common of these are terbutaline, albuterol, and metaproterenol. The inhaled antiinflammatory glucocorticoids (e.g., triamcinolone, beclomethasone) are also widely used. Cromolyn sodium is a nonsteroidal antiinflammatory agent that is used for prophylaxis in patients who have allergen-induced asthma. Cromolyn stabilizes mast cell membranes and prevents the histamine release which can produce bronchoconstriction. Theophylline was very popular some years ago but is now clearly a second line agent behind the inhaled medications listed above. Patients who present with a severe episode of bronchoconstriction are commonly treated with intravenous methylprednisolone or hydrocortisone. After disease stabilization, the patient is provided with 40–60 mg of oral prednisone which is tapered over the course of 2–3 weeks. Some patients will require chronic therapy with oral glucocorticoids. These patients may be at increased risk for gestational diabetes mellitus, intrauterine growth restriction, and preterm premature rupture of the membranes.

Bacterial or viral pneumonia is considered a fairly common infectious complication of pregnancy. A recent case series noted the incidence of pneumonia complicating pregnancy to be 1.2 cases per 1,000 deliveries. The usual criteria for diagnosis include fever, a productive cough, and clinical findings consistent with pneumonia. Chest x-ray (with abdominal shielding) is important to confirm the clinical impression. Pneumonia may engender a higher risk to the pregnant patient. Factors that may place the pregnant patient at increased risk for developing pneumonia include tobacco abuse, asthma, heart disease, anemia, HIV seropositivity, or immunosuppressive medications. Even in the era of multiple antibiotics and intensive care units maternal mortality secondary to pneumonia continues to be reported. Most cases of pneumonia during pregnancy will not be bacteriologically characterized. The most common agents of pneumonia in pregnancy are *Streptococcus pneumoniae* (the pneumococcus), *Hemophilus influenzae,* Mycoplasma and Legionella, influenza A, varicella, various fungi or protozoa, *Escherichia coli,* and *Klebsiella pneumoniae.* The pneumococcus is responsible for about 25% of the cases of community-acquired pneumonias diagnosed during pregnancy. It presents in the same manner as in the nonpregnant state with shaking chills, fever, dyspnea, sharp chest pain, and a cough that produces yellow-green sputum. The chest x-ray will commonly note a pleural effusion with lobar consolidation. Blood cultures will be positive in about 25% of cases. Typically, the sputum will demonstrate gram-positive organisms in chains or clusters. The atypical organisms (Mycoplasma or Legionella) produce a pneumonia of more insidious onset. The patient will commonly complain of having the flue for 1–2 weeks associated with a low-grade fever. The chest x-ray will often demonstrate patchy infiltrates with or without a pleural effusion. Most infectious disease experts consider that for a community acquired pneumonia the pregnant patient should be hospitalized and treated with antibiotics that will cover the pneumococcus, the atypical organisms, and *H. influenzae.* The most commonly selected antibiotics will include a second-generation cephalosporin and erythromycin. For a hospital-acquired pneumonia the patient will also require the gram-negative coverage afforded by a third-generation cephalosporin or an aminoglycoside (gentamycin).

There is controversy regarding influenza vaccination during pregnancy. This is a killed virus vaccine and is unlikely to have a significant degree of teratogenic potential. Many pregnant women died during the influenza epidemics of 1917–1918 and 1957–1958. This viral pneumonia appears to be especially dangerous during the third trimester of pregnancy. Women who are immunosuppressed or those who work in an environment where they are expected to come into frequent contact with this virus (e.g., nurses and physicians) are frequently encouraged to receive the vaccine after the first trimester has been completed. The patient with pneumonia secondary to influenza A will present with high fevers, chills, headaches, and myalgia. They will often relate a history of 4 to 7 days of upper respiratory tract symptoms. Auscultation will reveal no evidence of consolidation but there may be wheezing, upper airways rhonchi, and crackles. This diagnosis is difficult to make without equivocation, as techniques for viral isolation are not widely available. Pregnant patients considered to have influenza A pneumonia may be treated with amantidine (pregnancy category C). Pregnant patients exposed to known cases of influenza A and who are considered to be at increased risk for pneumonia may be treated prophylactically with amantidine; this may prevent up to 70% of infections. The dose for prophylaxis is 200 mg daily for 10 days.

Varicella is a DNA virus of the herpes family which may cause a life-threatening pneumonia in the pregnant patient. Varicella pneumonia is much more likely to develop in the pregnant patient who smokes tobacco. Patients should be queried regarding a history of chicken pox when they present for antenatal care. Those patients who have never had primary varicella and who are negative for varicella IgG are at risk. A pregnant woman who is varicella IgG seronegative and who has a known exposure to a case of chicken pox should receive intramuscular varicella-zoster immune globulin (VZIG) as a prophylactic treatment. Pregnant women most commonly contract the disease from exposure to a child with chicken pox. If pneumonia develops it is usually noted about 5 days after the typical exanthem. The patient will present with fever, rash, dyspnea, cough, and chest pain. Immediate hospitalization is warranted and intravenous acyclovir therapy is initiated. Treatment is otherwise supportive. A congenital varicella syndrome may be seen in about 2% of neonates whose mothers had varicella in the first 20 weeks of pregnancy.

Patients with immunosuppression are at risk for opportunistic pulmonary infections. In patients with the acquired immunodeficiency syndrome (AIDS) the most common of these opportunistic infections is *Pneumocystis carinii* pneumonia (PCP). Patients whose CD4 cell counts are $<200/mm^3$ are generally provided prophylaxis against PCP. This is most commonly accomplished by oral trimethoprim/sulfamethoxazole or by inhaled pentamidine. Patients with immunosuppression are also at risk for the fungal pneumonias such as those due to *Coccidioides immitis* (coccidiomycosis) or *Histoplasma capsulatum.* Most often these infections will require treatment with amphotericin B.

Tuberculosis is a disease that has been known for many centuries. Within the last two decades a resurgence has been noted in the United States secondary to the immunosuppression of HIV as well as to the immigration of individuals from countries where this malady is endemic. The etiologic agent is *Mycobacterium tuberculosis.* This is an insidious disease that may present as a syndrome of chronic fatigue, weight loss, night sweats, cough, and hemoptysis. Many pregnant patients with tuberculosis are only mildly symptomatic or are asymptomatic. There is evidence that pregnancy or delivery accelerates the disease process in infected individuals. Conversely, if appropriately treated, tuberculosis should have no detrimental effects on pregnancy outcome. In some U.S. clinics, all pregnant women are tested for tuberculosis with the Mantoux skin test. This purified protein derivative is injected intradermally (0.1 ml) and is read 48–72 hours later. It is important to measure only the amount of induration, and not of erythema, when the test is read. The Centers for Disease Control and Prevention uses three levels of induration ($\geq$5 mm, $\geq$10 mm, and $\geq$15 mm) to consider a test positive depending on the risk factors for the specific patient. Low-risk patients require $\geq$15 mm of induration while patients at high risk (those with HIV or with recent close contact with an active case) require only $\geq$5 mm of induration for the test to be considered positive.

Pregnant patients with a positive purified protein derivative (PPD) but without symptoms are considered to have been infected with *M. tuberculosis* even though they may be entirely without symptoms. These women will then proceed to chest x-ray. Guidelines for pharmacologic treatment of a pregnant patient will depend on the chest x-ray (normal versus abnormal), the patient's age, whether the patient's PPD has recently converted, and on other high-risk factors such as HIV seropositivity or the finding of acid-fast bacilli on sputum smears or sputum cultures. Pregnant patients who are considered to have active (symptomatic) tuberculosis will require pharmacotherapy. If there is no suspicion of a drug-resistant strain, the patient will be treated with isoniazid, rifampin, and pyridoxine. If there is a possibility of a drug-resistant strain, ethambutol is usually added until culture and sensitivity results are known. If a drug-resistant strain of *M. tuberculosis* is strongly suspected pyrazinamide is added to the treatment regimen and the patient should be followed by local infectious disease experts.

Cystic fibrosis is the most common autosomal recessive disease in the white population. Tremendous advances have been made in the treatment of patients with this disease and many women now live through adolescence and into adulthood and become pregnant. This is a systemic disease, but the major derangements include pancreatic exocrine deficiency and chronic bronchopulmonary disease. Pancreatic disease may cause a secondary diabetes mellitus. However, it is the pulmonary disorder that most often causes life-threatening morbidity and mortality. Women with cystic fibrosis will often present in the office of an obstetrician-gynecologist for a preconception counseling appointment. Assessment of risk is dependent upon evaluation of the patient's nutritional status and pulmonary function. These women will often have a persistent bronchial infection with *Pseudomonas aeruginosa*. These patients should undergo serial pulmonary function testing because prepregnancy FEV_1 is a helpful predictor of outcomes in women with cystic fibrosis. If the FEV_1 is <60% of the predicted value, the patient will be at risk for adverse pregnancy outcome as well as progressive deterioration of pulmonary function during gestation. If a patient's lung disease has progressed to the point of pulmonary arterial hypertension, she should be counseled against pregnancy. These patients may have a deficiency in their ability to digest dietary fats and may be poorly able to absorb the fat-soluble vitamins. Nutritional status is assessed by maternal weight. These patients' weight should be within 10%–15% of ideal body weight for an optimal outcome.

Anesthesia-related deaths comprise a significant proportion of maternal mortality. Thankfully, the number of anesthesia-related deaths has declined in recent years. The leading cause of these anesthetic deaths is airway problems such as aspiration of gastric contents, problems with induction of anesthesia or with intubation, inadequate ventilation, and respiratory failure. It is clear that medical efforts should be directed at preventing aspiration prior to surgery. A clear, nonparticulate antacid should be taken orally by the patient prior to any anesthetic procedure, including regional analgesia for labor. If general anesthesia is required it is prudent to apply continuous cricoid pressure during intubation to prevent the reflux of gastric contents through the esophagus. If aspiration does occur it will be less serious if the contents are not particulate and not of strongly acidic nature. Measures for treating aspiration include immediate clearance of the airway, adequate oxygenation, use of bronchodilators, and suctioning of foreign materials, if possible. Most of these patients will require treatment with antibiotics for the expected bacterial superinfections which commonly develop. Mechanical ventilation using positive end-expiratory pressure is often required for adequate oxygenation in patients who have aspirated gastric materials.

The adult respiratory distress syndrome (ARDS) is a clinical scenario that may be reached by any number of routes. It is a syndrome of pulmonary capillary permeability which leads to increased amounts of lung fluid. The most common signs are nonspecific and include tachypnea, dyspnea, and tachycardia. There should be no evidence of left heart failure or fluid overload. Clearly, excluding pulmonary edema secondary to heart failure from ARDS is oftentimes difficult and will frequently require the use of a flow-directed pulmonary artery catheter for the measurement of pulmonary capillary occlusive pressure ("wedge pressure"). The wedge pressure should be less than 18 mm Hg (ideally, <12 mm Hg) for the diagnosis of ARDS to be entertained. Other criteria for the diagnosis includes a PaO_2 of <50 mm Hg with an FiO_2 of >60%, an alveolar-arterial gradient (A-a gradient) of ≥350 mm Hg on 100% O_2, and evidence of decreased pulmonary compliance and intrapulmonary shunting. Many different stimuli may damage the pulmonary vascular endothelium, which will then allow a capillary leak. In pregnancy ARDS may be promoted by serious infections (e.g., pyelonephritis, septic abortion, endometritis, viral or bacterial pneumonias), aspiration of gastric contents, or by the severe hemorrhage associated with abruptio placenta. Preeclampsia and eclampsia are also common obstetric conditions which have been associated with ARDS. Early recognition and effective treatment may decrease the expected mortality of ARDS, which varies from 30% to 70%.

Therapy is aimed at the underlying cause of the ARDS (e.g., treating sepsis) while appropriately oxygenating the patient. This will usually require using the least amount of positive end-expiratory pressure (PEEP) and the lowest concentrations of FiO_2 that will maintain appropriate oxygenation. Elevated levels of PEEP may decrease venous return and cardiac output, while prolonged use of high levels of FiO_2 may result in oxygen toxicity. It is certainly recommended that obstetricians-gynecologists seek consultation from pulmonologists or intensivists for patients with ARDS.

General
1. Elkus R, Popovich J. Respiratory physiology in pregnancy. *Clin Chest Med* 1992; 13:555.
   An excellent general reference that reviews the pregnancy-induced changes in respiratory physiology.
2. Brancazio LR, Laifer SA, Schwartz T. Peak expiratory flow rate in normal pregnancy. *Obstet Gynecol* 1997;89:383.
   A recent study that discusses one of the most important parameters for pulmonary assessment of the pregnant patient.
3. Crapo RO. Normal cardiopulmonary physiology during pregnancy. *Clin Obstet Gynecol* 1996;39:3.
   Another excellent general reference that discusses the cardiopulmonary changes engendered by pregnancy.

Asthma
4. Wendel PJ, et al. Asthma treatment in pregnancy: a randomized controlled study. *Am J Obstet Gynecol* 1996;175:150.
   The use of inhaled steroids was noted to improve the management of asthma during pregnancy in this study.
5. Barth WH. Severe acute asthma. In: Clark SL, et al., eds. *Critical care obstetrics*. Malden, Massachusetts: Blackwell Science, 1997.
   An excellent reference that discusses the management of severe asthmatic exacerbations in pregnant patients.
6. Mabie WC, et al. Clinical observations on asthma in pregnancy. *J Matern Fetal Med* 1992;1:45.
   A brief general reference describes the outcome of pregnant women with asthma.
7. Mabie WC. Asthma in pregnancy. *Clin Obstet Gynecol* 1996;39:56.
   A recent general reference describes the prenatal and intrapartum management of the pregnant patient with asthma.

8. Clark SL. Asthma in pregnancy. *Obstet Gynecol* 1993;82:1036.
   This review of asthma in pregnancy was produced by the National Asthma Education Program of the National Institutes of Health.

Pneumonia
9. Richey SD, et al. Pneumonia complicating pregnancy. *Obstet Gynecol* 1994; 84:525.
   The experience of a large urban teaching center with pneumonia in pregnancy is presented in this excellent paper.
10. Madinger NE, Greenspoon JS, Ellrodt AG. Pneumonia during pregnancy: has modern technology improved maternal and fetal outcome? *Am J Obstet Gynecol* 1989;161:657.
    There was a significant amount of preterm delivery and perinatal mortality in this case series of acute pneumonia in pregnancy.
11. Rigby FB, Pastorek JG. Pneumonia during pregnancy. *Clin Obstet Gynecol* 1996; 39:107.
    This reference discusses the epidemiology and bacteriology of pneumonia during pregnancy.
12. Albino JA, Shapiro JM. Respiratory failure in pregnancy due to *Pneumocystis carinii:* report of a successful outcome. *Obstet Gynecol* 1994;83:823.
    This case report discusses respiratory failure due to the most common opportunistic infection in the setting of AIDS.
13. Tewari K, Wold SM, Asrat T. Septic shock in pregnancy associated with legionella pneumonia: case report. *Am J Obstet Gynecol* 1997;176:706.
    This case report details a particularly difficult case of a community-acquired pneumonia during pregnancy.

Tuberculosis
14. Margono F, et al. Resurgence of active tuberculosis among pregnant women. *Obstet Gynecol* 1994;83:911.
    Statistics from New York City demonstrate the increasing trend in tuberculosis cases during pregnancy in the setting of HIV infection.
15. Miller KS, Miller JM. Tuberculosis in pregnancy: interactions, diagnosis, and management. *Clin Obstet Gynecol* 1996;39:120.
    An excellent general reference regarding the diagnosis and treatment of tuberculosis during pregnancy.
16. Centers for Disease Control. Initial therapy for tuberculosis in the era of multidrug resistance: recommendations of the Advisory Council for Elimination of Tuberculosis (ACET). *MMWR* 1993;42:1.
    This reference presents the drug regimens that should be used when there is suspicion of antituberculous drug resistance.

Cystic Fibrosis
17. Canny CJ, et al. Pregnancy and cystic fibrosis. *Obstet Gynecol* 1991;77:850.
    A series of 38 pregnancies in 25 patients with cystic fibrosis is presented. This case series provides important statistics for the preconception counseling of women with cystic fibrosis.
18. Edenborough RP, et al. Outcome of pregnancy in women with cystic fibrosis. *Thorax* 1995;50:170.
    A more recent series of pregnant patients with cystic fibrosis is presented in this report.
19. Hilman BC, Aitken ML, Constantinescu M. Pregnancy in patients with cystic fibrosis. *Clin Obstet Gynecol* 1996;39:70.
    This report offers a general overview of the outcomes which may be expected in patients with cystic fibrosis who wish to become pregnant.

Aspiration and ARDS
20. Hawkins JL, et al. Anesthesia-related deaths during obstetric delivery in the United States, 1979–1990. *Anesthesiology* 1997;86:277.

This paper offers the latest statistics regarding maternal mortality associated with anesthesia. Most of the deaths involved general anesthesia for cesarean delivery.
21. Deblieux PM, Summer WR. Acute respiratory failure in pregnancy. *Clin Obstet Gynecol* 1996;39:143.
    An excellent general reference that lists the main etiologies for respiratory embarrassment in pregnancy.
22. Tomlinson MW, et al. Does delivery improve maternal condition in the respiratory-compromised gravida? *Obstet Gynecol* 1998;91:108.
    Dramatic improvement was not noted with delivery in this case series of women who required intubation for severe pneumonia.
23. Mason BM, Hankins GDV. Acute respiratory distress syndrome. In: Clark SL, et al., eds. *Critical care obstetrics.* Malden, Massachusetts: Blackwell Science, 1997.
    This is an excellent general reference regarding ARDS in the pregnant patient.

13. CARDIOVASCULAR DISEASE IN PREGNANCY

Everett F. Magann

Cardiovascular disease is a major nonobstetric cause of maternal death in the United States and it remains as the fourth leading cause of maternal death overall. A dramatic shift has been observed in the etiology of cardiovascular disease over the past 30 years. The number of cardiovascular lesions secondary to rheumatic fever has declined significantly, while the percentage of women with cardiovascular disease secondary to congenital heart lesions has increased. The advances in cardiovascular surgery for women with congenital heart lesions has permitted many children who previously would not have survived to enter the workplace, marry, and desire to become parents. Even though the advances in surgical techniques have permitted prolonged survival, many of these women have persistent hemodynamic derangements, which are often exacerbated by the physiologic changes of pregnancy.

A number of physiologic changes take place during the course of a normal pregnancy. The systemic vascular resistance is reduced by 25%, early in pregnancy, to accommodate the 50% increase in plasma volume that peaks at 32 weeks and then remains stable until term. The red blood count (RBC) mass will increase by 20% by term. The discordance between the 20% increase in RBC mass and the 50% increase in plasma volume results in the physiologic anemia of pregnancy.

The cardiac output will increase by 30%–50% by 20–24 weeks resulting in a blood volume expansion from 4 to 6 L. Initially the cardiac output is increased by an expansion in stroke volume and later in gestation by an increase in heart rate to a mean of 92 beats per minute (BPM) beyond 34 weeks. These changes are generally well tolerated by the gravida with a normal cardiovascular system. But in those women with congenital heart disease, who have had previous surgical interventions, the residual hemodynamic alterations may make a pregnancy much more complicated.

Blood flow to the uterus, which is 25% of the cardiac output at term, must be maintained throughout the pregnancy. Studies have demonstrated the influence of position on uterine blood flow. The uterine blood volume is maximized in the knee-to-chest position and compromised by motionless standing which impacts on pregnancy as early as the second trimester. In the third trimester of pregnancy, supine hypotension which occurs when the patient lies flat on her back can cause decreased cardiac output as the weight of the uterus on the vena cava reduces venous return from the lower extremities. Cardiac output is further changed by uterine contractions. At the acme of a uterine contraction, an additional 300–500 ml of blood is added to the maternal circulation. This increase in blood volume is accompanied by a decrease in heart rate.

The degree of cardiac compromise of patients with heart disease has been classified by the New York Heart Association (NYHA) into four categories based on functional capacity. Class I is asymptomatic, class II is symptomatic with exertion, class III is symptomatic with normal activity, and class IV is symptomatic at rest. This classification is useful in pregnant women with heart disease because the patient's symptoms have been found to be directly proportional to perinatal outcome. However, it must be remembered that 40% of patients who develop congestive heart failure in pregnancy are class I at the beginning of their pregnancy.

The maternal mortality associated with pregnancy in women with cardiovascular disease may be divided into three groups. Group 1 has a mortality of <1% and includes atrial septal defect (ASD), ventricular septal defect (VSD), patent ductus arteriosus (PDA), pulmonic/tricuspid disease, corrected tetralogy of Fallot, bioprosthetic valve, and mitral stenosis (NYHA class I and II). Group 2 has a 5%–15% risk of maternal mortality and includes mitral stenosis (NYHA class III and IV), mitral stenosis with atrial fibrillation, aortic stenosis, coarctation of the aorta (without valvular involvement), uncorrected tetralogy of Fallot, a previous myocardial infarction (MI), and artificial valves. Group 3 has a 25%–50% maternal mortality and includes primary pulmonary hypertension, coarctation of the aorta (with valvular involvement), MI and delivery within 2 weeks, cardiomyopathy, and Marfan's syndrome with aortic involvement. In counseling these women, it is often useful to put the discussion of mortality during pregnancy into perspective for the patient. The overall risk of maternal mortality in pregnancy is nine per 100,000 live births. A woman with a 1% risk of maternal mortality during pregnancy has a 100-fold increase in her risk of dying and a woman with a 50% risk of mortality has a 5,000-fold increased risk of dying during the pregnancy compared to the baseline population.

Valvular heart diseases includes mitral stenosis, aortic stenosis, mitral regurgitation, and aortic regurgitation. All of these women will require subacute bacterial endocarditis prophylaxis at the time of delivery. Mitral stenosis is the most common type of valvular heart disease, which is the result of rheumatic heart disease. The decreased diastolic ventricular filling of mitral stenosis results in a relatively fixed cardiac output. In labor and delivery invasive monitoring is needed for NYHA classification III and IV, tachycardia should be avoided (decrease diastolic filling time) and the pulmonary capillary wedge pressure needs to be maintained in the normal to high range to insure adequate left ventricular filling. Aortic stenosis is uncommon until the fifth or sixth decade of life. Because of a relative fixed cardiac output with aortic stenosis the maternal symptoms in pregnancy include syncope and angina. A 17% risk of sudden maternal death with a 32% risk of fetal mortality has been reported. In labor and delivery hypotension should be avoided by keeping the pulmonary capillary wedge pressure (PCWP) at 16–18. Women with mitral regurgitation generally tolerate pregnancy well because of an adequate preload and decreased systemic vascular resistance. Aortic regurgitation is complicated by chronic volume overload and is treated in labor and delivery by decreasing the afterload.

Left to right shunts (patent ductus arteriosus, ventricular septal defects, atrial septal defects) are well tolerated during pregnancy as long as pulmonary hypertension is not present. Most have been corrected in childhood and only require antibiotic prophylaxis in labor and delivery.

Right to left shunts (tetralogy of Fallot, Eisenmenger syndrome, and coarctation of the aorta) have a maternal mortality of 25 50% and pregnancy is best avoided. Tetralogy of Fallot consists of a VSD, overriding aorta, right ventricular hypertrophy, and pulmonic stenosis. With surgical correction the maternal mortality is <1%, but without correction the maternal mortality is 4%–15% with a fetal loss rate of 30%. Eisenmenger s syndrome consists of primary pulmonary hypertension with a resulting right to left shunt (ASD, VSD, or PDA). The maternal mortality is 34% with a vaginal delivery and 75% with an abdominal delivery. The risk of fetal death is 50%. Coarctation of the aorta occurs in the area of the ligamentum arteriosum (PDA) and the maternal risk of death is increased from 5%–15% to 25%–50% if the aortic valve is involved. Fetal outcome in the right to left shunts has been linked to the maternal hematocrit with an HCT of >65% associated with a poor fetal outcome. Hypotension must be avoided with all of the right to left shunts.

Marfan's syndrome is an autosomal dominant disorder with variable penetrance and may be associated with joint laxity, ocular disorders, hernias, and aortic root dilation with valvular insufficiency. An aortic root diameter that exceeds 40 mm (normal root diameter is 22 mm) is associated with a maternal mortality exceeding 50%. Idiopathic hypertrophic subaortic stenosis (IHSS) is another autosomal dominant condition with variable penetrance and results in left ventricular outflow obstruction and mitral valve regurgitation. The hypertrophied ventricular septum causes the symptoms of syncope, dyspnea, and angina. Treatment consists of maintaining a high preload to maintain a full left ventricle and high systemic vascular resistance to maintain distension of the left ventricle during systole.

Cardiomyopathy is a diagnosis of exclusion. It is most commonly seen in the last month of pregnancy to 6 months postpartum with a peak incidence in the second month postpartum. The dilated poorly contractile heart is more common in older, multiparous, African-American women whose pregnancy has been complicated by twins or hypertension. Treatment consists of bed rest, digitalis, diuretics, sodium restriction, and ace inhibitors. Persistent cardiomegaly past 6 months has >50% mortality within 5 years. In subsequent pregnancies, if the heart has returned to normal size the maternal mortality is 11%–14%, while persistent cardiomegaly has a maternal mortality of 40%–80%.

The incidence of an acute MI in pregnancy is one per 10,000. The average age is 33 with only 13% having documented coronary disease prior to conception. The overall mortality is 37% but is less in older women (those older than 35) because of suspected development of collateral circulation. Women who are most at risk of dying are those who have an acute MI within 2 weeks of delivery; the reported maternal mortality is 50%.

Women with a congenital cardiac lesion have a 5%–10% risk of having a child with a congenital cardiac lesion. The maternal and fetal cardiac lesions are concordant only 50% of the time. A fetal echo is essential in these pregnancies at 18–22 weeks to detect these cardiac lesions.

Nearly all cardiac medications (digoxin, beta-blockers, diuretics, and antiarrhythmic medications) cross the placenta and are excreted in breast milk. Information regarding their use in pregnancy is incomplete, making recommendations difficult. If the drugs are needed for maternal safety during the pregnancy, then they should be used. Some exceptions do exist, such as ace-inhibitors, which have been associated with fetal renal failure and skull ossification defects and should be avoided if alternative medications are available.

Fetal surveillance is important in mothers with cardiac disease because intrauterine growth restriction and fetal death in utero often accompany these pregnancies. The use of antenatal testing and serial ultrasounds for growth is essential in antepartum management.

The management of cardiac patients during pregnancy often requires the assistance of a cardiologist, anesthesiologist, neonatologist, and maternal-fetal medicine specialist. Intensive hemodynamic monitoring may be necessary and should be available. Epidural anesthesia is the treatment of choice in most patients except those in which a fall in systemic vascular resistance (aortic stenosis, IHSS, and primary pulmonary hypertension) is contraindicated. A semisitting position appears to be optimal for most cardiac patients. Subacute bacterial endocarditis (SBE) prophylaxis, which consists of ampicillin 2 g IV plus gentamicin 1.5 mg/kg not to exceed 120 mg, should be started early in the course of labor or immediately prior to a cesarean delivery and continued for at least two doses 8 hours apart postpartum. In women allergic to penicillin, vancomycin 1 g given over 1–2 hours is substituted.

Sterilization should be offered to women with significant disease. Contraception for the postpartum cardiac patient may be difficult because of the relative contraindications of oral contraceptives and intrauterine devices. Norplant or Depo-Provera injections offer a safer alternative. Barrier contraception is safe but carries a high failure rate in the poorly motivated patient.

General
1. Cardiac disease in pregnancy. *ACOG Tech Bull* no. 168, 1992.
   The American College of Obstetrics and Gynecology guidelines for the evaluation and treatment of patients with cardiac disease in pregnancy.

2. Mendleson MA. Congenital cardiac disease in pregnancy. *Clin Perinatol* 1997; 24:467.
   A current review of congenital heart lesions in pregnancy and preconceptual counseling.

Physiology
3. Yeomans ER, Hankins GVD. Cardiovascular physiology and invasive cardiac monitoring. *Clin Obstet Gynecol* 1989;32:2.
   An overview of the physiologic changes that take place in the heart patient who is pregnant and cardiac monitoring is involved.
4. Clark SL, et al. Central hemodynamic assessment of normal term pregnancy. *Am J Obstet Gynecol* 1989;161:1439.
   The article focuses on the hemodynamics measured in normal pregnancies antepartum and postpartum using pulmonary capillary wedge pressure.

Specific Lesions
5. Nolan TE, Hankins GVD. Myocardial infarction in pregnancy. *Clin Obstet Gynecol* 1969;32:68.
   Management guidelines for the pregnant patient with a myocardial infarction.
6. McColgin SW, Martin JN, Morrison JC. Pregnant women with prosthetic heart valves. *Clin Obstet Gynecol* 1989;32:76.
   Extensive review of pregnancy in patients with prosthetic valves.
7. Yaryura RA, et al. Management of mitral valve stenosis in pregnancy: case presentation and review of the literature. *J Heart Valve Dis* 1996;5:16.
   Operative management of a patient with severe mitral stenosis during pregnancy is discussed and options for therapy are discussed.
8. Oakley CM. Valvular disease in pregnancy. *Curr Opin Cardiol* 1996;11:155.
   A comprehensive review of rheumatic valvular disease, prosthetic valves, and valvular disease caused by inherited disorders such as Marfan's syndrome.

Counseling
9. Whittemore R, Hobbins JC, Engle MA. Pregnancy and its outcome in women with and without surgical treatment of congenital heart disease. *Am J Obstet Cardiol* 1982;50:641.
   Counseling a patient with congenital heart disease prior to pregnancy and for a subsequent pregnancy.
10. Shime J, et al. Congenital heart disease in pregnancy: short and long-term implications. *Am J Obstet Gynecol* 1987;156:313.
    A review of the benefits of surgical correction of congenital heart disease in the cyanotic women prior to pregnancy.

14. DIABETES MELLITUS ASSOCIATED WITH PREGNANCY

Rick W. Martin

Diabetes mellitus is a metabolic disorder associated with hyperglycemia, which results in an increased rate of congenital malformations and perinatal morbidity and mortality. Gestational diabetes can occur in 3%–12% of all pregnancies, and this represents approximately 90% of all diabetes occurring during pregnancy. Fortunately, glycemic control reduces maternal and neonatal complications.

Outside of pregnancy, diabetic patients are typically classified as type I for insulin-dependent diabetes and type II, non–insulin-dependent diabetes mellitus. Although the type II patients may require insulin therapy, they are not usually prone to ketoacidosis. White's classification divides pregnant patients according to gestational versus preexisting diabetes and also classifies patients as to the age at onset and duration of diabetes as well as any systemic involvement. More recently, a simplified approach classifies pregnant diabetics according to the degree of glucose control and the presence of vascular complications.

Women known to have diabetes should undergo evaluation prior to pregnancy. The risk of congenital anomaly has been shown to increase with poor glucose control as reflected by hemoglobin A_{1c} levels. The most common malformations include cardiac and neural tube defects. Ideal metabolic control during pregnancy is generally accepted to be a fasting plasma glucose of 60–90 mg/dl and before-meal glucose of 60–105 mg/dl. Two-hour postprandial glucose levels should be <120 mg/dl. Most pregnant women require 30 kcal/kg ideal body weight, or approximately 2,200 calories divided among three meals and a bedtime snack. A mid-morning and mid-afternoon snack may also be prescribed. Insulin therapy is administered twice daily, and, as a rule, two-thirds of the insulin is given in the morning with one-third given in the evening. Combinations of intermediate-acting insulins such as neutral protamine Hagedorn (NPH) and a short-acting insulin such as regular insulin are prescribed. Usually, human insulin obtained from recombinant techniques is preferable to animal-derived insulin. Laboratory evaluation of the insulin-dependent diabetic includes an assessment for systemic involvement with a 24-hour urine for creatinine clearance and protein, an EKG, and urine culture. An ophthalmologic evaluation is performed in each trimester. Prenatal visits are scheduled every 1–2 weeks throughout pregnancy. At each clinical visit, the maternal weight gain is assessed. The physician reviews blood sugars obtained by reflectance meter that are performed at home four times daily. Serial sonography evaluates fetal growth. An alpha-fetoprotein level and targeted sonogram are performed in the second trimester to evaluate fetal anomalies that may occur. Antepartum fetal surveillance is usually begun at 32 weeks' gestation but may begin earlier in individual cases. If the nonstress test is to be used, it should be performed on a twice-weekly basis. Others prefer a combination of weekly nonstress test and contraction stress testing. Positive tests are evaluated by biophysical profile or the physician may decide to accomplish delivery, especially when the fetus is mature. Delivery is usually planned before the 40th week of gestation. Amniocentesis documents fetal lung maturity, especially in cases where glycemic control has been poor. Fetal lung maturation may not proceed as predicted in diabetic pregnancies and often a phosphatidal glycerol evaluation is performed in addition to the lecithin/sphingomyelin (L:S) ratio.

At the onset of labor, should induction be chosen, glucose control remains important. In order to maintain a maternal glucose at approximately 100 ml/dl, a continuous infusion of regular insulin is administered in a 5% dextrose solution. The mother's glucose is evaluated regularly throughout labor. Using this procedure will decrease the risk of neonatal hypoglycemia.

In the postpartum period, glucose control is relaxed somewhat with the aim being to prevent ketoacidosis. Glucose values of 150–200 mg/dl are acceptable. The amount of insulin is decreased significantly after delivery, as hypoglycemia frequently occurs at this time.

The detection of those women who will display diabetes during pregnancy involves screening those at risk. Typical risk factors of diabetes, family history of diabetes, obesity, maternal age of >25, or prior macrosomic infant will only detect half of those patients. Some prefer to test all women during pregnancy. The most commonly employed technique involves the use of a 50-g glucose drink administered orally with a plasma glucose determined after a 1-hour interval. Values of >140 mg/dl are then followed with a formal 3-hour glucose tolerance test. For this procedure, at least 3 days of unrestricted diet with >150 g of carbohydrate daily intake are recommended. With the patient at rest, a fasting, 1-, 2-, and 3-hour plasma glucose levels are obtained with the normals being <105, 190, 165, and 145 mg/dl, respectively. If the patient exhibits two or more values exceeding these levels, she is considered to have gestational diabetes. The gestational diabetic may be managed with diet alone but should be followed at 1–2-week intervals, and if fasting levels exceed 105 mg/dl, or the 2-hour postprandial glucose exceeds 120 mg/dl, the patient is placed on an insulin regimen similar to that of the patient who has preexisting diabetes. Fetal surveillance begins later for the non–insulin-dependent diabetic with no other risk factor for fetal compromise. The patient with diabetes should be monitored frequently for hypertension, as this may coexist with the diabetes. Although vaginal delivery may usually be accomplished, particular attention should be given to estimation of fetal weight, as fetal macrosomia and subsequent shoulder dystocia may occur.

Contraception for the diabetic patient is a difficult problem. The barrier methods are less effective but would not exert systemic effects as one might expect with oral contraceptives. Low-dose contraceptives are probably safe for diabetic women without vascular disease. Permanent sterilization at the completion of childbearing should also be discussed.

General
1. Management of diabetes mellitus in pregnancy. *ACOG Tech Bull* no. 200, December 1994.
   Overview of accepted classification of diabetes in pregnancy and recommended screening techniques. General guidelines as to pregnancy management are also given.
2. Landon MB. Diabetes mellitus and other endocrine disease. In: Gabbe SG, Niebyl JR, Simpson JL, eds. *Obstetrics: normal and problem pregnancies.* New York: Churchill Livingstone, 1996.
   Excellent summary of the problem of diabetes in pregnancy and a detailed algorithm of clinical management is presented.
3. American Diabetes Association. Report of the Expert Committee on the Diagnosis and Classification of Diabetes Mellitus. *Diabetes Care* 1997;30:1183.
   The terms "type I" and "type II" are retained. The term "gestational diabetes mellitus" is retained and current screening procedures followed with an exemption for certain low-risk patients.

Diabetes Screening
4. Cousins SL, et al. Screening recommendations for gestational diabetes mellitus. *Am J Obstet Gynecol* 1991;165:493.
   A screening threshold no higher than 140 mg/dl is recommended following the 50-g oral glucose challenge test.
5. Lindsay MK, Graves W, Klein L. The relationship on one abnormal glucose tolerance test value and pregnancy complications. *Obstet Gynecol* 1989;73:103.
   Pregnant women with one abnormal value on the oral glucose tolerance test were at risk for fetal macrosomia and preeclampsia.
6. Carr S, et al. Precision of reflectance meters in screening for gestational diabetes. *Obstet Gynecol* 1989;73:727.
   The use of reflectance meters for glucose screening is not appropriate and will lead to a greater number of women requiring a 3-hour oral glucose test.
7. Sacks D, et al. Do the current standards for glucose tolerance testing in pregnancy represent a valid conversion of O'Sullivan's original data? *Am J Obstet Gynecol* 1989;161:638.
   Plasma glucose values of 96, 172, 152, and 131 mg/dl are recommended for the fasting, 1- 2- and 3-hour values of the oral glucose tolerance test.

Management
8. Jovanovic-Peterson L, Kitzmiller JL, Peterson CM. Randomized trial of human versus animal species insulin in diabetic pregnant women: improved glycemic control, not fewer antibodies to insulin, influences birth weight. *Am J Obstet Gynecol* 1992;167:1325.
   The use of human insulin was associated with less maternal hyperglycemia and hypoglycemia, fewer macrosomic infants, fewer large-for-gestational-age infants, and less neonatal hyperinsulinemia.
9. Coustan DR, et al. A randomized clinical trial of insulin pump versus intensive conventional therapy in diabetic pregnancies. *JAMA* 1986;255:631.

Excellent glucose control was obtained with either the insulin pump or conventional therapy.
10. Barrett JM, Salyer SL, Boehm FH. The nonstress test: an evaluation of 1000 patients. *Am J Obstet Gynecol* 1981;141:153.
    Weekly nonstress testing was not adequate in patients with diabetes mellitus.
11. Landon MB, Gabbe SG, Sachs L. Management of diabetes mellitus in pregnancy: a survey of obstetricians and maternal-fetal specialists. *Obstet Gynecol* 1990; 75:635.
    Intensive fetal surveillance, elective delivery, and high cesarean rates are common in pregnancies complicated by insulin-dependent diabetes. Most clinicians practice universal screening for diabetes.
12. Coustan DR, Imarah J. Prophylactic insulin treatment of gestational diabetes reduced the incidence of macrosomia, operative delivery, and birth trauma. *Am J Obstet Gynecol* 1984;150:836.
    The incidence of fetal macrosomia was 7% in the insulin-treated group, 17.8% in the untreated group, and 18.5% in a diet-only treated group of women with gestational diabetes.
13. Schuster MW, et al. Comparison of insulin regimens and administration modalities in pregnancy complicated by diabetes. *J Miss State Med Assoc* 1988;39:208.
    Premixed insulin (NPH 70%/regular 30%) was comparable to self-mixed combinations of NPH and regular insulin for pregnant women with diabetes mellitus.
14. Kjos SL, et al. Insulin-requiring diabetes in pregnancy: a randomized trial of active induction of labor and expectant management. *Am J Obstet Gynecol* 1993;169:611.
    After 38 weeks, expectant management did not lower the cesarean rate. Large-for-date infants and shoulder dystocia were also increased.
15. Major CA, et al. The effects of carbohydrate restriction in patients with diet-controlled gestational diabetes. *Obstet Gynecol* 1998;91:600.
    Women with carbohydrate intake below 42% had less fetal macrosomia and were less likely to require insulin.
16. Conway DL, Langer O. Elective delivery of infants with macrosomia in diabetic women: reduced shoulder dystocia versus increased cesarean deliveries. *Sm J Obstet Gynecol* 1998;178:922.
    Elective cesarean of fetuses with an estimated weight greater than 4,250 g decreased the rate of shoulder dystocia from 2.4% to 1.1%, and increased the cesarean rate from 21.7% to 25.1%.

Complications
17. Miller E, et al. Elevated maternal hemoglobin A1c in early pregnancy and major congenital anomalies in infants of diabetic mothers. *N Engl J Med* 1981;304:1331.
    The risk of major congenital anomalies when the hemoglobin A_1c value was below 8.5% was 3.4%, and the risk was 22.4% when the value was >8.5%.
18. Elman KD, et al. Diabetic retinopathy in pregnancy: a review. *Obstet Gynecol* 1990;75:119.
    The authors discuss the effect of diabetic retinopathy in pregnancy and evaluate current treatment.
19. Mills JL, et al. Incidence of spontaneous abortion among normal women and insulin-dependent diabetic women whose pregnancies were identified within 21 days of conception. *N Engl J Med* 1988;319:1617.
    Diabetic women with poor control had a significantly increased risk of spontaneous abortion.
20. Ojomo EO, Coustan DR. Absence of evidence of pulmonary maturity at amniocentesis in term infants of diabetic mothers. *Am J Obstet Gynecol* 1990;163:954.
    Twenty-one percent of women with gestational diabetes were negative for the presence of phosphatidal glycerol in the amniotic fluid as late as 38 weeks' gestation.
21. Kjaer K, et al. Infertility and pregnancy outcome in an unselected group of women with insulin-dependent diabetes mellitus. *Am J Obstet Gynecol* 1992;166:1412.
    Insulin-dependent diabetic women had a normal ability to conceive but had fewer pregnancies and fewer births per pregnancy than controls.

22. Reece A, et al. Diabetic nephropathy: pregnancy performance and fetomaternal outcome. *Am J Obstet Gynecol* 1988;159:56.
   With current methods of management of insulin-dependent diabetes, women with diabetic nephropathy did not encounter an excessive risk of adverse outcome.
23. Diamond T, Kormas N. Possible adverse fetal effect of insulin lispro. *N Engl J Med* 1997;337:1009.
   A letter reports malformations in infants of women treated with insulin lispro. The response by the pharmaceutical company states that only one of 19 patients in original trials delivered an infant with anomalies.
24. Macklon NS, Hop WC, Wladimiroff JW. Fetal cardiac function and septal thickness in diabetic pregnancy: a controlled observation and reproducibility study. *Br J Obstet Gynecol* 1998;105:661.
   Altered fetal cardiac morphology early in pregnancy in well-controlled diabetic pregnancies.

15. THYROID DISEASE IN PREGNANCY

Brian K. Rinehart

The thyroid gland is altered by the metabolic and hormonal changes of pregnancy. Likewise, the reproductive outcome may be affected by diseases of this organ. Since all forms of thyroid disease are three to four times more common in women than in men, disorders of this gland are not uncommon during pregnancy.

The hormonal milieu of pregnancy complicates interpretation of thyroid function studies. The T_3 resin uptake (T_3RU) decreases secondary to the increase in carrier proteins (thyroid binding globulin, albumin, prealbumin). By creating a fraction of the normal for T_3RU (measured T_3RU over the mean of normal) and multiplying times T_4, the functional (free) T_4 can be estimated. An example of this is as follows: If the normal mean for T_3RU is 30% and the patient's T_3RU is 15%, then 15/30 times a T_4 of 16 μg/dl equals 8 μg/dl—a level that is within normal limits for free T_4. This can also be done for the T_3. For a T_3RIA (normal, 80–200 ng/dl), a nonpregnant value of 250 ng/dl is reduced to 125 ng/dl during pregnancy. These calculations are necessary to evaluate any patient in an increased estrogenic state, whether due to pregnancy or exogenous estrogen therapy. Tests that are the most important in diagnosing the various thyroid disease states are T_3RU, free T_4, free T_3, or free thyroid index and thyroid-stimulating hormone (TSH), a pituitary hormone that is not altered by changes in pregnancy hormone levels or carrier protein levels. TSH is most important in diagnosing and following hypothyroidism, whereas free T_4 is most important in diagnosing hyperthyroidism.

The placenta is essentially impermeable to T_4, T_3, and TSH but not to iodine, so that the fetal thyroid develops independently of the maternal system. During pregnancy, radioiodine uptake assessment of thyroid function is contraindicated because of resultant fetal hypothyroidism. Neonatal and fetal thyroid function laboratory values are slightly higher than maternal levels, with increased free T_4, T_3, and TSH levels that decrease by the fifth day postdelivery to normal nonpregnant adult values.

Maternal hypothyroidism is relatively uncommon in the pregnant patient because menstrual irregularities, oligovulation, and spontaneous abortion are hallmarks of this disorder. Hypothyroidism is generally thought to be an immunologic disease with a multifactorial inheritance found predominantly in females. One of the more common etiologies is iatrogenic, that is, patients are told to stop thyroid replacement medications to observe for possible resolution of this condition. The primary condition is usually associated with a goiter (owing to the gland's inability to produce T_4 and T_3, which results in hypertrophy of the organ). The goiter is generally multinodular and can enlarge to cause potential airway management problems. Primary hypothyroidism is usually secondary to chronic thyroiditis, prior radioactive iodine therapy, thyroidectomy (surgical or ^{131}I), or the ingestion of goitrogens (e.g., thiocyanate, lithium carbonate, amiodarone). Secondary hypothyroidism owing to chromophobe adenoma of the pituitary gland, Sheehan's syndrome, and so on is rare. Idiopathic hypothyroidism has a much more protracted onset and is usually related to Hashimoto's disease.

Complaints of fatigue, obesity, coarse skin, thinning of the hair (particularly the eyebrows), myxedematous changes (facial or tibial), macroglossia, and a subnormal body temperature are typical signs of this disorder. Paresthesias and delayed deep-tendon reflexes are early symptoms in about 75% of patients with hypothyroidism. Postpartum amenorrhea and galactorrhea may be presenting complaints of hypothyroidism after pregnancy has ended. Thyroid antibodies are frequently detected in these cases. This scenario occurs more commonly after parturition than in nonpregnant patients. Laboratory diagnosis of hypothyroidism rests on a reduction in T_4 and T_3RU, anemia, and an elevated TSH. Once the diagnosis of hypothyroidism has been made, therapy should be instituted. Care must be taken in the older patient to gradually increase the dose of thyroid hormone, since cardiovascular insults can occur when the thyroid deficiency is corrected too rapidly. Most patients with early hypothyroidism may be started on 50–100 μg/day of levothyroxine, increasing the dosage by 25 μg/day/week until the patient is euthyroid. Most patients will require 100–200 μg/day of thyroxine for maintenance therapy. Optimal maintenance therapy can be determined by clinical symptoms, TSH levels, and free thyroxine index. Prognosis for both mother and fetus is excellent with corrected hypothyroidism in pregnancy. Antepartum fetal assessment in the third trimester is indicated owing to a small increase in the stillbirth rate.

Maternal hyperthyroidism is not uncommon, ranging from 0.05% to 0.2% during pregnancy. Hyperthyroidism during pregnancy is associated with an increase in neonatal wastage and low-birth-weight infants. There is no evidence that the pregnancy per se makes the disease process more difficult to control, although there is a propensity for relapse during the postpartum period. The most common etiologies in order of frequency are toxic diffuse goiter (Graves' disease), acute thyroiditis, toxic nodular goiter (Plummer's disease), and toxic adenoma. Graves' disease occurs frequently with pregnancy and is usually diagnosed by the classic symptoms of weight loss, ocular signs, pretibial myxedema, a resting pulse rate above 100 that fails to slow during a Valsalva maneuver, muscular wasting, and nervousness. The serum T_4 is above normal pregnancy values (>12 μg/dl). Similarly, the T_3RU in the normal nonpregnant range is indicative of thyrotoxicosis during pregnancy.

Treatment during pregnancy is basically medical, with surgery infrequently indicated and radioactive iodine therapy contraindicated. All therapies of hyperthyroidism initially center around slowing the release or stopping the conversion of T_4 to T_3. In pregnancy, propylthiouracil (PTU) is the drug of choice. In severe hyperthyroidism, doses of 100–200 mg four times daily may be required. Mild hyperthyroidism will usually respond to 100 mg three times daily. Symptoms of hyperthyroidism will usually decrease 2–3 weeks following the institution of the least effective dose to maintain the T_4 at about 14 μg/dl (usually <200 mg per day). In the face of impending thyroid storm, therapy to avoid decompensation is important. Treatment of hyperthermia with acetaminophen suppositories (aspirin should be avoided because it can cause displacement of thyroxine from thyroxine-binding globulin [TBG]) and cooling blankets can be effective. General therapy should also include the use of intravenous multivitamin preparations, glucose as well as fluids, and electrolytes. The use of 100 mg of hydrocortisone intravenously every 6–8 hours may also be indicated. There is the additional benefit of the blocking of thyroxine to triiodothyronine conversion with corticosteroid use.

Propranolol has been the standard beta-blocking agent used because of its physiologic role in controlling heart rate as well as blocking peripheral conversion of T_4 to T_3. The dosage of propranolol for the patient in thyroid storm is 60–120 mg orally every 6 hours until a pulse rate of less than 90 is reached, at which time dosage can be halved. In the case of the patient who will need emergent cesarean section, the use of the intravenous formulation for rapid control is preferred. It is of utmost importance to remember that the intravenous preparation is extremely potent. The starting dose of propranolol is 0.5–1 mg followed by 2–3 mg every 10–15 minutes. Again, a heart rate of less than 90 is the desired end point. If the patient has a history of bronchospasm, the use of propranolol is contraindicated; in this situation, the use of metoprolol tartrate (Lopressor), a beta$_1$-blocking agent, should be substituted. The dosage for metoprolol is 5 mg every 2 minutes, to a maximum dosage of 15 mg.

Graves' disease is a cyclic disease and may subside spontaneously. With adequate treatment and follow-up, the long-term maternal prognosis is excellent. Fetal prognosis with well-controlled hyperthyroidism is also excellent. However, two fetal precautions are necessary. First, a few studies have reported an increased stillbirth rate with maternal hyperthyroidism, and antepartum fetal assessment is indicated in the third trimester. Second, a fetal goiter rarely may lead to face presentation at delivery, thus necessitating operative delivery. Skilled resuscitation of the newborn after delivery may be needed if the airway is obstructed by a goiter.

Neonatal hypothyroidism is a remediable condition that occurs in one in 4,000 deliveries. Early diagnosis and treatment are extremely important because the age of initiation of treatment affects the prognosis; thus, all neonates should be screened. Endemic cretinism occurs in areas of the world with iodine deficiency, but parents usually have evidence of a goiter. Replacement of thyroid hormone in the infant will return thyroid levels to normal but does not reverse the associated neurologic deficits (e.g., deaf-mutism and spasticity) acquired in utero that appear to be due to lack of iodine in the developing brain.

Patients who have taken PTU may give birth to infants with a small goiter, although there is no evidence that PTU or other drugs have a detrimental long-term effect as far as growth and development are concerned. In contrast, iodine ingestion by the mother has been associated with large neonatal goiters at birth. One of the most important problems caused by these large goiters is respiratory distress owing to laryngeal pressure. In most infants with goiters, a low serum T_4 (<9.5 µg/dl) and a normal T_3 resin uptake are diagnostic of hypothyroidism.

Thyrotoxicosis is even more common in the newborn than in the mother. Although some infants will receive the 7S immunoglobin (long-acting thyroid stimulator [LATS]) from the mother via placental transfer, diagnosis is usually made on the basis of the total clinical picture, which includes maternal symptoms of the disease in conjunction with goiter, tachycardia, increased T_4, and hyperirritability in the infant. Occasionally, serum T_4 and the goiter may be absent; thus, the positive assay for LATS is helpful in some infants. Cardiac decompensation, hepatosplenomegaly, and jaundice have also been seen in these infants. If the hyperthyroidism is mild, usually no treatment is needed. If treatment is necessary, Lugol's solution (one drop three times a day) or PTU (10 mg every 8 hours) is utilized. Propranolol is reserved for thyrotoxic infants with severe cardiac decompensation. The infants are usually treated for 3–6 weeks; after that period of time, they require no further treatment.

General
1. Kaplan M. Thyroid diseases. In: Gleicher N, ed. *Principles and practice of medical therapy in pregnancy.* East Norwalk, CT: Appleton & Lange, 1992.
    A comprehensive review of basic and clinical considerations regarding thyroid gland function during pregnancy. The effects of hypothyroid and hyperthyroid states on the neonate and fetus are discussed.
2. Endocrine disorders in pregnancy. In: Galway AB, Burrow GN, eds. *Medicine of the fetus and mother.* Philadelphia: Lippincott, 1992.
    A detailed review of the thyroid gland, including clinical assessment and treatment in the abnormal state in the nonpregnant and pregnant patient.

Etiology
3. Kennedy RL, et al. Thyrotoxicosis and hyperemesis gravidarum associated with a serum activity which stimulates human thyroid cells in vitro. *Clin Endocrinol* 1992;36:83.

This study is a detailed evaluation of the sera response in five patients with biochemical hyperthyroidism and hyperemesis. The stimulatory activity could not be neutralized by depleting the sera of human chorionic gonadotropin.

4. Hayskip CC, et al. The value of serum antimicrosomal testing in screening for symptomatic thyroid dysfunction. *Am J Obstet Gynecol* 1988;159:203.

   Samples were drawn from 1,034 consecutive women on their second postpartum day for antimicrosomal (AMA) and antithyroglobulin antibodies. Biochemical thyroid dysfunction developed in 34 of 51 (67%) of AMA-positive women.

5. Learoyd DL, et al. Postpartum thyroid dysfunction. *Thyroid* 1992;2:73.

   This is a review article which shows that approximately 5%–9% of women develop thyroid dysfunction in the postpartum period, which appears to be related to a rebound from the relative immune tolerance of pregnancy.

6. Othman S. Iodine metabolism in postpartum thyroiditis. *Thyroid* 1992;2:107.

   This is a prospective study of 1,996 women during the second trimester of pregnancy. It was noted that iodine excretion in the immediate postpartum period of 152 women matched with 235 antibody-positive women did not differ. Neither did the iodine excretion from the 73 women who developed postpartum thyroiditis compared to controls. Iodine intake is thus unlikely to affect the relevance of postpartum thyroiditis.

Diagnosis

7. Zimmerman P, et al. Ultrasonography of the thyroid gland in pregnancies complicated by autoimmune thyroid disease. *J Clin Ultrasound* 1993;21:109.

   A detailed review of the ultrasound findings in pregnancy and in disease states.

8. Gerstein H. Incidence of postpartum thyroid dysfunction in patients with type I diabetes mellitus. *Ann Intern Med* 1993;118:419.

   This is a prospectus study to look at postpartum thyroid dysfunction in women with type I diabetes. It was noted that postpartum thyroid dysfunction occurred in 10 of 40 patients for a 25% incidence. This strongly supports routine thyroid function screening at postpartum visits in type I diabetics.

9. Gerhard I, et al. Thyroid and ovarian function in infertile women. *Hum Reprod* 1991;6:338.

   This study is a prospectus to look at the impact of thyroid function and the pituitary-ovarian axis in infertile women. One hundred eighty five infertile women without clinical signs of thyroid dysfunction were given a TRH test. Seventy-four were found to be euthyroid, 31 with latent hyperthyroid, and 80 with preclinical hypothyroid.

10. Klein RZ, et al. Prevalence of thyroid deficiency in pregnant women. *Clin Endocrinol* 1991;35:41.

    This study was to determine the extent of gestational hypothyroidism and utilized 2,000 consecutive women in Maine tested for alpha-fetoprotein concentrations. Hypothyroidism was noted in 0.3% and hyperthyroidism in 0.3%.

11. Goodwin TM, et al. Transient hyperthyroidism and hyperemesis gravidarum: clinical aspects. *Am J Obstet Gynecol* 1992;167:648.

    Sixty-seven patients seen with the diagnosis of hyperemesis gravidarum were studied prospectively with a finding of 66% having biochemical hyperthyroidism. Clinically, this was self-limited, resolving by 18 weeks' gestation but they were shown to have a higher incidence of abnormal electrolytes and increased liver enzyme levels.

12. Perelman AH, et al. Intrauterine diagnosis and treatment of fetal goitrous hyperthyroidism. *J Clin Endocrinol Metab* 1990;71:618.

    Case study that showed the utilization of percutaneous umbilical blood sampling (PUBS) to diagnose hypothyroidism and to treat the fetus in vitro with intraamniotic injections of T_4 with resulting normal thyroid functions at birth with normal neonatal development.

13. Fort P, et al. Neonatal thyroid disease: differential expression in three successive offspring. *J Clin Endocrinol Metab* 1988;66:645.

    This is an interesting case of a mother with hyperthyroidism and the impact on three children with different forms of thyroid dysfunction at birth. The first child was clinically normal, the second child had transient neonatal hyperthyroidism, and the third child had neonatal hypothyroidism. This spectrum of neonatal thyroid disease differs depending on whether stimulating or blocking antibodies predominate in the mother.

Treatment
14. Cooper D. Antithyroid drugs: to breast-feed or not to breast-feed. *Am J Obstet Gynecol* 1987;157:234.
    A review article with 14 references that summarize the data known on the effect of antithyroid medicine in infants exposed by breast milk. PTU is the drug of choice in this situation, since it does not cross membranes readily and milk concentrations are low.
15. Messer PM, et al. Antithyroid treatment of Graves' disease in pregnancy: long-term effects on somatic growth, intellectual development and thyroid function of the offspring. *Acta Endocrinol* 1990;123:311.
    Comparison was made between 17 children of 13 hyperthyroid mothers receiving antithyroid drug treatment with 25 children of 15 mothers who were euthyroid. There were no adverse effects noted of an antithyroid drug treatment during pregnancy.
16. Hashizume K, et al. Effect of administration of thyroxine on the risk of post-partum recurrence of hyperthyroid Graves' disease. *J Clin Endocrinol Metab* 1992;75:6.
    It was found that T_4 administration during pregnancy and after delivery was effective in decreasing the level of antibodies to TSH receptors, and in prevention of postpartum recurrence of hyperthyroidism.
17. Leung AS, et al. Perinatal outcome in hypothyroid pregnancies. *Obstet Gynecol* 1993;81:349.
    Sixty-eight hypothyroid patients were divided into two groups: 23 with overt and 45 with subclinical hypothyroidism. It was noted that gestational hypertension and pregnancy hypertension were significantly more common in the overt and subclinical thyroid patients, with rates of 22%, 15%, and 7.5%. Low birth weight was higher due to delivery for pregnancy-induced hypertension or eclampsia.
18. Matsura N, et al. Transient hypothyroidism in infants born to mothers with chronic thyroiditis—a nationwide study of 23 cases. *Endocrinol Jpn* 1990;37:369.
    This study showed that mothers whose maternal thyroid function during pregnancy was mild or corrected had normal development contrasting to clinical impairment with abnormal maternal thyroid functions. This suggests that maternal thyroid function during pregnancy is an important factor in the prognosis of infants born to mothers with chronic thyroiditis.

Complications
19. Davis LE, et al. Thyrotoxicosis complicating pregnancy. *Am J Obstet Gynecol* 1989;160:63.
    This 12-year study involved 120,000 women, of whom 60 had overt thyrotoxicosis (1:2,000). Thirty-two women, were diagnosed during pregnancy and had the preponderance of morbidity in the mother, leading to the author's advice of aggressive medical therapy, particularly when pregnancy was advanced.
20. Tamaki H, et al. Evaluation of TSH receptor antibody by "natural in vivo human assay" in neonates born to mothers with Graves' disease. *Clin Endocrinol* 1989;30:493.
    Maternal serum thyroid antibodies indices showed highly significant correlations with the serum T_4 index and free T_3 index in neonates 5–10 days after birth. Further evaluation of the relationship between antibodies and the stimulation index showed that in vitro assays using the animal thyroid cells as an index of response are suitable for detecting circulating thyroid stimulating activity in vivo.
21. Page DV, et al. The pathology of intrauterine thyrotoxicosis: two case reports. *Obstet Gynecol* 1988;72:479.
    This reviews in detail autopsy findings on two infants of mothers with hyperthyroidism. The autopsy findings suggest intrauterine thyrotoxicosis secondary to transplacental thyroid-stimulating immunoglobulin.

V. MORE HIGH-RISK PREGNANCIES

16. PREGNANCY IN THE ADOLESCENT

Sister Clarice Carroll

Adolescent pregnancy and childbearing is a persistent problem in the United States. Each year more than 1.1 million adolescents (10% of female adolescents) become pregnant. The births resulting from these pregnancies account for 20% of the total births in the United States. Two fifths of all American adolescent girls will have conceived by the age of 19, and 400,000 will have an abortion. Despite the availability of contraceptive information and methods and the legalization of abortion, pregnancy prevention in adolescent girls has not been successful.

Adolescent pregnancy is no longer associated with the poor and undereducated and the ethnically disadvantaged. The incidence of adolescent pregnancy is not bound by social class or race but more by the socially and economically disadvantaged. It is a known and proven fact that adolescents living in poverty are more likely than their middle-class peers to become sexually active in their teen and preteen years.

Statistics have proven that 95% of adolescent pregnancies are unintended and unplanned. Many are unwanted as well. Adolescent pregnancy has a negative impact on the physical, social, emotional, educational, and economic conditions of the teenaged woman. Too early she becomes a child-mother with a vulnerable and perhaps neglected and abused newborn.

The change in the age of menarche from just over 14 years to 12.5 years, with fertility occurring by age 14, has influenced the high rate of adolescent pregnancy. Increased sexual activity at younger ages, with one fifth of adolescents having had intercourse by age 16 and two thirds by age 19, also has contributed to the increasing pregnancy rate. Many of these teenagers have misinformation on human anatomy and reproduction. They may be biologically immature, yet half of premarital first pregnancies occur in adolescent girls within 6 months of beginning sexual intercourse, and one fifth occur in the first month.

Preexisting psychological problems are frequently found in a family where adolescent pregnancy occurs. Preventive strategies should focus on measures that improve the health of the family unit. The psychologic factors associated with the motivation for pregnancy in the adolescent are complex. These may include a desire to establish identity as an "adult," escape from responsibility, rebellion against authority figures, and a desire for or the need to give love. Pregnancy also may temporarily bolster her self-esteem through peer acceptance, or serve as a mechanism through which a relationship with a significant male can be established or maintained. In addition, adolescents who become pregnant have a poor self-image and self-esteem. Their own identity is incomplete, and they do not have the necessary skills to form their baby's identity. Repeat pregnancy among adolescent mothers is a major problem. Immature child-mothers are poorly equipped to face the demands of caring for the newborn, much less several newborns. Burdened grandmothers are frequently unskilled and ill-educated themselves. There is evidence that the younger sisters of childbearing adolescents are at risk for adolescent childbearing as well. Explanations might include social modeling, shared parenting, and attention seeking. Adolescence is a period of maturational crisis in which the role of child must evolve into the role of adult. The familiar prepubescent body image must be revised to that of a woman accommodating the changes of normal hormonal development. Psychological inconsistency with unpredictable reactions is characteristic of adolescents, and this produces confusion and frustration both in themselves and in those around them. Experimentation is essential for the adolescent and may play a major role in pregnancy. Likewise, pregnancy also may be viewed as a maturational crisis in which the familiar role of a single individual is exchanged for the role of mother and provider. When pregnancy occurs during adolescence, the young person must address two maturational crises at the same time, and satisfactory resolution is seldom possible. A syndrome of failure associated with adolescent pregnancy has been described. It includes failure to (1) fulfill developmental tasks of adolescence, (2) remain in school, (3) limit family size, (4) establish stable families, (5) be self-supporting, and (6) have healthy children. Adolescent pregnancy has been associated with an increased incidence of both obstetric and social complications, twice that of women in their twenties. There is an increased risk of anemia, pregnancy-induced hypertension (PIH), perinatal death, sexually transmitted diseases, human immunodeficiency virus infection, and premature delivery. The increased risk of PIH is significant, especially if the pregnancy occurs within 24 months of menarche. There is an increased incidence of cephalopelvic disproportion in women younger than 15 years of age, which is related to the relative skeletal immaturity of the pelvis, leading to a higher incidence of cesarean delivery, a surgical procedure associated with greater maternal morbidity. Pregnant adolescents are also more likely to experience abnormal labor patterns such as prolonged or precipitous labors, and both may be associated with neonatal sequelae. These teenagers also may experience an increased incidence of postpartum infection and hemorrhage. Adolescent mothers also may have unhealthy habits. Smoking, alcohol consumption, and the use of drugs are common among pregnant teenagers and may lead to sudden infant death syndrome, growth retardation, and neurologic dysfunction.

Owing to the rapid growth and development of the body, adolescence is normally a period of high nutritional needs. Pregnancy imposes additional nutritional demands on the growing body and may rapidly deplete already-limited reserves. The increased incidence of poor nutrition among adolescents owing to limitations on economic resources, poor eating habits, and lack of knowledge regarding nutrition has been directly related to the increased incidence of low-birth-weight infants, who are themselves susceptible to increased mortality as well as developmental and neurologic handicaps. Pregnant adolescents may be deficient in calcium, iron, and vitamins A and C, although they usually have adequate calories, protein, and other vitamins. Because a high proportion of pregnant adolescents are nutritionally at risk and require nutritional intervention throughout their pregnancy and postpartum period, a nutrition consultant who can skillfully establish rapport with them is essential. The pregnant adolescent needs professional help in identifying food sources to supplement or improve her nutrient intake not only during her pregnancy but well into the postpartum period.

The long-term consequences to adolescent parents can be extremely costly to both society and the individuals involved. Extensive study has revealed that both adolescent mothers and fathers have substantially less education than their peers, and the degree of educational deprivation is related to the age of the parent at the time of the infant's birth. Teenagers who become pregnant prior to completing the 12th grade usually drop out of school and never return. The earlier she drops out of school, the less chance that the pregnant adolescent will complete her education.

Adolescent mothers account for 17% of parturients with 8 years of education or less. Adolescent parents are also much more likely to hold low-prestige jobs owing to their relatively low educational attainment. Reduced occupational attainment also means lower income and greater job dissatisfaction. A young pregnant teenager is not likely to support herself; she bears an unwanted child who is born into poverty and exposed to inadequate parenting. She is dependent on family and governmental agencies for monetary assistance and child-care support. The majority of adolescent pregnancies do not result in marriage, and those that do are frequently dissolved.

Factors that influence the reproductive behavior of adolescents are peers, sexual partners, family, religion, schools, media, and the health-care system. A poorly planned pregnancy occurring during the adolescent years also adversely affects intrapersonal relationships. Social skills as well as intrapersonal relationship skills may not develop adequately; both have long-term social ramifications. Relationships with family members as well as with men may be jeopardized, leading to the development of further social or psychological complications.

Delivery of health care to the adolescent presents a complex challenge. No single health-care provider can meet the many needs of the adolescent, but a team of health-care providers can be invaluable. Her primary medical care will not differ significantly from the prenatal care of other women, although she may need more privacy and confidentiality. She is more likely to keep prenatal appointments and comply with medical regimens if a trusting, nonjudgmental relationship has been established with the health-care provider. The pregnant adolescent will often delay prenatal care because of the many fears that she has developed: fear of being pregnant, fear of her family being informed, and fear of being examined. She sometimes delays because she hopes that a more meaningful relationship will develop between her and the father. Professionals who work with adolescents on health-care issues need to know about adolescent development, sexuality, and counseling. As part of the health-care team, a nutritionist is necessary to discuss the adolescent's body needs and food requirements peculiar to pregnancy, thereby helping to provide the nutritional requirements for both the mother's growth and the growth of her unborn baby. A social worker can provide referral information and counseling regarding pregnancy alternatives. Above all, the pregnant adolescent needs the cooperation and understanding of her parents and school authorities, so that it may be possible for her to receive early and comprehensive prenatal care.

Consideration and support also must be given to the adolescent father, so that he may be included in health-care decisions, labor and delivery, and care of the infant, if he so chooses. Contrary to popular belief, most infants born to teenagers are not fathered by teenagers; however, the exact number of adolescent fathers cannot be determined because many adolescent mothers refuse to give identifying information about the father.

Adolescent pregnancy is not solely a medical problem, and not all solutions can be found within the scope of medical practice. Prevention of this problem is an important goal and ultimately may be reached through comprehensive educational programs. Such educational programs need to be directed toward formation of healthy, mature attitudes about sexuality and childbearing. Courses should be integrated into the elementary school curriculum before the teen years and continued throughout childhood and adolescence. Basic information about human reproduction and conception, conception prevention, fetal growth, antenatal development, and intrapartum experiences, as well as infant care, should be included. Discussions between adolescents and parents within the structure of religious institutions and schools may prove beneficial in reducing misconceptions regarding sexuality and pregnancy.

Many adolescents engage in unprotected sex, and those who choose to use some protection use condoms and the pill. Reasons given for nonuse of contraceptive protection are beliefs that they are not safe and that they are not available. The effectiveness of school-based contraceptive clinic programs is mixed, and they have not been remarkably successful.

The consequences of childbearing for adolescent parents, their children, and society are severe. Much stress has been placed on the consequences of adolescent sexual activity, namely pregnancy. A more serious consequence is the acquisition of sexually transmitted diseases, particularly the acquired immunodeficiency syndrome. Information alone will not prevent teen pregnancy, nor will increased communication between parents and teenagers and between teachers and teenagers. Only abstinence of sexual activity can prevent adolescent pregnancy.

General
1. East PL, Felice ME. Pregnancy risk among the younger sisters of pregnant and childbearing adolescents. *J Dev Behav Pediatr* 1992;13:128.
   There is increasing evidence that the younger sisters of childbearing teenagers are at risk for adolescent childbearing.
2. Ringheim K. Ethical issues in social science research with special reference to sexual behaviour research. *Soc Sci Med* 1995;40:1691.
   Beginning with the philosophical origin of ethical principles that guide research, this paper discusses the key ethical issues to be considered when designing and conducting social science research. Included are special precautions for research on adolescents, the purpose and properties of an informed consent procedure, and the formation and function of an ethical review committee.

3. Fielding JE, Williams CA. Adolescent pregnancy in the United States: a review and recommendations for clinicians and research needs. *Am J Prev Med* 1991;7:47.
   Clinicians have an important role in providing guidance for teenagers and their parents as well as in influencing schools and community leadership in providing sex education.

4. Stevens-Simon C, White MM. Adolescent pregnancy. *Pediatr Ann* 1991;20:322.
   The United States must improve its efforts to reduce teen pregnancy.

5. O'Sullivan AL. Tertiary prevention with adolescent mothers: rehabilitation after the first pregnancy. *Birth Defects* 1991;27:57.
   A large number of diverse local programs and specific projects exist across the nation.

6. Nelson PB. Repeat pregnancy among adolescent mothers: a review of the literature. *J Natl Black Nurses Assoc* 1990;4:28.
   Repeat pregnancy among adolescent mothers is a major problem facing healthcare providers today.

7. Davis S. Pregnancy in adolescents. *Pediatr Clin North Am* 1989;36:665.
   The United States must improve its effort to reduce teen pregnancy.

8. McAnarney ER, Hendee WR. The prevention of adolescent pregnancy. *JAMA* 1989;7:262.
   Prevention of adolescent pregnancy is problematic because adolescents become biologically mature at an earlier age.

9. Bluestein D, Starling ME. Helping pregnant teenagers. *West J Med* 1994;161:140.
   Physicians who can effectively discuss these topics can help pregnant teenagers make informed decisions and improve their prospects for the future.

10. Stevens-Simon C, Reichert S. Sexual abuse, adolescent pregnancy, and child abuse. A developmental approach to an intergenerational cycle. *Arch Pediatr Adolesc Med* 1994;148:23.
    Experiences associated with childhood sexual abuse may affect the incidence and outcome of adolescent childbearing. Identification and treatment of previously abused adolescent prenatal patients may break this vicious intergenerational cycle of violence.

11. Shulman V, Alderman E, Ewig JM, Bye MR. Asthma in the pregnant adolescent: a review. *J Adolesc Health* 1996;18:168.
    Adolescent pregnancy has increased in the past decade, often in association with poverty, poor education, and inadequate prenatal care. Asthma is also becoming more common, with an incidence of at least 6.6% in 15- to 16-year-old girls. Poverty and living in the inner city are associated with increased morbidity and mortality from asthma.

Etiology

12. Sowers JG. Preventive strategies in education: history, current practices, and future trends regarding substance abuse and pregnancy prevention. *Bull NY Acad Med* 1991;67:256.
    The most effective prevention of adolescent pregnancies consists of positive life and health promotion strategies.

13. Smith L. A critique of family-focused tertiary prevention with the adolescent mother and her child. *Birth Defects* 1991;27:155.
    The complexity of problems related to pregnant adolescents requires a coordinated multidisciplinary approach.

14. Gordon DE. Formal operational thinking: the role of cognitive-developmental processes in adolescent decision-making about pregnancy and contraception. *Am J Orthopsychiatry* 1990;60:346.
    Adolescents who become pregnant have difficulty envisioning alternatives.

15. Creatsas GK. Sexuality: sexual activity and contraception during adolescence. *Curr Opin Obstet Gynecol* 1993;5:774.
    Considering that 95% of adolescent pregnancies are unintended, increased efforts to prevent these pregnancies are warranted.

Diagnosis
16. Perkins JL. Primary prevention of adolescent pregnancy. *Birth Defects* 1991;27:29.
    Programs that contribute to the prevention of adolescent pregnancy and an under-standing of life options for adolescents are counterbalanced by cost.
17. Raines TG. Family-founded primary prevention of adolescent pregnancy. *Birth Defects* 1991;29:87.
    There is a need for expertise and influence in the area of primary prevention of adolescent pregnancy.
18. Flick LH. A critique of community-based tertiary prevention with the adolescent parent and child. *Birth Defects* 1991;27:250.
    The characteristics and circumstances that increase the likelihood of early child-bearing also increase the chances of harmful consequences to the young mother, the child, and perhaps the father.
19. Kokotailo PK, Adger H Jr. Substance use by pregnant adolescents. *Clin Perinatol* 1991;18:125.
    Research is needed to determine the prevalence of substance abuse among pregnant adolescents.
20. Barnet B, et al. Depressive symptoms, stress, and social support in pregnant and postpartum adolescents. *Arch Pediatr Adolesc Med* 1996;150:64.
    Results indicate that depressive symptoms are common among pregnant teenagers and postpartum adolescents. Identifying those teenagers with high stress and conflict and low levels of support will help identify those who are at particular risk for depressive symptoms.
21. Stevens-Simon C, Lowy R. Teenage childbearing. An adaptive strategy for the socio-economically disadvantaged or a strategy for adapting to socioeconomic dis-advantage? *Arch Pediatr Adolesc Med* 1995;149:912.
    As much as the long-term socioeconomic sequelae of adolescent childbearing reflect factors that influence the judgments young people make about the costs and benefits of contraception and parenthood, adolescent childbearing is a means of adapting to urban poverty. Thus, postponing adolescent conceptions and parenthood may have a less important effect on the socioeconomic well-being of young Americans than expected.
22. Sheaff L, Talashek M. Ever-pregnant and never-pregnant teens in a temporary housing shelter. *J Commun Health Nurs* 1995;12:33.
    This study indicates that teen pregnancy is a major problem among adolescents in temporary housing shelters. Our findings provide guidance for clinical interventions and further research with this at-risk population.
23. Segel JS, McAnarney ER. Adolescent pregnancy and subsequent obesity in African-American girls. *J Adolesc Health* 1994;15:491.
    Adolescents who are obese prior to their first pregnancy often become even more obese an average of 3.3 years following pregnancy. Such adolescents may be at par-ticular risk of retaining gestational weight gain, and the consequences of their morbid obesity may be ultimately life-threatening.

Treatment
24. Zabin LS. Adolescent pregnancy: the clinician's role in intervention. *J Gen Intern Med* 1990;5[Suppl]:81.
    This report reviews research on adolescent development and sexual behavior.
25. Stahler GJ, DuCette J, McBride D. The evaluation component in adolescent pregnancy care projects: is it adequate? *Fam Plan Perspect* 1989;21:123.
    This is a review of the activities promoted by the adolescent Family Life Act— projects designed to care for pregnant teenagers.
26. Stephenson JN. Pregnancy testing and counseling. *Pediatr Clin North Am* 1989; 36:681.
    Pregnancy testing and counseling are increasingly accepted as necessary services for adolescents.
27. Nutrition management of adolescent pregnancy: technical support paper. *J Am Diet Assoc* 1989;89:105.

A high proportion of pregnant teens are nutritionally at risk and require nutrition intervention.

28. Stevens-Simon C, Wallis J, Allen-Davis J. Which teen mothers choose Norplant? *J Adolesc Health* 1995;16:350.
    These data do not support the study hypothesis and are encouraging because they suggest that Norplant may reduce repeat pregnancy among adolescent parents.

29. Scholl TO, Hediger ML, Belsky DH. Prenatal care and maternal health during adolescent pregnancy: a review and meta-analysis. *J Adolesc Health* 1994;15:444.
    Although future research efforts will need to address the issues of bias inherent in much of the published research, the published literature suggests that prenatal care regimens which provide social and behavioral services along with medical care could improve both the health of the mother and the outcome of her pregnancy.

30. Agyei WK, Mukiza-Gapere J, Epema EJ. Sexual behaviour, reproductive health and contraceptive use among adolescents and young adults in Mbale District, Uganda. *J Trop Med Hygiene* 1994;97:219.
    Many adolescents still engaged in unprotected sexual relations. The most commonly used methods of contraception were the condom and the pill. Issues discussed included the safety of contraceptives and their nonavailability.

31. Carter DM, et al. When children have children: the teen pregnancy predicament. *Am J Prev Med* 1994;10:108.
    Clinical interventions, such as school-linked clinics to provide contraception and prenatal care programs to reduce perinatal morbidity, have varied in their approaches and their subsequent success.

32. Morris DL, et al. Comparison of adolescent pregnancy outcomes by prenatal care source. *J Reprod Med* 1993;38:375.
    Although teen clinic participants began prenatal care earlier and had more visits than traditional care participants, both groups had similar pregnancy outcomes. Groups receiving prenatal care had better prenatal outcomes (Apgar scores, preterm births, low and very low birth weight) than did those who received no care.

33. Jaccard J. Adolescent contraceptive behavior: the impact of the provider and the structure of clinic-based programs. *Obstet Gynecol* 1996;88[Suppl]:57.
    There is little convincing evidence that the presence of adolescent clinics promotes sexual activity.

34. Frost JJ, Forrest JD. Understanding the impact of effective teenage pregnancy prevention programs. *Fam Plan Perspect* 1995;27:188.
    Two programs significantly decreased the proportion of adolescents who became pregnant; these programs were the two that were most active in providing access to contraceptive services.

35. Romans SE, Martin JL, Morris EM. Risk factors for adolescent pregnancy: how important is child sexual abuse? Otago Women's Health Study. *N Engl J Med* 1997;110:30.
    Adolescent pregnancy does not occur randomly in the community but was found in women who came from families with preexisting psychosocial problems. This suggests that preventive strategies aiming to reduce adolescent pregnancy should focus on measures that improve the general functioning of family units, in addition to providing good sexual information.

Complications

36. Stevens-Simon C, Roghmann KJ, McAnarney ER. Repeat adolescent pregnancy and low birth weight: methods issues. *J Adolesc Health Care* 1990;11:114.
    The results of birth order and birth weight studies conducted among adolescent mothers is conflicting.

37. Hechtman L. Teenage mothers and their children: risks and problems: a review. *Can J Psychiatry* 1989;34:569(abst).
    To identify positive instrumentation, factors that influence the physical and psychologic health of adolescents must be recognized.

38. Slap GB, Schwartz JS. Risk factors for low birth weight to adolescent mothers. *J Adolesc Health Care* 1989;10:267.

The authors report the results of a study of mothers under 20 years of age who delivered babies weighing 2,500 g or less.

39. Furstenberg FF Jr, Brooks-Gunn J, Chase-Lansdale L. Teenaged pregnancy and childbearing. *Am Psychol* 1989;44:313.
   This study supports evidence that there is a need for more integration and availability of services to the adolescent needy.

40. Silva MO, Cabral H, Zuckerman B. Adolescent pregnancy in Portugal: effectiveness of continuity of care by an obstetrician. *Obstet Gynecol* 1993;81:142.
   Pregnant adolescents in this study received care from the same obstetrician and were followed in a special clinic. Maternal weight gain and infant weights were greater than those noted for controls, and the number of prenatal visits in the study group was twice that in the control group.

41. Creatsas GC. Adolescent pregnancy in Europe. *Int J Fertil Menopausal Stud* 1995;40[Suppl 2]:80.
   Although the medical complications of pregnancy and birth in adolescents can be minimized with good management and follow-up, the social and psychological implications continue to take a toll. Sex-education programs are one means of reducing the rate of adolescent pregnancy. For adolescents who do become pregnant, however, psychological and social support must be provided in addition to medical care.

42. Rainey DY, Stevens-Simon C, Kaplan DW. Are adolescents who report prior sexual abuse at higher risk for pregnancy? *Child Abuse Neglect* 1995;19:1283.
   Further study is needed to determine why a disproportionate number of sexually abused adolescents desire pregnancy. The efficacy of adolescent pregnancy prevention programs may be improved by identifying previously abused adolescents and by designing educational interventions that specifically address their desire to conceive.

43. Barnet B, et al. Association between postpartum substance use and depressive symptoms, stress, and social support in adolescent mothers. *Pediatrics* 1995; 96(Pt 1):659.
   This study indicates that alcohol and drug use are common among this sample of postpartum teenage mothers and that depression, stress, high support need, and peer group drug use are associated factors. Although this study cannot determine whether depression and stress precede or result from use of substances, attention to these factors appears warranted in the care of adolescent mothers.

---

17. ADVANCED MATERNAL AGE AND MANAGEMENT OF THE GRAND MULTIPARA

Michel E. Rivlin

Between 1970 and 1990, the rate of first births for women 30 to 39 years of age increased by 100%, and the rate for those 40 to 44 years of age increased by 50%. It is estimated that by the year 2000, 8.6% of births in the United States will involve women 35 to 49 years of age.

The wide availability of safe and effective contraceptives has allowed these women to delay childbearing. Other factors accounting for advanced maternal age include pursuit of a career, lack of a suitable partner, the beginning of a second marriage, and a desire for greater financial security. Furthermore, recent advances in assisted reproductive technologies have improved pregnancy rates among those with involuntary infertility.

The nature of counseling in women over 35 years of age differs from that in younger women. Fertility decreases with age, and many of these women have less time for the evaluation of problems that may arise. The incidence of chromosomal anomalies, including Down syndrome, in live-born infants increases to about one in 20 in mothers 45 years of age or older. Genetic counseling is discussed in Chapter 44. The incidence of spontaneous abortion also rises with increased maternal age. Many of these women have concerns about the effect of age on their pregnancy and the impact of an abnormal pregnancy on their careers and personal lives.

Various medical diseases such as diabetes and hypertension are more common as age increases. The risk of diabetes is 6% for women over 35, compared with 3% in younger age groups. Hypertension affects approximately 6% of women over 35, whereas, in general, chronic vascular disease complicates less than 2% of gestations. In most patient series, no difference in perinatal outcome with advancing maternal age has been noted, unless there is associated diabetes, hypertension, or obesity. However, the parity of the more mature woman does seem to have a bearing on the obstetric outcome. One epidemiologic study revealed that there was more intrauterine growth retardation and lower developmental scores in this group, but only in primiparas. Several researchers have noted prolonged labor to be associated with increasing maternal age. In particular, there is a greater incidence of secondary arrest and a longer second stage. Primary cesarean delivery rates are consistently higher in this age group, even when the data are controlled for such factors as fetal distress. One factor that may be responsible for this is increased physician attentiveness to problems in this age group and more aggressive management of these problems.

Maternal mortality appears to be increased in pregnant women older than 35 years, compared to their nonpregnant counterparts. In one large study, the leading causes for maternal death were obstetric hemorrhage and embolism. Other studies have shown an increase in maternal mortality owing to pregnancy-induced hypertension, placenta previa, and postpartum hemorrhage. In particular, the mortality at age 45 years may be as high as 200 times that of younger pregnant patients. The figures also show that race is an important factor; the mortality in black women 35 years or older is higher than that in whites in the same group. Additionally, underlying maternal conditions such as hypertension and diabetes greatly increase the chances for maternal death.

Fetal risks seem more related to maternal disease states than to maternal age alone, although vascular changes such as sclerotic lesions in the myometrial arteries are found more frequently in older patients. Intrapartum deaths do not seem to be increased in association with advanced maternal age; however, some studies suggest that antepartum fetal loss may be more common. There is a slight increase in birth weight with advanced maternal age, and the childhood IQ scores in the offspring of parturients in this group are higher.

Although probably the best approach to contraception in this age group of women is permanent sterilization, many (especially those of lower parity) may not have completed their families. The older patient is more likely to be in a stable relationship and presumably has a better understanding of barrier devices; therefore, this method is also most suitable. For similar reasons, the intrauterine device provides another alternative method. Oral contraceptive agents with less than 50 μg of estrogen also may be suitable, as long as the patient has no risk factors (e.g., smoking, obesity).

The definition of the grand multipara is a woman who has given birth seven times or more to an infant or infants weighing at least 500 g. Many early reports warned of increases in hypertension, abruptio placentae, malpresentation, cesarean delivery, and postpartum hemorrhage. Thus, because of the increased rate of maternal mortality in this group, sterilization was advocated. The findings from more recent surveys have contradicted these findings, however, with no maternal deaths encountered in one series consisting of more than 5,000 grand multiparas. One would expect such conditions as diabetes and hypertension, which primarily affect the older population, to be more prevalent in grand multiparas, but there appears to be no significant difference in their incidence versus that in younger patients.

Many physicians anticipate obstetric problems in the grand multipara. Because the uterus contains less muscle and more connective tissue with increased parity, uterine inertia and abnormal presentations would be expected to be more likely, but this is not the case. Instead, multiple gestation is increased 2.5 times in these grand multiparas, compared with that in mothers of lower parity.

According to the findings from older studies, the risk of uterine rupture in the grand multipara appeared to be 20 times that of the woman of lower parity, but the findings from recent studies do not confirm this. Nevertheless, the use of oxytocin in these patients is controversial. Although there are case reports of rupture with oxytocin use in the grand multipara, the results of most series do not substantiate this. Judicious administration of dilute oxytocin by means of a controlled infusion device in conjunction with internal uterine pressure monitoring provides an adequate defense against uterine rupture.

In summary, the aging of the obstetric population brings new problems for the obstetricians involved. Most pregnancies in older parturients are safely negotiated. Although in general the average parity is decreasing, the grand multipara occasionally requires the attention of practitioners who are less experienced with the obstetric management required. However, the individual patient can be reassured by the modern advances in obstetric care. The outcome in such women now appears to be no different from that in women of lower parity.

Maternal Age
1. Bianco A, et al. Pregnancy outcome at age 40 and older. *Obstet Gynecol* 1996;87:917.
   Maternal morbidity was increased, but overall neonatal outcome was unaffected.
2. Ekbald U, Vilpa T. Pregnancy in women over forty. *Ann Chir Gynaecol Suppl* 1994;208:68.
   The most common complications were prematurity (11%) and gestational diabetes (8%). Cesarean deliveries were performed in 26% and 36% of primipara women.
3. Bobrowski RA, Bottoms SF. Underappreciated risks of the elderly multipara. *Am J Obstet Gynecol* 1995;172:1764.
   The greatest age-related increase in risks was in multiparous rather than in nulliparous women.
4. Buehler JW, et al. Maternal mortality in women aged 35 years or older: United States. *JAMA* 1986;255:53.
   During a 5-year period beginning in 1974, the leading causes of maternal death in women aged 35 and older were obstetric hemorrhage and embolism.
5. Fretts RC, et al. Increased maternal age and the risk of fetal death. *N Engl J Med* 1995;333:953.
   Even when controlled for coexisting conditions, women over 35 had a risk of fetal death twice as high as that in younger women.
6. Cnattingius S, et al. Effect of age, parity, and smoking on pregnancy outcome: a population-based study. *Am J Obstet Gynecol* 1993;168(Pt 1):16.
   Older smokers are at high risk for small-for-gestational-age births, and parous smokers are at high risk for low birth weight and preterm delivery.
7. Gordon D, et al. Advanced maternal age is a risk factor for cesarean delivery. *Obstet Gynecol* 1991;77:493.
   Advanced maternal age alone may influence a physician's decisions, thereby placing some women at an unnecessary risk of cesarean delivery.
8. Peipert JF, Bracken MB. Maternal age: an independent risk factor for cesarean delivery. *Obstet Gynecol* 1993;81:200.
   Advanced maternal age was found to be an independent risk factor for cesarean delivery.
9. Ananth CV, et al. Effect of maternal age and parity on the risk of uteroplacental bleeding disorders in pregnancy. *Obstet Gynecol* 1996;88(Pt 1):511.
   Increasing maternal age was associated independently with an increased risk of placenta previa, but not with abruption or bleeding of unknown etiology.
10. Friedman EA, Sachtleben MR. Relation of maternal age to the course of labor. *Am J Obstet Gynecol* 1965;91:915.
    Secondary arrest of labor and a prolonged second stage of labor were observed with increasing maternal age.

11. Schwartz D, Mayaux MJ. Female fecundity as a function of age. *N Engl J Med* 1982;306:404.
    The fertility in women undergoing artificial insemination with no diagnosis other than oligospermia in their partners was found to be decreased with greater maternal age.

12. Maroulis GB. Effect of aging on fertility and pregnancy. *Semin Reprod Endocrinol* 1991;9:165.
    Increased pregnancy wastage after age 40 is due to abnormal embryogenesis as evidenced by the high incidence of aneuploidy in offspring and abortuses of women in this age range.

13. Sauer MV, Paulson RJ, Lobo RA. Pregnancy after age 50: application of oocyte donation to women after natural menopause. *Lancet* 1993;341:321.
    Many children have been raised by grandparents. The option of oocyte donation should not be withheld from women who are medically and psychologically suitable.

14. Hook EB. Rates of chromosomal abnormalities at different maternal ages. *Obstet Gynecol* 1981;58:282.
    The estimated rates of chromosomal abnormalities for a range of maternal ages are the standards used for counseling most women before amniocentesis.

15. Davies BL, Doran TA. Factors in a woman's decision to undergo genetic amniocentesis for advanced maternal age. *Nurs Res* 1982;31:56.
    The major concern of women undergoing amniocentesis was concern about the effect of maternal age on the developing child.

16. Mishell DR. Use of oral contraceptives in women of older reproductive age. *Am J Obstet Gynecol* 1988;158:1652.
    There is no increased risk of cardiovascular disease in patients taking low-dose oral contraceptives except in those women with other risk factors and those who smoke.

Grand Multiparity

17. Goldman GA, et al. The grand multipara. *Eur J Obstet Gynecol Reprod Biol* 1995;61:105.
    With good perinatal care, grand multiparity no longer needs to be considered a high risk obstetric category.

18. Toohey JS, et al. The dangerous multipara: fact or fiction? *Am J Obstet Gynecol* 1995;172(Pt 1):683.
    In a largely Hispanic population, grand multiparity was not associated with an increased incidence of intrapartum complications.

19. Jouppila P, Jouppila R. The intensity of labor pain in grand multiparas. *Acta Obstet Gynecol Scand* 1996;75:250.
    The majority of parturients, including grand multiparas, suffered from intense pain during labor. A significant number of grand multiparas felt that they did not receive sufficient pain relief.

20. Kallen K. Parity and Down syndrome. *Am J Med Genet* 1997;70:196.
    There appears to be a positive correlation between grand multiparity and Down syndrome.

21. Selo-Ojeme DO, Okonofua FE. Risk factors for primary postpartum haemorrhage. A case control study. *Arch Gynecol Obstet* 1997;259:179.
    Grand multiparity was not significantly associated with postpartum hemorrhage.

22. Dyack C, Hughes PF, Simbakalia JB. Vaginal delivery in the grand multipara following previous lower segment cesarean section. *J Obstet Gynaecol Res* 1997;23:219.
    Sixty percent of women had a successful uncomplicated vaginal delivery. There was a relatively high incidence of serious complications.

23. Miller DA, et al. Intrapartum rupture of the unscarred uterus. *Obstet Gynecol* 1997;89(Pt 1):671.
    In this series of 10 cases, grand multiparity was an associated factor in two.

18. MULTIFETAL GESTATIONS

William E. Roberts

The disproportionately high perinatal morbidity and mortality associated with multifetal gestations underscores its importance as a significant obstetric challenge. The incidence of twins in the United States is about one in 90 live births (11–12 per 1,000 live births), whereas the incidence of triplets is about one in 8,000 live births. However, early use of ultrasonography in pregnancy indicates that the incidence of twin conceptions is higher than expected and is often associated with the unrecognized loss of one twin. When compared with whites, multiple births occur more frequently in blacks and less frequently in Asians. Increasing maternal age as well as parity are also associated with higher rates of twinning. Other situations associated with a higher incidence of multifetal gestations include (1) women who are themselves a dizygotic twin, (2) women who conceive within 1 month of cessation of oral contraceptives, (3) women who have undergone ovulation induction with gonadotropin therapy (20%–40% incidence) or clomiphene (13%), and women whose pregnancy results from in vitro fertilization. Nowadays, in triplet or higher-order pregnancies, less than one in three occur naturally, whereas the remainder result from the use of potent ovulation-induction agents and the development of other assisted reproductive technologies.

Multiple gestations can arise from one or more ova. The division of a single fertilized ovum into two embryos is termed *monozygotic*, or identical twinning. If the fertilized ovum divides within the first 72 hours after fertilization, a diamniotic, dichorionic monozygotic twin pregnancy will develop and will have either two distinct placentas or a single-fused placenta. The most common time (70%) for ovum division is between the 4th and 8th days of development and produces a diamniotic, monochorionic, monozygotic twin pregnancy. The least frequent time for ovum division (5%) is after the 8th day. At this time of gestation, the amniotic cavity is already established, and embryo division results in a monoamniotic, monochorionic, monozygotic twin pregnancy. Varieties of conjoined twins result if division occurs after formation of the embryonic disk at 13 days of gestation.

Placental examination at delivery assists in the determination of zygosity. The existence of either one sac (one chorion, one amnion), or a monochorionic placenta with only amnions forming the intervening membrane are evidence of monozygosity. If neonates are of the same sex, blood-group testing or human leukocyte antigen typing is useful for determination of zygosity. The frequency of monozygotic twins remains constant worldwide at one in 250 births, whereas the frequency of dizygotic twins is influenced by maternal age, race, parity, and fertility therapy.

Dizygotic twins result from the maturation and fertilization of two ova from either the same or different ovaries. The two placentas, whether proximate or distinct, have separate amniotic and chorionic membranes (diamniotic-dichorionic). A superfecundation is the fertilization of two ova from more than one act of coitus in the same menstrual cycle. Superfetation is the fertilization of two ova from different menstrual cycles and is rare in humans. A third type of twinning is theoretic and occurs when a single ovum is fertilized by two sperm with subsequent zygote division.

The enlarged multifetal uterine mass is frequently associated with maternal discomfort, aortocaval compression, peripheral-dependent edema, varicosities, anemia, and fatigue. Uterine overdistension may contribute to the high frequency of premature labor, abnormal labor with hypotonic uterine dysfunction, and uterine atony with postpartum hemorrhage. Hydramnios is also more likely to occur in multifetal gestations. The acute form is more common in monozygotic twin pregnancy, often occurs secondary to extensive twin-to-twin transfusion, generally occurs remote from term, and is associated with a high fetal loss rate. Hydramnios occurring later in pregnancy usually indicates a congenital anomaly of one fetus, especially if it is confined to only one amniotic sac. Pregnancy-induced hypertension (PIH) occurs three times more often in twin pregnancies without regard to zygosity. Glucose intolerance is also more frequently observed in multifetal gestations.

In the United States, the perinatal death rate in twin gestations averages 15%, a rate 10 times that of singleton pregnancies. Spontaneous abortion is also increased, and preterm birth occurs in half of all multifetal gestations. Normal duration of pregnancy for twins is 261 days versus 280 in singletons, with a mean birth weight of 2,395 g in twins versus 3,377 g in singletons. Due to an estimated 50% mortality rate in monoamniotic twins secondary to intertwining umbilical cords as well as the excessive mortality associated with twin-to-twin transfusion syndrome, monozygotic twins have a 2.5 times greater overall perinatal death rate than dizygotic twins. As the number of fetuses in a pregnancy increase, the duration of gestation and birth weight decrease while the degree and overall incidence of fetal growth restriction increases. The frequency of malformations in the twin pregnancy is generally twice that of singletons, with malformations in monozygotic twins exceeding that in dizygotic twins. Even so, reduction of the high perinatal mortality of multifetal gestations is best achieved with a decrease in the incidence of preterm birth.

The most important step in the antenatal care of patients with a multifetal gestation is early diagnosis. Suggestions of a multifetal gestation include family history; recent administration of clomiphene, gonadotropins, or oral contraceptives; and a larger-than-expected uterine size. Clinical signs of a multifetal gestation include an increased transverse abdominal girth, multiple small palpable fetal parts, distinctly different fetal heart rates, a small fetal head in a large uterus, maternal anemia unresponsive to customary oral iron, PIH, and preterm labor.

The increased use of early gestational ultrasonography for pregnancy evaluation and gestational age assessment has led to a declining incidence of undiagnosed multifetal gestations. By the end of the first trimester of pregnancy, separate fetal heads can be identified by abdominal real-time ultrasonography. Using transvaginal ultrasonographic scanning, two gestational sacs can be identified by 5 to 6 weeks, with fetal body and heart motion detected by 7 to 8 weeks. As the number of fetuses above two increases, the accuracy of diagnosis relative to the number of fetuses as well as the technical difficulties in obtaining accurate fetal gestational age parameters become more difficult. The inability via ultrasonography to distinguish between the fetal bodies, the identification of more than three vessels in a single umbilical cord, the lack of a separating membrane, or the presence of fetal anomalies should heighten the suspicion of conjoined twins. In the absence of real-time ultrasonography, a confirmatory x-ray of the maternal abdomen after 18 weeks of gestation is suggested to determine fetal number. There is no biochemical test that can accurately discriminate multiple from singleton gestations. In multifetal pregnancies, each amniotic sac can be sampled for genetic studies with minimal complication. Dilute indigo carmine injected into the first amniotic sac after sampling permits assurance that one has sampled the second sac if clear amniotic fluid is obtained.

Some clinicians advocate consideration of selective pregnancy reduction in triplet and higher order gestations. It is well established that the incidence of both perinatal morbidity and mortality as well as maternal complications are directly related to an increase in fetal number. Although multifetal pregnancy reduction is a complex moral and ethical issue, available data indicate that transvaginal embryo aspiration at 7 to 8 weeks' gestation or transabdominal fetal reduction at 9 to 14 weeks improves overall perinatal performance in quadruplet pregnancies with a low procedure-related loss rate.

Management goals with multifetal gestation include (1) early diagnosis; (2) an optimal intrauterine environment; (3) prevention of preterm labor and delivery; (4) close fetal surveillance to detect malformations, deficient or discordant fetal growth, and other signs of fetal compromise; (5) atraumatic delivery; and (6) immediate expert neonatal care. Frequent periods of lateral recumbent rest and cessation of full-time employment are encouraged to promote fetal growth. Dietary requirements are increased by increments of 300 calories per day for each fetus in addition to folate and iron supplementation. In an attempt to reduce the incidence of preterm labor, frequent prenatal visits are scheduled to detect premature cervical dilatation, to educate the patient to signs and symptoms of preterm labor, and to assess uterine activity. Prophylactic cervical cerclage procedures, prophylactic tocolytic administration, and routine progestin administration have not been shown to be efficacious and are generally not recommended. Preterm premature rupture of the fetal membranes is usually managed conservatively as in a singleton pregnancy.

Serial sonography is performed to diagnose and verify gestational age in early pregnancy. In the late second and early third trimesters of pregnancy, serial sonography is initiated every 3 to 4 weeks to assess appropriate and concordant fetal growth. If discordant fetal growth is suggested by a biparietal diameter (BPD) difference of ≥5 mm or an abdominal circumference of ≥30 mm, estimation of fetal weight between or among fetuses should be undertaken, with discordance generally defined as a ≥20% difference when the weight of the larger fetus is used as the denominator.

Weekly nonstress testing (NST) beginning at 30 to 32 weeks is generally recommended to ensure fetal well-being. Due to its high false-positive rate coupled with a fear of initiating preterm labor, contraction stress testing should be avoided in multifetal gestations except to evaluate a nonreactive NST or other worrisome clinical or ultrasonographic finding. Biophysical profile and assessments of umbilical systolic/diastolic ratios are additional tools for fetal surveillance to alert the clinician to incipient fetal problems. Assessment of fetal lung maturation in the absence of labor is performed from a single sac if the BPDs of both fetuses are commensurate or if the second sac cannot be safely sampled. A lecithin:sphingomyelin ratio of 2.0:1 or more is expected by 32 to 33 weeks' gestation in a twin pregnancy.

The intrapartum management of multiple gestation remains controversial. If preterm labor is detected, if the cervix is ≤4 cm dilated, and if clinical evidence of compromising maternal or fetal disease is lacking, tocolytic agents with lateral recumbent bed rest and appropriate hydration are used to delay delivery and for consideration for glucocorticoid therapy to accelerate fetal lung maturity. Magnesium sulfate is the tocolytic agent of choice in multifetal gestations because beta-mimetic agents carry a greater risk of maternal pulmonary edema.

Optimally, the gravida with a laboring multiple gestation is referred to a tertiary perinatal care center for maternal, fetal, and subsequent neonatal care. Monitoring of both fetal heart rates is essential. A well-functioning intravenous line with a large-bore catheter is used, with blood transfusion capability readily available in case of postpartum hemorrhage. Determination of gestational age as well as fetal position and presentation will influence the mode of delivery. Vertex-vertex presentations usually allow safe vaginal delivery, whereas other combinations result in a higher incidence of abdominal delivery. The presenting twin's birth weight often bears no relationship to the weight of the second twin. Liberal use of low-vertical cesarean section, often in conjunction with a low-vertical abdominal incision, is recommended for gross fetal size discrepancies, in cases of nonreassuring fetal heart rate monitoring, umbilical cord prolapse, severe preterm PIH, a contracted cervix following the first twin delivery, a gestation of three or more fetuses, or a first twin breech presentation. Either skillfully executed conduction anesthesia by epidural catheter or general anesthesia is used for multifetal delivery. In all cases, sound medical judgment of the individual patient is essential for optimal results.

General
1. Devoe LD, et al. Antenatal assessment of twin gestations. *Semin Perinatol* 1995;19:413.
   This critical review addresses the individual and combined application of standard tests used for evaluation of intrauterine health in single pregnancies and how the tests should be modified in the multifetal gestation.
2. Fleming AD, et al. Perinatal outcomes of twin pregnancies at term. *J Reprod Med* 1990;35:881.
   This is a review of antepartum and postpartum complications encountered in twin gestations after 36 weeks' gestation.
3. Friedman SA, et al. Do twins mature earlier than singletons? Results from a matched cohort study. *Am J Obstet Gynecol* 1997;176:1193.

This matched cohort study of 112 sets of twins failed to demonstrate any accel-erated maturation or improved neonatal outcome when compared with matched singleton infants.

4. Herruzo AJ, et al. Perinatal morbidity and mortality in twin pregnancies. *Int J Gynaecol Obstet* 1991;36:17.
   Thorough discussion of antenatal, intrapartum, and postpartum complications in the multifetal gestation along with a review of early neonatal morbidity and mortality.
5. Lantz ME, et al. Multiple pregnancy. *Curr Opin Obstet Gynecol* 1993;5:657.
   This review article focuses on new interventions and techniques to improve out-comes in multifetal gestations.
6. Minakami H, et al. When is the optimal time for delivery? Purely from the fetuses' perspective. *Gynecol Obstet Invest* 1995;40:174.
   This extensive population survey reveals the optimal time for delivery of a multifetal gestation is 37 weeks' gestation.
7. O'Grady JP. Twins and beyond: management guide. *Contemp Obstet Gynecol* 1991;36:45.
   Covering every important aspect of twinning, this concise article contains the full range of pertinent considerations from physiology to diagnosis and delivery.

Etiology
8. Bassil S, et al. Predictive factors for multiple pregnancy in in vitro fertilization. *J Reprod Med* 1997;42:761.
   This retrospective study suggests that the best reproductive prognosis is achieved by replacing only two embryos of good quality.
9. Benirschke K. Multiple gestation: incidence, etiology, and inheritance. In: Creaky R, Resnik R, eds. *Maternal-fetal medicine: principles and practice,* 3rd ed. Philadelphia: WB Saunders, 1994.
   The author presents a thorough inclusive review of physiologic principles and clinical practice regarding multifetal gestations.

Diagnosis
10. Aisenbrey GA, et al. Monoamniotic and pseudomonoamniotic twins: sonographic diagnosis, detection of cord entanglement, and obstetric management. *Obstet Gynecol* 1995;86:218.
    This series of seven nonconjoined monoamniotic twin pregnancies demonstrates reliable methods to detect cord entanglement and presents a reasonable obstetric management protocol.
11. Divon MY, et al. Ultrasound in twin pregnancy. *Semin Perinatol* 1995;19:404.
    This comprehensive review evaluates the role of ultrasound in twin gestation. It in-cludes the indication for first-trimester scanning as well as the use of ultrasound in determining the type of placentation. The need for serial sonography late in pregnancy along with the ability of Doppler evaluation is discussed.
12. Goldenberg RL, et al. The preterm prediction study: risk factors in twin gesta-tions. National Institute of Child Health and Human Development Maternal-Fetal Medicine Units Network. *Am J Obstet Gynecol* 1996;175:1047.
    This extensive prospective study analyzes the association between the presence of bac-terial vaginosis, fetal fibronectin, and a short cervix and the risk of spontaneous preterm birth of twins.
13. Kushnir O, et al. Transvaginal sonographic measurement of cervical length. Evaluation of twin pregnancies. *J Reprod Med* 1995;40:380.
    This investigation studies transvaginal ultrasonographic measurement of the cervix throughout twin gestations and compares these findings with those in singleton pregnancies. The authors conclude from their data that the cervical length in twins was significantly shorter than the cervical length in matched singleton pregnancies.
14. Landy HJ, et al. The vanishing twin: ultrasonographic assessment of fetal dis-appearance in the first trimester. *Am J Obstet Gynecol* 1991;78:739.

The true incidence of multiple gestation in the first trimester ranges from 3.3% to 5.4%; one in five will vanish subsequently in association with vaginal bleeding with a good prognosis for the remaining twin.

15. Magann EF, et al. Amniotic fluid volume of third-trimester diamniotic twin pregnancies. *Obstet Gynecol* 1995;85:957.

    This study defines the normal range of amniotic fluid volume in third-trimester diamniotic twin gestations by using a dye dilution technique.

16. Ohno Y, et al. The value of Doppler ultrasound in the diagnosis and management of twin-to-twin transfusion syndrome. *Arch Gynecol Obstet* 1994;255:37.

    This longitudinal evaluation of 33 pairs of twins included 5 sets with twin-to-twin transfusion syndrome (TTTS). In cases of TTTS, the pulsatility index (PI) between the twin cohorts was greater than 0.5. In discordant twins without TTTS, the PI was less than 0.5.

17. Pruggmayer MRK, et al. Genetic amniocentesis in twin pregnancies: results of a multicenter study of 529 cases. *Ultrasound Obstet Gynecol* 1992;2:6.

    In this multicenter study, the abortion rate after genetic amniocentesis was 3.7%. Although this rate is higher than the 1.7% reported in singleton gestations, the authors did not feel it was substantially higher than the normal biologic rate in twin pregnancies.

18. Sebire NJ, et al. Intertwin disparity in fetal size in monochorionic and dichorionic pregnancies. *Obstet Gynecol* 1998;91:82.

    This prospective study reports sonographic findings of 123 monochorionic and 416 dichorionic twin pregnancies followed from 10 to 14 weeks' gestation. The findings of the study failed to demonstrate any significant intertwin disparity in fetal size for monochorionic and dichorionic twin pregnancies.

19. Sherer DM, et al. Fetal growth in multifetal gestation. *Clin Obstet Gynecol* 1997;40:764.

    This review depicts various sonographic methods to detect altered fetal growth in multifetal gestation along with obstetric strategies to determine cause.

20. Vetter K. Considerations on growth discordant twins. *J Reprod Med* 1993;21:267.

    This article presents the pathophysiologic basis of growth discordancy in twins along with sonographic methods to improve detection of discordant twin pairs.

Treatment

21. Boggess KA, et al. Delivery of the nonvertex second twin: a review of the literature. *Obstet Gynecol Surv* 1997;52:728.

    Approximately 40% of twin gestations enter labor in vertex-nonvertex presentations. Although there is agreement regarding the safety of vaginal delivery for twins when both are vertex, controversy exists over the intrapartum management when the second twin is nonvertex. This article reviews the obstetric literature to determine whether breech extraction or external cephalic version is associated with increased morbidity over cesarean delivery.

22. Chauhan SP, et al. Delivery of the nonvertex second twin: breech extraction versus external cephalic version. *Am J Obstet Gynecol* 1995;173:1015.

    The intrapartum course of 284 consecutive twin gestations are analyzed to compare the maternal and perinatal outcome of vertex-nonvertex presentations. The data presented demonstrate that total breech extraction is associated with less fetal distress and fewer emergent abdominal deliveries than external cephalic version.

23. Elliott JP, et al. Biophysical profile testing as an indicator of fetal well-being in high-order multiple gestations. *Am J Obstet Gynecol* 1995;172:508.

    The purpose of this investigation was to determine the utility of biophysical profile testing in the prevention of intrapartum death in patients with higher-order multiple gestations. The data and protocol used demonstrate that the biophysical profile is a reliable antepartum test of fetal well-being in triplet and quadruplet pregnancies.

24. Fasouliotis SJ, et al. Multifetal pregnancy reduction: a review of the world results for the period 1993–1996. *Eur J Obstet Gynecol Reprod Biol* 1997;75:183.
    This work evaluates the world literature on multifetal pregnancy reduction from 1993 to 1996. The total pregnancy loss rate in 1,453 completed cases was 12.2%. The review also offers some analyses of the ethical dilemmas associated with multifetal pregnancy reduction.

25. Hales KA, et al. Intravenous magnesium sulfate for premature labor: comparison between twin and singleton gestations. *Am J Perinatol* 1995;12:7.
    This investigation was conducted to determine the efficacy and safety of intravenous magnesium sulfate tocolysis in twin gestations using dosing regimens developed for singletons. The data presented verify that the dosing schedule for magnesium sulfate to treat preterm labor in singletons is equally safe and effective for twin gestations.

26. Houlihan C, et al. Intrapartum management of multiple gestations. *Clin Perinatol* 1996;23:91.
    This up-to-date article reviews the use of ultrasonography in the intrapartum management of multiple gestations. In addition, controversial topics such as external cephalic version versus breech extraction are discussed. Finally, future areas of research, such as the use of intravenous nitroglycerin for uterine relaxation to facilitate uterine manipulation of the second twin, are presented.

27. Roberts WE, et al. Risk of preterm delivery from preterm labor in high-risk patients. *J Reprod Med* 1995;40:95.
    This investigation focuses on high-risk factors for preterm delivery in more than 17,000 patients. Included in this series are women with multiple gestations, of whom 73% deliver preterm.

28. Rust OA, et al. Twins and preterm labor. *J Reprod Med* 1997;42:229.
    This retrospective, analytic study demonstrates that intensive prenatal surveillance, which includes home uterine activity monitoring, results in improved reproductive performance in twin pregnancies.

Complications

29. Bider D, et al. Combined vaginal-abdominal delivery of twins. *J Reprod Med* 1995;40:131.
    This article reviews the intrapartum events that precipitated the need for emergent cesarean delivery for the second twin. From this review, a management protocol is presented.

30. Kurzel RB, et al. Cesarean section for the second twin. *J Reprod Med* 1997;42:767.
    The purpose of this study was to determine the reason for cesarean section for the second twin following vaginal delivery of twin A. Umbilical cord prolapse of twin B and the inability to successfully perform a breech extraction or external cephalic version accounted for 81.5% of the cesarean sections.

31. Lee CY. Management of monoamniotic twins diagnosed by ultrasound. *Am J Gynecol Health* 1992;6:25.
    Criteria for antenatal diagnosis, details of prenatal care, and recommendations for operative delivery highlight this presentation of multifetal gestation's most dangerous circumstance.

32. Porreco RP, et al. Delayed-interval delivery in multifetal pregnancy. *Am J Obstet Gynecol* 1998;178:20.
    The authors present a management protocol for the selection of suitable cases for delayed-interval delivery in multifetal pregnancy along with an in-depth analysis of nine such cases.

33. Weiner CP. Challenge of twin-twin transfusion syndrome. *Contemp Obstet Gynecol* 1992;37:83.
    A plea is made for an accurate diagnosis by performance of invasive procedures. An algorithm for antenatal evaluation of a monochorionic twin gestation complicated by acute hydramnios and a stuck twin is presented.

19. RH ISOIMMUNIZATION

Kenneth G. Perry Jr.

Isoimmunization refers to the development of antibodies in response to isoantigens. If the isoantigens are of fetal erythrocyte origin, hemolytic disease of the newborn (HDN) can occur. Hemolytic disease of the newborn was first described in France during the seventeenth century. However, it was not until the 1940s that the association of the Rh antibodies (anti-D) and erythroblastosis was established. Despite the introduction of Rh immunoglobulin in 1966 and subsequent aggressive preventative programs, Rh isoimmunization continues to be the single most common cause of HDN. Nonetheless, the prevalence of Rh isoimmunization has declined over the past 50 years. This has led to a relative increase in isoimmunization due to other, less common, erythrocyte antigens (c, Kell, Fyᵃ, Jkᵃ, etc.). Approximately 15% of whites, 8% of African Americans, and 2% of Asians are Rh negative. Because only 40% of white men are Rh negative, Rh-negative women have about a 60% chance of having an Rh-positive fetus. Fortunately, only a small minority of such incompatible pregnancies will result in maternal sensitization.

For Rh isoimmunization to occur during pregnancy, the fetus must have Rh-positive erythrocytes (inherited from the father) and the mother must have Rh-negative erythrocytes. The mother, when exposed to Rh-positive erythrocytes as a result of either antepartum or intrapartum fetal-maternal hemorrhage or a prior blood transfusion, mounts an immune response with the production of antibodies against the D antigen. These immunoglobulin G antibodies are capable of transplacental passage and can cause fetal red blood cell hemolysis. The degree of hemolysis depends on the quantity of the antibody transferred from the mother to the fetus as well as the affinity of the antibody for the fetal erythrocyte. If excessive red blood cell destruction occurs, the fetus can become significantly anemic, stimulating compensatory extramedullary hematopoiesis. Extramedullary hematopoiesis occurs predominantly in the fetal liver and if profound can lead to portal hypertension and hepatic dysfunction, with subsequent hypoproteinemia, ascites, and ultimately fetal hydrops. Because bilirubin is easily metabolized by the placenta, the release of bilirubin from the destruction of red blood cells has minimal effect on the fetus in utero. However, hyperbilirubinemia can develop rapidly after birth and if not aggressively managed may be incorporated into the heavily myelinated cells of the brain, resulting in kernicterus.

At the initial prenatal visit, every patient should have her ABO blood group, Rh type, and antibody screen (indirect Coomb's) checked. If the patient is Rh negative or DU negative and has a negative antibody screen she is a candidate for Rh immunoglobulin (300 μg) at 28 to 32 weeks' gestation and again postpartum if she delivered an Rh-positive or DU-positive infant. Rh immunoglobulin is usually successful in the prevention of sensitization to the Rh antigen in subsequent pregnancies. When Rh immunoglobulin is administered within 72 hours of delivery, less than 1% of treated individuals develop subsequent sensitization. The dose of immune globulin required can be determined using the Kleihauer-Betke assay for fetal erythrocytes in the maternal circulation. In addition, Rh immunoglobulin should be administered to all Rh-negative unsensitized patients who undergo an abortion, ectopic pregnancy, amniocentesis, chorionic villus sampling, cordocentesis, or external cephalic version. Patients who experience antepartum hemorrhage or maternal trauma with a positive Kleihauer-Betke assay result should also receive Rhogam.

When a D antibody is detected in the mother and the titer is greater than 1:4, the pregnancy is Rh sensitized. If this is the first sensitized pregnancy, the antibody titer can give an estimate of the risk of erythroblastosis. In general, pregnancies are considered at risk for HDN if the anti-D titers are ≥1:16, and this indicates the need for amniocentesis. Antibody titers in the first sensitized pregnancy that are less than the threshold for HDN should be repeated at 20 weeks' gestation and every 4 weeks thereafter. In contrast, antibody titers are of no clinical value in patients having had a previously affected pregnancy and therefore should not be used to initiate amniocentesis. Regardless of antibody titers, the severity of the hemolytic disease in these gestations is usually equal to or greater than that of their prior affected pregnancy, making the obstetric history an important guide in their management. For example, if fetal hydrops developed at 30 weeks' gestation in a prior pregnancy, it is likely to develop at or before that gestational age in any subsequent gestation.

The father's Rh genotype can be helpful in the management of the Rh-sensitized pregnancy. If the father is Rh negative, then the fetus is not at risk for erythroblastosis. On the other hand, if the father is heterozygous for the D antigen, then there is a 50% probability that the fetus is Rh negative. In that case, if fetal Rh determination by cordocentesis or DNA analysis of amniocytes indicates that the fetus is Rh negative, then no further intervention is necessary.

Amniocentesis is the accepted method for assessing the severity of erythroblastosis in utero. As fetal hemolysis increases, the level of bilirubin in the amniotic fluid increases. Spectrophotometric examination of amniotic fluid containing bilirubin will cause a shift in the optical density at 450 nm (ΔOD_{450}). The ΔOD_{450} when plotted against the gestational age on the Liley graph can be used to indirectly estimate the degree of fetal erythrocyte hemolysis. Because the ΔOD_{450} trend is more reliable than a single value, amniocenteses are usually initiated at 24 to 28 weeks' gestation and repeated at 1- to 4-week intervals depending on which zone on the Liley graph the ΔOD_{450} is located. In general, zone I values require repeat amniocentesis at 2- to 4-week intervals, whereas zone II values are repeated in 7 to 14 days. Values in upper zone II and zone III indicate a fetus possibly at risk of hydrops or intrauterine fetal demise, and cordocentesis with an intrauterine blood transfusion or delivery should be considered depending on the gestational age and the documentation of fetal lung maturity. Regardless of the ΔOD_{450} value, isoimmunized pregnancies are at risk of chronic hypoxia. Therefore, daily fetal kick counts as well as weekly assessments with nonstress tests or biophysical profiles are indicated during the third trimester.

Ultrasonography is useful in the management of the Rh-isoimmunized pregnancy, especially in conjunction with amniocentesis, cordocentesis, and intrauterine fetal transfusion. Accurate dating is critical, and early ultrasonography for gestational age determination should be performed on all sensitized pregnancies. Ultrasonographic findings that have been associated with fetal compromise, such as hydramnios, placental hypertrophy, splenomegaly, and abnormal Doppler flow wave forms, are not sensitive indicators of early fetal deteriorization. Moreover, fetal hydrops is a late ultrasonographic finding and when present indicates an extremely anemic fetus. Despite recent advances, ultrasonographic technology has been unable to accurately determine the severity of fetal hemolysis and should not be used alone to dictate therapy in the isoimmunized pregnancy.

The timing of delivery in the isoimmunized patient is based on fetal status (ΔOD_{450} trend), gestational age, fetal lung maturity, and need for subsequent transfusion. In general, those pregnancies with ΔOD_{450} trends in zone I or lower zone II should be delivered at 37 to 40 weeks' gestation. Patients in mid-zone II should be delivered at 36 to 38 weeks' gestation once fetal lung maturity is documented. Those pregnancies in upper zone II or zone III or those having undergone intrauterine transfusions should be delivered at 34 to 36 weeks' gestation. A trial of labor is indicated in most cases of Rh isoimmunization, but judicious clinical judgment should be used.

Continuous electronic fetal monitoring during the intrapartum period allows for the detection of a compromised fetus. Most hydropic or severely anemic fetuses do not tolerate labor and should be delivered by cesarean section. A pediatric provider should be available in the delivery room so that appropriate care can be initiated immediately after birth. In cases where the fetus is hydropic or severely anemic, O-negative packed red blood cells cross-matched to the mother should be available at the time of delivery for possible transfusion in the delivery room.

General
1. Bowman J. The management of hemolytic disease in the fetus and newborn. *Semin Perinatol* 1997;21:39.

The author provides an excellent review of hemolytic disease in the fetus that outlines current diagnostic and treatment modalities.

2. Tannirandorn Y, Rodeck CH. New approaches in the treatment of hemolytic disease of the fetus. *Ballieres Clin Haematol* 1990;3:289.
   The articles found in this series review all aspects of isoimmunization.
3. Stangenberg M, et al. Rhesus immunization: New perspectives in maternal fetal medicine. *Obstet Gynecol Surv* 1991;16:189.
   The authors present an excellent review article detailing antenatal screening for isoimmunization, diagnostic assessment for fetal hemolytic disease, treatment of hemolytic disease of the newborn, and prophylaxis.
4. Management of Isoimmunization in Pregnancy. ACOG Educational Bulletin #227 [replaces #148], August 1996.
   This bulletin provides up-to-date diagnostic and management advice regarding Rh isoimmunization.

Etiology

5. Tovey LA. Haemolytic disease of the newborn—the changing scene. *Br J Obstet Gynaecol* 1986;93:960.
   With the introduction of Rh immunoglobulin, the number of sensitized pregnant women has decreased by 70% and fetal death has decreased 96%. Isoimmunization from antigens other than Rh(D) now exceeds those from Rh(D).
6. Bowman JM. Treatment options for the fetus with alloimmune hemolytic disease. *Transfus Med Rev* 1990;4:191.
   The Rh blood group system is actually made up of at least five antigens that can cause isoimmunization. The most common and significant antigen is D, and currently it is the only one that can be prevented. Other antibodies to antigens within the Kell, Kidd, Duffey, and MNS blood group systems have been associated with severe hemolysis. Currently prophylaxis is unavailable for these antigens.

Diagnosis

7. Wang XH, Zipursky A. Maternal erythrocytes in the fetal circulation. *Am J Clin Pathol* 1987;88:346.
   Maternal-fetal hemorrhage can be documented in 14% of Rh-negative infants born to Rh-positive mothers. This may explain some cases of sensitization in primigravid women.
8. Polesky HF, Sebring ES. Evaluation of methods for detection and quantitation of fetal cells and their effects on Rh IgG usage. *Am J Clin Pathol* 1981;76:525.
   An accurate index of the amount of fetomaternal hemorrhage is necessary to know how much Rh immunoglobulin to administer. If the amount of hemorrhage is not quantitated, a single injection may be inadequate and may result in treatment failures.
9. Hyland CA, Wolter LC, Saul A. Identification and analysis of RH genes: application of PCR and RFLP typing tests. *Transfus Med Rev* 1995;9:289.
   This article reviews the advances in polymerase chain reaction technique in isolating Rh antigens.
10. Reece EA, et al. Diagnostic fetal umbilical blood sampling in the management of isoimmunization. *Am J Obstet Gynecol* 1988;159:1057.
    The authors managed Rh isoimmunization in five patients by fetal umbilical blood sampling using PUBS. Their diagnostic accuracy was increased, and their complication rate did not rise with continued experience.
11. Van den Veyver IB, Moise KJ Jr. Fetal RhD typing by polymerase chain reaction in pregnancies complicated by rhesus alloimmunization. *Am J Obstet Gynecol* 1996; 88:1061.
    The authors review the specificity and sensitivity of a diagnostic technique for the determination of fetal RhD status.

Management

12. Parer JT. Severe Rh isoimmunization—current methods of *in utero* diagnosis and treatment. *Am J Obstet Gynecol* 1988;158:1323.

*Severely isoimmunized patients now have greater than a 90% chance of success-
ful pregnancy outcome when managed with high-resolution ultrasonography, cordocentesis, intravascular fetal transfusion, and meticulous fetal surveillance.*

13. Berkowitz RL, et al. Intravascular monitoring and management of erythroblastosis
    fetalis. *Am J Obstet Gynecol* 1988;158:783.
    *Percutaneous transfusions or exchange transfusions with ultrasonic guidance
    were successful in 87% of patients.*
14. Moise KJ Jr, et al. The predictive value of maternal serum testing for detection
    of fetal anemia in red blood cell alloimmunization. *Am J Obstet Gynecol* 1995;
    172:1003.
    *Three maternal serum tests are assessed for their usefulness in predicting fetal
    anemia.*
15. Voto LS, et al. High-dose gammaglobulin (IVIG) followed by intrauterine trans-
    fusions (IUTs): a new alternative for the treatment of severe fetal hemolytic disease.
    J Perinatol Med 1997;25:85.
    *The use of high-dose gammaglobulin and intrauterine transfusions for the treat-
    ment of severe fetal anemia is described.*
16. Ronkin S, et al. Intravascular exchange and bolus transfusion in the severely
    isoimmunized fetus. *Am J Obstet Gynecol* 1989;160:407.
    *Rh-sensitized fetuses were treated with 31 intravascular transfusions (PUBS).
    Bleeding from the puncture site was found in one third, but this was without
    apparent maternal or fetal consequence.*
17. Gollin YG, Copel JA. Management of the Rh-sensitized mother. *Clin Perinatol*
    1995;22:545.
    This article is an excellent review of the management of Rh isoimmunization.
18. Spinnato JA, et al. Hemolytic disease of the fetus: a comparison of the Queenan
    and extended Liley methods. *Obstet Gynecol* 1998;92:441.
    *This article compares the clinical utility of the Liley and Queenan methods to
    monitor hemolytic disease.*

Complications
19. Frigoletto FD Jr, et al. Intrauterine fetal transfusion in 365 fetuses during fifteen
    years. *Am J Obstet Gynecol* 1981;139:781.
    *Reviewing 365 consecutive cases of fetuses who received intrauterine fetal transfusion
    from 22 to 32 weeks, 45% survived. Direct ultrasonographic guidance offers increased
    success in this procedure.*
20. Grannun PAT, Copel J. A prevention of Rh isoimmunization and treatment of the
    compromised fetus. *Semin Perinatol* 1988;12:324.
    *This article is replete in detailing the use of Rh immunoglobulin and has a nice
    table on the various doses of the drug to use for each condition. It likewise has
    a well-organized treatment approach to the severely affected fetus.*

Prophylaxis
21. Wegmann A, Gluck R. The history of rhesus prophylaxis with anti-D. *Eur J
    Pediatr* 1996;155:835.
    A historical overview of the development of Rh immunoglobulin is detailed.
22. Prevention of D isoimmunization. ACOG Technical Bulletin No. 147, October 1990.
    *Current recommendations of the American College of Obstetricians and Gyne-
    cologists concerning the administration of Rh immunoglobulin are detailed.*
23. Bowman JM. Antenatal suppression of Rh alloimmunization. *Clin Obstet Gynecol*
    1991;34:296.
    *Routine use of antenatal Rh immunoglobulin at 28 to 30 weeks' gestation and
    again 12 weeks later if the patient is undelivered resulted in the incidence of
    Rh(D) isoimmunization declining from 1.8% to 0.1%. This method of adminis-
    tration is cost-effective and apparently safe for mother and fetus.*
24. Urbaniak SJ. Consensus conference on anti-D prophylaxis, April 7 & 8 1997: final
    consensus statement. *Transfusion* 1998;38:97.
    *A recent consensus statement based on published research and expert opinions
    regarding anti-D prophylaxis is presented.*
25. Robson SC, Lee D, Urbaniak SJ. Anti-D immunoglobulin in RhD prophylaxis. *Br
    J Obstet Gynaecol* 1998;105:129.
    This commentary outlines the use of Rh immunoglobulin during pregnancy.

20. POSTTERM PREGNANCY

James Nello Martin Jr.

A postterm pregnancy is one that truly extends beyond 42 weeks of confirmed gestational age. Proper clinical and ultrasonographic dating are required for accurate diagnosis. This is important because the 5% to 8% of pregnancies that actually exceed this limit are at increased maternal and perinatal risk. The primary maternal risks include an increased incidence of cesarean delivery, vaginal trauma from the delivery of large babies, hemorrhage from uterine atony, postpartum infections, wound complications, and prolonged hospitalization. Compared with 40 weeks' gestation, perinatal mortality is doubled by 42 weeks and quadrupled by 44 weeks. Primary contributors to this are complications of placental insufficiency, oligohydramnios, birth trauma from macrosomia, and meconium aspiration syndrome. Approximately 10% of fetuses in postterm pregnancies develop dysmaturity, a condition of growth retardation engendered by uteroplacental insufficiency that if undetected could progress to asphyxial damage and possible stillbirth.

Accurate, proper dating of all prenatal patients is imperative so that the postterm pregnancy can be diagnosed correctly. The best clinical predictor of gestational age is patient recall of the exact date her last menses began. Nagele's rule is invoked using this information to estimate the date of delivery at 40 weeks, adding 7 days to the date of menses onset and subtracting 3 months. Other useful clinical parameters include first-trimester pelvic examination, date of first positive pregnancy test, first fetal heart tones by Doppler (10–12 weeks), date of uterine fundus reaching the umbilicus (20 weeks), and quickening (16–20 weeks). In the absence of reliable clinical data or to confirm this information, ultrasonography can be used to estimate gestational age, with a maximum error of 1 week when performed in the first trimester, 2 weeks in the second trimester, and 3 to 4 weeks in the third trimester. Because a screening ultrasonogram at 16 to 20 weeks facilitates better review of fetal anatomy than first-trimester sonography, it is the most cost-effective period for ultrasonographic dating.

Weekly cervical examination from 38 weeks onward to strip or sweep membranes away from the internal os appears to be a safe method to shorten the length of term gestation and reduce the incidence of postterm pregnancy. Knowledge of placental position away from the lower uterine segment and a fetal vertex position well applied to the pelvis are prerequisites.

When the well-dated pregnancy reaches 41 weeks, the cervical status should be checked and induction considered if the Bishop score exceeds 7. This is undertaken to reduce the possibility of macrosomia and cephalopelvic disproportion due to continued fetal growth and to eliminate the remote (0.5–1.0:1,000) possibility of unexplained stillbirth if the pregnancy progressed further. If cervical ripeness or favorability for induction is not present, the clinician has two major management options: expectancy (await spontaneous labor while fetal status is monitored for reassurance) or delivery (proceed with some form of cervical ripening followed by induction of labor). Either approach to management is acceptable.

In view of increasing perinatal mortality beyond 40 weeks' gestation, when the management option of expectancy is chosen, it is recommended that some form of antenatal surveillance of fetal well-being (or a combination) should be initiated during the 41st week of pregnancy to supplement ongoing patient assessment of fetal movement and physician assessment of cervical status. Fetal heart rate testing (nonstress test or contraction stress test), ultrasonographic evaluation of amniotic fluid volume, biophysical profile, or a combination of these tests is used on a weekly or twice-weekly basis depending on the clinical situation. Oligohydramnios (an amniotic fluid index of 5 cm or less) is an important development in the postterm pregnancy that can become manifest as quickly as 3 to 4 days after a normal ultrasonographic study. Delivery is usually indicated if the results of fetal testing are not reassuring or once oligohydramnios develops. Even if the results of fetal testing are reassuring and oligohydramnios has not yet developed, when 42 confirmed weeks are reached, induction of labor can be undertaken. Delivery by the 43rd week at the latest is recommended.

If induction of labor at 41 weeks is undertaken instead of expectancy, cervical ripening using prostaglandin gel or a mechanical dilator such as laminaria or a Foley balloon can be helpful. Prostaglandin ripening, however, should be used with caution in this late pregnancy patient group with equivocal antepartum testing because uterine hyperstimulation can be seen occasionally. Failure of the cervix to ripen in postdate pregnancy is a high-risk factor for cesarean delivery. Routine induction of labor at 41 weeks has been found to reduce perinatal mortality, cesarean delivery, and meconium staining compared with expectant management.

Because the major complications of the intrapartum period for postterm pregnancies are fetal intolerance to labor, meconium passage, and macrosomia, management includes (1) careful fetal surveillance, (2) amnioinfusion to dilute meconium and suctioning of meconium-stained fluid at birth to prevent its aspiration, and (3) identification of macrosomia with prevention of trauma to the very large fetus. Fetal intolerance to labor with intrapartum asphyxia is more common in the postterm pregnancy due probably to a combination of placental deterioration, long labor, and oligohydramnios with cord compression. If persistent late decelerations are associated with decreased variability or an elevated baseline fetal heart rate, delivery is indicated. Likewise, variable decelerations that are worsening with slow return to baseline, blunting in shape, and overshooting the baseline after recovery may reflect developing fetal hypoxia. Due to a longer time in utero and a diminishing amniotic fluid volume, meconium is four times more common in the postterm pregnancy than in term gestations. Although the use of amnioinfusion with normal saline and thorough DeLee suctioning of the nasopharynx and oropharynx before delivery of the shoulders reduce the number of postterm infants with meconium below the cords, these measures do not prevent pulmonary injury in the rare fetus asphyxiated in utero prior to the onset of labor. If clinical and ultrasonographic estimates of fetal weight suggest a macrosomic infant of more than 4,000 g, mid-pelvic operative vaginal delivery should be avoided and preparations to properly manage shoulder dystocia should be made. Cesarean delivery without induction of labor should be considered for the postterm fetus estimated to weigh more than 4,500 g, the mother with a marginal pelvis, or the mother who suffered a prior difficult vaginal delivery with the same- or smaller-sized infant.

General
1. ACOG Criteria Set No. 10. Postterm pregnancy. August 1995.
   This is a one page outline of important aspects of management of the postterm pregnancy.
2. Campbell MK, Ostbye T, Irgens LM. Post-term birth: risk factors and outcomes in a 10 year cohort of Norwegian births. *Obstet Gynecol* 1997;89:543.
   Increased perinatal mortality was associated with small-for-gestational-age infants and maternal age over 35 years. Large-for-date infants were associated with obstetric trauma and dysfunctional labor.
3. Gardosi J, Vanner T, Francis A. Gestational age and induction of labour for prolonged pregnancy. *Br J Obstet Gynaecol* 1997;104:792.
   The number of inductions was increased when there was uncertainty in gestational dating. Dating all pregnancies using mid-trimester sonography can reduce the number of pregnancies referred to as postterm.
4. Ingermarsson I, Kallen K. Stillbirths and rate of neonatal deaths in 76,761 postterm pregnancies in Sweden. *Acta Obstet Gynecol Scand* 1997;76:658.
   Although the neonatal death rate with postterm pregnancy was increased for multiparas and primiparas, intrauterine fetal demise was increased only in primiparas.
5. Weinstein D, Ezra Y, Picard R, et al. Expectant management of post-term patients: observations and outcome. *J Matern Fetal Med* 1996;5:293.
   Expectant management of postterm pregnancies resulted in an outcome similar to that of control group between 37 and 41 weeks' gestation.

6. Divon MY, Marks AD, Henderson CE. Longitudinal measurement of amniotic fluid index in postterm pregnancies and its association with fetal outcome. *Am J Obstet Gynecol* 1995;172(Pt 1):142.

   A reduction in the amniotic fluid index (AFI) in postterm pregnancies was not associated with adverse outcome so long as the AFI was greater than 5 cm.

7. Tongsong T, Srisomboon J. Amniotic fluid volume as a predictor of fetal distress in postterm pregnancy. *Int J Gynaecol Obstet* 1993;40:213.

   Amniotic fluid volume along with nonstress test (NST) better predicted fetal distress in labor than the NST alone.

8. Henriksen TB, Wilcox AJ, Hedegaard M, Secher NJ. Bias in studies of preterm and postterm delivery due to ultrasound assessment of gestational age. *Epidemiology* 1995;6:533.

   Factors that reduce fetal size such as female sex and maternal smoking may introduce bias into the ultrasonographic prediction of gestational age.

9. Arabin B, et al. Prediction of fetal distress and poor outcome in prolonged pregnancy using Doppler ultrasound and fetal heart rate monitoring combined with stress tests (II). *Fetal Diagn Ther* 1994;9:1.

   The ratio of resistance indices of the fetal carotid / umbilical artery along with NST were predictive of fetal distress in labor.

10. Weiner Z, Reichler A, Zlozover M, et al. The value of Doppler ultrasonography in prolonged pregnancies. *Eur J Obstet Gynecol Reprod Biol* 1993;48:93.

    Doppler velocimetry alone was not useful for follow-up of postterm gestations, but was a useful adjunct to other antepartum tests.

11. Druzin ML, et al. Prospective evaluation of the contraction stress and nonstress tests in the management of post-term pregnancy. *Surg Gynecol Obstet* 1992; 174:507.

    More than 800 patients with prolonged pregnancy were evaluated with nonstress test and contraction stress test (CST). There were no differences in outcome in the group with abnormal CST when compared to those with an NST that was reactive.

12. Mannino F. Neonatal complications of postterm gestation. *J Reprod Med* 1988; 33:271.

    Postterm infants that do not suffer asphyxia have normal growth and intellectual development.

13. Freeman RK, et al. Postdate pregnancy: utilization of contraction stress testing for primary fetal surveillance. *Am J Obstet Gynecol* 1981;140:128.

    A total of 679 patients were evaluated with contraction stress test for postterm pregnancies without a single perinatal death.

14. Niswander KR. EFM and brain damage in term and postterm infants. *Contemp Obstet Gynecol* 1991;36:39.

    Abnormal electronic fetal monitoring tracing is a poor prediction of cerebral palsy in the newborn. Several fetal heart rate patterns may be suggestive of an infant with existing fetal brain damage.

Management

15. Berghella V, Rogers RA, Lescale K. Stripping of membranes as a safe method to reduce prolonged pregnancies. *Obstet Gynecol* 1996;87:927.

    Weekly membrane stripping beginning at 38 weeks was safe and reduced the incidence of prolonged pregnancies.

16. Kaplan B, et al. The outcome of postterm pregnancy. A comparative study. *J Perinatol Med* 1995;23:183.

    The authors advocate active management of prolonged pregnancy over expectant management using ultrasonography, electronic fetal monitoring, and cervical ripening.

17. Shaw KJ, Medearis AL, Horenstein J, et al. Selective labor induction in postterm patients. Observations and outcomes. *J Reprod Med* 1992;37:157.

    Women with postdate pregnancies and a Bishop score greater than 6 underwent either induction of labor or expectant management. The cesarean rate was lower in the induction group.

18. Hannah ME, Huh C, Hewson SA, Hannah WJ. Postterm pregnancy: putting the merits of a policy of induction of labor into perspective. *Birth* 1996;23:13.
    Data from the Canadian Multicenter Postterm Pregnancy Trial favor the early induction of labor on pregnancies of at least 41 weeks' gestation.
19. The NICHD Network of Maternal-Fetal Medicine Units. *Am J Obstet Gynecol* 1994;170:716.
    In uncomplicated pregnancies of greater than 41 weeks gestation, either expectant management or induction of labor appears acceptable.
20. McColgin SW, et al. Stripping membranes at term: can it safely reduce the incidence of postterm pregnancies? *Obstet Gynecol* 1990;76:678.
    Women who had received treatment with membrane stripping beginning at 38 weeks had earlier deliveries and fewer postterm deliveries than did those in a control group. The effect was most notable in nulliparous women.
21. Rayburn W, Husslein P. Use of prostaglandins for induction of labor. *Semin Perinatol* 1991;15:173.
    The authors provide an overview of prostaglandin use for cervical ripening.
22. Rayburn WF. Prostaglandin E$_2$ gel for cervical ripening and induction of labor: a critical analysis. *Am J Obstet Gynecol* 1989;160:529.
    This report summarizes 3,313 pregnancies in 59 clinical trials evaluating prostaglandin E$_2$ gel for cervical ripening.

21. ANEMIAS AND HEMOGLOBINOPATHIES IN PREGNANCY

Dom A. Terrone

Anemia is one of the most common disorders of young women, especially during pregnancy. In the second trimester, a relative anemia develops in most pregnancies secondary to a proportionately larger increase in the plasma volume relative to the red blood cell (RBC) mass. Pathologic anemias occur because of decreased erythrocyte production, increased RBC destruction, or blood loss. Second only to blood loss, the most common cause of anemia is decreased erythrocyte production. These are collectively referred to as hypoproliferative anemias. They usually stem from deficiency of essential subcellular substrates, such as iron, folic acid, or vitamin B$_{12}$. Although the vast majority of anemias are acquired, anemia may be congenital, as in the hemoglobinopathies. These are genetically defined disorders in which there is a malfunction at the molecular level, and they affect either the production rate (thalassemia) or the structural integrity of the hemoglobin (Hb) molecule (sickle cell Hb). Homozygous sickle cell anemia (Hb SS), Hb SC disease, and Hb S-thalassemia constitute a potentially devastating disorder known as sickle cell disease (SCD). The incidence of SCD is from one in 400 to one in 600 patients.

Although there is a 50% increase in maternal plasma volume, there is an increase in RBC mass of only 25%, yielding a relatively dilutional anemia. These changes commonly resolve by 6 weeks after delivery. The exact laboratory value at which a pregnant patient is considered anemic varies among researchers, but generally an Hb of less than 11.0 gm/dl or a hematocrit (HCT) of less than 32% are considered abnormal. Whether anemia causes poor perinatal outcomes is controversial. However, there is evidence that anemic parturients are more likely to deliver prematurely and give birth to infants that are small for gestational age. Additionally, these patients have longer recuperation periods and are more likely to experience postpartum complications.

The laboratory evaluation for the anemic patient is guided by the results of the complete blood count (CBC). The mean corpuscular volume (MCV), which is a portion of the CBC, can indicate whether a patient has a normocytic (MCV 80–100 fl), a macrocytic (MCV >100 fl), or a microcytic (MCV <80 fl) anemia. A peripheral blood smear can further support this diagnosis. Microcytic anemias are by far the most common, and the evaluation focuses primarily on iron deficiency and hemoglobinopathies. A hemoglobin electrophoresis and iron studies will help differentiate the diagnosis. A macrocytic anemia is commonly the result of folate deficiency, with or without a deficiency of vitamin B_{12}. A normocytic anemia is frequently associated with a mixed picture of iron and folate or B_{12} deficiency.

Iron deficiency anemia (IDA) can be implicated in up to 75% of all anemias that occur during pregnancy. The total iron requirement during a normal gestation is approximately 1,000 mg, exceeding the amount available from even the best diets. Based on this information, some researchers recommend iron supplementation for all pregnant patients. The diagnosis of IDA is dependent on a number of laboratory studies. A peripheral blood smear shows hypochromic microcytic red cells. The first changes that occur in IDA are a depletion of the body's iron stores. This is reflected by a decrease in serum iron (<60 mg/dl) and a decrease in the saturation of transferrin (<16%). Total iron binding capacity (TIBC) increases as a reflection of an increase in unbound transferrin. The TIBC, however, has a high false-positive rate in pregnancy and is therefore an unreliable marker. The serum ferritin levels can vary significantly from day to day, but they do provide the best predictor of the severity of IDA. The treatment for IDA entails administration of 60 mg of elemental iron (325 mg of ferrous sulfate) three times daily. The absorption of iron is improved in an acidic environment, for example, when taken with orange juice, and is impaired if taken with antacids.

Folic acid deficiency is responsible for 20% to 22% of the cases of anemia during pregnancy. Therefore, folic acid deficiency and IDA together account for approximately 97% of all anemias that occur in reproductive age women. Laboratory findings suggesting folate deficiency include hypersegmented neutrophils and macrocytic, hyperchromic red cells on peripheral blood smears. Additionally, a low serum folate level is encountered in these patients. Studies have demonstrated that folic acid supplementation prior to conception can reduce the incidence of neural tube defects (NTDs). Because the neural tube closes by the 28th day after conception, supplementation prior to conception is imperative. Current recommendations include 0.4 mg daily for all women (as can be obtained in most standard multivitamins), and 4 mg daily for those women who have had a previously affected pregnancy. These interventions when begun 2 months prior to pregnancy and continued through the first trimester can reduce the incidence of first NTDs by 50% and recurrent NTDs by more than 70%. Supplementation of staple foods can provide nearly 0.2 mg daily; however, this is less than the recommended daily dose. Prenatal vitamins provide 1 mg per day of folic acid, an adequate amount for most singleton gestations.

Anemias associated with the defective production of erythrocytes are numerous, but they are rarely seen clinically. Various toxins may give rise to an aplastic anemia, whereas antiinflammatory drugs or acute infections may be toxic to the bone marrow. A mortality rate as high as 75% has been reported in patients with aplastic anemia, but pregnancy itself does not impact on the outcome. Chronic medical conditions such as autoimmune disorders and cancer can be an etiologic factor in anemia.

Hemolytic diseases of pregnancy include those in which RBCs are destroyed prematurely. With spherocytosis and porphyria, family history and past medical history may prove quite informative. Diseases particular to pregnancy, such as a form of preeclampsia known as HELLP (hemolysis, elevated liver enzymes, and low platelets) syndrome, as well spherocytosis and porphyria, exhibit blood smears that demonstrate bizarrely shaped RBCs.

Heterozygotes for hemoglobinopathies such as thalassemia or patients with sickle cell trait may have a mild anemia, but the majority of pregnancies proceed routinely. Patients with sickle cell trait are at increased risk for complications stemming from urinary tract infections and therefore should have a urine culture performed each trimester. In contrast, patients with SCD face a significant risk for maternal and perinatal morbidity and mortality. There is an increased incidence of vasooclusive crisis caused by hydrophobic bonding of the sickle Hb in patients with SCD. This condition is aggravated by infections, pregnancy, hypoxia, and acidosis.

Advances in diagnosis and therapy, and improvements in patient care have improved maternal and fetal outcomes in patients with SCD. There has been a dramatic decrease in the number of premature and low-birth-weight infants born to mothers with SCD when intensive medical therapy is provided. Some researchers favor the use of prophylactic partial exchange transfusions on a regular basis to prevent complications, whereas others prefer to use blood component therapy only when symptoms are severe. If transfusions are used in either setting, the patient must be counseled about their potential risks, including hepatitis, transfusion reaction, formation of red cell antibodies, and potential exposure to the human immunodeficiency virus. Both management strategies can provide good maternal and fetal outcomes, but exchange transfusion reduces the frequency of vasoocclusive crisis. Buffy-coat poor washed RBCs are administered on an ambulatory basis by erythrocytophoresis. A reduction in the Hb S concentration to less than 50% and a concomitant increase in Hb A concentration to at least 40% is the goal. In most cases this will yield an HCT level of greater than 30%.

The method of follow-up of these patients is fairly standardized. Evaluation of hemoglobin electrophoresis every 2 weeks is used to assess changes in the Hb S and Hb A concentrations. Most authors agree that repeated transfusion is indicated if the Hb A concentration falls below 20%. Antisickling agents such as urea, thiocyanate, and adipimidates have not been extensively studied in pregnancy and therefore cannot be recommended. Folic acid supplementation at a dose of 1 mg daily is recommended in patients with SCD, and iron therapy is appropriate in the nearly two thirds of sickle cell patients with concomitant IDA.

It is important to keep in mind the special need of the patient with SCD during labor. Although regional anesthesia appears to be an excellent option for these patients, care must be taken to prevent the hypotension and resultant tissue hypoxia that can accompany their administration because it can lead to sickling. Continuous electronic fetal monitoring along with supplemental oxygen (4 L/min) are appropriate in these patients. Cesarean section is reserved for obstetric indications, and labor augmentation is without additional risk in this population. Postpartum care should include intensive surveillance for infections. The hospital stay is not necessarily prolonged unless there is evidence of infections.

Genetic counseling and patient education are of paramount importance in patients with SCD. Therapeutic abortion for maternal reasons is usually not necessary unless severe maternal disease is present. The father of the baby should undergo a hemoglobin electrophoresis to provide information as to the risk of the fetus being affected. It is possible to offer prenatal diagnosis for hemoglobinopathies through chorionic villus sampling, amniocentesis, or periumbilical blood sampling. Coordination of care with a hematologist can optimize patient care during and after pregnancy.

General
1. Morrison JC, Gookin KS. Anemia associated with pregnancy. In: Sciarra JJ, ed. *Gynecology and obstetrics.* Vol. 3. Philadelphia: JB Lippincott, 1988.
   This is an in-depth review of the various causes of anemia and how they relate to pregnancy. A nice section is also included on laboratory determinations.
2. Samson D. The anemia of chronic disorders. *Postgrad Med* 1983;59:543.
   Chronic disease such as infection, inflammatory disease, or malignancy is the most common known cause of normochromic, normocytic anemia. This article classifies the methods of diagnosis as well as the clinical manifestations and contains more than 50 references.
3. Sergeant GR. Sickle haemoglobin and pregnancy. *Br Med J* 1983;287:628.
   This timely overall review of the subject by a noted authority with 25 years of experience is concise, to the point, and good basic reading for the person interested in sickle cell hemoglobinopathies.
4. Savitt TL, Goldberg MF. Herrick's 1910 case report of sickle cell anemia. The rest of the story. *JAMA* 1989;261:266.
   This special communications article is a lucid report on the first publication involving sickle cell anemia. Eighty-two references of very early medical works make it must reading for those interested in this subject.

5. Institute of Medicine (U.S.). Subcommittee on Nutritional Status and Weight Gain During Pregnancy. *Nutrition during pregnancy*. Washington, DC: National Academy Press, 1990.
   This in-depth text provides practical guidelines on nutrition in pregnancy.
6. Mani S, Duffy TP. Anemia of pregnancy. *Clin Perinatol* 1995;22:593.
   This is a comprehensive review of all causes of anemia with emphasis on diagnosis and contains an excellent diagnostic algorithm.

Etiology
7. Pryor JA, Morrison JC. Nutritional anemia. In: Bern M, Frigoletto F, eds. *Hematologic contribution to fetal health*. New York: Liss, 1989.
   This is a review of the etiology, diagnosis, complications, and treatment of nutritional anemia, with 37 references.
8. Steinberg MH, Hebbel RP. Clinical diversity of sickle cell anemia: genetic and cellular modulation of disease severity. *Am J Hematol* 1983;14:405.
   Various cellular and genetic factors may play a role in modulating clinical effects of the sickle Hb gene, which may explain the clinical spectrum ranges from incapacitating problems to an absence of clinical symptomatology.

Diagnosis
9. Roberts WE, Morrison JC, Blake PG. Evaluation of anemia in pregnancy. In: Kitay DZ, ed. *Hematologic problems in pregnancy*. New York: Grune & Stratton, 1985.
   This chapter describes the essentials in the diagnosis of anemia during pregnancy in the setting of all acquired disorders. Thirty-three references are included.
10. McClure S, Custer E, Bessman JD. Improved detection of early iron deficiency in nonanemic subjects. *JAMA* 1985;253:1021.
    The RBC distribution width was 100% sensitive in correlating with decreased serum iron saturation in nonanemic subjects.
11. Butler E. The common anemias. *JAMA* 1988;259:2433.
    This concise review of the common anemias includes an especially applicable discussion of the diagnosis of iron-deficiency anemia and many recent references.
12. Alter BP. Prenatal diagnosis of hemoglobinopathies: development of methods for study of fetal red cells and fibroblasts. *Am J Pediatr Hematol Oncol* 1983;5:378.
    Prenatal testing for hemoglobinopathies has been performed since 1974, with 2,000 cases studied by fetal globin synthesis and approximately 100 by restriction enzyme techniques.
13. Hogge WA. Prenatal diagnosis of sickle cell anemia. *Contemp Obstet Gynecol* 1989;33:21.
    This is a short but well-defined article with good diagrams illustrating how the prenatal diagnosis of sickle cell anemia is undertaken.
14. Osborne PT, et al. An evaluation of red blood cell heterogeneity (increased red blood cell distribution width) in iron deficiency of pregnancy. *Am J Obstet Gynecol* 1989;160:336.
    Early iron deficiency without anemia is infrequently identified by classic means. A new classification, making use of the mean corpuscular volume, was evaluated in 331 patients in this study and did not improve the diagnostic accuracy among those without frank anemia.

Treatment
15. Morrison JC, Martin JN Jr, McKay ML. DIC, ITP and hemoglobinopathies. In: Knuppel RA, ed. *High risk obstetrics: a team approach*. Philadelphia: WB Saunders, 1986.
    Causes of anemia that are related to various pathologic disorders in obstetrics are detailed and their treatment is elucidated.
16. Food and Nutrition Board, National Research Council. *Recommended dietary allowances*. Washington, DC: National Academy of Sciences, 1980.
    This is a detailed listing of nutritional requirements.
17. IV iron dextrose therapy. Drug information bulletin. Vol. 18, No. 3, March-April 1984.

This is a review of the indications, techniques, and complications of parenteral iron therapy.

18. Morrison JC, et al. Prophylactic transfusions in pregnant patients with sickle hemoglobinopathies: benefit versus risk. *Obstet Gynecol* 1980;56:274.
    Analyses of 75 patients with severe sickle cell hemoglobinopathies who received prophylactic exchange transfusions are outlined.

19. Perry KG Jr, Morrison JC. The diagnosis and management of hemoglobinopathies during pregnancy. *Semin Perinatol* 1990;14:90.
    The authors present a review of the physiology, diagnosis, and appropriate therapeutic interventions in pregnant patients with a hemoglobinopathy.

20. Embury SH. Effects of oxygen inhalation on endogenous erythropoietin kinetics, erythropoiesis, and properties of blood cells in sickle-cell anemia. *N Engl J Med* 1984;311:291.
    The effect of continuous oxygen during crises with SCD was tested. The number of irreversibly sickled cells increased after the cessation of oxygen therapy (rebound effect). Oxygen should be administered intermittently rather than continuously.

21. James J, Oakhill A, Evans J. Preventing iron deficiency in at-risk communities. *Lancet* 1989;1:40.
    The authors offer tips on how to appropriately counsel patients about dietary indiscretions that may lead to iron deficiency anemia. They were able to reduce the frequency of iron deficiency anemia in patients who participated in nutritional counseling.

22. Huch A, et al. Recombinant human erythropoietin in the treatment of postpartum anemia. *Obstet Gynecol* 1992;80:127.
    A comparative study of women with postpartum anemia. This article contains a succinct review and discussion of erythropoietin and its effectiveness in the postpartum anemic patient.

23. Whitehead R, Bates C. Recommendations of folate intake. *Lancet* 1997;350:1642.
    Current recommendations for folate and biochemical processes it plays a role in.

24. Daly S, et al. Minimum effective dose of folic acid for food fortification to prevent neural-tube defects. *Lancet* 1997;350:1666.
    The role of food supplementation and its importance in prevention of neural tube defects are discussed.

25. Simon TL, et al. Practice parameter for the use of red blood cell transfusions. *Arch Pathol Lab Med* 1998;122:130.
    The College of American Pathologist's transfusion guidelines include a section concerning hemoglobinopathies and transfusion in pregnancy, as well as a large reference section.

26. Koshy M, et al. Prophylactic red-cell transfusions in pregnant patients with sickle cell disease. A randomized cooperative study. *N Engl J Med* 1988;319:1447.
    Pain crises were reduced, but the authors felt that omitting exchange transfusions did not harm patients.

Complications

27. Agarwal RMD, Tripathi AM, Agarwal KN. Neonatal hematological values in maternal anemia. *Indian J Pediatr* 1983;20:369.
    Details and neonatal hematologic profiles in the offspring of anemic and nonanemic parturients are presented. The parameters were significantly higher in the newborns of anemic mothers through the first 7 days on the basis of mild chronic hypoxia even though the maternal anemia was mild.

28. Reid CD. The national sickle cell disease program. *Am J Hematol* 1983;14:265.
    Data on specific symptomatology in those with SCD are offered. Particularly interesting are the data on infection as they relate to patients with SCD.

29. Pastorek JG, Seiler B II. Maternal death associated with sickle cell trait. *Am J Obstet Gynecol* 1985;151:295.
    A patient with sickle cell trait can be at risk for severe morbidity and death if faced with a condition that aggravates intravascular sickling.

30. MRC Vitamin Study Research Group. Prevention of neural tube defects: results of the medical research council vitamin study. *Lancet* 1991;338:131.

The results and discussion of a randomized double-blind prevention trial of folic acid in high-risk patients for NTD.
31. Committee on Obstetrics: Maternal and Fetal Medicine. Folic acid for the prevention of recurrent neural tube defects. ACOG Committee Opinion No. 120, 1993. *Recommendations concerning the use of folic acid in patients at high risk for NTD.*

22. PRETERM LABOR

Everett F. Magann

Preterm delivery occurs in 8% to 10% of all births, and that rate has remained unchanged over the past 40 years. Some recent reports have even suggested that the rate has increased slightly. Preterm delivery, even though it affects fewer than 10% of all births, is responsible for more than 50% of all cases of perinatal morbidity and mortality. The risk factors associated with preterm delivery include African-American race, low socioeconomic status, maternal age under 20 for any pregnancy and over 35 for the first pregnancy, maternal weight of under 50 kg at the onset of pregnancy, poor maternal weight gain during pregnancy, previous preterm birth (reoccurrence risk is 17%–47%), previous second-trimester abortion, uterine anomalies, strenuous physical work, smoking, pyelonephritis, multiple gestation (up to 50% deliver prior to 37 weeks), fetal congenital anomalies, hydramnios, unexplained elevation of maternal serum alpha fetoprotein, maternal infection, illicit drug use, and preterm premature rupture of membranes. Several investigators have developed scoring systems to detect preterm birth. Once women with risk factors were identified, they were placed in special clinics with enhanced education, frequent clinic visits, and periodic cervical examination. These programs have been particularly successful in France, showing a decline in preterm births in the years in which the programs were implemented. Typically, approximately 10% of pregnant women who are at risk are identified; however, only 30% of these women so identified will actually develop preterm labor.

The diagnosis of preterm labor is determined by the presence of regular uterine contractions accompanied by a change in effacement or dilatation of the cervix. If there has been no cervical change, then the patient does not have preterm labor and should not be treated with tocolytic therapy. Labor can also be diagnosed if there are greater than four contractions in 20 minutes, eight contractions in an hour, there is rupture of membranes, or the cervix on initial examination is at least 2 cm dilated and 80% effaced. The health-care provider must keep in mind that uterine activity increases as pregnancy progresses, with an average of four contractions per hour at 36 weeks, and that women only perceive 15% of their contractions. Patients dilated less than 2 cm on initial presentation also may be observed serially over time to determine if they are in labor by watching for cervical change prior to the initiation of tocolytics with no difference in outcome. If the initial examination of the cervix is more than 4 cm dilated and 80% effaced, tocolytics are of limited effectiveness. The two most reliable indicators for women presenting with preterm contractions to predict delivery within 7 days are rupture of membranes and cervical effacement that is ≥80%.

Two new tests currently used to assist in the diagnosis of preterm labor include fetal fibronectin and cervical length. Fetal fibronectin is an isoform of fibronectin that resides at the choriodecidual interface and is usually not found in cervicovaginal secretions at 20 to 37 weeks' gestation. In women with a positive fetal fibronectin test result after 20 weeks' gestation in secretions taken from the posterior vaginal fornix, 60% will deliver within 1 week. The greatest use of fetal fibronectin is not its presence but its absence. If the fetal fibronectin test result is negative, 99.3% of pregnancies will not deliver within 7 days. Knowledge of the presence or absence of fetal fibronectin allows the physician to hospitalize and aggressively treat patients with positive fetal fibronectin test results and discharge early those with negative results. If the cervical length is less than the 10th percentile (25 mm) or there is evidence of funneling or beaking of the amniotic fluid at the internal os, the patient is at risk for preterm delivery and must be managed aggressively.

Contraindications to tocolysis include acute fetal distress, severe hypertensive crises, fetal anomaly incompatible with life, fetal demise, severe maternal hemorrhage, fetal maturity, and known chorioamnionitis. Relative contraindications to tocolysis are rupture of membranes, cardiac disease, and diabetes mellitus. A number of treatments commonly used but which have not shown benefit in prospective assessments include bed rest and absence of coitus in the woman with intact membranes and without vaginal bleeding. Prophylactic tocolytics in women with a history of preterm delivery and in multiple gestations have not been shown to be helpful. Hydration has been used in preterm labor and is sometimes effective for the patient in false labor but not for patients in preterm labor. Sedation is also frequently used but is not helpful in the woman in preterm labor and can be harmful in preterm gestations. Documentation of gestational age is very important. An early examination, reliable last menstrual period, and ultrasonography prior to 20 weeks are all helpful in establishing gestational age. Amniocentesis is sometimes indicated to document fetal pulmonary maturity. Each hospital must establish its own threshold for treatment. Many hospitals have chosen 34 weeks as a time period when the risks of tocolysis exceed the benefits of treatment. The beta-agonist drugs and magnesium sulfate are the most commonly used medications for tocolysis. Ritodrine is the only drug approved by the U.S. Food and Drug Administration (FDA) for tocolysis. The initial dosage is 50 to 100 μg/min intravenously, increased by 50 μg/min every 10 minutes until contractions cease or until a maximum of 350 μg/min dosage is obtained. Ritodrine is noted for its cardiovascular effects, and maternal pulse and blood pressure should be monitored frequently. Fetal tachycardia also may occur. Intravenous ritodrine therapy is usually followed by oral ritodrine given 10 mg every 2 hours for the first 24 hours followed by 10 to 20 mg every 4 to 6 hours. The physician should be particularly cautious with the use of ritodrine in the presence of multifetal gestation or pyelonephritis because pulmonary edema can occur. Another beta-agonist, terbutaline, remains to be approved by the FDA for use in preterm labor. Many protocols use 2.5 μg/min as an intravenous drip and increase to a maximum of 20 μg/min or 0.25 mg subcutaneously every 20 minutes for three doses and then 0.25 mg subcutaneously every 3 hours, keeping the maternal pulse below 130 beats per minute. Oral terbutaline, 5 mg every 4 to 6 hours, may follow the use of intravenous terbutaline. Complications associated with the use of terbutaline include chest pain, cardiac arrhythmias, glucose intolerance, and, in women with borderline hyperthyroidism, thyroid storm. Although magnesium sulfate is not approved by the FDA for use as a tocolytic drug, it is also an effective tocolytic agent and seems to have fewer cardiovascular side effects than the beta-agonists. Magnesium sulfate has been available for the treatment of preeclampsia for many years, and obstetricians are therefore familiar with its use. The usual dosage of magnesium sulfate is a 4- to 6-gram loading dose followed by an infusion of 1 to 4 g/h. Because the kidneys excrete magnesium, normal renal function should be documented and urine output recorded regularly. Oral maintenance following magnesium sulfate therapy is usually provided with a beta-agonist drug or oral magnesium. Magnesium gluconate may be given as 2 g orally every 4 hours. Gastrointestinal side effects may occur with oral magnesium compound. Tocolytic drugs are most effective when given before marked cervical dilatation has occurred. Oral doses of both terbutaline and magnesium sulfate are frequently administered after labor has been stopped with intravenous or subcutaneous agents despite any prospective randomized trial demonstrating benefit when compared with a placebo. Magnesium must be used with caution in pregnancies complicated by renal disease or hypocalcemia and should not be used in pregnancies complicated by myasthenia gravis.

Newer agents are usually considered as second-line therapy for preterm labor. Indomethacin has had good results and is usually administered as a 50-mg rectal suppository followed by an oral dose of 25 mg every 4 to 6 hours. The prolonged use of indomethacin is discouraged because oligohydramnios can occur. The drug is used with caution beyond 27 weeks and is not recommended beyond 32 weeks' gestation because of concerns about premature closure of the fetal ductus arteriosus. Contraindications to the use of indomethacin use include a history of asthma, gastrointestinal bleeding, and coronary artery disease. Calcium channel-blocking drugs, such as nifedipine, also have been used as second-line therapy. Nifedipine may be administered as an oral dose of 10 to 20 mg initially followed by 10 to 20 mg every 6 hours. Nifedipine should be used with caution in women with a history of liver disease. When preterm delivery is anticipated, glucocorticoids should be administered for all fetuses in which delivery may be anticipated between 24 and 34 weeks to reduce the risk of respiratory distress syndrome, intraventricular hemorrhage, and necrotizing enterocolitis. Other widely used regimens include betamethasone in two doses of 12 mg given 24 hours apart or dexamethasone in four doses of 6 mg given every 12 hours.

Should efforts to delay delivery fail, intrapartum management becomes very important. Most clinicians would agree that electronic fetal heart rate monitoring of the fragile preterm fetus is desirable. Vaginal birth seems appropriate for the vertex preterm infant as long as there are no signs of fetal distress. Most clinicians would perform cesarean section for the preterm breech infant. Should a cesarean section be required, special attention should be focused on an adequate incision for delivery because the lower uterine segment is often thick and may cause trauma to the infant. Many clinicians suggest a low segment vertical incision prior to 32 weeks because of the poorly developed lower uterine segment. Neonatal physicians and the newborn intensive care unit should be available to assist in the care of preterm infants.

General
1. Kramer MS. Preventing preterm birth: are we making progress? *Prenat Neonat Med* 1998;3:10.
   A review of preterm labor over the past 20 years shows that rates of preterm birth have not only failed to decrease but have even increased slightly.
2. Preterm Labor. ACOG Technical Bulletin No. 206, June 1995.
   Infant survival as related to gestational age is discussed. Common tocolytic drug therapy is presented.
3. Beckmann CA, Beckmann CR, Stanziano GJ. Accuracy of maternal perception of preterm uterine activity. *Am J Obstet Gynecol* 1996;174:672.
   This is a brief review of the subject of prematurity. Ethical and financial issues are also discussed.
4. Gibbs RS, et al. A review of premature birth and subclinical infection. *Am J Obstet Gynecol* 1992;166:1515.
   The authors conclude that preterm birth results in part from infection caused by genital tract bacteria.
5. Amon E, Nshyken JM, Sibai BM. How small is too small and how early is too early? A survey of American obstetricians specializing in high-risk pregnancies. *Am J Perinatol* 1992;9:17.
   Four hundred five maternal-fetal medicine specialists were surveyed to determine their clinical opinions regarding intrapartum management of the severely preterm fetus.
6. Keirse MJ. New perspectives for the effective treatment of preterm labor. *Am J Obstet Gynecol* 1995;173:618.
   Preterm births account for the vast majority of neonatal morbidity and mortality. Specific treatments for infections and selective tocolytics offer the best hope for altering the rate of preterm delivery.
7. Gibbs RS, et al. A review of premature birth and subclinical infection. *Am J Obstet Gynecol* 1992;166:1515.
   This is a comprehensive analysis of the role of infection and preterm birth.

Risk Assessment
8. Creasy RK. Preterm birth prevention: Where are we? *Am J Obstet Gynecol* 1993;168:1223.
   This overview of preterm birth discusses the problems associated with diagnosis and management.

9. Creasy RK, Gummer BA, Liggins GC. System for predicting spontaneous preterm birth. *Obstet Gynecol* 1980;55:692.
   A risk scoring system is presented that selects approximately 10% of patients. Only one third of the patients identified actually developed preterm labor.
10. Morrison JC, et al. Oncofetal fibronectin in-patients with false labor as a predictor of preterm delivery. *Am J Obstet Gynecol* 1993;168:538.
    A positive fetal fibronectin result in women who have false labor indicated a significant risk for preterm labor and early delivery.
11. Lockwood CJ, et al. Fetal fibronectin in cervical and vaginal secretions as a predictor of preterm birth. *N Engl J Med* 1991;325:669.
    The presence of fetal fibronectin in the cervico-vaginal secretions of women between 20 and 37 weeks of pregnancy identifies these women as at risk for a preterm delivery.
12. Grimes DA, Schulz KF. Randomized controlled trials of home uterine activity monitoring: a review and critique. *Obstet Gynecol* 1992;79:137.
    The authors questioned the efficacy of home uterine monitoring.
13. Berghella V, et al. Cervical ultrasonography compared with manual examination as a predictor of preterm delivery. *Am J Obstet Gynecol* 1997;177:723.
    Cervical length measurement by ultrasonography is a better predictor of preterm delivery than is the length measured manually.

Treatment

14. Lewis DF, Bergstedt S, Edwards MS. Successful magnesium sulfate tocolysis: is weaning the drug necessary? *Am J Obstet Gynecol* 1997;177:742.
    The weaning of magnesium sulfate increases health care cost without benefit.
15. Gibbs RS, Eschenbach DA. Use of antibiotics to prevent preterm birth. *Am J Obstet Gynecol* 1997;177:375.
    Antibiotic therapy appears to now be indicated in selected patients to prolong pregnancy and prevent maternal-neonatal complications.
16. Macones GA, Berlin M, Berlin JA. Efficacy of oral beta-agonist maintenance therapy in preterm labor: a meta-analysis. *Obstet Gynecol* 1995;85:313.
    Current data do not support a role for oral beta-agonist therapy following the resolution of an acute episode of preterm labor.
17. Papatsonis DN, et al. Nifedipine and ritodrine in the management of preterm labor: a randomized multicenter trial. *Obstet Gynecol* 1997;90:230.
    Nifedipine is well tolerated and is associated with fewer side effects and longer postponement to delivery than ritodrine.
18. Lewis R, et al. Oral terbutaline after parenteral tocolysis: a randomized, double-blinded, placebo-controlled trial. *Am J Obstet Gynecol* 1996;175:834.
    Maintenance oral terbutaline therapy is not associated with pregnancy prolongation or a reduction in the incidence of recurrent preterm labor.
19. Macones GA, Robinson CA. Is there justification for using indomethacin in preterm labor? *Am J Obstet Gynecol* 1997;177:819.
    The benefits of indomethacin outweigh the risks at less than 32 weeks' gestation.

Neonatal Problems

20. Verma U, et al. Obstetric antecedents of intraventricular hemorrhage and periventricular leukomalacia in the low-birth-weight neonate. *Am J Obstet Gynecol* 1997;176:275.
    The incidence and severity of intraventricular hemorrhage and periventricular leukomalacia are increased in premature rupture of membranes and preterm labor. Accompanying chorioamnionitis increases the incidence and severity of these lesions.
21. Halsey CL, Collin MF, Anderson CL. Extremely low-birth-weight children and their peers. A comparison of school-age outcomes. *Arch Pediatr Adolesc Med* 1996;150:790.
    Extremely low-birth-weight infants are significantly disabled, with one out of every two requiring special educational services.
22. Allen MC, Donohue PK, Dusman AE. The limit of viability: neonatal outcome of infants born at 22 to 25 weeks gestation. *N Engl J Med* 1993;329:1597.

The authors discuss the perplexing medical-ethical problems associated with births on the borderline of neonatal viability.

23. Martin GI, Sindel BD. Neonatal management of the very low birth weight infant: the use of surfactant. Clin Perinatol 1992;19:461.
   The authors present a review of the administration of surfactant for the prevention of respiratory distress syndrome.

24. Robertson PA, et al. Neonatal morbidity according to gestational age and birth weight from five tertiary care centers in the United States, 1983 through 1986. Am J Obstet Gynecol 1992;166:1629.
   The incidence of respiratory distress syndrome and patent ductus arteriosus is decreased with increasing gestational age and birth weight. Severe intraventricular hemorrhage, necrotizing enterocolitis, and sepsis diminish markedly after 34 weeks.

25. Escobar GJ, Littenberg B, Petitti DB. Outcome among surviving very low birth weight infants: a meta-analysis. Arch Dis Child 1991;66:204.
   An analysis of more than 26,000 births worldwide of infants weighing less than 1500 grams was performed. Forty-one percent of the infants died and 25% of the survivors were noted to have a disability.

23. PREMATURE RUPTURED MEMBRANES

Brian K. Rinehart

Premature rupture of the fetal membranes (PROM) occurs prior to the onset of labor in up to 8% of pregnancies at term. PPROM is the rupture of fetal membranes prior to the onset of labor in a pregnancy that is less than 37 weeks' gestation. This occurs in approximately 33% of preterm births and is a major contributor to perinatal and neonatal morbidity and mortality. PROM and PPROM should be considered as separate entities because the etiology and associated morbidities differ widely.

When rupture of membranes occurs prior to term (37 weeks' gestation) the risk of maternal morbidity and fetal morbidity and mortality increases substantially. Risk factors that may help predict PPROM include lower socioeconomic status, vaginal bleeding, cervicitis, sexually transmitted infections, prior preterm delivery, prior cervical surgery for dysplasia, trauma, uterine anomalies, cigarette smoking, emergent cerclage, preterm labor, multifetal gestation, and hydramnios. However, cases of PPROM often occur in pregnancies without identifiable risk factors, and the presence of risk factors does not often allow for intervention or prevention except in the case of cervical or vaginal infections.

Once PPROM has occurred, most pregnancies will terminate in preterm delivery within 7 days. Associated fetal morbidity includes the recognized sequelae of prematurity consisting of increased risk of respiratory distress syndrome, retinopathy of prematurity, necrotizing enterocolitis, and intraventricular hemorrhage. In addition, these infants are at an increased risk for neonatal sepsis due to their higher rate of intraamniotic infection (up to 50%). Abruption will occur in up to 7% of these patients. The incidence of fetal malpresentation increases with decreasing gestational age. The incidence of umbilical cord prolapse is increased in both PPROM and fetal malpresentation.

After PPROM, timely evaluation of the patient is of utmost importance. This evaluation includes a thorough history and physical examination with the purpose of determining gestational age and excluding intrauterine infection. The history is directed to ascertain the onset and duration of rupture of membranes, any color or odor associated with the amniotic fluid, and any coincident symptoms. Physical examination should include assessment of maternal temperature, uterine tenderness and/or contractions, and fetal heart rate pattern because elevated temperature, uterine activity or tenderness, and fetal tachycardia can all be indicators of chorioamnionitis. The pelvic examination should never include a digital examination because this has been shown to increase the risk of intrauterine infection and decrease the latency period. Cervical dilation can be assessed by sterile speculum examination and at the same time fluid from the posterior fornix should be collected for fern and nitrazine tests. Cervical cultures for gonorrhea and chlamydia also may be collected, and a swab of the vagina and rectum should be obtained to evaluate for group B *Streptococcus* colonization. Fluid from the vaginal vault can be collected for fetal lung maturity assay in patients of appropriate gestational age. Ultrasonographic examination to determine fetal presentation, residual amniotic fluid volume, and estimated fetal weight also should be performed because these parameters will affect management and outcome.

The diagnosis of rupture of membranes is confirmed by a positive nitrazine test and evidence of ferning or arborization of the fluid collected from the posterior fornix when it is examined after drying on a microscope slide. The nitrazine test should not be used alone for confirmation due to a high rate of false-positive results due to contamination with blood or vaginal infection. If there is no fluid in the vaginal vault, having the patient lie in the Valsalva position will often cause an efflux of fluid, which visually confirms membrane rupture. In patients whose history is suspicious, but the diagnosis cannot be confirmed, a tampon test may be performed by injecting a 1:10 dilution of indigo carmine by amniocentesis and then having the patient ambulate with a tampon in the vagina to check for escape of the blue dye.

Once the diagnosis is confirmed, a plan of management should be determined based on gestational age and the presence of chorioamnionitis. In the presence of intrauterine infection, expectant management should never be initiated; the patient should be delivered regardless of gestational age or fetal lung maturity. This is due to the increased rate of both maternal endomyometritis and sepsis and neonatal sepsis associated with intrauterine infection. Antibiotic coverage may be instituted to cover gram-positive and gram-negative organisms, and ampicillin and gentamycin are the gold standard. Vaginal delivery should be pursued unless there are maternal or fetal indications for cesarean delivery.

If PPROM occurs at less than 24 weeks' gestation, the likelihood of successful neonatal outcome is extremely low. Evaluation of the patient can be conducted as described above. If there is no evidence of intrauterine infection, expectant management may be used with surveillance for infection and a brief course of broad-spectrum antibiotics such as ampicillin/sulbactam. After 24 to 48 hours of in-hospital observation and continuing counseling, the amniotic fluid volume can be reassessed. In patients with persistent oligohydramnios there is an extremely high rate of neonatal morbidity and mortality. These patients may be offered expectant management or pregnancy termination. In patients who opt for expectant management and who have no evidence of chorioamnionitis after a short hospital course, outpatient management with bed rest and daily surveillance of clinical signs of infection can be considered. Patients who are managed on an outpatient basis should be evaluated frequently and offered readmission to the hospital if a gestational age consistent with fetal viability is reached.

In gestations of less than 32 to 34 weeks' duration, without evidence of chorioamnionitis, expectant management should be used. This includes continuing surveillance for developing intrauterine infection, periodic assessment of fetal well-being, short-term treatment with a broad-spectrum antibiotic such as ampicillin/sulbactam, and corticosteroid therapy. These interventions have been shown to be safe and effective in increasing the latency period from membrane rupture to delivery and decreasing the complications of prematurity. However, once evidence of chorioamnionitis becomes evident, the fetus should be delivered. The efficacy of expectant management of PPROM beyond 32 to 34 weeks' gestation has not been demonstrated, and the risk of neonatal morbidity from infectious complications most likely outweighs the risk of prematurity, and these patients should be delivered.

At term, the management of PROM is less complex. Patients presenting with rupture prior to the onset of labor should be thoroughly evaluated, as in PPROM patients. However, assessment of fetal lung maturity is not performed and, if delivery is anticipated, digital examination of the cervix is not contraindicated. If the membranes have been ruptured for more than 18 hours, group B *Streptococcus* prophylaxis should be initiated. One of two management schemes can then be used. The first is to expectantly observe the patient for 12 to 72 hours, realizing that 95% of patients will deliver within 28 hours. Induction of labor should be initiated upon evidence of intrauterine infection or at the end of the predetermined period. The second option is to begin induction immediately after evaluation of the patient. In the patient with an unfavorable cervix, this can be accomplished with oxytocin, or intravaginal or intracervical prostaglandins. If the cervix is favorable, pitocin induction may be used. The risk of abdominal delivery is not increased in either group, nor is the risk of neonatal infection; however, the risk of maternal infection appears to be greater in the expectantly managed group.

Both PROM and PPROM remain significant obstetric problems. The appropriate evaluation and management of these patients can decrease both maternal and fetal morbidity.

General
1. Hertz RH, Rosen MG. Clinical management of premature rupture of the membranes. In: Sciarra JJ, ed. *Gynecology and obstetrics*. Vol. 2. Hagerstown, MD: Harper & Row, 1985.
   A very practical effort in addressing the problems in diagnosis and management of PROM is presented.
2. Schutte MF, et al. Management of premature rupture of membranes: the risk of vaginal examination to the infant. *Am J Obstet Gynecol* 1983;146:395.
   The authors present outcome with conservative management concerning 6,160 infants born after PROM. The risk of infection was related to gestational age and vaginal examination but not to length of membrane rupture.
3. Cox SM, et al. The natural history of preterm ruptured membranes: what to expect of expectant management. *Obstet Gynecol* 1988;71:558.
   The outcome of expectant management in PROM prior to 34 weeks was reviewed in an indigent population. Only 7% of patients in this group were not in labor within 48 hours. The incidence of PROM in this population before 34 weeks was 1.7% but accounted for 20% of the perinatal deaths.
4. ACOG Practice Bulletin No. 1. Premature rupture of membranes. June 1998.
   This is an excellent review of the current literature pertaining to PROM and PPROM and includes evaluation of prospective trials and meta-analyses as well as management protocols.
5. Duff P. Premature rupture of membranes at term. *Semin Perinatol* 1996;20:401.
   The authors present a review of the epidemiology and management of term rupture of membranes.

Etiology
6. Lenihan JP Jr. Relationship of antepartum pelvic examinations to premature rupture of the membranes. *Obstet Gynecol* 1984;63:33.
   The incidence of PROM in 349 patients near term was greater if weekly pelvic examinations were performed.
7. Shubert PJ, et al. Etiology of preterm premature rupture of membranes. *Obstet Gynecol Clin North Am* 1992;19:251.
   An excellent summary of the multiple etiologies presumed to contribute to the development of PROM: biochemical changes, mechanical factors, infection, pH, nutrition, smoking, bleeding, incompetent cervix, and coitus.
8. Lonky NM, Hayashi RN. A proposed mechanism for premature rupture of membranes. *Obstet Gynecol Surv* 1988;43:22.
   A good review of the different factors currently thought to play an important part in PROM. The potential impact of smoking, infection, and coitus and the balance between proteases and antiproteases are discussed.
9. McGregor JA. Prevention of preterm birth: new initiatives based on microbial-host interactions. *Obstet Gynecol Surv* 1988;43:1.

The authors present an outstanding review of the role of bacteria and the resultant host reaction to infection in relation to PROM. The complex role of prostaglandins is discussed. Potential areas for future treatment and prevention of PROM are addressed.

Diagnosis

10. Reece EA, et al. Amniotic fluid arborization: effect of blood, meconium, and pH alterations. *Obstet Gynecol* 1984;64:248.

    The effects of blood meconium and pH alterations were tested on the ability of the fern test to diagnose PROM. Ferning was unaffected by meconium or alteration in the pH but was absent when blood was mixed with amniotic fluid in equal amounts.

11. Barber HRK. Diagnosis of premature rupture of the membranes (PROM). *Diagn Gynecol Obstet* 1982;4:3.

    The principal assessment techniques for diagnosis of PROM are listed by the author in a "cookbook" style. This is a handy procedure manual.

12. Eriksen NL, et al. Fetal fibronectin: a method for detecting the presence of amniotic fluid. *Obstet Gynecol* 1992;80:451.

    The presence of fetal fibronectin in the posterior fornix is a sensitive test to detect subtle ruptured membranes.

13. O'Keefe DF, et al. The accuracy of estimated gestational age based on ultrasound measurement of biparietal diameter in preterm premature rupture of the membranes. *Am J Obstet Gynecol* 1985;151:309.

    Estimating gestational age using the biparietal diameter after PROM is probably inadequate and will likely lead to underestimation. Head circumference or long bone measurements will be more accurately correlated with true gestational age.

14. Gembruch U, Hansmann M. Artificial instillation of amniotic fluid as a new technique for the diagnostic evaluation of cases of oligohydramnios. *Prenat Diagn* 1988;8:33.

    The use of ultrasound to direct transabdominal instillation of electrolyte solution is presented as an approach for diagnosing the etiology of severe oligohydramnios. Unsuspected PROM may be found. The ability to obtain fetal fibroblasts for chromosomal analysis is discussed, as is the major complication of the techniques.

Treatment

15. Moller M, et al. Rupture of fetal membranes and premature delivery associated with group B streptococci in urine of pregnant women. *Lancet* 1984;1:69.

    Of 2,745 women, there was a greater incidence of PROM and premature delivery occurred more often in those colonized (urine) with group B streptococci. A urine culture in women with PROM for group B streptococci may be indicated.

16. Duff P, Huff RW, Gibbs RS. Management of premature rupture of membranes and unfavorable cervix in term pregnancy. *Obstet Gynecol* 1984;63:697.

    The authors treated 134 patients at term with PROM and an unfavorable cervix either aggressively with induction after 12 hours or by observation. In the intervention group, a longer labor and higher incidence of cesarean birth and intraamniotic infection were noted.

17. Curet LB, et al. Association between ruptured membranes, tocolytic therapy, and respiratory distress syndrome. *Am J Obstet Gynecol* 1984;148:263.

    The association between PROM, tocolytic therapy, and neonatal respiratory distress syndrome (RDS) was studied in 297 patients. PROM and tocolytic therapy each had a lower incidence of RDS individually; however, when both were present in the same patient, there was actually a higher incidence of RDS.

18. Moretti M, Sibai BM. Maternal and perinatal outcome of expectant management of premature rupture of membranes in the midtrimester. *Am J Obstet Gynecol* 1988;159:390.

    The outcome of PROM at less than 23 weeks' gestation is reviewed in 118 patients. The perinatal survival rate was 13.3%, of which approximately two thirds were subsequently developing normally. There was one maternal death owing to sepsis.

Complications
19. Nimrod C, et al. The effect of very prolonged membrane rupture on fetal development. *Am J Obstet Gynecol* 1984;148:540.
   A retrospective study of 100 patients with PROM for more than 1 week was compared to 100 control patients with intact membranes. Pulmonary hypoplasia was increased when PROM occurred at less than 26 weeks' gestation, and there was a threefold increase in positional deformities.
20. Hardt NS, et al. Influence of chorioamnionitis on long-term prognosis in low birth weight infants. *Obstet Gynecol* 1985;65:5.
   Long-term infant outcome of mothers who had chorioamnionitis was compared with those who did not. The potential advantage of leaving infants in utero after PROM may be offset by the disadvantage of chorioamnionitis with respect to future development in surviving infants.
21. Weitzel HK, et al. Clinical aspects of antenatal glucocorticoid treatment for prevention of neonatal respiratory distress syndrome. *J Perinatol Med* 1987; 15:441.
   The indications and contraindications for the use of glucocorticoids are discussed with reference to several key articles on the subject, including a collaborative study. The use of steroids was not believed to be indicated with PROM since there is no clear benefit and the maternal infectious morbidity rate may double.
22. Roberts AB, et al. Fetal breathing movements after preterm premature rupture of membranes. *Obstet Gynecol* 1991;164:821.
   A significant reduction in fetal breathing was found the first 2 weeks after PROM. This finding is hypothesized to play a role in the development of pulmonary hypoplasia if PROM occurs before 24 weeks.
23. Brown CL, et al. Cervical dilation: accuracy of visual and digital examinations. *Obstet Gynecol* 1993;81:215.
   Visual examination to determine cervical dilation with PROM correlated well with digital examination.
24. Carlan SJ, et al. Preterm premature rupture of membranes: a randomized study of home versus hospital management. *Obstet Gynecol* 1993;81:61.
   Although very few patients with PROM met strict criteria for home management, there was no difference in perinatal outcome compared with hospital management.

Management
25. Mercer BM, et al. Induction versus expectant management in premature rupture of the membranes with mature amniotic fluid at 32-36: a randomized trial. *Am J Obstet Gynecol* 1993;169:775.
   This randomized trial indicated that PPROM patients with mature fetal lung profiles had decreased hospital stays and lower neonatal and maternal infection rates.
26. Natale R, et al. Management of premature rupture of membranes at term: randomized trial. *Am J Obstet Gynecol* 1994;171:936.
   This randomized trial indicated that early labor induction does not increase the abdominal delivery rate in term PROM.
27. Hannah ME, et al. Induction of labor compared with expectant management for prelabor rupture of the membranes at term. *N Engl J Med* 1996;334:1005.
   This prospective randomized trial indicated that aggressive induction of labor in term PROM does not increase adverse outcomes and is more favorably perceived by the patient.
28. Lewis DF, et al. Latency period after preterm premature rupture of membranes: a comparison of ampicillin with and without sulbactam. *Obstet Gynecol* 1995; 86:392.
   This small randomized trial supported the efficacy of broad-spectrum antibiotics in increasing the latency period in PPROM.
29. Hadi HA, Hodson CA, Strickland D. Premature rupture of the membranes between 20 and 25 weeks gestation: role of amniotic fluid volume in perinatal outcome. *Am J Obstet Gynecol* 1994;170:1139.

This retrospective series revealed an association with residual amniotic fluid volume after membrane rupture at 20 to 25 weeks' gestation and perinatal morbidity and mortality. These results are useful in counseling patients with PPROM in the late second trimester.

30. Mercer BM, Arheart KL. Antimicrobial therapy in expectant management of preterm premature rupture of the membranes. *Lancet* 1995;346:1271.
   The authors present a meta-analysis of the effect of antibiotic use on latency period and maternal and infant morbidity in PPROM patients.

31. Lewis DF, et al. Effects of digital vaginal examination on latency period in preterm premature rupture of membranes. *Obstet Gynecol* 1992;80:630.
   This prospective randomized trial implicates digital cervical examination as a major risk factor for reduced latency period in PPROM patients.

32. Mercer BM. Antibiotic therapy for preterm rupture of membranes. *Contemp Obstet Gynecol* 1997;42(3):7.
   This is a great general review of the efficacy of antibiotic use in PPROM.

33. Naef RW, et al. Premature rupture of membranes at 34 to 37 weeks' gestation: aggressive versus conservative management. *Am J Obstet Gynecol* 1998;178:126.
   This prospective randomized trial compares expectant management with immediate induction in PPROM after 34 weeks. The results support aggressive induction of labor.

---

24. FETAL DEMISE

Garland D. Anderson

In about 1% of pregnancies, the mother and the obstetrician are jolted by the realization that the fetus has died in utero. Antepartum fetal demise may occur any time during pregnancy. Early intrauterine death is suspected when the fetus is small for dates and fetal heart tones are not heard. After mid-pregnancy, loss of viability is often heralded by loss of both subjective fetal activity as well as fetal cardiac activity.

Since the advent of ultrasonography, the confirmation of intrauterine death is much less difficult. A sonogram performed early in pregnancy may show disruption of the gestational sac or an absence of fetal echoes. Later in pregnancy, there is absence of fetal cardiac activity and collapse of the fetus, if a sufficient interval has elapsed since death.

Intrapartum fetal death can occur during labor, with an absence of fetal heart tones, as revealed by scalp electrode recording or ultrasonographic imaging, confirming the diagnosis. If fetal death is a strong possibility, caution is necessary because the maternal electrocardiogram can be transmitted through the fetus. Any heart activity that is attributed to the fetus must not be synchronous with that of the mother. If there is any question of fetal viability, the presence or absence of fetal heart activity can be determined by real-time ultrasonography.

Management of antepartum fetal death is simplified if the uterus is 14 weeks size or less because suction curettage is indicated at this time, although coagulation studies should be performed beforehand. When the uterus is greater than 14 weeks size, there are several management options: observation only, prostaglandin E_2 vaginal suppositories, prostaglandin E_1 (misoprostil) analog, intravenous oxytocin, intraamniotic PGF_{2a} (carboprost), and on rare occasion hysterotomy.

Those clinicians who advocate expectant therapy (observation only) know that 80% of the patients will go on to experience spontaneous labor and delivery within 2 to 23 weeks of intrauterine fetal demise. Unfortunately, intrauterine demise represents a great emotional burden for the mother, and this approach to management is unacceptable to most patients. Although it involves great stress, a woman with a fetal death may agree to expectant therapy. The key to convincing her is the physician's ability to deal with the couple and not offer delivery immediately in response to the woman's grief. The patient who wants immediate delivery after the diagnosis of fetal demise may benefit from a brief period of time to deal with her loss before induction of labor. A 48-hour wait before induction of labor gives the woman time to gather her family together for emotional support. Before induction is begun, what is to be expected should be fully discussed with the woman and her family. For example, they should know that when gestations are less than 24 weeks along, with induction accomplished by prostaglandin E_2 suppositories, the woman will very likely deliver in bed. Besides the emotional component, another drawback to observation is the potential for development of a coagulopathy. A woman is at risk for coagulopathy if the gestation is 16 weeks or greater and if she has retained a dead fetus for more than 4 weeks. At 5 weeks after fetal demise, there is a 25% chance of significant hypofibrinogenemia developing; the subsequent risk increases with the duration of fetal retention. Hypertonic saline injected intraamniotically has been an effective abortifacient. This method is contraindicated, however, in patients with renal or cardiovascular disease, and its use may increase the risk of a coagulation defect. Intraamniotic administration of carboprost 1 mg under ultrasonographic guidance has been used with minimal complication. Carboprost is contraindicated in patients with asthma and certain cardiac conditions. Intravenous oxytocin has had the widest use for this purpose and is an agent familiar to all obstetricians. Unfortunately, the preterm uterus is relatively insensitive to the effects of oxytocin, even though high dosages (up to 1,000 mU/min) have been used. Water intoxication resulting from the antidiuretic effect of oxytocin, uterine rupture, and cardiac arrhythmias have been reported with its use.

Vaginal suppositories containing prostaglandin E_2 (Prostin E_2) have been approved by the U.S. Food and Drug Administration for use in the patient with intrauterine fetal demise at less than 28 weeks' gestation, and many practitioners use them later in pregnancy. They are easy to administer, and the side effects (nausea, vomiting, diarrhea, and temperature elevation) are transient. The present dosage consists of half of a 20-mg suppository administered initially and then a full suppository administered every 4 hours until delivery. Delivery will usually occur within 12 to 24 hours, and ripening of the cervix with Laminaria or prostaglandin gel (2 mg) may be helpful. Recently, misoprostil (synthetic E_1 analog) has been successfully used to achieve delivery with fewer adverse effects than with prostaglandin E_2. Misoprostil 50- to 100-μg tablets are inserted into the posterior vaginal vault every 6 hours. Heavy sedation is usually not needed during labor.

The key to successful intervention is an individualized approach. For the patient with a gestation of 14 weeks or less, suction curettage is the treatment of choice. In the second trimester, prostaglandin E_2 vaginal suppositories, intraamniotic carboprost, or misoprostil are usually used. After 28 weeks' gestation, the choice is between intravenous oxytocin, prostaglandin E_2 suppositories, and misoprostil. After 36 weeks' gestation, oxytocin induction is almost always used. Hysterotomy is reserved for the unusual patient in whom other options have failed. A special case is the patient who has had a previous cesarean delivery and whose uterus is too large for suction curettage. Use of prostaglandins, hypertonic saline, and oxytocin pose the threat of causing uterine rupture, but if the cesarean birth was performed in the lower segment, labor is usually allowed. An internal-pressure cannula may be placed to monitor uterine contractions. If these conditions cannot be met, hysterotomy is indicated.

Before any mode of therapy is initiated, coagulation studies should be performed. In the rare patient with hypofibrinogenemia, heparin may be indicated if there is no bleeding, and a 1- to 2-day course (1,000 U/h) will increase the fibrinogen concentration to acceptable levels (>200 mg/dl) before attempts to empty the uterus are made. Cryoprecipitate or fresh-frozen plasma is used for the treatment of patients with bleeding hypofibrinogenemia.

Management responsibilities do not cease when the fetus has been delivered. Further goals are emotional support for the parents and a search for the cause of the intrauterine death. It is now recognized that the parents experience a grief reaction similar to that occurring with the loss of other family members; thus, there is a definite need for effective bereavement counseling. The stages of grief reaction (shock, anger, questioning, depression, and acceptance) must be resolved by the parents. During delivery, the shock stage is usually dominant. The physician will need to repeat information and explanations. The parents are encouraged to see the baby, and many like a memento of the neonate, such as a photograph or lock of hair. In addition to the grief, there is frequently an element of inappropriate guilt. One or both parents may search at length for something that they did wrong to cause the fetal death. All members of the perinatal team should learn the dynamics of the grief-guilt process, avoid intellectualization, and know the practical aspects involved, such as the proper written forms to use, the arrangements for hospital disposal versus burial, and how to go about requesting postmortem studies. If there is no obvious reason for the fetus' death, the parents should be so counseled. Both parents also should be told that the grief process is a normal reaction, and they should discuss their feelings with each other. They should be seen frequently in the office after discharge to see how they are coping with the grief process. The findings from autopsy reports should be discussed at length with both parents as soon as possible after the event. Parents should be encouraged to join support groups.

It is imperative that a cause be sought. Chromosome studies, complete autopsy, total body x-ray films, and full-body photographs should be considered in the evaluation of fetal deaths, when appropriate. Many cases of intrauterine fetal demise are a result of fetal-maternal hemorrhage. This is detected by examining maternal blood for the presence of fetal erythrocytes.

Intrauterine death remains a sad reality. The obstetrician must apply both science and art to ensure safe management of the mother's condition and emotional support for the couple. In subsequent pregnancies, the woman who has suffered a previous intrauterine loss must be considered a high risk. She will need to be seen more frequently and her pregnancy monitored more aggressively.

General

1. Paul RH, Gauthier RJ, Quilligan EJ. Clinical fetal monitoring. The usage and relationship to trends in cesarean delivery and perinatal mortality. *Acta Obstet Gynecol Scand* 1980;59:289.
   The impact of fetal monitoring on the prevention of intrapartum deaths is discussed. An extensive bibliography is available regarding all aspects of this problem.
2. Stierman ED. Emotional aspects of perinatal death. *Clin Obstet Gynecol* 1987;30:352.
   The emotional and psychologic responses of parents who experience fetal death are reviewed.
3. Lake MF, et al. Evaluation of a perinatal grief support team. *Am J Obstet Gynecol* 1987;157:1203.
   Positive evaluations of a perinatal grief team are presented.
4. Vance JC, et al. Early parental responses to sudden infant death, stillbirth or neonatal death. *Med J Aust* 1991;155:292.
   The authors discuss the initial emotional response of parents to the death of an infant or to a stillbirth.
5. Lemmer CM. Parental perceptions of caring following perinatal bereavement. *West J Nurs Res* 1991;13:475.
   Parents discuss their perceptions of the events that happen with the death of a fetus or infant.
6. Pauw M. The social worker's role with a fetal demise or stillbirth. *Health Soc Work* 1991;16:291.
   The authors discuss the social worker's role in helping parents who have experienced perinatal loss.
7. Brenner B, Blumenfeld Z. Thrombophilia and fetal loss. *Blood Rev* 1997;11:72.
   This article reviews the recent knowledge relating thrombophilia with fetal loss.

Etiology

8. Quinn PA, et al. A prospective study of microbial infection in stillbirths and early neonatal death. *Am J Obstet Gynecol* 1985;151:238.

This study illustrates that, particularly in the case of stillbirths that occur for no related cause, infection (most commonly genital Mycoplasma *infection) may be associated with the majority of cases.*

9. Liban E, Salzberger M. A prospective clinicopathological study of 1108 cases of antenatal fetal death. *Isr J Med Sci* 1976;12:34.
This is a good review of the etiologic factors contributing to antenatal fetal death.
10. Fay RA. Feto-maternal hemorrhage as a cause of fetal morbidity and mortality. *Br J Obstet Gynaecol* 1983;90:443.
A significant number of stillborns may be due to fetal-maternal hemorrhage.
11. Hovatta O, et al. Causes of stillbirth: a clinico-pathological study of 243 patients. *Br J Obstet Gynaecol* 1983;90:691.
The etiology of fetal death is examined in a large number of stillborns.
12. Freeman RK, et al. The significance of a previous stillbirth. *Am J Obstet Gynecol* 1985;151:7.
A previous stillbirth is a predictive event when associated with intrauterine growth retardation or hypertension in a current gestation.
13. Branch DW. Immunologic disease and fetal death. *Clin Obstet Gynecol* 1987; 30:295.
This article presents the immunologic causes of fetal death and includes 124 references.
14. Ingemarsson I, Kallen K. Stillbirths and rate of neonatal deaths in 76,761 post-term pregnancies in Sweden, 1982–1991: a register study. *Acta Obstet Gynecol Scand* 1997;76:658.
The authors report the frequency and cause of stillbirths from the Swedish Medicine Birth Registry.

Diagnosis
15. Barr M Jr, Burdi AR. Evaluation of the abortus and stillborn infant. *J Reprod Med* 1982;27:601.
The authors outline the steps that should be taken in evaluating the abortus or stillborn infant in order to counsel the parents regarding future pregnancies.
16. Woods DL, Draper RR. A clinical assessment of stillborn infants. *S Afr Med J* 1980;57:441.
The authors emphasize the clinical assessment of stillborn infants. The figures they provide are of assistance in predicting recurrence rates.
17. York AC, Rettenmaier MA. An unusual complication of delayed management in the case of fetal death. *Am J Obstet Gynecol* 1984;150:101.
The authors point out that one of the dangers from delayed management of fetal demise is misdiagnosis of an abdominal pregnancy.
18. Meier PR, et al. Perinatal autopsy: its clinical value. *Obstet Gynecol* 1986;67:349.
The positive value of autopsy in assisting or correcting diagnoses in 139 perinatal deaths is noted.
19. Carey JC. Diagnostic evaluation of the stillborn infant. *Clin Obstet Gynecol* 1987;30:342.
The author describes the evaluative procedures in stillborn infants.
20. Hammersley L, Drinkwater C. The prevention of psychological morbidity following perinatal death. *Br J Gen Pract* 1997;47:583.
This article documents the high incidence of psychological morbidity following perinatal death and interventions that may reduce the morbidity rate.

Treatment
21. Southern EM, et al. Vaginal prostaglandin E_2 in the management of fetal intrauterine death. *Br J Obstet Gynaecol* 1978;85:437.
The authors describe results in 709 cases of a missed abortion or intrauterine fetal demise actively managed with prostaglandin E_2 vaginal suppositories.
22. Romero R, et al. Prolongation of a preterm pregnancy complicated by death of a single twin in utero and disseminated intravascular coagulation. Effects of treatment with heparin. *N Engl J Med* 1984;310:772.

The use of intravenous heparin to reverse disseminated intravascular coagulation allowed the authors to prolong to the time of viability a twin gestation that was complicated by fetal demise.

23. Spinnato JA, et al. Aggressive intrapartum management of lethal fetal anomalies: beyond fetal beneficence. *Obstet Gynecol* 1995;85:89.

    The authors report on four women who had fetuses with lethal anomalies and requested intrapartum management.

24. Fox R, et al. The management of late fetal death: a guide to comprehensive care. *Br J Obstet Gynaecol* 1997;104:4.

    This is an in-depth review of management of fetal deaths that occur at term.

Complications

25. Graham MA, et al. Factors affecting psychological adjustment to a fetal death. *Am J Obstet Gynecol* 1987;157:254.

    These authors found that less depression was experienced by women if they were kept informed of problems, received sympathy from medical personnel, and were allowed to see the infant.

26. Taylor PB, Gideon MD. Crisis counseling following the death of a baby. *J Reprod Med* 1980;24:208.

    Practical advice about effective crisis counseling is provided—a must for those professionals desiring to provide emotional support for the bereaved parents.

27. Callan NA, Colmorgen GH, Weiner S. Lung hypoplasia and prolonged preterm ruptured membranes: a case report with implications for possible prenatal ultrasonic diagnosis. *Am J Obstet Gynecol* 1985;151:756.

    Lung hypoplasia complicating prolonged premature rupture of the membranes is documented by sonographic evidence.

28. Goldenberg RL, et al. Pregnancy outcome following a second-trimester loss. *Obstet Gynecol* 1993;81:444.

    Pregnancy loss at 13 to 24 weeks was associated with a 39% risk of preterm delivery, a 5% risk of stillbirth, and a 6% risk of neonatal death in the next pregnancy.

---

25. SURGERY AND TRAUMA IN PREGNANCY

Michel E. Rivlin

The evaluation and treatment of the obstetric patient with a disease requiring surgical intervention or one who has sustained recent trauma are modified by the physiologic and anatomic factors related to pregnancy. Accidental injury occurs in approximately 7% of pregnant women, and at least 1% of parturients will undergo a surgical procedure other than cesarean delivery. This sizable group of patients presents management difficulties for the practitioner who must balance maternal and fetal concerns.

Consideration of the teratogenic effect of drugs and diagnostic procedures predominates in the treatment plans in early gestation. Drug exposure in the 2 weeks after conception results either in an intact fetus or in abortion, the so-called all-or-none principle. The period of organogenesis from weeks 4 to 12 (menstrual age) follows. It is during this time that the fetus is most susceptible to damage. For surgical patients, some commonly prescribed analgesics such as codeine should be avoided. Meperidine, morphine, and acetaminophen are acceptable. The antibiotic tetracycline may produce bone and teeth problems in the offspring as well as hepatic toxicity in the mother. Sulfonamides administered in the third trimester may interfere with the protein binding of bilirubin, and kernicterus may result in the newborn. Vaccines that contain live viruses should be avoided in early pregnancy, except when there is a great maternal risk of disease. Toxoids or killed vaccines such as tetanus toxoid, however, can be administered in pregnancy. Most anesthetic agents produce no demonstrable teratogenic effects, although the findings from retrospective studies do point to a higher rate of abortion when anesthesia is given in the first and second trimesters. There is the possibility that ionizing radiation at any level may increase the risk of future malignancies in the offspring. Childhood leukemia is particularly worrisome. The teratogenic effects of diagnostic x-ray studies are not detected when the dose to the fetus is low. Currently, a dose of 5 rad (equivalent to that in an intravenous pyelogram) delivered directly to the fetus is considered safe, but abdominal shielding should be used when possible.

Pregnancy alters the nature of the laboratory evaluation in the patient requiring a surgical procedure. Many measurements will reflect the increase in plasma volume, which is 50% greater than that in the nonpregnant patient. A white blood cell count of less than 15,000/ml is normal. The red blood cell mass is increased by 30%, but, secondary to the proportionately greater increase in the plasma volume, the hematocrit decreases slightly during pregnancy. The alkaline phosphatase level may be elevated, owing to the placental contribution to this enzyme. The erythrocyte sedimentation rate is mildly elevated. The measurement of thyroid and adrenal hormones is altered by protein binding. The concentrations of most of the clotting factors are elevated in pregnancy. The modest enhanced coagulability increases the risk of thrombosis, especially during and after surgical procedures. The increased respiratory rate and tidal volume lower the partial pressure of carbon dioxide and thus cause a mild compensated respiratory alkalosis. These respiratory events alter the dosage of anesthetic gases used in pregnancy.

Anatomic variations also change the way in which patients are evaluated. The enlarging uterus is responsible for many of the alterations. In the supine position, vena caval compression may cause hypotension and shortness of breath in the mother and may diminish blood flow to the fetus. The effect is most pronounced during conduction or general anesthesia, unless the gravida is placed in a left lateral tilt position. The obstruction of venous return from the lower extremities is responsible for the edema that many women experience. As the gravid uterus fills the abdomen, the likelihood of esophageal reflux is greater, with an accompanying risk of aspiration of gastric contents. The enlarged uterus also displaces the other organs from their normal positions. The appendix is pushed into the right upper quadrant, and the heart is rotated and appears enlarged on a chest roentgenogram. Because the uterus lifts the parietal peritoneum away from the underlying structures, the pain of a small bowel obstruction or appendicitis may be diminished. Ureteral compression at the pelvic brim is more pronounced on the patient's right side, owing to the dextrorotation of the uterus and enlargement of the pelvic vasculature.

Surgical conditions of the maternal abdomen present a difficult challenge for the obstetrician-gynecologist, mainly because of concerns about disturbing the preterm fetus or uterus. Appendicitis is the most common nonobstetric reason for a laparotomy. The most common signs during pregnancy are a vague pain in the right side of the abdomen and anorexia. If the pain felt by the patient when examined in the supine position is reproduced in the same region of the abdomen when the patient is rolled onto her side (Alder sign), the source of the abdominal discomfort is likely to be extrauterine and possibly caused by appendicitis. If the location of the pain shifts with movement of the uterus, the pain is most likely uterine or adnexal. When laparotomy is performed, a midline incision is recommended during the first trimester. Later in gestation, the incision is usually made over the point of maximal tenderness.

Gallbladder disease is the second most common surgical condition of pregnancy. Cholecystitis is associated with cholelithiasis in 90% of cases. The hormonal changes that take place in pregnancy are responsible for a decreased contractility of the gallbladder, an elevated biliary cholesterol level, and an increasing gallbladder capacity, which combined predispose to stone formation. Pain, with inspiratory arrest, may be evoked while palpating over the gallbladder (Murphy sign). Medical therapy consisting of intravenous fluids and nasogastric suction is usually successful, with a positive response within 24 to 48 hours. Surgical intervention is most often implemented in patients when medical management fails, the gallbladder becomes perforated, jaundice arises because of a common duct stone, significant obstruction occurs, or the associated complication of pancreatitis intervenes.

Small-bowel obstruction is encountered usually (1) during months 4 and 5, when the uterus becomes an abdominal organ; (2) during months 8 and 9, when the fetal head descends into the pelvis; or (3) during delivery and the puerperium, when there is a sudden change in uterine size that alters the relationship of adhesions and the surrounding bowel. The treatment is surgical. A high index of suspicion is required on the part of the physician to avoid delay and increased mortality.

The presence of a persistent adnexal mass is a cause for concern, owing to the associated risks of an underlying malignancy in approximately 6% of such patients. Other risks include the possibility of rupture, torsion, or hemorrhage resulting from such a mass. In the asymptomatic patient, surgical intervention may be postponed until the second trimester, because the chance for adverse effects on pregnancy is less at that time.

Trauma in pregnancy is most commonly incurred in a motor vehicle accident. In fact, automobile collisions are the leading nonobstetric cause of maternal death in the United States. Pregnant women should be encouraged to wear seat belts. The shoulder harness provides the best protection, not only by preventing the mother from being thrown from the automobile but also by distributing the forces of impact over a larger area. When seat belts are not used, the most common cause of maternal death is head trauma associated with expulsion from the automobile. Fetal death is most commonly due to death of the mother. Second in incidence is abruptio placentae. Although delayed abruption has occurred sometimes days after the event, most researchers recommend fetal monitoring for 4 hours initially after moderate to severe trauma. Although a positive Kleihauer-Betke test result may indicate maternal-fetal hemorrhage in cases of abruption, clinical correlation is required. A useful adjunct in the evaluation of such patients is paracentesis. Positive findings include the aspiration of grossly bloody fluid, a red blood cell count greater than $100,000/\mu l$, a white blood cell count greater than $500/\mu l$, or an amylase level greater than 175 IU/dl.

The pregnant trauma patient also may be the victim of a stabbing incident or gunshot wound. Especially later in gestation, the enlarged uterus protects other abdominal organs. Although cushioned in amniotic fluid, the fetus can be injured. A projectile may be localized by fetogram or ultrasonography. In cases of peritoneal penetration, an exploratory laparotomy is indicated. That portion of the small bowel that is compressed superiorly by the gravid uterus is most likely injured when the projectile enters the upper abdomen.

Thermal injury and electrical shock may adversely affect the pregnancy. Fetal loss is greatest in the setting of first-trimester maternal burns, but later fetal loss depends on the gestational age and the extent of the maternal injury. Even when there does not appear to be an injury from electrical shock, intrauterine growth retardation has been observed in exposed fetuses. Careful follow-up using serial sonography is necessary.

As many as 10% of pregnant women may be the victims of physical abuse. It is essential that the practitioner consider this possibility whenever a trauma patient is evaluated. In one series, these women were more likely than control subjects to be divorced or separated, to be of lower socioeconomic status, and to have emotional problems. Many of these women present with chronic psychosomatic complaints. Pregnancy may lead to increased stress and an increase in violent behavior in these families.

In most situations, the well-being of the fetus will parallel that of the patient. Assessment of the fetus when the mother has been traumatized or is to undergo operation is important. Maintenance of the left lateral decubitus position and avoidance of hypotension in the mother are essential to ensuring fetal health. The fetus should be monitored electronically from the outset of the maternal evaluation. Newer technology has enabled the surgeon to monitor the status of the fetus during the surgical procedure, if this is germane to an individual case. Cesarean delivery is not always necessary when exploring the abdomen, and correction of hypovolemia may alleviate an abnormal fetal heart rate. After operation, use of tocolytic drugs should be considered, but they should not be prescribed routinely. Pregnancies complicated by peritonitis or abdominal procedures performed in the third trimester are at greatest risk for preterm labor. Magnesium sulfate, with its fewer cardiovascular effects than the beta-mimetic drugs, is preferred for tocolysis. Adjunctive progesterone therapy is considered when the corpus luteum is removed in early pregnancy.

General

1. Duncan PG, et al. Fetal risk of anesthesia and surgery during pregnancy. *Anesthesiology* 1986;64:790.
   There was no increase in the cases of congenital anomalies in the offspring of women undergoing general anesthesia in the first two trimesters. More spontaneous abortions occurred in the treatment group (relative risk, 1.58).

2. Petrikovsky SM, Vintzileos AM. Fetal heart rate monitoring during obstetrical operations: a review. *Obstet Gynecol Surv* 1988;43:721.
   These authors offer a review of the worldwide literature concerning fetal heart rate monitoring during and after obstetric operations. They outline a clinical management protocol.

3. Nathan L, Huddleston JF. Acute abdominal pain in pregnancy. *Obstet Gynecol Clin North Am* 1995;22:55.
   It is vital to differentiate surgical, gynecologic, medical, and obstetric causes of acute abdominal pain in pregnancy.

Surgical Disorders in Pregnancy

4. Coleman MT, Trianfo VA, Rund DA. Nonobstetric emergencies in pregnancy: trauma and surgical conditions. *Am J Obstet Gynecol* 1997;177:497.
   Early suspicion and serial examination may result in appropriate interventions for appendicitis, cholecystitis, pancreatitis, and bowel obstruction.

5. Fallon WF, et al. The surgical management of interabdominal inflammatory conditions during pregnancy. *Surg Clin North Am* 1995;75:15.
   The sonographic findings of cholelithiasis, wall thickening, pericholecystic fluid, and ultrasonographic Murphy's sign are reliable in 90% of cases in pregnancy.

6. Connolly MM, Unti JA, Nova PF. Bowel obstruction in pregnancy. *Surg Clin North Am* 1995;75:101.
   Most cases are due to adhesions from previous surgery or pelvic inflammatory conditions, with volvulus (25%) and intussusception (5%) also major causes.

7. Dias MS, Sekhar LN. Intracranial hemorrhage from aneurysms and arteriovenous malformations during pregnancy and the puerperium. *Neurosurgery* 1990;27:855.
   Operative clipping for aneurysmal hemorrhage is beneficial in pregnancy, and the usual neurosurgical indications for operation for malformations may also apply in pregnancy.

8. Reedy MB, et al. Laparoscopy during pregnancy. A survey of laparoendoscopic surgeons. *J Reprod Med* 1997;42:33.
   This article addresses the safety and complications of laparoscopy in pregnancy. The most common procedures were cholecystectomy, appendectomy, and surgery for adnexal masses.

Trauma in Pregnancy

9. Eposito TJ. Trauma during pregnancy. *Emerg Med Clin North Am* 1994;12:167.
   Traumatic abruptio may follow an increase in intraamniotic pressure that deforms the elastic uterus around the inelastic placenta, initiating a shearing effect of the placenta from the decidua.

10. Lavery JP, Staten-McCormick M. Management of moderate to severe trauma in pregnancy. *Obstet Gynecol Clin North Am* 1995;22:69.
    Head injuries and hemorrhagic shock are implicated in the majority of maternal deaths.

11. Buchsbaum HJ. Diagnosis and management of abdominal gunshot wounds during pregnancy. *J Trauma* 1975;15:425.
    Rarely is the pregnant uterus spared with a gunshot wound to the abdomen late in gestation. The fetal mortality rate is high in the setting of such injuries.

12. Deitch EA, et al. Management of burns in pregnant women. *Surg Gynecol Obstet* 1985;161:1.
Burns in the first trimester were associated with a high rate of fetal loss. Before 28 weeks, fetal survival was related to maternal survival, but less so after 32 weeks.

13. Sakala EP, Kort DD. Management of stab wounds of the pregnant uterus: a case report and review of the literature. *Obstet Gynecol Surv* 1988;43:319.
Only 19 cases of stab wounds to the pregnant uterus have been reported. The management of such injuries is discussed.

14. Schoenfeld A, et al. Vehicular trauma in pregnancy: an algorithm for diagnosis and fetal therapy. *Fetal Ther* 1987;2:51.
A useful clinical approach is given for the management of the pregnant trauma patient.

15. Petersen R, et al. Violence and adverse pregnancy outcomes: a review of the literature and directions for future research. *Am J Prev Med* 1997;13:366.
Violence is estimated to occur in 0.9% to 20.1% of pregnant women in the United States. There appears to be an association with adverse outcomes of the pregnancy.

16. McFarlane J, et al. Assessing for abuse during pregnancy. Severity and frequency of injuries and associated entry into prenatal care. *JAMA* 1992;267:3176.
Physical abuse occurred in 17% of the pregnancies, and 60% of these women reported more than a single episode.

17. Holland JG, Hume AS, Martin JN Jr. Drug use and physical trauma: risk factors for preterm delivery. *J Miss State Med Assoc* 1997;38:301.
Screening results were positive for alcohol, cocaine, or marijuana use in 11% of women with physical trauma in pregnancy, and there was a 21% incidence of preterm birth.

18. O'Brien JA, et al. Prepartum diagnosis of traumatic fetal-maternal hemorrhage. *Am J Perinatol* 1985;2:214.
A test for maternal-fetal hemorrhage is recommended in cases of maternal trauma.

19. Rothenberger DA, et al. Diagnostic peritoneal lavage for blunt trauma in pregnant women. *Am J Obstet Gynecol* 1977;129:479.
The technique and criteria for the assessment of peritoneal lavage are discussed.

20. Pearlman MD, Tintinalli JE, Lorenz RP. A prospective controlled study of outcome after trauma during pregnancy. *Am J Obstet Gynecol* 1990;162:1502.
Fetal-maternal hemorrhage occurred in 30.6% of the pregnancies complicated by trauma, and was more common in the anterior placenta. Electronic fetal monitoring is recommended for 4 hours as a screening tool for adverse perinatal outcome.

21. Jacob S, et al. Maternal mortality in Utah. *Obstet Gynecol* 1998;91:187.
Trauma, pulmonary embolism, and cardiac disease are the most common identifiable causes of maternal death.

26. HYPEREMESIS GRAVIDARUM

Sister Clarice Carroll

Hyperemesis gravidarum is defined as excessive vomiting and nausea occurring before the 20th week of gestation. It is a condition that usually necessitates hospitalization and is complicated by weight loss, dehydration, ketonuria, and sometimes by serious psychological disturbances. It is a complication that can lead to severe maternal nutritional deprivation and can threaten fetal well-being.

Morning sickness must be distinguished from hyperemesis. Nausea and vomiting are the most common symptoms of early pregnancy, second only to amenorrhea. They can appear within 2 weeks after a missed period and usually diminish by the 14th week of gestation in up to 50% of pregnant women. These symptoms were described by the Egyptians as early as 2000 B.C. Although a certain degree of nausea and vomiting is to be expected, they are usually the first symptoms of pregnancy and are self-limiting, abating by 12 to 14 weeks' gestation. If the symptoms persist and become more severe, however, fluid and electrolyte imbalance can result. If left untreated, the results can be fatal. If nausea and vomiting are present (particularly if they begin after the 12th week of pregnancy) a medical or surgical condition may be responsible.

Hyperemesis gravidarum occurs in up to 2% of pregnancies, although the diagnosis is not well defined because the diagnostic criteria used differ from one geographic area to another. However, if the vomiting is severe enough to require hospitalization, the diagnosis is usually applied.

Although the cause of hyperemesis remains unclear, the etiologic factors include (1) vitamin B_6 deficiency, owing to a change in protein metabolism; (2) impaired function of the adrenal cortex; (3) hyperthyroidism and excess human chorionic gonadotropin secretion; (4) psychopathologic and emotional factors; (5) alterations in gastrointestinal physiology; (6) a hypersensitivity reaction; and (7) poor nutrition.

The primary clinical manifestation of hyperemesis is frequent and sustained vomiting (usually 4–8 weeks in duration), resulting in significant weight loss and dehydration. Other signs of starvation that gradually develop include metabolic acidosis, ketonuria, hypokalemic alkalosis, oliguria, hemoconcentration, and constipation. In diagnosing and treating hyperemesis, other disorders must be excluded. Hydatidiform mole, gastroenteritis, multiple gestation, hepatitis, cholecystitis, peptic ulcer, hyperthyroidism, hiatal hernia, gastric carcinoma, and intestinal obstruction may all be mimicked by hyperemesis. Severe forms of hyperemesis involving weight loss of greater than 5% of prepregnant weight has been associated with poor fetal growth and outcome. Continued vomiting and dehydration also can lead to the formation of brainstem lesions resembling those characteristic of Wernicke's encephalopathy.

The prognosis in these patients is excellent, provided proper treatment is given. The principal underlying treatment of hyperemesis gravidarum is to prevent dehydration and starvation, and recognizing any psychologic component that may be present. Treatment includes hospitalization in a quiet room (isolation may be required for some patients) and a complete physical examination, including documentation of a verbal history that may be helpful in revealing any emotional problems. Physical and laboratory determinations, such as temperature, pulse, respiration, blood pressure, weight on admission and daily weight, urinalysis, and strict fluid assessment (intake and output) are usually performed. Laboratory evaluation of the electrolyte status, including the potassium, sodium, blood urea nitrogen, glucose, and serum creatinine levels, should be obtained.

In some cases, parenteral nutrition is required to maintain or restore an anabolic state. Parenteral nutrition has improved from its previous regimen of dextrose and sodium chloride to one consisting of either short- or long-term nutritional maintenance including the recommended dietary allowances of carbohydrates, amino acids, electrolytes, preparations of fat emulsions, vitamins, and trace elements. The number of calories per day must be determined so that a balance of carbohydrates, fat, and proteins can be administered.

In most cases gastric rest, gained by not allowing oral intake, is helpful. Nutritional assessment of each patient suffering from hyperemesis must be established because all pregnant women do not have the same nutritional requirements. Simple baseline parameters should include height and weight.

Antiemetics or mild sedatives such as intramuscularly administered promethazine (Phenergan, 25–50 mg) or orally administered phenobarbital (16–32 mg), 1 hour before meals and at bedtime, also may be used. However, because some drugs may have teratogenic effects if given in the first 12 weeks of pregnancy, scrutiny of all medications is wise. Vitamin B complex, vitamin C, and vitamin B_6 (100 mg) added to intravenous solutions may be useful. Psychiatric consultation is sometimes necessary, and isolation from family and relatives is helpful in some cases.

Some physicians suggest that, when the patient begins to respond to intravenous therapy (as indicated by cessation of vomiting, return of the electrolyte balance to normal, and an increase in urinary output), small sips of water, 1 ounce (30 ml) hourly, can be initiated. As soon as the patient can tolerate food, she should be given small, frequent meals consisting of fairly dry and easily digested high-energy foods in the form of carbohydrates and liquids, such as fruit drinks, tea, and milk. Intravenous therapy should be discontinued as soon as possible, and the diet should progress from liquids to semisolids (e.g., boiled eggs, cooked cereals, toast, and dry crackers) before solids are introduced. Similarly, vitamin, antiemetic, and sedative therapy can be tapered or discontinued. One study identified steroid therapy as a successful management of hyperemesis.

Moderate activity should gradually be initiated, and the patient's weight recorded biweekly. The weight chart, more than any other guide, will document the progress of the patient. In severe cases, the use of total parenteral nutrition is necessary to ensure maternal weight gain. Because the psychological component can be significant, the patient should be given an opportunity to discuss any problems and should possibly be referred for psychiatric consultation. The patient may be safely discharged from the hospital after the nausea and vomiting have ceased and she begins to gain weight. Continued intensive outpatient follow-up is necessary.

There is little evidence that the patient with hyperemesis gravidarum will deliver a small-for-gestational-age or intrauterine-growth-retarded baby, except in the event of severe hyperemesis. Similarly, there appears to be no increased risk of congenital malformations associated with the condition. Ketonuria, however, should be prevented, because fetal abnormalities are increased if this persists. Maternal complications resulting from persistent vomiting include hemorrhagic retinitis, rupture of the esophagus, aspiration pneumonitis, electrolyte depletion, acid-base disturbance, and dental erosion. Complications of antiemetic therapy include jaundice, irregular jerky movements, and opisthotonos owing to the administration of phenothiazines. The association of transient hyperthyroidism with hyperemesis gravidarum has been investigated. In this situation, a short course of antithyroid therapy readily reverses the cause of the disease, while resolving the hyperemesis as well.

General
1. Cunningham FG, et al. Gastrointestinal disorders. In: *Williams obstetrics.* Norwalk, CT: Appleton-Century-Crofts, 1993.
   This is a review of the diagnosis and treatment of nausea and vomiting in pregnancy.
2. Kayuppila A, Huhtaniemi I, Ylikorkala O. Raised serum human chorionic gonadotrophin concentrations in hyperemesis gravidarum. *Br Med J* 1979;1:1670.
   An extensive review with 26 references that examines the psychologic, social, and biologic aspects of hyperemesis gravidarum. The effect of body type and psychologic gain is emphasized.
3. Kallen B. Hyperemesis during pregnancy and delivery outcome: a registry study. *Eur J Obstet Gynecol Reprod Biol* 1987;26:291.
   The authors present the results of a study of 3,068 pregnancies with the diagnosis of hyperemesis recorded in a Swedish Birth Registry for the years 1973 to 1981.
4. Tsang IS, Katz VL, Wells SD. Maternal and fetal outcomes in hyperemesis gravidarum. *Int J Gynaecol Obstet* 1996;55:231.
   Hyperemesis was defined as excessive nausea and vomiting resulting in dehydration, extensive medical therapy, and / or hospital admission. Women with hyperemesis have similar demographic characteristics to the general obstetric population, and have similar obstetric outcomes.
5. Trovik J, et al. Nasoenteral tube feeding in hyperemesis gravidarum. An alternative to parenteral nutrition. *Tidsskr Nor Laefeforen* 1996;116:2442.
   A severe form of hyperemesis gravidarum involving maternal weight loss greater than 5% of the prepregnant weight occurs in up to 0.1% to 0.2% of all pregnancies and may lead to retarded fetal growth.
6. Tareen AK, et al. Thyroid hormone in hyperemesis gravidarum. *J Obstet Gynaecol* 1995;21:497.
   Thyroid hormone levels were significantly altered and the extent of increase or decrease in their level correlated well with the severity of symptoms in the study subjects.

7. Gulley RM, Vander PN, Gulley JM. Treatment of hyperemesis gravidarum with nasogastric feeding. *Nutr Clin Pract* 1993;8:33.

Hyperemesis gravidarum, an antepartum disorder characterized by severe nausea and vomiting, is usually a benign condition with a favorable outcome.

Etiology

8. Burrows GN, Ferris TF. Nausea and vomiting of pregnancy and hyperemesis gravidarum. In: Burrows GN, Ferris TF, eds. *Medical complications during pregnancy.* Philadelphia: WB Saunders, 1988.
   This is a comprehensive review of the topics of nausea, vomiting, and hyperemesis gravidarum.
9. Mori M, et al. Morning sickness and thyroid function in normal pregnancy. *Obstet Gynecol* 1988;72:355.
   The authors measured thyroid levels in 132 normal women in early pregnancy and in 20 nonpregnant women. They could not find any correlation between either these levels or the human chorionic gonadotropin titers and the occurrence of hyperemesis.
10. Cowan MJ. Hyperemesis gravidarum: implications for home care and infusion therapies. *J Intrav Nursing* 1996;19:46.
    Nausea and vomiting afflict up to 80% of pregnancies, with the more severe form, hyperemesis, complicating about 1%. Hyperemesis in pregnancy causes fluid volume deficit, starvational ketoacidosis, and, at times, metabolic alkalosis with hypokalemia. Significant weight loss may occur and may reflect fluid as well as lean tissue loss. The cause is unknown, and although prognosis is generally good with aggressive fluid replacement and nutritional support, there is the potential for decreased birth weight. Management strategies for hyperemesis gravidarum, including hydration, enteral and parenteral nutrition, antiemetic therapies, monitoring needs, and psychosocial concerns, are discussed with applications made to the home care setting.

Diagnosis

11. Juras N, Banovac K, Sekso M. Increased serum reverse triiodothyronine in patients with hyperemesis gravidarum. *Acta Endocrinol* 1983;102:284.
    A study of 33 patients with hyperemesis gravidarum revealed elevated T3 levels.
12. Levine MG, Esser D. Total parenteral nutrition for the treatment of severe hyperemesis gravidarum: maternal nutritional effects and fetal outcome. *Obstet Gynecol* 1988;72:102.
    This article outlines a clinical management plan that relies principally on psychosocial support and nutritional counseling for the mother.
13. Borgeat A, Fathi M, Valiton A. Hyperemesis gravidarum: is serotonin implicated? *Am J Obstet Gynecol* 1997;176:476.
    Hyperemesis gravidarum is not associated with an increase of serotonin secretion.

Treatment

14. Adno J. Treatment of hyperemesis gravidarum. *S Afr Med J* 1986;69:110.
    A local ethnic food that is difficult to regurgitate was used experimentally to treat hyperemesis gravidarum.
15. Rafla N. Limb deformities associated with prochlorperazine. *Am J Obstet Gynecol* 1987;156:1557.
    This author reports on two cases of congenital abnormalities that may have resulted from using an antiemetic only.
16. Boyce RA. Enteral nutrition in hyperemesis gravidarum: a new development. *J Am Diet Assoc* 1992;6:733.
    Enteral nutrition in the treatment of hyperemesis gravidarum is an effective and safe technique.
17. Stellato TA, Danziger LH, Burkons D. Fetal salvage with maternal total parenteral nutrition: the pregnant mother as her own control. *JPEN J Parenter Enter Nutr* 1988;12:412.

The authors found that fetal outcome was normal in mothers with severe hyperemesis when total parenteral nutrition is used. Care must be taken in working with such a severely nutritionally depleted patient because total parenteral nutrition also has risks.

18. Walters WAW. The management of nausea and vomiting during pregnancy. *Med J Aust* 1987;147:290.
   The author provides details on a series of patients with hyperemesis gravidarum who were treated using his clinical approach, consisting of both supportive and therapeutic measures.

19. van Stuijvenberg ME, et al. The nutritional status and treatment of patients with hyperemesis gravidarum. *Am J Obstet Gynecol* 1995;172:1585.
   The hyperemetic pregnant patient is at nutritional risk; prompt initiation of corrective therapy is recommended.

20. Taylor R. Successful management of hyperemesis gravidarum using steroid therapy. *Q J Med* 1996;89:103.
   High-dose prednisolone therapy is effective in suppressing symptoms of intractable hyperemesis gravidarum and allowing normal maternal nutrition.

21. Hsu JJ, et al. Nasogastric enteral feeding in the management of hyperemesis gravidarum. *Obstet Gynecol* 1996;88:343.
   Enteral feeding via nasogastric tube seems to be effective in relieving intractable nausea and vomiting and in providing adequate nutritional support. Enteral nutrition should be considered as an alternative to total parenteral nutrition in the management of hyperemesis gravidarum.

22. Johnson DR, et al. Dehydration and orthostatic vital signs in women with hyperemesis gravidarum. *Acad Emerg Med* 1995;2:692.
   Women who present to the emergency room with hyperemesis gravidarum experience measurable improvement in postural pulse rate and systolic blood pressure changes with rehydration.

23. Anderson AS. Managing pregnancy sickness and hyperemesis gravidarum. *Professional Care Mother Child* 1994;4:13.
   Hyperemesis gravidarum—severe vomiting in pregnancy—requires management in hospital to restore electrolyte balance and prevent severe dehydration.

Complications

24. Colin JF, et al. Hyperthyroidism: a possible factor of cholestasis associated with hyperemesis gravidarum of prolonged evolution. *Gastroenterol Clin Biol* 1994; 18:378.
   The association of jaundice and hyperthyroidism suggests that hyperthyroidism is a possible factor of cholestasis in patients with hyperemesis gravidarum.

25. Lao RR, Chin RKJ, Chang AMZ. The outcome of hyperemetic pregnancies complicated by transient hyperthyroidism. *Aust N Z J Obstet Gynaecol* 1987;27:99.
   A study of 39 patients with hyperemesis gravidarum, in 17 of whom transient hyperthyroidism developed. There was no adverse effect on pregnancy outcome.

27. INTRAUTERINE GROWTH RESTRICTION

Dom A. Terrone

Intrauterine growth restriction (IUGR) is a term applied to infants whose birth weights are much lower than one would expect for their gestational age. These infants may be born prematurely, at term, or postterm. These pregnancies are of concern because their perinatal rate of mortality is 10 times greater than the baseline. The neonate with IUGR is generally identified by a birth weight that is at or below the

10th percentile for that expected at a given gestational age. Using this criterion, one in 10 babies will be so designated, with 70% of fetuses that meet the definition of being normal or constitutionally small. The difficulty in managing these pregnancies is differentiating the fetus that is truly at risk from the fetus that is merely small for gestational age (SGA). In addition, some of these infants appear to have an increased incidence of neurologic impairment during infancy and childhood. The IUGR infant is also more likely to have congenital anomalies, in utero hypoxia, meconium aspiration, cold stress, hypoglycemia, hypocalcemia, hyperviscosity syndrome, respiratory distress, and pulmonary hemorrhage.

If an infant is identified as IUGR, various etiologic factors may be responsible. Approximately 10% of these infants will have an abnormal karyotype, with another 10% being associated with intrauterine infections (e.g., herpes, rubella, cytomegalovirus, toxoplasmosis, or syphilis). Maternal conditions such as essential hypertension, diabetes mellitus, chronic renal disease, cyanotic heart disease, and hemoglobinopathies also place the fetus at risk for IUGR. In addition, the maternal nutritional status, socioeconomic level, smoking habits, and use of alcohol and other drugs may adversely affect fetal growth. Placental abnormalities associated with IUGR include previa, chronic abruption, multiple gestations, and placental tumors. Despite these numerous, recognized etiologic factors, as many as 50% of cases of IUGR have no clearly identifiable cause.

Because intrauterine fetal weight cannot be easily or accurately measured and because gestational age is often not precisely known, the prenatal diagnosis of IUGR presents a formidable obstetric challenge. Some pregnancies at risk for IUGR can be suspected by maternal history and complications. For example, having previously given birth to a growth-restricted baby is a strong predictor of risk for subsequent pregnancies. Clinical information such as maternal weight gain and the serial measurement of uterine fundal height are the only screening tools. Unfortunately, their lack of sensitivity and positive predictive value make them poor screening tools. This serves to emphasize the importance of identifying patients at risk.

There are several parameters that are useful in the diagnosis and management of IUGR. For example, an accurate determination of gestational age is of critical importance. Correlation of normal and clearly recalled menstrual data with a pelvic examination prior to 12 weeks and heart tones heard by a standard fetoscope by 20 weeks provides an accurate estimation of gestational age (± 7 days). Ultrasonography can enhance and complement these clinical tools. The most accurate method of assessing gestational age is to measure fetal crown-rump lengths during the gestational interval between 8 and 12 weeks (± 5 days). The most commonly used ultrasonic technique for gestational age determination, however, is biparietal diameter (BPD) measurements or femur length (FL) assessment at 16 to 24 weeks (± 10 days). In addition to BPD and femur length, the head circumference (HC), abdominal circumference (AC) and other biometric data are good estimates of gestational age if performed before the third trimester, when there is more variation (± 21 days).

Estimation of fetal weight by ultrasonography using the multiple biometric parameters appears to provide the closest estimation of actual fetal weight, and therefore should represent the primary diagnostic modality. Serial evaluations of growth are most often performed every 2 to 3 weeks. Of the individual parameters, the AC is the most sensitive marker for IUGR. The presence of slowed abdominal growth may herald impending IUGR and has been referred to by some researchers as AC lag. In an effort to more accurately identify the fetus truly at risk, additional ultrasonographic parameters have been used. These include calculation of the HC:AC ratio, which is increased in the growth-restricted fetus; and FL:AC ratio, which when greater than 23.5:1 is consistent with IUGR. The role of Doppler velocimetry in these patients is somewhat controversial. Although measuring uterine artery blood flow does not appear to be a useful tool, umbilical artery systolic:diastolic (S:D) ratios can be an excellent additional test. Elevated Doppler S:D ratios, when found in conjunction with other markers of fetal stress, may assist the clinician in planning to move toward delivery. If, however, there is absent or reversed end-diastolic flow, the fetus is clearly in jeopardy and surveillance must be increased (with a low tolerance for delivery). In addition, oligohydramnios is often found in conjunction with IUGR, serving as an indicator of chronic hypoxia. Oligohydramnios predisposes the fetus to um-bilical cord compression and may herald fetal deterioration.

Once a fetus has been diagnosed as having decreased growth, obstetric manage-ment should be directed at modifying any associated factors that can be changed. For example, nutrition can be improved, cigarette smoking discontinued, and alcohol use abandoned. Treatment of a pregnancy with IUGR has usually meant striving to ame-liorate underlying causes whenever possible. New data, however, have introduced two interesting treatment interventions. Low-dose aspirin has been shown in some re-ports to decrease the incidence of IUGR in patients at high risk. The evidence is not definitive, but is encouraging. Maternal hyperoxygenation, although apparently not a long-term solution, can improve the intrauterine environment so that cortico-steroids to advance fetal lung maturity can be administered. Bed rest in the left lat-eral position will increase uterine blood flow and, it is hoped, can improve oxygena-tion of the fetus. Because these fetuses are at risk for uteroplacental insufficiency, serial fetal assessments should be performed. These can be in the form of twice-weekly nonstress testing or biophysical profile, or weekly contraction stress testing. Continued surveillance to detect oligohydramnios is indicated.

There are no data to support early delivery of infants with IUGR in the absence of documented uteroplacental insufficiency as assessed by the aforementioned tests or oligohydramnios. During either spontaneous or induced labor, a patient with an IUGR fetus should be monitored electronically and observed carefully for fetal intol-erance of labor. This may take the form of recurrent severe variable or late decelera-tions unresponsive to treatment (lateral positioning, oxygen, and correction of hy-potension or hypovolemia). Delivery should be effected safely and expeditiously, most often by cesarean birth. If the amniotic fluid is meconium-stained, neonatal meconium aspiration can be minimized by suctioning the oropharynx prior to delivery of the shoulders. Amnioinfusion also has been demonstrated to be of use in these cases.

After delivery, cold stress must be avoided, blood glucose measured, and the hy-perviscosity syndrome and respiratory distress treated if they occur. In addition, these neonates must be evaluated carefully for the presence of congenital anomalies and in utero infections. Therefore, these pregnancies are optimally delivered in a facility that can provide intensive monitoring during labor and delivery as well as subsequent care and evaluation in the neonatal period.

The data concerning the subsequent growth and development of these infants should be viewed in light of the heterogeneity of the group. If infants with chromoso-mal abnormalities, congenital anomalies, and infections are excluded, the prognosis is generally good for subsequent normal physical development and neurologic out-come. Prevention and treatment of hypoxia during labor and the appropriate man-agement of neonatal problems will decrease the risk of morbidity and mortality in this group of high-risk pregnancies.

General

1. Brenner WE, Edelman DA, Hendricks CH. A standard of fetal growth for the United States of America. *Am J Obstet Gynecol* 1976;126:155.
   The 10th, 25th, 50th, and 75th percentiles of fetal weight were calculated from 8 to 20 menstrual weeks. The derived growth curves are often used clinically and for investigational purposes.

2. Seeds JW. Impaired fetal growth: Definition and clinical diagnosis. *Obstet Gynecol* 1984;64:303.
   This landmark article reviews the significance, clinical definition, and diagnos-tic tests used in the problem of impaired fetal growth.

3. Spinnato JA, et al. Inaccuracy of Dubowitz gestational age in low birth weight infants. *Obstet Gynecol* 1984;63:491.
   This study shows that all infants labeled as SGA or IUGR may simply have an error in the neonatal gestational age score (Dubowitz) assigned by the pediatri-cian. This variable has important clinical implications.

4. Brar HS, Rutherford SE. Classification of intrauterine growth retardation. *Semin Perinatol* 1988;12:2.
   This excellent review offers not only a classification for growth retardation but also an anthology of normal growth. It also proffers 125 references.

Etiology

5. Wen SW, et al. Intrauterine growth retardation and preterm delivery: prenatal risk factors in an indigent population. *Am J Obstet Gynecol* 1990;162:213.
   Prenatally assessed risk factors for low birth weight were investigated in 17,000 indigent women. Smoking, short stature, low weight and low weight gain showed the greatest correlation to IUGR.
6. Carlson EE. Maternal diseases associated with intrauterine growth retardation. *Semin Perinatol* 1988;12:17.
   The various maternal complications by system and their effect on fetal growth are detailed in this excellent article. Sixty updated references are listed.
7. Lee K-S, et al. Maternal age and incidence of low birth weight at term: a population study. *Am J Obstet Gynecol* 1988;158:84.
   Sociodemographic factors and advancing maternal age are associated with a decreased potential for fetal growth and an increased risk of maternal complications that might lead to IUGR.
8. Li CQ, et al. The impact on infant birth weight and gestational age of cotinine-validated smoking reduction during pregnancy. *JAMA* 1993;269:1519.
   Cotinine-validated smoking reduction rates were positively associated with increased infant birth weight. Women who stopped smoking had the most improvement in birth weight, but decreasing smoking also was associated with significantly increased birth weight.
9. Econommides DL, Nicolaides K. Blood glucose and oxygen tension levels in small-for-gestational age fetuses. *Am J Obstet Gynecol* 1989;160:385.
   These authors found no significant influence from maternal-fetal glucose gradient and hypoxia between umbilical venous and arterial samples in SGA babies, indicating that a major cause for hypoglycemia in these neonates is reduced supply rather than increased consumption.

Diagnosis

10. Rosendahl H, Rivinen S. Routine ultrasound screening for early detection of small for gestational age fetuses. *Obstet Gynecol* 1988;71:518.
    Real-time ultrasonographic screening examinations were performed in 3,208 unselected singleton pregnancies at 17 and 34 weeks to detect fetuses with IUGR; 4.9% were SGA.
11. Vintzileos AM, et al. Value of fetal ponderal index in predicting growth retardation. *Obstet Gynecol* 1984;67:584.
    There was relatively poor correlation between fetal and neonatal ponderal indices. Although the ponderal index may be useful in ruling out IUGR, it was not very useful in making the diagnosis of IUGR because of the high false-positive rate.
12. Divon MY, et al. Intrauterine growth retardation—a prospective study of the diagnostic value of real-time sonography combined with umbilical artery flow velocimetry. *Obstet Gynecol* 1988;72:611.
    The best predictor of IUGR was estimated fetal weight less than the 10th percentile for gestational age.
13. Berkowitz GD, et al. Sonographic estimation of fetal weight and Doppler analysis of umbilical artery velocimetry in the prediction of intrauterine growth retardation: a prospective study. *Am J Obstet Gynecol* 1988;158:1149.
    This is a report of 168 patients at risk for IUGR who were evaluated by Doppler velocimetry studies compared with sonographic prediction of intrauterine growth retardation. The sensitivity of the systolic to diastolic ratio of the umbilical artery was lower than the sonographic estimation (55% versus 75%); however, the umbilical artery studies had a higher specificity (92% versus 80%).
14. Pardi G, et al. Diagnostic value of blood sampling in fetuses with growth retardation. *N Engl J Med* 1993;328:692.
    No fetuses with normal heart rates and normal umbilical artery velocimetry had hypoxia or acidosis. If the fetal heart rate and velocimetry were abnormal, 64% had lactic acidosis, low blood oxygen, or low pH values as determined by fetal umbilical cord sampling.

15. Minior VK, Divon MY. Fetal growth restriction at term: myth or reality? *Obstet Gynecol* 1998;92:57.
    A comparative analysis of the term IUGR infant compared with appropriate-for-gestational-age controls demonstrating increased morbidity in the IUGR group.

Treatment

16. Cox WL, et al. Physiology and management of intrauterine growth retardation: a biologic approach with fetal blood sampling. *Am J Obstet Gynecol* 1988;159:36.
    Data are presented from fetal blood sampling in 24 cases of IUGR. An elevated white blood cell count (12 of 24), mean corpuscular volume (22 of 24), and a pH below the normal range (7 of 24) were found. Lactic dehydrogenase levels were markedly elevated in most cases, and the glutamyl transferase levels were greatly increased in all but six fetuses.
17. Block BSB, Llanos AJ, Creasy RK. Responses of the growth-retarded fetus to acute hypoxemia. *Am J Obstet Gynecol* 1984;148:878.
    Fetuses who are growth-retarded are more likely to be affected by acute hypoxemia during labor. Although this study was performed with fetal lambs, it was elegantly controlled and the data appear to be applicable to humans.
18. Wallace RL, Schifrin BS, Paul RH. The delivery route for very-low-birth-weight infants. A preliminary report of a randomized, prospective study. *J Reprod Med* 1984;29:736.
    The delivery route for small babies was studied in this prospective report. The difficulty in accurately diagnosing fetal weight was encountered by the investigators, but it did not appear that abdominal delivery was of advantage in low-birth-weight babies (<1,500 g).
19. Wallenburg HCS, Rotmans N. Prevention of recurrent idiopathic fetal growth retardation by low-dose aspirin and dipyridamole. *Am J Obstet Gynecol* 1987;157:1230.
    Controlled, nonrandomized trial of 24 multigravida women with at least two previous pregnancies complicated by IUGR, who received 1 to 1.6 mg/kg aspirin and 225 mg dipyridamole daily from 16 to 34 weeks' gestation. IUGR occurred in 61% of control pregnancies and in 13% of treated pregnancies.
20. McCormick MC. The contribution of low birth weight to infant mortality and childhood mortality. *N Engl J Med* 1985;312:82.
    This article details the effect of low birth weight in infants on subsequent mortality during childhood. It graphically illustrates that babies who are SGA have a proportionately higher risk of dying during childhood compared with their normal-birth-weight counterparts.
21. Platt LD. Genetic factors in intrauterine growth retardation. *Semin Perinatol* 1988;12:11.
    When growth retardation is diagnosed, the possibility of genetic problems should be entertained. The involvement of consultants in a baby who is growth retarded at delivery is an important first step in making the diagnosis.
22. van Zeben-van der Aa TM, et al. Morbidity of very low birth weight infants at corrected age of two years in a geographically defined population. Report from project on preterm and small for gestational age infants in the Netherlands. *Lancet* 1989;1:253.
    In a very homogeneous population with 97% follow-up, a major handicap was found in 4.4% of low-birth-weight infants. This rate is much lower than what has been published in the Netherlands (30%).
23. Low JA, et al. Intrauterine growth retardation: a study of long-term morbidity. *Am J Obstet Gynecol* 1982;142:670.
    Prospective follow-up study of 76 IUGR children and 88 children with weights appropriate for gestational age. There was no significant difference in the incidence of motor and cognitive handicap or developmental delay, language developmental delay, and tests of vision and hearing between the children of the IUGR and control groups.

24. Cacciatore B, et al. Effects of transdermal nitroglycerin on impedance to flow in the uterine, umbilical, and fetal middle cerebral arteries in pregnancies complicated by preeclampsia and intrauterine growth retardation. *Am J Obstet Gynecol* 1988; 179:140.
    A small study using nitroglycerin patches to treat pregnancies complicated by IUGR and associated preeclampsia.
25. Gulmezoglu M, de Onis M, Villar J. Effectiveness of interventions to prevent or treat impaired fetal growth. *Obstet Gynecol Surv* 1997;52:139.
    A review of multiple modalities aimed at treating or reducing the incidence of IUGR.
26. Leitich H, et al. A meta-analysis of low dose aspirin for the prevention of intrauterine growth retardation. *Br J Obstet Gynaecol* 1997;104:450.
    A meta-analysis reporting that early treatment with aspirin may reduce the incidence of IUGR.

VI. FETAL MALPOSITIONS

28. BREECH PRESENTATION

James A. Bofill

Breech presentation is defined as the entrance of the fetal buttocks or the lower extremities into the maternal pelvic inlet. The incidence of singleton breech presentation at term gestation is 3% to 4%. This incidence is dependent on gestational age; about 25% of fetuses are in a breech presentation at 28 weeks of gestation. Breech presentations are characterized as either frank, complete, or incomplete (footling). The *frank breech* fetus has both hips sharply flexed with the thighs on the abdomen and both knees in the extended position. In this position the fetal feet are in close proximity to the fetal head. The *complete breech* has both hips and both knees in flexion, with the buttocks being the presenting part. The *incomplete* or *footling breech* has one or both hips in the extended position such that a foot (or both feet) is (are) the presenting part(s). Overall, the frank breech is the most common (65%) of these presentations, followed by the footling breech (about 25%), with the remainder presenting as a complete breech (10%).

Several conditions may predispose to breech presentation. Prematurity is the most commonly observed association. During the second and early third trimesters the ratio of the intrauterine volume to the size of the fetus is large, and this predisposes the pregnancy to breech presentation. Breech presentation is also frequently seen in twin or higher-order multifetal gestations. Other factors that may predispose to breech presentation include fetal aneuploidy, disorders of amniotic fluid volume (hydramnios or oligohydramnios), fetal anomalies (hydrocephalus or anencephaly), uterine structural abnormalities, high maternal parity, or abnormalities of placentation (placenta previa or a fundal-cornual placenta). However, in more than half the cases, the cause of breech presentation is not known.

The diagnosis of breech presentation is usually suspected when Leopold's maneuvers identify the fetal head in the uterine fundus and the breech in the pelvis. Alternatively, when the fetal heart rate is heard best above the umbilicus, a breech presentation may be suspected. Routine cervical examination may reveal a breech presentation. Occasionally, the breech may be confused with a face or shoulder presentation during cervical examination. The breech may be differentiated from the face presentation because the anal orifice forms a straight line with the ischial tuberosities, whereas the fetal mouth in a face presentation is not in line with the malar eminences. In modern day obstetric units the breech presentation is confirmed using bedside ultrasonography. If a breech presentation is confirmed, sonography may then be used for fetal biometry (to estimate the fetal weight) as well as to exclude fetal malformations. Additionally, ultrasonography also may be used to exclude hyperextension of the fetal head.

It is certainly preferable to make the diagnosis of breech presentation in the antenatal clinic prior to labor rather than when the patient presents in active labor. The diagnosis of breech presentation prior to labor allows for a planned attempt at external cephalic version (ECV). The early diagnosis of a breech presentation also allows for a thorough discussion of all of the risks and benefits, both maternal and fetal, of cesarean delivery versus a trial of labor. Most physicians will attempt ECV at 36 to 37 weeks' gestation because although it may be more successful at earlier gestational ages, there is also a higher rate of spontaneous reversion to breech presentation. Furthermore, if fetal distress requiring a cesarean delivery supervenes during an attempt at ECV, a fetus at 36 to 37 weeks' gestation would be expected to do well. ECV performed after 36 weeks is permanently successful in approximately 65% of cases. A reactive fetal heart rate tracing is a prerequisite for ECV, and terbutaline-induced relaxation is commonly used prior to the procedure. Some researchers have used fetal vibroacoustic stimulation and epidural analgesia to improve ECV success rates. ECV appears to be safe for both the mother and the fetus and may be used in the presence of a previous low-segment transverse cesarean section scar.

In the past 30 years, the rate of cesarean birth performed for breech delivery has increased tremendously. In the United States, about 90% of term breech infants are now delivered by cesarean. Most physicians recommend abdominal delivery for women with breech presentations of large (>3,600 g) or premature (<2,000 g) infants. The use of oxytocin for augmentation or induction of breech labor is controversial. Some physicians will not allow a trial of labor for the primigravida with a breech presentation. Incredibly, there have been only two prospective and randomized clinical trials of breech vaginal delivery versus planned cesarean delivery. Although there were no differences in the rates of neonatal morbidity and mortality, the total numbers of patients studied was small. For this reason, most discussions of maternal and fetal outcomes in vaginal versus cesarean delivery for breech presentation include studies of retrospective design. Two recent meta-analyses have documented that although neonatal morbidity and mortality due to delivery trauma is low in breech vaginal delivery, it appears to be significantly more frequent than with planned cesarean delivery. It is estimated that serious birth injury or death will occur in 1.23% of vaginally delivered infants, whereas this rate is 0.9% with cesarean delivery. Cesarean birth, however, is associated with a significantly lower rate of neonatal morbidity and mortality in those infants with birth weights between 1,000 and 2,000 g. Total breech extraction, in which the obstetrician grasps the fetal feet, provides traction, but performing maneuvers in an attempt to provide a rapid delivery is associated with higher perinatal morbidity and mortality. Breech extraction, which can result in fetal central nervous system injuries, should be reserved for emergency situations such as umbilical cord prolapse and should be performed only by the most experienced practitioners. In modern practice total breech extraction is almost exclusively reserved for the breech-presenting second twin. After the vertex delivery of the first twin, a total breech extraction may be performed if the second twin is in a complete or footling breech presentation and the fetal feet can be easily reached. If a total breech extraction is performed just after the vertex delivery of the first twin, the maternal cervix will still be completely dilated and the procedure can usually be readily accomplished.

It is absolutely crucial for each delivery service to have a plan in place to deal with the contingency of a patient presenting at term, in labor, with a breech presentation. There should be clear criteria delineated for allowing a trial of breech labor. Many obstetric services use X-ray or computed tomography for pelvimetry as well as to assess the attitude of the fetal head prior to allowing a trial of breech delivery. The patient whose fetus has a hyperextended head (the stargazing fetus) is not considered for a breech vaginal delivery, and cesarean delivery is promptly accomplished. Most commonly, a biischial diameter of 10 cm is used as a criterion for an adequate pelvis. Some obstetric services also measure the anteroposterior and transverse diameters of the pelvic inlet to document an adequate pelvis. Sonography is liberally used to estimate the fetal weight as well as to exclude obvious congenital anomalies. Most protocols for breech vaginal delivery will allow frank or complete breech fetuses that are estimated to weigh between 2,000 and 3,600 g a trial of labor if pelvimetry is adequate and there is no evidence of fetal jeopardy. Appropriate informed consent is of utmost importance. The benefits to the mother of a vaginal delivery must be weighed against the possible risks to the fetus; this is the essence of the informed consent process. The decision to allow a vaginal delivery or to proceed with cesarean delivery should be made without procrastination. The patient who is allowed a trial breech vaginal delivery should be carefully observed during labor. A considerable proportion of women who attempt a breech vaginal delivery will require a cesarean delivery for non-reassuring fetal status or protracted labor. These labors should be assessed by continuous electronic fetal monitoring as well as uterine contraction monitoring. If there is progressive cervical dilatation and normal descent of the presenting part, the labor is allowed to continue. Because of the possibility of umbilical cord prolapse, the membranes are usually kept intact as long as possible. Any evidence of non-reassuring fetal status or of a prolapsed cord mandates cesarean birth. As mentioned above, the use of oxytocin in breech labor is controversial, and some physicians would opt for cesarean delivery rather than augment a protracted breech labor.

Consultation with the obstetric anesthesia team is important, and, most often, a continuous segmental epidural is chosen for labor analgesia. When this is not available a pudendal block may provide adequate pain relief at the time of delivery of the breech. A liberal episiotomy is performed as the breech is crowning. The breech is allowed to deliver spontaneously until the umbilicus appears; the obstetrician then gently assists the delivery of the fetal legs, trunk, and arms. The aftercoming head may be delivered either by the Mauriceau-Smellie-Veit maneuver or using Piper forceps. Many obstetricians have abandoned breech vaginal deliveries specifically for the fear of entrapment of the aftercoming head. If the fetal head becomes entrapped and the fetus is undeliverable, an immediate laparotomy is performed for abdominal rescue. Incisions of the cervix (Duhrssen's incisions) to allow vaginal delivery are rarely used in modern obstetrics. As long as there has not been excessive traction on the fetal neck in an effort to effect delivery, abdominal rescue for an entrapped aftercoming head will usually produce a normal infant.

In summary, vaginal breech delivery can be performed in carefully selected patients who make adequate progress and display no signs of fetal compromise. Cesarean delivery should be performed if the clinical circumstances do not favor a vaginal delivery. As data have accumulated, the increased rate of cesarean delivery for breech presentation has been associated with a decreased incidence of perinatal mortality and morbidity, particularly in preterm infants. Nevertheless, the decision regarding the management of breech presentation at term should be individualized and based on clinical grounds.

General
1. Gimovsky ML, McIlhargie CJ. Breech presentation. In: O'Grady JP, Gimovsky ML, McIlhargie CJ: *Operative obstetrics.* Baltimore, MD: Williams & Wilkins, 1995.
   The number of skilled operators with the ability to safely deliver singleton breech fetuses continues to dwindle.
2. Gilstrap LC. Breech delivery. In: Hankins GDV, Clark SL, Cunningham FG, Gilstrap LC, eds. *Operative obstetrics.* Norwalk, CT: Appleton & Lange, 1995.
   The neonatal outcome of the nonvertex twin delivered after 35 weeks of gestation is not affected by the route of delivery.
3. Kunzel W. Recommendations of the FIGO committee on perinatal health on guidelines for the management of breech delivery. *Int J Gynecol Obstet* 1994; 44:297.
   International recommendations may not be applicable to the United States.
4. Eller DP, VanDorsten JP. Route of delivery for the breech presentation: a conundrum. *Am J Obstet Gynecol* 1995;173:393.
   The safety-of-trial-of-labor conundrum will probably never be adequately addressed.

Series
5. Cheng M, Hannah M. Breech delivery at term: a critical review of the literature. *Obstet Gynecol* 1993;82:605.
   The increased cesarean rate has not been associated with differential improvement in neonatal outcome.
6. Gifford DS, et al. A meta-analysis of infant outcome after breech delivery. *Obstet Gynecol* 1995;85:1047.
   The authors report on the increased maternal risk from cesarean delivery and the increased risk of neonatal morbidity after trial of labor.

Studies of Breech Deliveries
7. Collea JV, Chein C, Quilligan EJ. The randomized management of term frank breech presentation: a study of 208 cases. *Am J Obstet Gynecol* 1980;137:235.
   No difference in fetal risk was observed between a selected trial of labor and elective cesarean section.
8. Gimovsky ML, et al. Randomized management of the non-frank breech presentation at term: a preliminary report. *Am J Obstet Gynecol* 1983;146:34.

Approximately one half of trial-of-labor cases may deliver vaginally and with neonatal morbidity similar to cesarean delivery.
9. Schiff E, et al. Maternal and neonatal outcome of 846 term singleton breech deliveries: seven-year experience at a single center. *Am J Obstet Gynecol* 1996;175:18.
   The authors discuss balancing the risk to the mother and fetus in obstetric decisions concerning route of delivery for the breech presentation.

Procedures
10. Johnson RL, Elliot JP. Fetal acoustic stimulation, an adjunct to external cephalic version: a blinded, randomized crossover study. *Am J Obstet Gynecol* 1995;173:1369.
    ECV can reduce the neonatal and maternal morbidity associated with breech presentation.
11. Schorr SJ, et al. A randomized trial of epidural anesthesia to improve external cephalic version success. *Am J Obstet Gynecol* 1997;177:1133.
    Transient fetal heart rate abnormalities are common following ECV, and the subsequent fetal outcome appears to be unrelated to these abnormalities.
12. Landy HJ, Zarate L, O'Sullivan MJ. Abdominal rescue using the vacuum extractor after entrapment of the aftercoming head. *Obstet Gynecol* 1994;84:644.
    Replacement of the fetus into the uterus for abdominal delivery in cases of failed vaginal delivery is termed the Zavanelli *maneuver.*

---

29. NONBREECH ABNORMAL PRESENTATIONS, POSITIONS, AND LIES

Michel E. Rivlin

In about 5% of cases, near term, a deviation from the normal vertical lie, cephalic presentation, and well-flexed attitude of the fetal head occurs, and such deviation constitutes a fetal malpresentation. In these instances, there is an increased risk to both the mother and the fetus. Malpresentations are often associated with fetal malformation and abnormal placentation, which require timely diagnostic exclusion. In general, closely monitored labor and vaginal delivery are possible with most malpresentations, but if normal progress in labor is not observed, cesarean section is usually indicated. The malpresentations reviewed in this chapter are transverse lie, face and brow presentation, compound presentations, and occipitoposterior position.

The lie of the fetus is the orientation of the fetal spine to the maternal spine. If these axes cross, the fetus is in a transverse or oblique lie, which would result in a shoulder or arm presentation. If the fetus is very mobile, the lie is unstable. Longitudinal lie occurs in 99% of laboring patients. An abnormal fetal lie is more common before term, occurring in about 2% of pregnancies at 32 weeks. If an abnormal lie persists beyond 37 weeks, rupture of membranes may result in cord prolapse.

Etiologic factors include great parity, prematurity, pelvic contracture, abnormal placentation, uterine malformation, hydramnios, and fetal anomalies. In twin gestations, 16% of the second twins are transverse during labor. Diagnosis is by abdominal palpation or vaginal examination and is confirmed via ultrasonography. The perinatal mortality rate varies from 3.9% to 24%. Fetal loss is associated with prolapsed cord (20 times as common as with cephalic presentation) or traumatic delivery. Maternal deaths may occur secondary to abnormal placentation, infection after premature rupture of membranes, or secondary to operative intervention or traumatic delivery.

A transverse/oblique or unstable lie late in pregnancy necessitates ultrasonography to exclude major fetal malformations and abnormal placentation: 10% to 15% of abnormal lies are associated with a low-lying or placenta previa. Expectant management is associated with significant risk, including cord prolapse, so that active intervention beyond 37 weeks, once lung maturity is confirmed, may be of benefit. External cephalic version (ECV) with subsequent induction of labor may be successful. The success of ECV is increased by the use of tocolytics, but abnormal bleeding, premature rupture of the membranes, and a previously scarred uterus are relative contraindications. Intrapartum ECV is also often successful, reducing the necessity for cesarean delivery by 50% in these patients. However, in the singleton pregnancy, if ECV fails beyond 39 weeks, or in labor, cesarean delivery is recommended. If membranes have ruptured, cesarean delivery is indicated and vaginal delivery is permitted only when the conceptus is small and nonviable. Internal podalic version and breech extraction may be indicated after ECV has failed in twin pregnancies, when the second fetus is transverse and greater than 1,500 g, but there is no place for this approach in singleton pregnancies because of the unacceptably high rate of fetal and maternal complications.

In cases of neglected transverse lies, the shoulder may become wedged in the pelvic canal with an arm prolapsed in the vagina. If left untreated, a pathologic uterine contraction ring (Bandl's ring) may form and the uterus may rupture. Immediate abdominal delivery is indicated to prevent maternal and fetal death. The choice of incision for cesarean section is affected by an abnormal axial lie. In general, a vertical incision is indicated, often extending into the upper uterine cavity as a classical cesarean incision; this is especially necessary if membranes are ruptured. This incision is chosen because the lower uterine segment is often poorly developed and to enable easy and atraumatic delivery of the fetus, which may become trapped if the customary lower segment transverse incision is attempted.

Full extension of the fetal head on the neck results in a face presentation. The fetal chin is the point of designation. The incidence is about one in 500 live births, with a perinatal mortality rate of 2% to 3%. As many as 60% are malformed, with anencephaly the cause of about one third of face presentations, and cephalopelvic disproportion is present in 10% to 40% of cases. Diagnosis is by vaginal examination and may be confirmed by ultrasonography or x-ray.

Mentum anterior (MA) occurs in 60% to 80%, mentum transverse (MT) in 10% to 12%, and mentum posterior (MP) in 20% to 25%. In the absence of disproportion, MA cases will deliver vaginally, most MT cases will rotate to MA and deliver vaginally, but only 25% to 33% of MP cases will rotate to MA and deliver vaginally. Persistent MP cases generally will not deliver vaginally, and cesarean section may be necessary. Overall, 12% to 30% of face presentations are delivered abdominally.

Prolonged labor is common, and abnormal fetal heart rate (FHR) patterns occur with increased frequency. If internal monitoring is used, careful placement of the electrode, preferably on the fetal chin, is required. Oxytocin is not contraindicated unless macrosomia or a small pelvis is identified. Outlet forceps delivery for the MA position is acceptable.

A brow presentation is midway between full flexion and full extension of the cephalic attitude (military position). The frontal bones are the point of designation. Incidence is about one in 1,500 deliveries, with a perinatal mortality rate of 1% to 8%. Etiologic factors in up to 60% include cephalopelvic disproportion, grand multiparity, and prematurity. Diagnosis is usually by vaginal examination (with x-ray or ultrasonographic confirmation), with frontum anterior the most common position. A persistent brow, that is, one that does not convert by flexion to vertex or extension to face, requires engagement and descent of the largest (mentooccipital) diameter of the head (14 cm). This could only occur with a small infant and a large pelvis. Trial of labor with close monitoring may be appropriate, and oxytocin is not contraindicated in the well-selected patient. Prolonged labor is common, and fewer than half of the infants with persistent brow presentations deliver spontaneously. If brow presentation persists with a large baby, cesarean delivery is indicated. Manipulation of the brow to a more favorable position is not recommended.

A compound presentation is diagnosed whenever an extremity is found prolapsed beside a major presenting fetal pole. The combination of an upper extremity and the vertex is the most common combination. An incidence ranging from one in 377 to one in 1,213 deliveries is quoted. Diagnosis is by vaginal examination, and prematurity is the most common etiologic factor. Perinatal mortality is increased, with fetal risk due to cord prolapse (11%–20%) and birth trauma, the latter usually involving neurologic and musculoskeletal damage to the prolapsed extremity. Most of these women may be delivered vaginally with close fetal monitoring and nonmanipulation of the extremity. Indications for cesarean delivery include cord prolapse, fetal distress, and failure to progress. Vaginal delivery is more often successful with a small infant, with cesarean delivery frequently necessary for the term-sized infant.

The occipitoposterior (OP) position is the most common malposition, with 5% of deliveries occurring as persistent OP. However, 87% of fetuses that enter labor as OP rotate into an occipitoanterior (OA) position and deliver without significant prolongation of labor. The android or anthropoid pelvic shapes predispose to OP, and the android and platypelloid shapes predispose to the occipitotransverse (OT) position. The second stage of labor is frequently prolonged, but the rates of perinatal morbidity and mortality are no different from those of the OA position. The diagnosis is made by vaginal examination. In the event of persistent OP or OT positions and a prolonged second stage, manual rotation of the occiput to OA may be attempted. Frequently, the fetus will deliver OP with the aid of an episiotomy and adequate anesthesia. Forceps rotation with specialized forceps (Kjelland, Barton's) or with the Scanzoni maneuver (rotation from OP to OA with forceps reapplication) is seldom used except by those experienced with the technique and in the absence of any cephalopelvic disproportion. Vacuum extraction is another option. If a trial of forceps fails, cesarean section is indicated.

Transverse Lie
1. Hankins GDV, et al. Transverse lie. *Am J Perinatol* 1990;7:66.
   In parturients at term who presented in active labor with a transverse lie, the incidence of fetal acidosis and trauma was found to be increased. Active intervention consisting of external version followed by labor induction (or cesarean delivery for version failures) was advocated beyond 38 weeks' gestation.
2. Edwards RI, Nicholson HO. The management of the unstable lie in late pregnancy. *J Obstet Gynaecol Br Commonw* 1969;76:713.
   Abdominal binders may help prevent spontaneous return to an abnormal lie after ECV and induction of labor.
3. Pelosi MA, et al. The intra-abdominal version technique for delivery of transverse lie by low segment cesarean section. *Am J Obstet Gynecol* 1985;135:1009.
   The authors describe a technique of intraabdominal version for delivery of the infant in the transverse lie, to avoid using the classic cesarean delivery and permit the more desirable low transverse cervical cesarean incision to be made.
4. Bethune M, Permezel M. The relationship between gestational age and the incidence of classical caesarean section. *Aust N Z J Obstet Gynecol* 1997;37:153.
   Most women having a classical cesarean section at term had either a transverse lie or a major degree of placenta previa.
5. Dildy GA, et al. Very advanced maternal age: pregnancy after age 45. *Am J Obstet Gynecol* 1996;175(Pt 1):668.
   Cesarean section rate was 31.7%; the most frequent indication was abnormal lie.
6. Thorp JM, Jenkins TJ, Watson W. Utility of Leopold maneuvers in screening for malpresentation. *Obstet Gynecol* 1991;78:394.
   Systematic abdominal palpation (Leopold maneuvers) for fetal lie and presenting part provide an excellent screening tool, and may indicate the need for sonography to confirm the initial findings.

Face and Brow
7. Cruikshank DP, Cruikshank JE. Face and brow presentation: a review. *Clin Obstet Gynecol* 1981;24:333.
   In 91% of brow presentations with an adequate pelvis, conversion to face or vertex leads to vaginal delivery. In the presence of pelvic contracture, only 20% deliver vaginally.

8. Levy DL. Persistent brow presentation—a new approach to management. *South Med J* 1976;69:191.
   Fewer than 50% of brow presentations are detected before the second stage of labor, and many only during delivery.
9. Watson WJ, Read JA. Electronic fetal monitoring in face presentation at term. *Milit Med* 1987;152:324.
   The incidence of abnormal FHR patterns is up to 53% with face presentations.
10. Neuman M, et al. Intrapartum bimanual tocolytic-assisted reversal of face presentation: preliminary report. *Obstet Gynecol* 1994;84:146.
    Conversion of mentoposterior to occipitoanterior, followed by vaginal delivery, was successful in 10 of 11 women in whom cesarean section was not possible.

Compound
11. Breen JL, Wiesmelen E. Compound presentation—a survey of 131 patients. *Obstet Gynecol* 1968;32:419.
    The authors reported a 2% cesarean rate, whereas others have reported rates as high as 25%.
12. Cruikshank DP, White CA. Obstetric malpresentations—twenty years experience. *Am J Obstet Gynecol* 1973;116:1097.
    Seventy-five percent of vertex/upper extremity combinations deliver spontaneously.
13. Ang LT. Compound presentation following external version. *Aust N Z J Obstet Gynaecol* 1978;19:213.
    The author discusses the unusual complication of external version.

Occipitoposterior/Occipitotransverse
14. Gardberg M, Laakkonen E, Salevaara M. Intrapartum sonography and persistent occiput posterior position: a study of 408 deliveries. *Obstet Gynecol* 1998;91 (Pt 1):746.
    In most cases persistent occipitoposterior (OP) presentation develops through a malrotation and only in about one-third of cases through absence of rotation from an initially OP position.
15. Gardberg M, Tuppurainen M. Persistent occiput posterior presentation—a clinical problem. *Acta Obstet Gynecol Scand* 1994;73:45.
    The authors report a frequency of 4.7%, higher birth weight, and longer labor, less than half delivered without operative intervention.
16. Kuo YC, Chen CP, Wang KG. Factors influencing the prolonged second stage and the effects on perinatal and maternal outcomes. *J Obstet Gynaecol Res* 1996; 22:253.
    Persistent OP presentation is significantly associated with a prolonged second stage of labor.
17. Hawkins JL, et al. A reevaluation of the association between instrument delivery and epidural analgesia. *Reg Anesth* 1995;20:50.
    Transverse and OP positions are independently associated with an increase in the incidence of instrument delivery independent of epidural use.

---

30. HYDRAMNIOS AND OLIGOHYDRAMNIOS

Richard L. Rosemond

Hydramnios (polyhydramnios) is an excessive amount of amniotic fluid, whereas oligohydramnios is an abnormally low volume of amniotic fluid. The uterus at term contains 800 to 1,000 ml of fluid. Volumes of greater than 2,000 ml or less than 400 ml are abnormal and indicate a pregnancy at risk for adverse outcome.

The incidence of *hydramnios* ranges from 0.4% to 1.5%. The volume of amniotic fluid depends on the relative rates of production from the fetal kidneys and transudation through the fetal skin, versus consumption through the process of fetal swallowing and reabsorption in the lungs. Most explainable causes of hydramnios result from an excess urine production or decreased absorption by the gastrointestinal system. Approximately 20% of the cases of hydramnios are associated with congenital malformations. These include (1) central nervous system disorders (52%; i.e., anencephaly); (2) cardiovascular disorders (30%; i.e., arrhythmia, coarctation, and hydrops); (3) gastrointestinal tract disorders (47%; i.e., facial clefts, duodenal atresia, diaphragmatic hernia, and abdominal wall defects); (4) respiratory disorders (i.e., cystic adenomatoid malformation and pulmonary sequestration); (5) musculoskeletal defects (19%; i.e., thanatophoric dwarf); and (6) genitourinary anomalies (16%; i.e., ureteropelvic junction obstruction and posterior urethral valves). Another 25% of the cases of hydramnios are associated with diabetes mellitus. Multiple gestation and isoimmunization each account for 10% of the cases; however, the most common cause of hydramnios remains idiopathic (35%).

Chromosomal abnormalities have been reported in mothers with hydramnios, but at this time there is not enough evidence to support routine karyotype testing in these patients, unless associated with other anomalies, IUGR, or abnormal Doppler findings.

Hydramnios should be suspected whenever the uterus is larger than expected for a particular gestational age, there is difficulty palpating the fetus, or the fetal heart tones are difficult to hear with the fetoscope. The volume of amniotic fluid should then be assessed ultrasonographically. There is controversy regarding the best technique to use for confirming the diagnosis. The most common methods are subjective impression, measuring the largest vertical pocket, and calculating an amniotic fluid index. The last technique involves dividing the uterus into four quadrants, using the umbilicus as the center point, and then measuring the largest vertical pocket of each quadrant in centimeters and adding the four values. This index is then compared with a table of normal values, and hydramnios is diagnosed if the index value is greater than the 95th percentile for that gestational age. In sheep models, this was found to be 88% accurate, with intraobserver and interobserver errors averaging 1 and 2 cm, respectively.

Maternal complications associated with hydramnios include preterm labor, premature ruptured membranes, maternal discomfort, and respiratory compromise. The incidence of these complications is even greater when the evolution of the hydramnios is acute (days) rather than chronic (weeks).

The treatment of hydramnios should be directed at the underlying cause, when this is known. Correction of a fetal arrhythmia or improvement in maternal glycemic control are examples of directed therapy. When a specific cause is not identified, generally no treatment is indicated unless maternal complications develop (i.e., premature labor or respiratory compromise). Treatment is either surgical or medical. Surgical therapy consists of amniocentesis, with removal of sometimes tremendous quantities of amniotic fluid. Care is taken not to decompress the uterine cavity so rapidly as to cause an abruption. From personal experience, removal of 1,000 ml of fluid over 10 to 15 minutes seems safe. This procedure can be repeated many times; however, each additional procedure carries an additional risk of precipitating preterm labor, premature ruptured membranes, abruption, and amnionitis. In addition, maternal discomfort and the cost of the procedure should be considered.

Medical therapy consists of the administration of indomethacin (25 mg orally every 6 hours). The mechanism of action appears to be a decrease in urine output and subsequent decrease in the amniotic fluid volume. It has the added benefit of being an effective tocolytic agent; however, there are risks and contraindications to consider. Indomethacin should not be given to any woman beyond 34 weeks' gestation because the risk of fetal ductal constriction increases after this time. Similarly, fetuses should be screened for any kind of ductal-dependent heart defect prior to administration. The fluid volume usually decreases steadily when this treatment is used, but it may be several days or even weeks before the desired level is reached. Monitoring during this time should include weekly fluid volume assessment and Doppler evaluation of ductal flow.

Multiple gestation can pose a unique problem to the obstetrician, in that hydramnios of one twin can exist simultaneously with oligohydramnios of the other. This represents the stuck twin phenomenon, and may reflect the twin-twin transfusion syndrome. Although this generally carries a poor prognosis, one study revealed favorable outcomes following serial therapeutic amniocentesis.

In summary, patients identified with hydramnios should undergo a careful anatomic ultrasonographic examination to detect any structural abnormalities and rule out macrosomia. The diabetes mellitus status of the patient should be assessed, and treatment should be instituted if a cause is found or if maternal complications warrant. Amniocentesis is offered if other anomalies or abnormal Doppler velocimetry is found.

Oligohydramnios may be suspected when the size of the uterus is less than that expected for a particular gestational age, when there is evidence of fetal crowding, or when variable decelerations appear during fetal monitoring. The diagnosis is confirmed by ultrasonography. Again, oligohydramnios can be determined either by a subjective assessment of the fluid volume, or by an objective one, using the 5th percentile of the amniotic fluid index as the cutoff.

Oligohydramnios occurs in approximately 4% of pregnancies. The most common causes include ruptured membranes, intrauterine growth restriction (IUGR), postdates syndrome, and fetal anomalies. The presence of oligohydramnios together with ruptured membranes may be associated with a decreased latency period and an increased risk of infection; however, this is not necessarily an indication for delivery. As the placental blood flow to an IUGR fetus decreases, the blood in the fetus is shunted away from the kidneys and urine output decreases. The presence of oligohydramnios, therefore, is a marker for the more severe forms of IUGR. Abnormal Doppler flow measurements of the umbilical and uterine system may identify the fetus at greater risk for an adverse outcome in this scenario. If oligohydramnios occurs before the third trimester, or there is no explanation for the decreased placental function, chromosome analysis should be considered. Fetal anomalies known to cause oligohydramnios include renal obstruction or agenesis. The absence of fetal kidneys is called Potter syndrome and results in typical facies and skeletal malformations as well as lung hypoplasia. This is a fatal condition. When there is urinary obstruction and subsequent oligohydramnios, delivery may be indicated, except in the very premature fetus, which might benefit from an in utero shunt procedure.

The fetus in an environment of oligohydramnios is at risk for cord compression and subsequent demise. If diagnosed before term, careful fetal ultrasonographic assessment with biometry, anomaly screening, and Doppler velocimetry should be performed followed by aggressive fetal monitoring (nonstress tests and/or biophysical profiles, one to two times per week) and consideration of delivery when fetal maturity is present. The development of oligohydramnios at term and beyond is an indication for delivery. Patients who present in labor with significant variable decelerations have been treated with amnioinfusion, with resolution of the variable decelerations in some cases. Amnioinfusion is performed by placement of an intrauterine pressure catheter and infusion of 500 ml of warmed normal saline or lactated Ringer solution, followed by continuous infusion at a rate of 100 to 200 ml/h. Overdistention of the uterus must be avoided. This technique also has been used to decrease the incidence of meconium aspiration syndrome. Amnioinfusion (via amniocentesis) also has been used to improve visualization for the anatomic evaluation of a fetus with oligohydramnios.

In summary, oligohydramnios can be associated with ruptured membranes, anomalies, aneuploidy, or uteroplacental insufficiency; however, frequently, no cause is discovered. Regardless, the pregnancy is considered high risk and needs to be monitored aggressively. When discovered at the extremes of gestational age (i.e., <22 weeks and >41 weeks), delivery can be considered.

General
1. Bruce RA. Physiology of amniotic fluid volume regulation. *Clin Obstet Gynecol* 1997;40:280.
   A basic overview of amniotic fluid production and regulation.

2. Moise KJ. Polyhydramnios. *Clin Obstet Gynecol* 1997;40:266.
   An excellent review of the subject covering definition, evaluation, therapy, and complications. Sixty-five references are cited.
3. Peipert JF, Donnenfeld AE. Oligohydramnios: a review. *Obstet Gynecol Surv* 1991;46:325.
   This is a comprehensive review of the topic of oligohydramnios covering diagnosis, prognosis, and management, and including more than 150 references.

Etiology
4. Barnhard Y, Bar-Hava I, Hivon MY. Is polyhydramnios in an ultrasonographically normal fetus an indication for genetic evaluation? *Am J Obstet Gynecol* 1995; 173:1523.
   The authors concluded that patients with hydramnios and IUGR or structural anomalies need genetic evaluation but not if the fetus is sonographically normal.
5. Landy HJ, Isada NB, Larsen JW Jr. Genetic implications of idiopathic hydramnios. *Am J Obstet Gynecol* 1987;157:114.
   Hydramnios is often associated with chromosomal abnormalities.
6. Hendricks SK, et al. Diagnosis of polyhydramnios in early gestation: indication for prenatal diagnosis? *Prenat Diagn* 1991;11:649.
   Of 138 cases of polyhydramnios, there were seven involving chromosomal abnormalities; all were associated with other ultrasonographic findings. The authors doubt the need for amniocentesis after the diagnosis of early polyhydramnios.
7. Hickok DE, et al. Unexplained second trimester oligohydramnios: a clinical pathologic study. *Am J Perinatol* 1989;6:8.
   The authors emphasize the importance of oligohydramnios in the absence of fetal malformations as a cause of adverse pregnancy outcome. Hypoplastic lungs as well as cord accidents were more common.
8. Many A, Lazebrik N, Hill LM. The underlying cause of polyhydramnios determines prematurity. *Prenat Diagn* 1996;16:55.
   Preterm delivery occurred in 36% of fetuses with malformations, 27% with diabetes, and only 14% if the hydramnios was unexplained.
9. Bruner JP, Rosemond RL. Twin-to-twin transfusion syndrome: a subset of the twin oligohydramnios-polyhydramnios sequence. *Am J Obstet Gynecol* 1993; 169:925.
   True twin-twin transfusion existed in only 44% of those pregnancies initially fulfilling clinical criteria for the diagnosis.

Diagnosis
10. Quetal TA, et al. Amnioinfusion: an aid in the ultrasonic evaluation of severe oligohydramnios in pregnancy. *Am J Obstet Gynecol* 1992;167:333.
    The diagnostic capability was improved in 13 patients who presented with early oligohydramnios by the transabdominal infusion of warmed saline and indigo-carmine dye.
11. Phelan JP, et al. Amniotic fluid index measurements during pregnancy. *J Reprod Med* 1987;32:601.
    The technique for quantitative assessment of amniotic fluid volume is detailed in this report.
12. Moore TR. Superiority of the four-quadrant sum over the single deepest pocket technique in ultrasonic identification of abnormal amniotic fluid volumes. *Am J Obstet Gynecol* 1990;163:762.
    Maximum vertical pocket measurements failed to identify 58 percent of the cases of oligohydramnios identified by the amniotic fluid index.
13. Lombardi SJ, Rosemond RL, Ball R. Umbilical artery velocimetry as a predictor of adverse outcome in pregnancies complicated by oligohydramnios. *Obstet Gynecol* 1989;74:338.
    The findings from umbilical Doppler flow studies were found to be predictive of an adverse outcome in patients with unexplained oligohydramnios.

Treatment
14. Wenstrom F, Andrews WW, Maher JE. Amnioinfusion survey: prevalence, protocols, and complications. *Obstet Gynecol* 1995;86:572.
   A survey of the techniques and complications of amnioinfusion. Complications were observed in 1% to 14% of patients.
15. Elliott JP, Urig MA, Clewell WH. Aggressive therapeutic amniocentesis for treatment of twin-twin transfusion syndrome. *Obstet Gynecol* 1991;77:537.
   The authors report on 17 cases of twin-twin transfusion, with a remarkable 79% perinatal rate of survival.
16. Moise KJ. Indomethacin therapy in the treatment of symptomatic polyhydramnios. *Clin Obstet Gynecol* 1991;34:310.
   Indomethacin treatment was successful in 36 of 38 cases, with attainment of normal fluid volume in 4 to 20 days.
17. Vergani P, Ceruti P, Strobelt N. Transabdominal amnioinfusion in oligohydramnios at term before induction of labor with intact membranes: a randomized clinical trial. *Am J Obstet Gynecol* 1996;175:465.
   The incidences of abnormal fetal heart rate tracings and cesarean section for fetal distress were lower in the treatment group.

Complications
18. Lawrence S, Rosenfeld CR. Fetal pulmonary development and abnormalities of amniotic fluid volume. *Semin Perinatol* 1996;10:142.
   This is a review of the pathophysiologic characteristics of lung hypoplasia in the setting of oligohydramnios and includes data from both animal and human studies.
19. Vintzileos AM, et al. Degree of oligohydramnios and pregnancy outcome in patients with premature rupture of the membranes. *Obstet Gynecol* 1985;66:162.
   These authors showed that oligohydramnios, occurring after premature rupture of membranes that lasted for more than several days, correlated with a poor outcome in the fetus.
20. Major CA, Kitzmiller JL. Perinatal survival with expectant management of midtrimester rupture of membranes. *Am J Obstet Gynecol* 1990;163:838.
   The authors report on the improved perinatal survival rates as neonatal care has become more sophisticated. This report gives survival statistics that can be used in counseling patients.
21. Kilpatrick SJ. Therapeutic interventions for oligohydramnios: amnioinfusion and maternal hydration. *Clin Obstet Gynecol* 1997;40:328.
   This report summarizes the efforts that have been made to improve the amniotic fluid volume, including risks, benefits, and complications.

VII. LABOR AND DELIVERY

31. ANALGESIA AND ANESTHESIA FOR LABOR AND DELIVERY

L. Wayne Hess, Randall C. Floyd, Robert F. Fraser II,
and Susan E. Winkelmann

The use of medications during the intrapartum period must be carefully assessed because they may potentiate the physiologic effects of pregnancy in the mother and may adversely affect the fetus. It is important to conduct antepartum and intrapartum risk assessment to detect maternal and fetal complications before introducing other variables such as analgesia and anesthesia. Although there is a trend toward a more family-oriented and natural approach to the birth process, many patients elect to receive analgesia or anesthesia during labor and delivery. Additionally, litigation has ensued when adequate pain relief has been refused to a patient during labor. The type of analgesia or anesthesia can be selected only after the history, physical findings, obstetrics conditions, and desires of the patient are evaluated in the context of the practices and philosophy of the obstetrician and anesthesiologist. Although many patients and physicians prefer regional anesthesia, systemic analgesics are the primary form of pain relief used in the practice of obstetrics in the United States, and most of this analgesia is provided by obstetricians.

Careful analgesia and anesthesia risk assessment in the antenatal period is particularly important for those gravidas at particular risk for adverse events. Referral to an anesthesiologist for consultation much in advance of labor and delivery is preferential. This allows a careful evaluation and thoughtful planning for labor and delivery pain relief. It also allows discussion with the gravida concerning her diagnosis and the risks, benefits, alternatives, indications, prognosis, and expected outcome of the various methods of pain relief. All patients with morbid obesity (weight greater than 250–275 pounds, in whom difficult intubation is a major risk), major illnesses, difficulty with prior anesthesia, spinal injury at risk for autonomic hyperreflexia, and so forth should be referred for antepartum anesthesia consultation.

Almost every drug used for analgesia in the mother during labor crosses the placenta and can affect the fetus. Most analgesic agents are small in molecular weight (<1,000 daltons), are lipid soluble, and have a high negative logarithm of the dissociation constant (pKa), thus allowing for easy transit across the placenta. Narcotic agents, principally meperidine (Demerol), are the most common type of analgesic administered during pregnancy. In most cases, meperidine, given in 25- to 50-mg increments every 2 to 4 hours, is sufficient for pain relief during labor and has little effect on the fetus other than decreasing the beat-to-beat variability of the fetal heart. At these dosage levels, if the fetus is depressed at birth, invariably it is not due to the analgesic. Although neurobehavioral changes have been associated with meperidine usage, the effects are self-limited and have no long-term consequences. Additionally, some clinicians have interdicted meperidine just before parturition because of the risk of fetal depression. However, most agree that the drug should not be withheld because the patient is going to deliver within the next 1 to 2 hours.

Regional anesthesia is used more today in obstetrics than ever before. The use of segmental epidural blocks has gained wide popularity in the United States. Intrathecal narcotics (with or without bupivacaine) and epidural narcotics (with or without bupivacaine) have also gained wide acceptance for pain relief with labor. Epidural analgesia using the amide derivative drugs (lidocaine and bupivacaine) may selectively block uterine pain during labor and has the advantage of also being able to render satisfactory anesthesia for delivery. Complications include inadvertent entry into the spinal canal and hypotension. Paresthesia, an infrequent complication, usually occurs with the ester-based local anesthetics (2-chloroprocaine). Direct toxicity with high percentage bupivacaine (0.75%) has been observed after epidural anesthesia. In addition, many obstetricians believe that the use of conduction anesthesia prolongs labor and leads to an increased incidence of fetuses in the transverse (vertex) position and the subsequent need for mid-forceps rotation or cesarean section. The adverse effects on the mother and fetus in this setting, however, are generally outweighed by the benefits of this type of anesthesia.

Psychoprophylaxis (prepared childbirth) also has gained wide acceptance in this country as a method of analgesia in labor and, if successful, is very rewarding for the parturient and her support person. If unsuccessful, small doses of analgesic agents can be administered, and this permits the parturient to still actively participate in the birth process. It is necessary to tailor psychoprophylaxis to each patient rather than to enforce a rigid protocol of analgesia versus no analgesia because hyperventilation with resultant hypocapnia and epinephrine release may result in fetal hypoxia directly related to natural childbirth.

Sedatives and hypnotics are now used infrequently in labor and delivery suites. Barbiturate usage, at least during the active intrapartum phase of labor, is almost entirely limited to the induction of general anesthesia for cesarean birth. For vaginal deliveries, these agents are best avoided because they are ineffective analgesic agents and there are disadvantages associated with their use in both the mother and fetus.

The Duke inhaler, the intermittent administration of anesthetic gases such as methoxyflurane or nitrous oxide, and twilight sleep (morphine and scopolamine) are not popular and are now considered inadvisable for use in intrapartum analgesia. Once popular narcotic analgesics such as alphaprodine (Nisentil) and anileridine (Leritine) are no longer marketed in the United States. Other marketed narcotics such as fentanyl (Sublimaze), sufentanil (Sufenta), codeine, buprenorphine (Buprenex), oxymorphone (Numorphan), and hydromorphone (Dilaudid) are not approved by the U.S. Food and Drug Administration, nor are they recommended by the manufacturers for use as intrapartum analgesics.

Anesthesia for vaginal delivery now rarely includes low spinal (saddle block) anesthesia. This method provides good relaxation for a forceps delivery, if this proves necessary. Hypotension is the principal problem that may arise and must be prevented by ensuring adequate hydration and wedging the patient to prevent development of the supine hypotensive syndrome. The use of local agents such as lidocaine provides analgesia to the episiotomy site and allows for episiotomy repair. Pudendal anesthesia is also frequently used but carries a high degree of partial effects even in the best hands.

Anesthesia for cesarean delivery can be accomplished by general or regional means. Regional anesthesia includes the epidural or spinal techniques. For cesarean birth, regional anesthesia up to the T10 dermatome is the objective. For both regional techniques, hypotension is the principal danger, but it can be prevented by maintaining adequate hydration and by wedging (tilting) the patient to prevent the supine hypotension syndrome from developing. Balanced endotracheal anesthesia using rapid induction, in which intravenous barbiturates and a muscle relaxant are given, is equally efficacious for providing anesthesia in abdominal deliveries. If the patient's case is uncomplicated, the team gathered for the procedure (anesthesiologists, pediatrician, and obstetrician) can usually allow the patient to choose the method of anesthesia. In complicated cases, the obstetric anesthesiologist in consultation with the perinatologist and neonatologist should decide the best method of anesthesia for delivery.

The use of new agents (such as transcutaneous nerve stimulation) holds promise for the future. Other analgesia and anesthesia techniques include hypnosis and acupuncture. These techniques, although demonstrated effectively in some studies, have not generally been accepted by the medical community. Additionally, patient-controlled analgesia is becoming increasingly popular for labor analgesia.

General
1. Bonica JJ, McDonald JS. *Principles and practice of obstetric analgesia and anesthesia,* 2nd ed. Malvern, PA: Williams & Wilkins, 1995.
   This is the definitive textbook for pain relief during labor, delivery, or surgery with pregnancy.

2. Cohen S. Strategies for labor pain relief—past, present and future. *Acta Anaesthesiol Scand Suppl* 1997;110:17.
   The is a comprehensive review of labor pain relief.
3. Faure EA. The pain of parturition. *Semin Perinatol* 1991;15:342.
   A general review of the physiology of pain during labor.
4. Samuels P. Advances in anesthesia and pharmacology in the puerperium. *Curr Opin Obstet Gynecol* 1991;3:773.
   This is an excellent review of the pharmacology of labor analgesia.
5. Ranta P, et al. Paracervical block—a viable alternative for labor pain relief? *Acta Obstet Gynecol Scand* 1995;74:122.
   This is a comprehensive review of paracervical block.
6. Rosaeg OP, Yarnell RW, Lindsay MP. The obstetrical anaesthesia assessment clinic: a review of six years experience. *Can J Anaesth* 1993;40:346.
   The authors review antepartum anesthesia consultation and its benefits.

Parenteral Analgesia
7. Kuhnert BR, et al. Disposition of meperidine and normeperidine following multiple doses during labor. I. Fetus and neonate. *Am J Obstet Gynecol* 1985;151:410.
   The administration of multiple doses of meperidine with a long drug-to-delivery interval results in the accumulation of normeperidine in fetal tissues and subsequent neonatal depression.
8. Gambling DR, White PF. Role of patient-controlled epidural analgesia in obstetrics. *Eur J Obstet Gynecol Reprod Biol* 1995;59[Suppl]:39.
   This is a review of patient-controlled epidural analgesia.
9. Ward ME. Acute pain and the obstetrics patient: recent developments in analgesia for labor and delivery. *Int Anesthesiol Clin* 1997;35:83.
   The author reports on new methods of analgesia with labor.
10. Dan U, et al. Intravenous pethidine and nalbuphine during labor: a prospective double-blind comparative study. *Gynecol Obstet Invest* 1991;32:39.
    The authors report on a comparison of Demerol and Nubain for analgesia.
11. Berg TG, Rayburn WF. Effects of analgesia on labor. *Clin Obstet Gynecol* 1992;35:457.
    This is a review of the possible risks of analgesia during labor.

Regional Analgesia and Anesthesia
12. Eddleston JM, et al. Comparison of the maternal and fetal effects associated with intermittent or continuous infusion of extradural analgesia. *Br J Anaesth* 1992; 69:154.
    Minimal fetal effects are associated with epidural anesthesia.
13. Curran MJ. Options for labor analgesia: techniques of epidural and spinal analgesia. *Semin Perinatol* 1991;15:348.
    This is a general review of the regional methods used to achieve analgesia for labor.
14. Goins JR. Experiences with mepivacaine paracervical block in an obstetric private practice. *Am J Obstet Gynecol* 1992;167:342.
    Introduction of a paracervical block during labor appears beneficial and is associated with minimal risks.
15. Morgan B. Combined spinal and epidural blockade for analgesia in labour. *Eur J Obstet Gynecol Reprod Biol* 1995;59[Suppl]:59.
    The author reports on combined spinal and epidural anesthesia.
16. Morgan P. Spinal anaesthesia in obstetrics. *Can J Anaesth* 1995;42:1145.
    A comprehensive review of spinal anesthesia in obstetrics.
17. Lyon DS, et al. The effect of instituting an elective labor epidural program on the operative delivery rate. *Obstet Gynecol* 1997;90:135.
    The operative delivery rate was not increased with epidural use in labor.
18. Ramin SM, et al. Randomized trial of epidural versus intravenous analgesia during labor. *Obstet Gynecol* 1995;86:783.
    Epidural anesthesia increased the risk of uterine infection and prolonged labor, and necessitated more operative deliveries in this study.

Psychologic Analgesia
19. Bernat SH, et al. Biofeedback assisted relaxation to reduce stress in labor. *J Obstet Gynecol Neonat Nurs* 1992;21:295.
    This is a review of the various relaxation techniques to decrease the pain of labor.
20. Hodnett E. Nursing support of the laboring woman. *J Obstet Gynecol Neonat Nurs* 1996;25:257.
    The importance of nursing support during labor is discussed.

General Anesthesia
21. Yam I, Rubin AP. Emergency caesarean section. *Br J Hosp Med* 1992;48:244.
    The methods of anesthesia for emergency delivery are reviewed.
22. Dick W, et al. General anesthesia versus epidural anesthesia for primary caesarean section—a comparative study. *Eur J Anaesthesiol* 1992;9:15.
    The comparative risks of general versus regional anesthesia during labor are analyzed.
23. Marx GF, Katsnelson T. The introduction of nitrous oxide analgesia into obstetrics. *Obstet Gynecol* 1992;80:715.
    The authors provide a historic review of balanced anesthesia in labor.
24. Finster M, et al. Obstetric anesthesia. *Minerva Anestesiol* 1992;58:853.
    A review of general anesthesia in labor is given.

Complications
25. Rasmussen GE, Malinow AM. Toward reducing maternal mortality: the problem airway in obstetrics. *Int Anesthesiol Clin* 1994;32:83.
    The authors offer tips for the problem airway.
26. Norman PF, Eichhorn JH. Management of anesthetic complications and emergencies in the obstetric patient. *Obstet Gynecol Clin North Am* 1995;22:1.
    The complications of obstetric anesthesia and their management are discussed.
27. Willatts S. Anaesthetic lessons to be learnt from confidential inquiries into maternal death. *Acta Anaesthesiol Scand Suppl* 1997;110:25.
    The author presents a review of anesthetic maternal death.

32. FORCEPS AND VACUUM EXTRACTION

Richard L. Rosemond and Rudolph P. Fedrizzi

The American College of Obstetricians and Gynecologists has defined the following categories of forceps operations. An *outlet forceps delivery* is one in which (1) the skull is visible at the introitus without separating the labia, (2) the fetal skull has reached the pelvic floor, (3) the sagittal sutures are in the anteroposterior position, and (4) the fetal head is at or on the perineum. According to this definition, rotation cannot exceed 45 degrees. The application of forceps when the leading point of the skull is at +2 station or more, but other criteria for outlet forceps extraction are not met, is termed a *low-forceps delivery*. The low-forceps delivery has two subdivisions: (1) rotation 45 degrees or less (e.g., left occiput anterior to occiput anterior and left occiput posterior to occiput posterior) and (2) rotation more than 45 degrees. The application of forceps when the head is engaged but the leading point of the skull is above the +2 station is called a *mid-forceps delivery*. Under unusual circumstances, such as the sudden onset of severe fetal or maternal compromise, application of forceps above the +2 station but below or equal to the zero station may be attempted while simultaneously initiating preparation for cesarean delivery in the event that the forceps maneuver is unsuccessful. Forceps should not be applied to an unengaged head or when the cervix has not completely dilated.

The forceps instrument is described in terms of its design with special reference to the blade (solid or fenestrated), the pelvic curve (straight or curved), the cephalic curve (wide or narrow), the shanks (separate or overlapping), the lock (English or sliding), and the handle. There are many different models of forceps from which to choose, and each has its own particular application. The Simpson, Elliott, and Tucker-McLean instruments are classic outlet forceps. The latter two are used primarily for the unmolded head, with the difference being that the blade on the Elliott forceps is fenestrated and the blade of the Tucker-McLean forceps is not. Simpson forceps are preferred for the larger molded head. Specialized forceps such as the Kielland and Barton are used primarily for rotation. The Keilland has an absent pelvic curve, and the resulting rotational motion is much like the action of a key in a lock. The Barton forceps are used to deliver the head through a platypelloid pelvis. Piper forceps are used for the aftercoming head in a breech delivery.

The indication for the use of forceps should be clearly documented in the patient's chart. Accepted indications include the presence of maternal diseases (cardiac, cerebrovascular, or pulmonary), which may worsen with prolonged pushing or maternal exhaustion, or an inability to push effectively secondary to excessive analgesia or lack of cooperation. Fetal indications include fetal distress, malposition, asynclitism, and deflexion. Another indication is a prolonged second stage, which is defined as greater than 2 hours in the nulliparous patient and greater than 1 hour in the parous patient. An additional hour is added if conduction anesthesia is used. However, before an operative vaginal delivery is attempted because of a prolonged second stage, the operator must be sure that cephalopelvic disproportion is not present. There is hardly a worse scenario than to forcibly deliver the head and have a shoulder dystocia occur.

Prerequisites for applying forceps include (1) complete cervical dilatation, (2) ruptured membranes, (3) an engaged head, (4) known fetal position, (5) adequate analgesia, (6) assessment of the maternal pelvis–fetal size relationship, (7) capability for performing a cesarean section, (8) empty bladder and rectum, and (9) presence of an experienced operator. Deviations from these requirements can result in a poor outcome.

Controversy regarding the safety of forceps-assisted deliveries persists to the present time. However, a large study conducted by the Collaborative Perinatal Project involving approximately 30,000 babies, all undergoing periodic examinations for up to 4 years, failed to reveal any evidence that forceps operations increased the hazard of neonatal death or were associated with subsequent neurologic impairment of the neonates. Another large retrospective study from Israel revealed no physical or cognitive differences at 17 years of age among those born by instrumental vaginal, spontaneous vaginal, or cesarean section delivery. Conflicting data also surround midforceps delivery. This problem exists because some forceps operations are easy, whereas others are difficult; and a fair comparison cannot be made between the two. Regardless, persisting in attempts to effect vaginal delivery when it is obviously difficult may lead to unfavorable results. The maternal pelvic tissue is more frequently injured during these types of deliveries.

Over the past decade, there has been a decline in the frequency of forceps-assisted vaginal delivery and a reluctance to use mid-forceps extraction. According to a recent survey of residency programs, 36% do not even teach the techniques of mid-forceps delivery. This is alarming, for almost every obstetrician has been in a situation where fetal distress is present and a cesarean delivery is not immediately possible. A skillful forceps delivery in this scenario can be lifesaving.

Whereas forceps have been used in obstetrics for over four centuries, the vacuum extractor has been in use for only four decades. This device consists of a metal or plastic cup through which a vacuum suction is created after application to the fetal head. Traction is then applied during contractions. The force of suction should not exceed 0.8 kg/cm^2.

A definitive study comparing vacuum extraction to forceps delivery suggests that vacuum extraction is associated with decreased maternal morbidity. Other advantages include its ease of application and the need for less anesthesia. The vacuum extractor also can be applied without decreasing the station of the head. It takes up very little space in the vagina and does not cause deflexion of the head. It also can be used in special circumstances such as when fetal distress occurs in a second vertex twin when the station precludes the use of forceps, or for delivery of the fetal head through the uterine incision during a cesarean section.

Disadvantages include causing increased scalp trauma to the fetus and increased failure-to-deliver rate. Fortunately, most of the trauma is mild in nature and rarely clinically serious. The artificial caput (chignon) that is created usually resolves within several hours, but may persist for 1 to 2 days. More important complications include subgaleal and retinal hemorrhages.

The indications for vacuum extraction are the same as those for forceps delivery. It is contraindicated for face or brow and breech presentations, if there is a suspected fetal coagulation defect, and if fetal scalp blood sampling has been performed.

Many clinicians find the use of this device frustrating because there are no clear standards for its use. For example, how many pulls can be safely attempted, how many times can the device pop off the fetal head before the procedure should be abandoned, and what is the safe total time limit to effect delivery? These are questions that need to be addressed in the literature.

In summary, the same indications and requirements that pertain to forceps deliveries apply to the use of the vacuum extractor. Obstetricians need to be trained in the use of both modalities, and selection should be based on individual patient needs and circumstances. Every operator has his or her own preference, and there is something to be said for using an instrument with which one is comfortable; however, this should not be an excuse for a lack of skill in the full range of operative vaginal delivery techniques.

General
1. ACOG Committee on Obstetrics: Maternal and fetal medicine. Obstetric forceps. ACOG Committee Opinion No. 71, August 1989.
   The entire classification of forceps has been revised to include new definitions for outlet-, low-, and mid-forceps procedures.
2. Dennen PC. *Dennen's forceps deliveries,* 3rd ed. Philadelphia: FA Davis, 1989.
   This is a well-illustrated, readable primer on the history, instruments, and techniques of forceps use.
3. Laufe LE, Berkus MD. *Assisted vaginal delivery.* New York: McGraw-Hill, 1992.
   With an emphasis on forceps delivery, this authoritative book reviews all instrument-assisted vaginal delivery techniques.
4. Bofill JA, et al. Forceps and vacuum delivery: a survey of North American residency programs. *Obstet Gynecol* 1996;88:622.
   The authors provide a survey of delivery practices in teaching institutions.

Techniques and Indications
5. Boehm FH. Vacuum extraction during cesarean section. *South Med J* 1985; 78:1502.
   The author describes the use of the vacuum extractor during cesarean section to facilitate the delivery of the presenting vertex.
6. Boyd ME, et al. Failed forceps. *Obstet Gynecol* 1986;68:779.
   This large investigation (>6,000 patients) assessed the reasons for failed forceps deliveries and noted that birth trauma was not increased in the setting of mid-forceps delivery, when it was successful.
7. Bofill JA, et al. A randomized prospective trial of the obstetric forceps versus the m-cup vacuum extractor. *Am J Obstet Gynecol* 1996;175:1325.
   The authors compare the forceps to the vacuum extractor and conclude that both are equally efficacious but that maternal trauma is increased with the forceps and fetal trauma is increased with the vacuum extractor.
8. Morales R, et al. Vacuum extraction of preterm infants with birth weights 1500–2499 grams. *J Reprod Med* 1995;40:127.
   The authors suggest that vacuum extraction is safe even in low-birth-weight infants.
9. Dell DL, Slightler SE, Plauche WC. Soft cup vacuum extraction: a comparison of outlet delivery. *Obstet Gynecol* 1985;66:624.
   One hundred patients were randomly assigned to undergo a forceps delivery, a Silastic vacuum extraction delivery, or delivery using the Mityvac vacuum extractor. All three instruments were considered effective for outlet delivery.

10. Schifrin BS. Polemics in perinatology: disengaging forceps. *J Perinatol* 1988; 8:242.
    The author's comments regarding forceps are set in a practical manner; this is a must-read article for persons who use forceps.
11. Williams MC, et al. A randomized comparison of assisted vaginal delivery by obstetric forceps and polyethylene vacuum cup. *Obstet Gynecol* 1991;78:789.
    This prospective, randomized study revealed no significant differences in the safety or efficacy between these two modalities in a population undergoing predominantly low-pelvic assisted delivery.
12. Yeomans ER, Hankins GDV. Operative vaginal delivery in the 1990's. *Clin Obstet Gynecol* 1992;35:487.
    The authors provide contemporary guidelines for the proper conduct of instrumental delivery, including both forceps and vacuum extraction.

Complications
13. Punnonen R, et al. Fetal and maternal effects of forceps and vacuum extraction. *Br J Obstet Gynaecol* 1986;93:1132.
    In this large series, vacuum extraction and forceps delivery were compared, and there was a reduced incidence of low Apgar scores and a reduced amount of birth trauma associated with the latter.
14. Robertson PA, Laros RK, Zhao R. Neonatal and maternal outcome in low-pelvic and midpelvic operative deliveries. *Am J Obstet Gynecol* 1990;162:1436.
    This is a retrospective analysis using the updated American College of Obstetricians and Gynecologists classifications of operative vaginal deliveries, which cautions against the use of midforceps or midvacuum delivery unless the maternal benefit is balanced carefully with the fetal risk.
15. Seidman DS, et al. Long-term effects of vacuum and forceps deliveries. *Lancet* 1991;337:1583.
    A retrospective review of more than 2,600 instrumental vaginal deliveries compared with spontaneous vaginal delivery and cesarean section revealed no evidence of physical or cognitive impairment at 17 years of age associated with instrumental delivery.
16. Hankins GDV, Rowe TF. Operative vaginal delivery—year 2000. *Am J Obstet Gynecol* 1996;175:275.
    The authors suggest that forceps deliveries involving greater than 45 degrees rotation should be abandoned.
17. Teng FY, Sayre JW. Vacuum extraction: does duration predict scalp injury? *Obstet Gynecol* 1997;89:281.
    The authors report that the incidence of cephalohematoma increases with increasing application-to-delivery times.

---

33. CESAREAN BIRTH

Steven A. Culbert

Cesarean birth is the delivery of an infant through an incision in the abdominal and uterine walls. It has become the most commonly performed hospital-based operative procedure in the United States, accounting for approximately 25% of live births. Although cesarean delivery, with the expectation of survival of both the mother and the fetus, was proposed in the late eighteenth century, the first operation was not performed until the early nineteenth century. The technique was not widely used until the 1920s. Improved surgical and anesthesia skills, antibiotics, aseptic techniques, and blood product availability have decreased the risks of this procedure. However, cesarean birth still holds a much greater risk for the mother, with a maternal mortality rate of 20 per 100,000 births in the United States compared with a maternal mortality rate from vaginal delivery of 2.5 per 100,000 births. Indications for performing a primary cesarean section include dystocia (29%), breech or other abnormal presentation (15%), fetal intolerance of labor (5%), and other maternal-fetal indications (45%).

Types of uterine incisions used in cesarean delivery are low cervical (transverse or vertical) and classical. Currently, more than 90% of cesarean births use a low transverse incision. Low cervical incisions are made into the portion of the uterus that is less muscular than the contractile portion of the uterus. This allows the physician to deliver the infant through an area of the uterus that is less likely to rupture with subsequent pregnancies, more likely to heal without significant complications, and usually more hemostatic during the procedure. The low vertical incision is usually employed in cases of breech or other malpresentations. The classical uterine incision is a vertical incision that involves the upper uterine segment. Although this incision allows rapid uterine entry, complications encountered include increased blood loss and a greater risk of uterine rupture prior to or during labor in a subsequent pregnancy.

Extraperitoneal cesarean section was first described by Frank in 1907. Prior to the availability of antibiotics, this technique was used to minimize the occurrence of peritonitis. This procedure is still occasionally used to decrease the amount of serious postoperative infections when severe amnionitis is present at the time of delivery. However, since the increase in availability and efficacy of antibiotic therapy, there is some controversy over whether this procedure is still needed.

Cesarean hysterectomy is a hysterectomy performed at the time of cesarean delivery. It is usually an emergent procedure. The indications for emergency cesarean hysterectomy include placenta accreta (45%), uterine atony (20%), intractable hemorrhage (15%), uterine rupture (10%), placenta percreta (5%), large leiomyoma (3%), and infection (1%). Elective cesarean hysterectomies are performed in gravidas with underlying gynecologic indications for hysterectomy. Cesarean hysterectomy as a means to achieve sterilization is generally felt to carry excessive risks because of increased operative morbidity, and is rarely warranted. Although cesarean hysterectomy is a more difficult operation, in experienced hands it has been shown to be safe and may play a significant role in the overall management of obstetric patients in selected cases.

Elective cesarean sections are the major cause of iatrogenic preterm delivery in the United States. Some studies have indicated that 1% to 20% of hyaline membrane disease (HMD) cases are products of elective cesarean delivery. When abdominal delivery must be performed prior to fetal maturity, it is imperative to document, confirm, or be assured of pulmonary maturity. Assurance of pulmonary maturity may be done through early ultrasonography (first trimester is best for dating), reliable last menstrual period, quickening movements, auscultation of fetal heart tones with a fetoscope at 20 weeks, or early uterine examinations. Elective cesarean delivery no earlier than 39 weeks is advised by the American College of Obstetricians and Gynecologists. If the patient has insulin-requiring diabetes mellitus during pregnancy, or dating cannot be firmly established, an amniocentesis is recommended to confirm lung maturity via a series of lung phospholipid studies if delivery is to be undertaken prior to 39 weeks' gestation.

Anesthesia for cesarean birth is usually divided into two categories: general endotracheal technique and regional anesthesia. Regional techniques usually entail either spinal or epidural blocks. Regional anesthesia provides pain control with minimal risk of aspiration to the patient. The advantage of epidural over spinal anesthesia is that epidural anesthesia gives a continuous dosage of anesthetic, thereby allowing the surgeon not to be concerned about the length of the operation. It also can be used for postoperative pain management. General anesthesia is frequently used in emergency situations. The major disadvantages of general anesthesia are the risk of aspiration and possible neonatal suppression from induction agents. The advantages include reliability, expeditious induction, and the avoidance of maternal hypotension. Regardless of the technique, it is important that the anesthesiologist be experienced in dealing with the physiologic changes in pregnancy and be aware of fetal considerations.

For the past decade, rising cesarean section rates have been the subject of much attention by the medical, professional, and lay communities. In 1965 the cesarean birth rate was 4.5 per 100 births; by 1988 it had increased to 24.7 per 100 births. Because approximately 25% of cesarean sections in this country are repeat procedures, vaginal births after cesarean section (VBAC) have become increasingly supported by the medical community. The success rate for VBAC has been reported to be from about 60% for patients who were previously delivered for pelvic dystocia to more than 70% for patients who were delivered by cesarean birth for nonrecurring conditions, such as breech presentation or fetal distress.

The advantages of vaginal birth include decreased maternal and neonatal morbidity as well as decreased hospital time for both mother and baby. The use of oxytocin or epidural anesthesia is not contraindicated in VBAC. A trial of labor should be offered for all women with a nonclassical uterine incision. The risk of uterine rupture for which the dictum "once a cesarean section, always a cesarean section" was once used has been noted to be approximately 0.5%, as compared with 10% in patients with prior classical incisions. Prenatal education regarding risks and benefits, access to blood bank, and anesthesia, as well as the capability for rapid cesarean delivery, are recommended for the trial of labor. Some researchers have recommended a separate informed consent for patients undergoing a trial of labor after cesarean delivery.

Although maternal morbidity has decreased significantly with cesarean section, it is still between eight and 12 times higher than for a vaginal birth. Postoperative febrile morbidity (10%–50%), depending on whether the cesarean birth is performed electively or during labor with ruptured membranes, is markedly decreased with vaginal delivery (1%–3%). Prophylactic antibiotic use can reduce postoperative infection by 50% in the high-risk patient. Risk factors for postoperative infection include maternal obesity, duration of operation more than 1 hour, blood loss more than 800 cc, prolonged ruptured membranes, multiple pelvic examinations, and general anesthesia. This increase in maternal morbidity, along with prolonged hospital stay, adds to the increased expenses of health care, which are of concern to the patient and the public.

Although cesarean section rates have increased, the incidence of cerebral palsy has remained constant. Whereas some studies suspect fetal monitoring as a reason for the overall increase in cesarean section, other data indicate that fetal monitoring is not responsible. Changes in the management of breech presentation, a reluctance to perform difficult forceps deliveries, and a more aggressive approach to the high-risk obstetric patient, combined with the increased safety of the procedure and the changing medicolegal climate, have all contributed significantly to the increase in cesarean birth.

Risks to the fetus from cesarean birth, including neonatal depression from anesthesia, incisional trauma to the fetus while entering the uterus, fetal blood loss while transversing an anterior placenta, and injury to the fetus during extraction procedures, as well as increased transient respiratory distress syndrome, are increased when compared with infants delivered vaginally.

General

1. Taffel SM, et al. 1989 U.S. cesarean section rate steadies—VBAC rate rises to nearly one in five. *Birth* 1991;18:2.
   This study suggests that the 25-year increase in the cesarean section rate may have plateaued as the vaginal birth rate has increased.
2. Porreco RP. High cesarean section rate: a new perspective. *Obstet Gynecol* 1985;65:307.
   Using specific management criteria for common abdominal delivery indications, a primary cesarean birth rate of 5.7% was achieved with no difference in Apgar scores or neonatal mortality from other studies with higher cesarean rates.
3. Beguin EA. Vaginal birth after cesarean section: what are the risks? *Female Patient* 1988;13:16.
   This is an excellent general reference that summarizes the place of vaginal birth after cesarean in the obstetrician's armamentarium. Recommendations for use are given.
4. Fraser W, et al. Temporal variation in rates of cesarean section for dystocia: does "convenience" play a role? *Am J Obstet Gynecol* 1987;156:300.

The authors found that more cesarean sections were performed in the evening after office hours but that this timing of cesarean birth did not have an overall effect on cesarean birth or dystocia.

5. Shiono PH, et al. Recent trends in cesarean birth and trial of labor rates in the United States. *JAMA* 1987;257:494.
   An excellent general reference regarding the number of cesarean births and the reasons for which they are performed.

6. Ophir E, et al. Trial of labor following cesarean section: dilemma. *Obstet Gynecol Surv* 1988;44:19.
   This fine article boasts 49 references covering all aspects of this very complicated subject. Their conclusions allow the clinician to more effectively manage patients undergoing vaginal birth after cesarean section.

7. Leveno KJ, Cunningham FG, Pritchard JA. Cesarean section: The House of Horne revisited. *Am J Obstet Gynecol* 1989;160:78.
   The authors note that although the cesarean birth rate is higher in the United States compared with that in Ireland, the similar perinatal mortality rates are accounted for by the United States' hospitals having almost five times the low-birth-weight rate. When the populations are equalized, the increase in cesarean section rate appears to assist the infant.

Etiology

8. Rosen MG, et al. NIH Consensus Development statement on cesarean childbirth. *Obstet Gynecol* 1981;57:537.
   A 2-year report concerning a consensus development statement on cesarean section by the National Institutes of Health (NIH) is summarized in this article. It is must reading for all those interested in the increase in the rate of cesarean sections in our society.

9. Rosen MB, Chik L. The effect of delivery route on outcome in breech presentation. *Am J Obstet Gynecol* 1984;149:909.
   No significant association was found between outcome and birth route, except in the footling breech, if the infant was alive at the start of labor and had no major abnormalities.

10. Oshan AF, et al. Cesarean birth and neonatal mortality in very low birth weight infants. *Obstet Gynecol* 1984;64:267.
    After adjustment for birth weight, presentation, and place of birth, cesarean birth was not associated with a decreased mortality rate in the very-low-birth-weight infants.

11. Phelan JP, et al. Twice a cesarean, always a cesarean? *Obstet Gynecol* 1989;73:161.
    In an effort to increase the number of vaginal births after cesareans, the authors looked at more than 6,250 women who had cesarean sections. Of these, 1,088 had two previous cesarean sections and underwent a trial of labor, with 69% delivering vaginally. They also believed that oxytocin was integral to a successful vaginal-birth-after-cesarean rate.

12. Gould J, Davey B, Stafford R. Socioeconomic differences in rates of cesarean section. *N Engl J Med* 1989;321:233.
    Several reports suggest that the rate of cesarean section is increased in direct proportion to the patient's socioeconomic status.

Diagnosis

13. Read JA. The scheduling of repeat cesarean section operations: prospective management protocol experience. *Am J Obstet Gynecol* 1985;151:557.
    In a controlled environment (Army Medical Corps), a protocol to delineate previous cesarean sections with good dates was used to schedule delivery without amniocentesis or labor. Almost half the patients managed by this method delivered electively without problems for the mother or the baby.

14. Gilstrap LC III, Hauth JC, Toussaint S. Cesarean section: changing incidence and indications. *Obstet Gynecol* 1984;63:205.
    Meticulous monitoring and rapid responses to dystocia and fetal distress may help decrease the incidence of primary cesarean section.

15. Lonky NM, Worthen N, Ross MG. Prediction of cesarean section scars with ultrasound imaging during pregnancy. *J Ultrasound Med* 1089;8:15.
    The authors examined by ultrasound 47 women with previous cesarean sections. Scars were visualized well in 28%; this may be helpful in patients with an unknown incision who are considering vaginal birth after a cesarean.

Treatment
16. Ayers JWT, Morley GW. Surgical incision for cesarean section. *Obstet Gynecol* 1987;70:706.
    The authors describe operative morbidity in relationship to the abdominal incision. They conclude that as long as the incision is adequate, the type of incision does not play a role in morbidity in the mother or baby.
17. Flamm BL, et al. Oxytocin during labor after previous cesarean section: results of a multicenter study. *Obstet Gynecol* 1987;70:709.
    This large series (776 patients) demonstrates that oxytocin is safe to use in patients with previous cesarean births.
18. Flamm BL, et al. Vaginal birth after cesarean section: results of a multicenter study. *Am J Obstet Gynecol* 1988;158:1079.
    This is the largest series of patients undergoing labor after previous cesarean birth (4,929 patients); the authors did not find a single instance of maternal or perinatal mortality related to uterine scar rupture.
19. Haynes DM, Martin BJ. Cesarean hysterectomy: a twenty-five year review. *Am J Obstet Gynecol* 1979;134:393.
    This 25-year review of 149 cesarean hysterectomies suggests that cesarean hysterectomy should remain a part of the obstetrician's repertoire, but that it may not be advisable for strictly elective indications.

Complications
20. Gibbs RS, Blanco JD, St. Clain PJ. A case-control study of wound abscess after cesarean delivery. *Obstet Gynecol* 1983;62:498.
    This is an excellent review of the complications associated with abscess.
21. Duff P. Pathophysiology and management of postcesarean endomyometritis. *Obstet Gynecol* 1986;67:269.
    This article describes the pathophysiology and management of postcesarean endomyometritis and is an excellent review of the subject.
22. Emmons SL, et al. Development of wound infections among women undergoing cesarean section. *Obstet Gynecol* 1988;72:559.
    In more than 1,000 women undergoing cesarean birth, wound infections were most often related to Staphylococcus aureus, and the attack rate was not related to prolonged labor or other factors during labor.
23. Stanco LM, et al. Emergency peripartum hysterectomy and associated risk factors. *Am J Obstet Gynecol* 1993;168:879.
    A review of 123 cases of emergency cesarean hysterectomy from 1985 to 1990 in a large university center.
24. Khan GQ, et al. Controlled cord traction versus minimal intervention techniques in delivery of the placenta: a randomized controlled trial. *Am J Obstet Gynecol* 1997;177:770.
    Data are presented here that support controlled cord traction to deliver the placenta at the time of cesarean delivery. There was a significantly decreased incidence of postpartum hemorrhage.
25. McMahon MJ, et al. Comparison of a trial of labor with an elective second cesarean section. *N Engl J Med* 1996;335:689.
    This is a controversial study that reports worse outcomes in patients with a failed trial of labor in comparison with those undergoing an elective repeat cesarean delivery.
26. Chapman SJ, Owen J, Hauth JC. One- versus two-layer closure of a low transverse cesarean: the next pregnancy. *Obstet Gynecol* 1997;89:16.
    This is a comparison of outcomes of future pregnancies of patients who had one- versus two-layer closure of the uterus at the time of a low transverse cesarean section.

27. Boyle JG, Gabbe SG. T and J vertical extensions in low transverse cesarean births. *Obstet Gynecol* 1996;87:238.
A description of complications in cases where the uterine incision is extended for a difficult delivery.

34. FAILURE TO PROGRESS IN LABOR

Michel E. Rivlin

The term *labor* refers to the progressive dilatation of the uterine cervix in the presence of repetitive uterine contractions. Failure to progress refers to lack of progressive cervical dilatation or descent of the fetal head. There are three stages of labor. The first stage of labor begins with the onset of labor and lasts to the time of full cervical dilatation. The second stage of labor follows, and continues until the delivery of the infant. The period after delivery of the infant until delivery of the placenta is the third stage of labor. The first stage of labor can be depicted graphically. If time is plotted on the abscissa and cervical dilatation on the ordinate, two phases are described, latent and active. The active phase of labor is further divided into the acceleration phase, which is the phase of maximum slope, and the deceleration phase. Active labor usually begins when the cervix is 3–4 cm dilated and the rate of cervical dilatation is also notably increased from the latent phase. Abnormal labor patterns have been characterized by Friedman. A prolonged latent phase lasts more than 20 hours in the nulligravida and 14 hours in the multipara. There are also protraction disorders of dilatation (less than 1.2 cm/hour, nulligravida; less than 1.5 cm/hour multigravida) and descent (change in station less than 1 cm/hour in the nulligravida; less than 2 cm/hour in the multipara in the second stage of labor). Arrest of dilatation is deemed to occur when cervical dilatation has ceased for more than 2 hours. Arrest of descent occurs after a 1-hour interval.

Arrest of cervical dilatation may be primary or secondary. A prolonged latent phase is often treated with a therapeutic rest, in which the mother is given sedation with morphine or meperidine. When the mother awakens from the sedation, the contractions will either have subsided, indicating that the patient was not in true labor, or the contractions will resume in a more effective manner. X-ray pelvimetry is rarely used today to assess pelvic size, but the pelvis should be assessed clinically. A clinical estimation of fetal weight should also be performed. Although an ultrasound-derived estimation of fetal weight is somewhat inaccurate, ultrasonography may be performed to help identify an extremely large fetus or fetal anomaly which might interfere with normal cervical dilatation. One simple method for determining the adequacy of the pelvis for vaginal delivery is the Müller-Hillis maneuver, which consists of exerting pressure on the fundus while performing a vaginal examination. An impression of easy downward movement of the presenting part suggests that the pelvis is adequate. Once the active phase of labor is reached and failure to progress has occurred, many authors prefer to rupture the membranes and insert an intrauterine pressure catheter for better evaluation of uterine activity. Although there is a wide range of uterine activity that is considered adequate, contractions of at least 50 mm Hg occurring every 2–3 minutes lasting 45–60 seconds are desirable.

Cephalopelvic disproportion is responsible for the arrest disorder in as many as 50% of the women, and these women require cesarean section for delivery. If it is the labor that is judged inadequate, gentle augmentation with an oxytocin infusion is recommended. An interval of 40–60 minutes after initiating an oxytocin infusion is required for a steady-state concentration to be reached. Oxytocin is administered in a balanced-salt solution via a controlled infusion device. Careful monitoring of the fetal heartbeat is advised, and the oxytocin infusion is discontinued if any signs of fetal distress appear. The patient must also be observed for possible uterine hyperstimulation. The infusion is increased 1–2 μ/min over a 30-minute interval until an adequate labor pattern is established. The findings from early studies suggested that perinatal morbidity was higher when the second stage of labor exceeded 2 hours. With the availability of fetal monitoring, a longer time is now allowable, as long as the fetal heart rate remains satisfactory. The effects of epidural anesthesia may lengthen the second stage of labor, and the use of forceps for delivery to shorten the second stage is also increased in this setting.

Dystocia is a diagnostic category that includes failure to progress in labor, prolonged labor, and dysfunctional labor. Numerous factors are associated with longer labors. These include advanced maternal age, nulliparity, maternal anxiety, multiple gestation, and fetal malposition. Epidural anesthesia prolongs both the first and second stages of labor and increases the need for oxytocin stimulation of labor. Labor may be shortened by amniotomy, oxytocin, emotional support, ambulation, and positional change. Instrumental delivery shortens the second stage of labor.

Dystocia is an important factor in rising cesarean section rates, which may exceed 20%. The active management of labor has been advocated in an attempt to reduce the rate of cesarean section. Active management includes strict criteria for the diagnosis of labor, early amniotomy, prompt intervention with high-dose oxytocin in the event of inefficient uterine action, and a commitment to never leave a woman in labor unattended.

In summary, the appropriate management of arrest or protraction disorders of labor requires careful attention to the progress of labor. Cervicographic analysis is often helpful for this purpose. Assessment of fetal size, pelvic dimensions, and uterine forces is necessary to achieve an optimal result for the mother and the baby.

Normal Labor / Cervicogram / Partogram
 1. Albers LL, Schiff M, Gorwoda JG. The length of active labor in normal pregnancies. *Obstet Gynecol* 1996;87:355.
    Active labor in healthy women lasted longer than is widely appreciated. Upward revision of clinical expectations for the length of active labor is warranted.
 2. Friedman EA. Normal and dysfunctional labor. In: Cohen WR, Acker DB, Friedman EA, eds. *Management of labor,* 2nd ed. Rockville, MD: Aspen Publishers, 1989;1–18.
    An excellent overview of normal and dysfunctional labor from the developer of the cervicogram.
 3. Dujardin B, et al. Value of the alert and action lines on the partogram. *Lancet* 1992;339:1336.
    Philpott's partogram includes an alert line set 4 hours to the right of the line, indicating normal progress, and an action line to the right of the former. This tool is widely used in less developed countries.
 4. Bernardes J, Costa-Pereira A. A multicentre comparative study of 17 experts and an intelligent computer system for managing labor using the cardiotocogram. *Br J Obstet Gynaecol* 1995;102:688.
    Computer-generated display of labor curves and management options.
 5. Khan KS, Rizvi A. The partograph in the management of labor following cesarean section. *Int J Gynaecol Obstet* 1995;50:151.
    Arrest of active phase and length of labor were related to uterine scar rupture.

Etiology
 6. Alexander JM, et al. The course of labor with and without epidural analgesia. *Am J Obstet Gynecol* 1998;178:516.
    Epidural anesthesia decreases uterine performance during oxytocin-stimulated labor, resulting in an increase in the length of the first and second stages of labor. Different guidelines for management should probably be adapted for the patient in labor with an epidural anesthetic.
 7. Gardberg M, Tuppuraimen M. Persistent occiput posterior presentation—a clinical problem. *Acta Obstet Gynecol Scand* 1994;73:45.

The most common fetal malposition causing prolonged labor; associated with android or anthropoid pelvic shape; diminished use of rotation forceps with increased use of cesarean section.

8. Piper JM, Bolling DR, Newton ER. The second stage of labor: factors influencing duration. *Am J Obstet Gynecol* 1991;165:976.
   A prolonged second stage of labor was associated with epidural anesthesia, a prolonged active-phase duration, lower maternal parity, excess maternal weight gain, and increasing fetal weight.

9. Morgan MA, Thurnau GR. Efficacy of the fetal-pelvic index in nulliparous women at high risk for fetal-pelvic disproportion. *Am J Obstet Gynecol* 1992;166:810.
   A combination of ultrasonography-derived estimation of fetal weight with x-ray pelvimetry was utilized to develop a fetal-pelvic index.

10. Johnson N, Johnson VA, Gupta JK. Maternal positions during labor. *Obstet Gynecol Surv* 1991;46:428.
    An interesting overview of the effect of maternal position on the fetus and labor progress.

11. Stephens MB, Ford RE. Intrathecal narcotics for labor analgesia. *Am Fam Physician* 1997;56:463.
    Intrathecal narcotics do not affect the natural progression of labor and are not associated with adverse fetal outcomes.

12. Strong TH Jr. The effect of amnioinfusion on the duration of labor. *Obstet Gynecol* 1997;89:1044.
    Amnioinfusion has no effect on the duration of labor.

Active Management

13. Peaceman AM, Socol ML. Active management of labor. *Am J Obstet Gynecol* 1996; 175:363.
    Active management of labor appears to shorten labor and maternal infectious morbidity, and may decrease operative deliveries for dystocia.

14. Malone FD, et al. Prolonged labor in nulliparas: lessons from the active management of labor. *Obstet Gynecol* 1996;88:211.
    Less advanced cervical dilation on admission and epidural use, especially when placed early, are strongly associated with prolonged labor.

15. Satin AJ, et al. High- versus low-dose oxytocin for labor stimulation. *Obstet Gynecol* 1992;80:111.
    High-dose oxytocin to augment ineffective labor minimized the number of cesarean sections for dystocia, but increased the cesarean rate for fetal distress.

16. Goffinet F, et al. Early amniotomy increases the frequency of fetal heart rate abnormalities. Amniotomy Study Group. *Br J Obstet Gynaecol* 1997;104:548.
    Reduction in labor duration but not of cesarean section incidence. Operative deliveries may increase based on electronic fetal monitoring, indicating fetal distress.

17. Zhang J, et al. Continuous labor support from labor attendant for primiparous women: a meta-analysis. *Obstet Gynecol* 1996;88:739.
    Labor support may have important positive effects on obstetric outcomes among young, disadvantaged women.

Outcome

18. Bottoms SH, Hirsch VJ, Sokol RJ. Medical management of arrest disorders of labor: a current overview. *Am J Obstet Gynecol* 1987;156:939.
    With medical management, arrest disorders were not associated with an increased risk of adverse perinatal outcome.

19. Chelmow D, Laros RK. Maternal and neonatal outcomes after oxytocin augmentation in patients undergoing a trial of labor after prior cesarean delivery. *Obstet Gynecol* 1992;80:966.
    The findings from this retrospective analysis support the use of oxytocin and epidural anesthesia to augment labor after a prior cesarean section.

20. Rosen MG, et al. Abnormal labor and infant brain damage. *Obstet Gynecol* 1992;80:961.

A diagnosis of failure to progress was not associated with increased neurologic abnormalities in infants. Neither the method of delivery nor the use of oxytocin were factors in the etiology of infant brain damage.

21. Reynolds JL. Post-traumatic stress disorder after childbirth: the phenomenon of traumatic birth. *CMAJ* 1997;156:831.

There is very little literature on this topic. The evidence available is from case series, qualitative research, and studies of women seeking elective cesarean section for psychologic reasons.

---

35. CEPHALOPELVIC DISPROPORTION

Baha M. Sibai, Farid Mattar, and Dorel Abramovici

Normal labor is characterized by the progressive effacement and dilation of the cervix, associated with descent of the fetal presenting part. During the cervical changes that begin either during or before the latent phase of labor, the cervix undergoes significant biochemical changes in the ground substance structure, reticulum, and water content. The rate of dilation accelerates rapidly during the active phase, is complete by the end of the first stage, and depends on uterine contractions of adequate intensity and frequency. Descent of the fetal head begins during the last deceleration phase of labor, and depends on uterine contractions, maternal pelvic capacity, and fetal factors.

Most labors progress in a normal fashion, leading to spontaneous vaginal delivery, but a small percentage manifest abnormal patterns of progress, in the form of protraction or arrest of dilatation, descent, or both, as measured by the Friedman labor curve or partogram. This dystocia represents a potential adverse effect on the fetus and mother. Consequently, it is prudent for all obstetric providers to recognize these abnormal patterns as early as possible, so that an orderly, systematic plan of management can be undertaken.

Cephalopelvic disproportion (CPD) is defined as the inability of the presenting part of the fetal head to pass through the maternal pelvis. CPD is responsible for most abnormal labor patterns if uterine activity, as measured by intrauterine pressure monitoring, is adequate. It occurs in about 1%–3% of all primigravidas and in 30% of those who have a protracted active phase of dilation or descent, while about 50% of these parturients have an arrest of descent. CPD is categorized into two sets of factors: (1) maternal factors, which include the size and shape of the bony pelvis as well as soft tissue resistance, and (2) fetal factors, which include size, presentation, position, and moldability of the fetal head. Clinical evaluation of pelvic capacity can be performed by digital examination during the first antepartum visit, and typing of the pelvis should be carried out according to the Caldwell-Moloy classification (i.e., gynecoid, android, or platypelloid). Attention must be directed to the diagonal conjugate, the inclination of the pelvic side walls, the prominence of the ischial spines, the shape of the sacrum, and the angle of the suprapubic arch. About 85% of the patients will have a clinically adequate pelvic capacity; 1% will have a clearly inadequate pelvis; and the remainder will have a borderline pelvis. The following findings indicate a possible contracted pelvis: (1) ability to touch the sacral promontory with the index finger; (2) significant convergence of the side walls; (3) forward inclination of a straight sacrum; (4) sharp ischial spines with a narrow interspinous diameter; (5) a narrow suprapubic arch; (6) a congenital sacral abnormality; (7) a history of difficult labor; (8) maternal disease, such as rickets or polio, and trauma; and (9) adolescent pregnancy. Digital pelvimetry should be repeated during the intrapartum period, with attention paid to fetal-pelvic relationship, so that the pelvic capacity can be gauged against the presenting fetal part.

The presence of abnormal progress in labor (dystocia) may be the first evidence of pelvic inadequacy. Because about 45% of patients who experience secondary arrest of dilation or descent, or both, have CPD, careful evaluation is mandatory before labor stimulation is utilized. Ultrasound imaging and x-ray pelvimetry to determine the fetal head size are used by some to compare pelvic capacity with the fetal vertex, but there is much controversy regarding the benefits of such techniques. Some clinicians believe that the benefits may far outweigh the theoretical risk from radiation exposure, whereas the majority believe that the knowledge imparted by these tests may not be helpful in clinical management.

Maternal risks associated with CPD include abnormal thinning of the lower uterine segment with possible uterine rupture, pressure necrosis of the bladder, pelvic lacerations associated with instrument delivery, postpartum hemorrhage, and increased postpartum uterine infections. Fetal risks include fetal distress (10%), cord prolapse, intracranial hemorrhage, skull fracture, and long-term neurologic abnormalities.

Proper management of CPD involves early recognition during labor, identification of the cause, and prompt institution of therapy. A good initial history and physical examination, with high index of suspicion in those with predisposing factors, is a most important initial step. Attention should be given to the position and presentation of the fetal head, as noted during a combined abdominal and pelvic examination, with special emphasis on the thrust of the fetal head into the birth canal during contractions or when applying fundal pressure (the Müller–Hillis maneuver).

In many cases, particularly in primigravidas, the active management of labor, which includes early amniotomy, use of oxytocin in the latent phase, and aggressive treatment of arrest or protraction disorders, may help in preventing the need for cesarean delivery previously deemed to be due to CPD. On the other hand, in cases of labor requiring oxytocin, the fetal head is poorly applied to the cervix, and the head-to-cervix force does not mirror the rise and fall in intrauterine pressure. The identification of dystocia, which assumes the form of protraction or arrest disorders, should be a warning sign of CPD. Dystocia is usually best detected by frequent assessment during labor and the use of a labor graph or partogram in each pregnancy.

In the face of controversial data, overwhelming managed care and medico-legal issues, and a poor understanding of the mechanisms of labor, aggressive management has yet to be established as a successful alternative to abdominal delivery. In recent literature, continuous emotional support during labor was found to be the only precept of active management consistently and significantly associated with decreased cesarean section rates. Conclusions should not be drawn until this factor is adequately addressed in future clinical trials of active treatment.

The association of documented CPD with abnormal patterns of progress, in the form of arrest of dilatation or descent, is an indication for cesarean birth without any further trial of labor. The use of oxytocin (Pitocin) stimulation or mid forceps procedures in the presence of probable CPD or arrest patterns of labor is usually unsuccessful. In other cases of borderline CPD with dystocia or in patients with inadequate labor, oxytocin stimulation may be indicated. Recent reports emphasize the importance of aggressively managed labor, with oxytocin stimulation an alternative to performing an abdominal delivery in those with borderline CPD. In addition, the use of an intrauterine catheter and pressure-curve integrator to measure uterine activity, coupled with a specific computer-defined goal of contractile activity, has made it much safer to use oxytocin stimulation in cases of borderline CPD. Such findings were refuted by other reports that failed to show a favorable effect on the cesarean section rates, operative delivery rates, or neonatal outcome. Once CPD is diagnosed, cesarean delivery is the treatment of choice.

General
1. American College of Obstetricians and Gynecologists. Shoulder dystocia. *ACOG Pract Patterns* no. 7, October 1997.
   Provides information from recent literature regarding the diagnosis, prevention, and management of shoulder dystocia.
2. Bowes WA. Clinical aspects of normal and abnormal labor. In: Creasy RK, Resnik R, eds. *Maternal fetal medicine: principles and practice.* Philadelphia: Saunders, 1999;541–568.

The physiology and normal progress of labor are detailed. Abnormal forms of labor during the first and second stages are described, and diagnosis and management of these abnormalities are detailed.

3. American College of Obstetricians and Gynecologists. Induction and augmentation of labor. *ACOG Tech Bull* no. 157, November 1991.

Details the indications for and contraindications to induction of labor and the methods used for oxytocin administration; new dosage schedules are recommended.

Etiology

4. Allman ACJ, et al. Head-to-cervix force: an important physiological variable in labour. 1. The temporal relation between head-to-cervix force and intrauterine pressure during labor. *Br J Obstet Gynaecol* 1996;103:763.

This is the first report of the temporal relation between intrauterine pressure and head-to-cervix force in labor. The authors found that the rise and fall in these two measured variables occur simultaneously in only 15% of cases. They suggested that in labors requiring oxytocin, the cervix was more frequently poorly applied to the fetal head between contractions. They concluded that measuring this temporal relation was of little value in determining whether a labor is likely to progress normally.

5. Fairlie FM, et al. An analysis of uterine activity in spontaneous labor using a microcomputer. *Br J Obstet Gynaecol* 1988;95:57.

A significant parity-related difference in the contraction frequency was observed in the first stage but not in the second stage (higher activity in the nulliparous). Epidural analgesia did not appear to influence uterine activity in the first stage but was associated with a lower mean active pressure, contraction frequency, and intensity in the second stage.

6. Fisk NM, Shweni PM. Labor outcome of juvenile primiparae in a population with a high incidence of contracted pelvis. *Int J Gynecol Obstet* 1989;28:5.

The authors compare the labor outcome of primiparous women younger than 17 years of age with that of the normal population. There was no difference in the rate of cesarean birth in this population but the incidence of operative delivery, low birth weight, and perinatal mortality were higher among the adolescents.

7. Thurnau GR, et al. Evaluation of the fetal-pelvic relationship. *Clin Obstet Gynecol* 1992;35:570.

This review provides a historical and analytic approach to the study of fetal-pelvic relationships. In addition, methods of evaluating the fetal-pelvic relationship as well as current concepts on this subject are described.

8. American College of Obstetricians and Gynecologists. Dystocia. *ACOG Tech Bull* no. 37, December 1989.

The etiology, diagnosis, and management of dystocia are summarized in detail.

9. Harbert GM Jr. Assessment of uterine contractility and activity. *Clin Obstet Gynecol* 1992;35:546.

The physiology as well as the methods of measuring uterine contractility and activity are detailed. Abnormal forms of uterine contractility leading to dysfunctional patterns of labor during the first and second stages of labor are reviewed, and clinical management of these patterns is described.

Diagnosis

10. Glantz JC, McNanley TJ. Active management of labor: a meta-analysis of cesarean delivery rates for dystocia in nulliparas. *Obstet Gynecol Surv* 1997;52:497.

In this meta-analysis of two prospective, randomized and three retrospective, non-randomized studies, the authors found a general tendency to show greater difference in an outcome when historical rather than randomized controls are used. When the three highest quality studies (two randomized and one nonrandomized) were included, the analysis revealed a 34% decrease in the odds of undergoing cesarean section delivery for dystocia in actively managed nulliparas, without compromising fetal status.

11. Olah KS, Gee H. Commentaries. The active management of labour. *Br J Obstet Gynaecol* 1996;103:729.

In reference to a meta-analysis of the available randomized studies on the active management of labor, the authors report that oxytocin augmentation does not improve cesarean section rates, operative delivery rates, or neonatal outcome. Amniotomy causes a small decrease in the duration of labor, without influencing perinatal outcome or operative delivery rates.

12. O'Brien WF, Cefalo RC. Evaluation of x-ray pelvimetry and abnormal labor. *Clin Obstet Gyencol* 1982;25:157.

    The authors review the history, anatomic basis, and current systems of x-ray pelvimetry. The risks and benefits are also summarized. They conclude that the use of intrapartum x-ray pelvimetry does not improve perinatal outcome, and its potential risks outweigh its benefits.

13. Yamazaki H, Uchida K. A mathematical approach to problems of cephalopelvic disproportion of the pelvic inlet. *Am J Obstet Gynecol* 1983;147:25.

    The authors describe a mathematical formula to calculate a pelvic index based on calculation of the ratio between an area of the pelvic inlet plane and a cross area of the fetal skull. They suggest that this index may serve as a guide to proper management of labor in patients with cephalopelvic disproportion.

14. Raman S, et al. A comparative study of x-ray pelvimetry and CT pelvimetry. *Aust NZ J Obstet Gynaecol* 1991;31:217.

    The results of conventional erect lateral x-ray pelvimetry were compared to those done by computed tomography (CT) pelvimetry in 24 patients who had cesarean section for various obstetric reasons. The risks and benefits are also summarized. The authors conclude that CT pelvimetry is preferred and should be performed postpartum in nulliparous women who were delivered by cesarean section for cephalopelvic disproportion or had difficult forceps delivery.

15. Morgan MA, Thurnau GR. Efficacy of the fetal-pelvic index in nulliparous women at high risk for fetal-pelvic disproportion. *Am J Obstet Gynecol* 1992;166:810.

    The fetal-pelvic index and two other methods of identifying fetal-pelvic disproportion (estimated fetal weight of more than 4,000 g by ultrasound and Mengert's index) were compared with respect to clinical outcome and the accuracy of predicting the presence of cephalopelvic disproportion (CPD) in 137 nulliparous women at high risk for CPD. The authors found the fetal-pelvic index to be more efficacious in determining the presence or absence of CPD than ultrasonography or x-ray pelvimetry.

Treatment

16. Frigoletto FD, et al. A clinical trial of active management of labor. *N Engl J Med* 1995;333:745.

    In this report, active management of labor did not reduce the rate of cesarean section in nulliparous women but was associated with a somewhat shorter duration of labor and less maternal fever.

17. Chazotte C, Cohen WR. Drug use selection for latent-phase labor. *Contemp Obstet Gynecol* 1987;30:73.

    Many drugs are available to influence contractility and to relieve pain during the latent phase of labor. This report reviews the benefits and side effects of the various drugs during this stage.

18. Bottoms SF, Hirsch VJ, Sokkol J. Medical management of arrest disorders of labor: current overview. *Am J Obstet Gynecol* 1987;156:935.

    This report analyzed the management and outcome in 5399 births selected to rule out risks clearly not caused by abnormal labor. Arrest disorders occurred in 11%, and medical management was used in 96% of these cases. Fifty percent of the patients in this group delivered without oxytocin, and only 21% in this group required cesarean section.

19. Satin AJ, et al. Factors affecting the dose response to oxytocin for labor stimulation. *Am J Obstet Gynecol* 1992;166:1260.

    The authors used a computerized data base to determine obstetric variables affecting the dose response to oxytocin for labor stimulation in 1,773 pregnancies. They found that gestational age, parity, and cervical dilation influenced the pregnancy response to oxytocin. However, they found considerable variability in response to oxytocin, suggesting that these factors were not useful in predicting the dose response to oxytocin for labor stimulation.

20. Muller PR, et al. A prospective randomized clinical trial comparing two oxytocin induction protocols. *Am J Obstet Gynecol* 1992;167:373.

    A total of 151 women were randomized into one of two oxytocin induction protocols: One protocol included gradual increase in the dose of 1–2 mU / minute at 30-minute intervals (n = 76) and the other protocol included doubling of the rate of oxytocin every 40 minutes (n = 75). The authors found that induction with larger-dose increments resulted in shorter time to adequate labor without an associated increase in uterine hyperstimulation or poor neonatal outcome. However, the larger-dose protocol was associated with higher frequency of altered fetal heart rate changes during the induction.

21. Owen J, Hauth JC. Oxytocin for the induction or augmentation of labor. *Clin Obstet Gynecol* 1992;35:464.

    Details the methods used for oxytocin administration; new dosage schedules are compared, and recommendations for induction and augmentation of labor are made.

22. Lopez-Zeno JA, et al. A controlled trial of a program for the active management of labor. *N Engl J Med* 1992;326:450.

    The authors describe a program for labor management that includes early amniotomy plus using oxytocin at an initial rate of 6 mU / minute that was subsequently increased by 6 mU / minute every 15 minutes (to a maximum of 36 mU / minute) until there are seven contractions every 15 minutes. This program reduced the incidence of dystocia and increased the rate of vaginal delivery without increasing maternal or neonatal morbidity.

Complications

23. Seitchik J, Holden AEC, Castillo M. Amniotomy and oxytocin treatment of functional dystocia and route of delivery. *Am J Obstet Gynecol* 1986;155:858.

    The authors describe the details of clinical management in 101 nulliparous patients with functional dystocia who underwent amniotomy and were treated with oxytocin in the first stage of labor. Sixty-eight delivered vaginally, and 33 were delivered by cesarean section.

24. Saunders NG, et al. Neonatal and maternal morbidity in relation to the length of the second stage of labour. *Br J Obstet Gynaecol* 1992;99:381.

    Maternal and neonatal morbidity were correlated to the duration of the second stage of labor in 25,069 women delivered of an infant of at least 37 weeks' gestation after spontaneous onset of labor. The risks of both postpartum hemorrhage and maternal infection were increased in relation to increased second stage of labor. In contrast, the duration of second stage of labor was not associated with poor neonatal outcome. The authors conclude that second-stage labors of up to 3 hours' duration are not associated with fetal risks.

25. Cahill DJ, et al. Does oxytocin augmentation increase perinatal risk in primigravid labor? *Am J Obstet Gynecol* 1992;166:847.

    Adverse maternal and perinatal outcomes were analyzed in 30,874 primigravid term deliveries in which high-dose oxytocin augmentation was used. The authors conclude that high-dose oxytocin to correct dystocia is safe for both mother and fetus.

---

36. FETAL DISTRESS IN THE INTRAPARTUM PERIOD

Michel E. Rivlin

Although the term *fetal distress* is used to describe a variety of fetal situations, most physicians associate this phrase with fetal asphyxia. Asphyxia generally refers to fetal hypoxia and metabolic acidosis. Because of the decreased uterine blood flow during contractions, labor is associated with a relative fetal hypoxia. Usually this is tolerated well by the normal fetus, and fetal heart rate (FHR) monitoring is the most widely used method to evaluate fetal status in labor. The FHR may be determined by simple auscultation with a fetoscope or by electronic monitoring. If auscultation is chosen, low-risk patients are monitored every 30 minutes during the active phase of labor and at least every 15 minutes in the second stage of labor. The intervals are decreased for high-risk patients, with auscultation performed every 15 minutes in the active phase of labor and every 5 minutes in the second stage of labor. The findings from current studies indicate that there is little difference in outcome regardless of whether electronic monitoring or auscultation is used, though many busy obstetric services find that they cannot perform auscultation according to the standards just described.

The normal FHR varies between 120 and 160 beats per minute, although rates slightly above and below this may be considered normal in the absence of ominous patterns. Accelerations of the fetal heart during contractions are generally considered to be a reassuring pattern. The short-term FHR variability (beat-to-beat) usually varies between 3 and 7 beats per minute. Loss of short-term variability may suggest fetal hypoxia, but other factors may also be responsible, such as the fetal sleep state or the effect of drugs administered to the mother.

Certain periodic changes in the FHR have been observed in association with uterine contractions. There are three classic types of changes: early, variable, and late decelerations. Early decelerations usually mirror the effect of uterine contraction on the FHR tracing, with the heart rate returning to baseline as the contraction is completed. Fetal head compression with descent into the birth canal is the usual explanation for the phenomenon. Variable decelerations occur at different times in association with uterine contractions. In these, there is a more rapid decrease in the rate and a quicker return to the baseline, and they are thought to be due to compression of the umbilical cord, as might occur in the presence of a nuchal cord or cord compression in the setting of oligohydramnios. Although mild variable decelerations are tolerated well, more severe ones may result in fetal acidosis. When the FHR pattern is symmetrical with the uterine contraction but returns to baseline only after completion of the contraction, this is deemed a late deceleration. Repetitive late decelerations may be associated with fetal distress approximately 50% of the time. A more ominous pattern is late decelerations in the presence of decreased beat-to-beat variability.

Certain measures may improve the fetal status if the FHR is abnormal. If oxytocic agents are being administered, they should be discontinued. Maternal hydration may improve intervillus perfusion and administering oxygen to the mother may enhance placental gas exchange. In addition, the mother should be placed in the lateral decubitus position to improve uterine blood flow. If the ominous FHR pattern is corrected, then further observation is indicated. In the presence of a nonreassuring FHR pattern, the physician must decide between immediate delivery by cesarean section or further observation. Because of the high false-positive rate with FHR monitoring, some physicians elect to perform fetal scalp pH sampling in this situation. This procedure is technically cumbersome, but values of more than 7.25 pH would permit further observation. A scalp blood pH of less than 7.20 is generally an indication for medical or surgical intervention.

Meconium-stained amniotic fluid occurs in approximately 7%–22% of live births. Older studies implicated the passage of meconium with fetal hypoxia, acidosis, or distress. However, recent investigations do not find a significant correlation between meconium and infant condition at birth, as reflected by such measures as the Apgar score, need for resuscitation, and umbilical cord acid-base measurements. Nevertheless, clinicians are concerned about the incidental physiologic presence of meconium in the setting of relative intrauterine hypoxia leading to fetal gasping and possible meconium aspiration syndrome. For this reason, transcervical amnioinfusion in the presence of heavy meconium staining is widely employed, together with aggressive infant tracheal suctioning, and has improved fetal outcome. Amnioinfusion has also been helpful in correcting variable decelerations due to cord compression associated with oligohydramnios.

At the time of delivery, the infant may have a low Apgar score, but this does not necessarily correlate with fetal acidosis. This is especially true in the preterm infant. Some recommend obtaining umbilical cord arterial blood gas measurements to better determine the neonatal status. Using the term *birth asphyxia* to refer to the diagnosis is not recommended, as it is an imprecise term. For a possible neurologic deficit to be associated with perinatal asphyxia, the following criteria should be met: (1) profound umbilical artery acidemia (pH of less than 7.0), (2) Apgar score of less than 3 after 5 minutes; (3) neonatal neurologic sequelae such as seizures, and (4) multiorgan system dysfunction, which may include cardiovascular, gastrointestinal, pulmonary, or renal difficulties.

General
1. Anonymous. Electronic fetal heart rate monitoring: research guidelines for interpretation. National Institute of Child Health and Human Development Research Planning Workshop. *Am J Obstet Gynecol* 1997;177:1385.
   Recommendations for interpreting fetal heart rate patterns with standardized and unambiguous definitions.
2. Quirk JG, Miller FC. FHR tracing characteristics that jeopardize the diagnosis of fetal well-being. *Clin Obstet Gynecol* 1986;29:12.
   Excellent review of available information on intrapartum fetal monitoring as it relates to perinatal death and fetal acid-base status.
3. Sykes GS, et al. Do Apgar scores indicate asphyxia? *Lancet* 1982;1:494.
   Only 19% of the babies with a 5-minute Apgar score of less than 7 had severe acidosis.
4. Hueston WJ, McClaflin RR, Claire E. Variations in cesarean delivery for fetal distress. *J Fam Pract* 1996;43:461.
   When adjusted for risk status, previous cesarean, nonwhite race, pitocin, length of labor site, and time of day (more between 9 p.m. and 3 a.m.), were significant predictors for cesarean for fetal distress.

Acid-Base Evaluation
5. Low JA, et al. The prediction of intrapartum fetal metabolic acidosis by fetal heart rate monitoring. *Am J Obstet Gynecol* 1981;139:299.
   The probability of fetal metabolic acidosis was 48% in the presence of late decelerations.
6. Assessment of Fetal and Newborn Acid-Base Status. *ACOG Tech Bull* no. 127, April 1989.
   The types of acidemia and the interpretation of umbilical cord gas values are reviewed. Umbilical artery pH values of less than 7.0 more realistically represent clinically significant acidosis.
7. Perkins RP. Perinatal observations in a high-risk population managed without intrapartum fetal pH studies. *Am J Obstet Gynecol* 1984;149:327.
   Intrapartum fetal scalp blood pH studies were not utilized in this institution. The rates of stillbirth, operative intervention, and neonatal compromise did not appear to be increased over those observed in institutions using this method.
8. Clark SL, Gimobsky ML, Miller MC. Fetal heart rate response to scalp blood sampling. *Am J Obstet Gynecol* 1982;144:706.
   Fetal heart rate accelerations in response to scalp blood sampling were associated with a scalp pH of more than 7.20.
9. Goldenberg RL, Huddleston JF, Nelson KG. Apgar scores and umbilical arterial pH in preterm newborn infants. *Am J Obstet Gynecol* 1984;149:651.
   In preterm infants, little correlation between the Apgar score and the umbilical cord pH was observed.
10. Page FO, et al. Correlation of neonatal acid-base status with Apgar scores and fetal heart rate tracings. *Am J Obstet Gynecol* 1986;154:1306.

The combination of fetal heart rate monitoring, cord blood pH, and Apgar assessment was better than any one technique alone in predicting fetal status after delivery.

Amniotic Fluid Meconium

11. Richey SD, et al. Markers of acute and chronic asphyxia in infants with meconium-stained amniotic fluid. *Am J Obstet Gynecol* 1995;172:1212.
    There was no correlation between any marker of asphyxia and the degree of thickness of meconium.

12. Ramin KD, et al. Amniotic fluid meconium: a fetal environmental hazard. *Obstet Gynecol* 1996;87:181.
    The authors suggest that physiologically passed meconium can become a hazard if fetal acidemia supervenes.

13. Hofmeyr GJ, et al. The collaborative randomised amnioinfusion for meconium project (CRAMP). 1. South Africa. *Br J Obstet Gynaecol* 1998;105:304.
    Patients receiving amnioinfusion have fewer low Apgar scores, less meconium below the cords, and a lower incidence of operative delivery, with no adverse effects.

In Search of a Better Mousetrap

14. Cibils LA. On intrapartum fetal monitoring. *Am J Obstet Gynecol* 1996;174:1382.
    Fetal heart rate monitoring is sensitive but nonspecific for detecting fetal compromise. Additional clinical information is needed to discern those fetuses not at risk for development of intrapartum acidosis to avoid unnecessary intervention.

15. Irion O, et al. Is intrapartum vibratory acoustic stimulation a valid alternative to fetal scalp pH determination? *Br J Obstet Gynaecol* 1996;103:642.
    Fetal heart rate (FHR) acceleration following acoustic stimulation was significantly associated with a normal scalp pH but offered no advantage over FHR tracings and could not replace fetal blood sampling.

16. Dildy GA. The relationship between oxygen saturation and pH in umbilical blood: implications for intrapartum fetal oxygen saturation monitoring. *Am J Obstet Gynecol* 1996;175:682.
    It appeared that a critical threshold for fetal arterial oxygen saturation by reflectance pulse oximetry (SpO_2) would be represented by a cutoff value of 30%.

17. Dildy GA, Clark SL, Loucks CA. Intrapartum fetal pulse oximetry: past, present, and future. *Am J Obstet Gynecol* 1996;175:1.
    Fetal oxygen saturation monitoring (pulse oximetry) is already widely used in anesthesiology, critical care, and newborn intensive care.

18. van Wijngaarden WJ, et al. Improved intrapartum surveillance with PR interval analysis of the fetal electrocardiogram: a randomized trial showing a reduction in fetal blood sampling. *Am J Obstet Gynecol* 1996;174:1295.
    The addition of fetal electrocardiogram analysis to electronic monitoring can reduce the need for scalp blood sampling without increasing adverse outcomes.

19. Nordstrom L, et al. Scalp blood lactate: a new test strip method for monitoring fetal wellbeing in labour. *Br J Obstet Gynaecol* 1995;102:894.
    Intrapartum scalp blood lactate was significantly correlated with scalp pH and umbilical artery lactate.

Neonatal Outcome

20. Perlman JM. Intrapartum hypoxic-ischemic cerebral injury and subsequent cerebral palsy: medicolegal issues. *Pediatrics* 1997;99:851.
    Abnormal fetal heart rate patterns and low Apgar scores are more often the consequence of early gestational brain damage or maldevelopment than of intrapartum ischemia and hypoxemia in children with cerebral palsy.

21. Helene TC, et al. Follow-up of children born with an umbilical arterial blood pH <7. *Am J Obstet Gynecol* 1995;173:1758.
    Umbilical artery pH at birth is not predictive of serious developmental delay, unless it is accompanied by clinical evidence of hypoxic encephalopathy.

22. Phelan JP, et al. Nucleated red blood cells: a marker for fetal asphyxia? *Am J Obstet Gynecol* 1995;173:1380.

When asphyxia was present, distinct nucleated red blood cell patterns were identified that were in keeping with the observed basis for the fetal injury.

23. Naeye RL, Localio AR. Determining the time before birth when ischemia and hypoxemia initiated cerebral palsy. *Obstet Gynecol* 1995;86:713.
    This time is critical in determining whether damage occurred in conjunction with obstetric interventions.

---

37. DELIVERY OF THE SMALL AND LARGE INFANT

Barbara B. Hogg and Debora F. Kimberlin

Both small-for-gestational age (SGA) and large-for-gestational age infants are subject to unique labor and delivery complications, ranging from intolerance of labor to shoulder dystocia. Accurate estimation of birth weight is important in order to identify the at-risk infant. However, the most reliable method of estimating fetal weight is unclear. Prospective trials of term infants that compare sonographic and clinical estimations of birth weight do not have consistent findings; however, it appears that estimates from abdominal palpation are at least as accurate as those derived by sonographic parameters with approximately 70% of estimates falling within 10% of the actual birth weight. For the term normally grown infant, neither method is superior. Both methods are prone to error and tend to overestimate the weight of small infants and underestimate the weight of large infants. In addition, sonographic estimates are notoriously inaccurate during labor, when the fetal position may preclude adequate measurements. The accuracy of fetal weight estimation by Leopold's maneuvers is not related to operator experience or amniotic fluid index.

Ultrasound and clinical estimates both overestimate the infant's actual birth weight with a smaller mean error by ultrasonographic evaluation. In the patient in whom an SGA infant is clinically suspected, the sonographic abdominal circumference and estimated fetal weight (EFW) are the best predictors of the SGA infant at birth. While an abdominal circumference below the tenth percentile will detect the highest percentage of SGA fetuses, the likelihood of SGA in an individual fetus is greatest when the sonographic EFW is below the tenth percentile. The role of umbilical artery and uteroplacental waveform indices for the prediction of SGA at birth is unclear.

The prediction of macrosomia is dependent upon the birth weight definition of this cohort of infants. In general, macrosomia is defined as a birth weight of more than 4,000 g. Both clinical and sonographic methods tend to underestimate the actual birth weight, with approximately 60% of macrosomic infants having a birth weight of ±10% of the predicted weight. In the prediction of macrosomia, the sensitivity and specificity of sonographic prediction depends on the birth weight cutoff, with a sensitivity of 65% and a specificity of 90% when a 4,000-g cutoff is utilized. In a large series from Quebec, only 43% of infants weighing more than 4,500 g were correctly identified prior to delivery. For every macrosomic infant identified in this cohort, nine others were incorrectly identified.

Both the appropriately grown preterm fetus and the SGA infant (EFW of less than the 10th percentile for gestational age) are at risk for unique intrapartum complications. These high-risk pregnancies require careful attention to a number of details by the obstetric care provider.

Aggressive attempts should be made to prevent delivery of the preterm infant if there are no maternal or fetal contraindications to tocolysis. In addition, every effort should be made to transport the high-risk maternal-infant pair to a tertiary care center with an experienced maternal-fetal medicine specialist and a well-staffed neonatal intensive care unit prior to delivery, as infants born in a tertiary care center have better outcomes than those transported after birth. Every effort should be made to administer corticosteroids to enhance fetal lung maturity when a preterm delivery is anticipated. Recently, the National Institutes of Health consensus panel recommended that either two doses of betamethasone (12 mg IM administered 24 hours apart) or four doses of dexamethasone (6 mg IM, 12 hours apart) be given 24–36 hours prior to delivery. The interval between courses and optimal number of courses have not been determined. In general, courses are given weekly and every attempt is made to minimize long-term maternal exposure to corticosteroids. Corticosteroid administration should be limited to clinical situations which suggest that preterm delivery is imminent. In the setting of preterm labor, corticosteroids are not felt to be beneficial prior to 24 weeks' or after 34 weeks' gestation and with preterm premature rupture of the membranes, corticosteroid administration is not recommended prior to 24 weeks' or after 30–32 weeks' gestation.

While in labor, continuous electronic fetal monitoring should be employed in the preterm appropriately grown infant and the SGA infant. Such techniques as external and internal fetal heart rate monitoring may enhance detection of hypoxia and acidosis, thus preventing prolonged in utero exposure to these stresses. While the rate of intraventricular hemorrhage does not appear to be associated with intrapartum acidosis, the severity of respiratory distress syndrome may be related.

In accordance with Centers for Disease Control guidelines, a management scheme (screening-based approach or risk-factor approach) for group B Streptococcus (GBS) prophylaxis should be adopted. The American College of Obstetricians and Gynecologists recommends that intrapartum antibiotic prophylaxis be given for high-risk pregnancies. Risk factors for GBS infection include (1) preterm labor, (2) premature rupture of the membranes, (3) prolonged (more than 18 hours) rupture of the membranes, (4) intrapartum maternal fever, or (5) prior infant affected by GBS infection. Current recommended regimens include either ampicillin (2 g IV then 1 g IV q 4 hours until delivery) or penicillin G (5 million units IV then 2.5 million units IV q 4 hours until delivery). The penicillin-allergic patient should receive either clindamycin 900 mg IV q 8 hours or erythromycin 500 mg IV q 6 hours until delivery. Compared to term infants, preterm infants have a markedly increased risk of early onset GBS infection (relative risk 7.3).

At the time of vaginal delivery, a liberal episiotomy should be performed if the perineum is not relaxed. However, there is no evidence that performing an extensive episiotomy reduces the rate of intraventricular hemorrhage. Although forceps deliveries are felt to be safe for the fetus, they need not be performed prophylactically. In general, use of the vacuum is contraindicated when the gestational age is less than 35 weeks or the EFW is less than 2,500 g. Appropriate pediatric personnel should be in attendance at the time of delivery.

Compared to the term infant, the preterm or SGA infant is more likely to be in a nonvertex presentation at the time of labor. Cesarean section should be performed for the viable fetus in a transverse, oblique, and/or incomplete breech presentation. The appropriate management of a fetus in frank or complete breech presentation, however, is more controversial. In general, breech vaginal delivery is an option when the EFW is at least 2,000 g. Patients should be counseled about the option of vaginal delivery if the obstetrician feels the patient is an appropriate candidate for a vaginal breech delivery. Such infants are at slightly higher risk for head entrapment due to the disproportionately large fetal head as compared to the breech. In the event of head entrapment, standard maneuvers including the use of Duhrssen's incisions are indicated. If the patient is not a candidate for vaginal breech delivery, cesarean section should be performed. The choice of uterine incision in the setting of the malpresenting preterm infant generally requires ascertainment of the development of the lower uterine segment and typically mandates a vertical or classical uterine incision in order to allow for easy delivery of the fetus.

The preterm or SGA infant is less likely to tolerate the stress of labor and may require cesarean delivery. Prophylactic cesarean sections, however, do not prevent intraventricular hemorrhage or improve perinatal outcome in the SGA or preterm fetus. In this population, cesarean delivery should be reserved for the usual obstetric indications.

Large for gestational age infants are those infants weighing more than the 90th percentile at birth. Clinically apparent differences in perinatal morbidity and mortality are evident when the fetal weight exceeds 4,000–4,500 g. Macrosomia is generally defined as a fetal weight of more than 4,000 g at the time of delivery and represents between 7% and 10% of term deliveries. Predicting which infants are excessively large is difficult. Maternal risk factors for macrosomia include diabetes, obesity, multiparity, a prior macrosomic infant, age of more than 35 years, and excessive pregnancy weight gain. Such infants are at greater risk for birth trauma including shoulder dystocia, brachial plexus injury with either short- or long-term impairment, and meconium aspiration. In general, these outcomes have not been improved by an increased cesarean section rate in this population. Clinical pelvimetry should be assessed carefully when considering a trial of labor in a woman with a macrosomic fetus, and prophylactic cesarean section should be considered in the diabetic patient with an EFW of more than 4,000 g and in the nondiabetic patient whose EFW is more than 4,500 g.

The risks to the macrosomic infant are those associated with the delivery process. Because macrosomia is difficult to accurately predict, the obstetrician should be familiar with the maneuvers that aid in expeditious delivery. The labor progress of a suspected macrosomic infant should be closely monitored with judicious use of oxytocin augmentation in the face of inadequate progress. Midforceps deliveries in this setting are clearly associated with increased perinatal morbidity and, in general, should not be performed.

Shoulder dystocia occurs when the fetal head is delivered on the perineum and the anterior shoulder fails to deliver with gentle downward traction. For patients considered to be at risk for shoulder dystocia, by either fetal weight estimates or maternal risk factors, the delivery should be performed with several additional personnel available and the patient should be placed in the dorsal lithotomy position. Excessive traction on the fetal head should be avoided at all times. Upon delivery of the fetal head, those infants with a shoulder dystocia often demonstrate a turtle sign where the fetal head initially extends and then flexes back toward the perineum. Upon recognizing the dystocia, suprapubic pressure (not fundal) should be performed by an attendant while the delivering physician applies gentle downward traction to the fetal head. The patient's legs should then be removed from the stirrups and flexed upon the abdomen by additional attendant personnel. This maneuver, called the McRoberts maneuver, allows the pelvis to rotate anteriorly and may allow for delivery of the impacted anterior shoulder. If the dystocia is not relieved by either of these maneuvers, the obstetrician should attempt either a Wood's corkscrew maneuver or delivery of the posterior shoulder. The Wood's corkscrew maneuver involves placing the operator's hand posterior to the fetal shoulder and gently rotating the baby in a corkscrew manner to relieve the impacted anterior shoulder. The posterior shoulder can be delivered by carefully sweeping the fetus' posterior arm across the chest and then delivering the arm. Both the Wood's corkscrew maneuver and delivery of the posterior arm require that the obstetrician be able to place his or her hand in the vagina. If an episiotomy is needed to allow the operator to perform these maneuvers, it should be performed. Additional maneuvers include intentional fracture of the clavicle, which is performed by placing the operator's fingers behind the clavicle and fracturing it away from the fetus, and the Zavanelli maneuver, which involves flexing the head and replacing the head into the pelvis and subsequently performing an emergent cesarean delivery.

Fetal Weight Estimation
1. Sherman DJ, et al. A comparison of clinical and ultrasonic estimation of fetal weight. *Obstet Gynecol* 1998;91:212.
   Clinical estimates of birth weight are similar to ultrasound estimates overall. Ultrasound is a better predictor at less than 2,500 g, clinical estimate is superior in the 2,500–4,000-g range, and the two are equivalent at more than 4,000 g.
2. Watson WJ, Soisson AP, Harlass FE. Estimated weight of the term fetus. *J Reprod Med* 1988;33:369.

There is no difference in clinical and ultrasound estimates of birth weight in the term fetus.

3. Chauhan SP, et al. Intrapartum clinical, sonographic, and parous patients estimates of newborn birth weight. *Obstet Gynecol* 1992;79:956.
   At term, parous patient birth weight estimates are equal to clinical and ultrasound predictors.

4. Benacerraf BF, Gelman R, Frigoletto FD. Sonographically estimated fetal weights: accuracy and limitation. *Am J Obstet Gynecol* 1988;159:1118.
   Ultrasound is limited in its ability to accurately predict birth weight.

5. Chang TC, et al. Prediction of the small for gestational age infant: which ultrasonic measurement is best? *Obstet Gynecol* 1992;80:1030.
   Abdominal circumference is the best predictor of small-for-gestational age infants.

Small for Gestational Age

6. Powell S, et al. Recent changes in delivery site of low-birth-weight infants in Washington: impact on birth weight-specific mortality. *Am J Obstet Gynecol* 1995;173:1585.
   Preventable neonatal mortality in the less-than-2,000-g infant is increased by nontertiary delivery.

7. NIH Consensus Development Panel. Effect of corticosteroids for fetal maturation on perinatal outcomes. *JAMA* 1995;273:413.
   This commentary outlines the risks, benefits, and indications for corticosteroid use to enhance fetal lung maturation.

8. Kimberlin DF, et al. Relationship of acid-base status and neonatal morbidity in <1000-g infants. *Am J Obstet Gynecol* 1996;174:382.
   Umbilical artery acidemia is associated with the severity of respiratory distress syndrome.

9. Centers for Disease Control. Handout for CDC GBS Prevention Update. November 8, 1995.
   Current Centers for Disease Control recommendations regarding group B Streptococcal *prevention.*

10. Eller DP, VanDorsten JP. Breech presentation. *Curr Opin Obstet Gynecol* 1993; 5:664.
    The route of delivery of the preterm breech is controversial.

11. Malloy MH, Onstad L, Wright E. The effect of cesarean delivery on birth outcome in very low birth weight infants. *Obstet Gynecol* 1991;77:498.
    Cesarean delivery does not lower perinatal mortality or rate of intraventricular hemorrhage in infants of <1,500 g.

Large for Gestational Age

12. Acker DB, Sachs BP, Friedman EA. Risk factors for shoulder dystocia. *Obstet Gynecol* 1985;66:762.
    Shoulder dystocia is associated with increasing infant birth weight, labor arrest, and maternal diabetes.

13. Langer O, et al. Shoulder dystocia: should the fetus weighing >4000 grams be delivered by cesarean section? *Am J Obstet Gynecol* 1991;165:831.
    Shoulder dystocia occurs more commonly in nondiabetic women with fetal weights of more than 4,500 g and diabetic women with fetal weights of more than 4,250 g.

14. Boyd ME, Usher RH, McLean FH. Fetal macrosomia: prediction, risks, proposed management. *Obstet Gynecol* 1983;61:715.
    Macrosomia is difficult to predict, and attendant morbidities are associated with the delivery process.

15. Gordon M, et al. The immediate and long-term outcome of obstetric birth trauma. *Am J Obstet Gynecol* 1973;117:51.
    Brachial plexus injuries rarely result in permanent paralysis.

16. Cunningham GF. Dystocia-abnormal presentation, position, and development of the fetus. In: Cunningham GF, et al. eds. *Williams obstetrics,* 20th ed. Stamford, CT: Appleton & Lange, 1997.
    The management of shoulder dystocia requires knowledge of the techniques outlined in this summary.

VIII. PUERPERIUM

38. LACTATION AND LACTATION SUPPRESSION

Harriette Hampton

Prolactin is the key hormone controlling milk production. The entire process of lacto-genesis, however, requires multiple hormonal interactions that affect the development of both the ductal and alveolar cells as well as modulate the nutritional content of milk. Growth of the epithelium comprising the duct system depends on estrogen, which is synergized by the presence of growth hormone, prolactin, and cortisol. Development of the lobular alveolar system requires both estrogen and progesterone in the presence of prolactin. The synthesis of milk protein and fat is regulated principally by prolactin and facilitated by insulin and cortisol.

Although estrogen and progesterone act to stimulate mammary development, these hormones inhibit the formation of milk during pregnancy, thereby reserving milk production for the postpartum state. High levels of estrogen and progesterone block prolactin action on the mammary target cells through antagonism of prolactin receptors. After delivery, estrogen and progesterone levels fall rapidly. This precipitous decline in the circulating hormone levels results in unopposed autoregulatory increases in the mammary prolactin receptor content. As prolactin receptors become abundant in glandular mammary tissue, milk production (lactogenesis) begins and is usually apparent in 3–4 days postpartum.

While the initiation of lactation depends on sex steroids and trophic hormone stimulation, its maintenance depends on unique neuroendocrine responses to mechanical stimulation of the nipple during suckling. Sensory signals originating in the nipple during stimulation are conveyed in a somatic afferent spinohypothalamic pathway to the periventricular and supraoptic nuclei of the hypothalamus. This neuronal system controls the release of oxytocin and prolactin. The myoepithelial cells contract the mammary alveolar duct and eject milk in response to oxytocin stimulation. Maternal-fetal play or the anticipation of feeding by the mother can produce an episodic release of oxytocin, clearly illustrating the involvement of higher centers in the neuroendocrine control of oxytocin secretion.

In addition to the oxytocin release that occurs with nursing, there is a prompt and dramatic release of prolactin that is temporally associated with, but independent of, the episodic oxytocin release. The transient increase in prolactin secretion is usually sufficient to maintain an adequate supply of milk for the infant until the next feeding time. In the first postpartum week, prolactin levels in breast-feeding women decline from pregnant levels of 200–300 ng/ml to approximately 100 ng/ml. The prolactin levels are then sustained to 40–50 ng/ml for the next 2 to 3 months, with transient 10- to 20-fold increases in the serum concentrations during suckling. In the first 3–4 months after birth, the basal prolactin levels fall to normal, but suckling still produces episodic releases, which are essential for continued milk production.

The composition of human milk has been analyzed extensively. Physiochemically, milk is an isotonic emulsion of fat and water. Mature human milk contains 3%–5% fat, 0.8%–1.2% protein, 6.8%–7.2% carbohydrates, and 0.2% mineral constituents. The energy content is 60–75 kilocalories per 100 ml. Colostrum, the secretory product of the breast before the initiation of lactogenesis, contains more protein and less carbohydrate than mature milk. The major proteins in milk are caseins, alpha-lactalbumin, lactoferrin, immunoglobulin A (IgA), lysozyme, and serum albumin. All vitamins, except vitamin K, are present in human milk, but in variable amounts. Human milk contains a low concentration of iron, although this iron is absorbed more readily than that from cow's milk. The immunologic advantage afforded by breast milk is not found in other milk sources. The immunoglobulins (especially secretory IgA), lactoferrin, and lysozyme found in breast milk are able to protect the neonate against infections.

The nutritional status of the mother during lactation is important. For each 20 calories of milk produced, the mother who breast-feeds must consume 30 calories.

A dietary caloric requirement of approximately 600 additional calories per day is observed in women who maintain their body weight while lactating. The energy cost of lactation is met in most, however, by the mobilization of fat stores laid down during pregnancy. Recommended daily dietary increases for lactation consist of a 20-g increase in protein, a 20% increment in all vitamins and minerals except folic acid, which should be increased by 50%, and a 33% elevation in the intake of calcium, phosphorus, and magnesium. Continuation of prenatal vitamin and iron supplementation usually meets these requirements.

Breast-feeding is not an instinctive art. A nurse or other practitioner is invaluable in helping the new mother position the baby and in offering support and encouragement. The most common problems encountered in breast-feeding are nipple soreness and engorgement, particularly in the early days of nursing. Reassurance from the physician that it is common and temporary is essential to the breast-feeding mother. Persistent nipple soreness does not result from the duration of breast-feeding but from an improper grasp of the nipple and areola. Allowing the nipples to air-dry after nursing can be of benefit when nipples are painful or cracking. The application of plain anhydrous lanolin may help, as long as moisture is not trapped beneath the ointment.

Engorgement of the breast involves lymphatic and vascular congestion as well as an accumulation of milk in the ductal system. The best management of engorgement, of course, is prevention, which can be most easily accomplished by having the infant nurse in an early, unscheduled, and frequent fashion. Treatment includes proper bra support and the application of cold packs after nursing. If the baby is nursing poorly, the problem should be addressed through manual pumping of the breast. The temporary use of analgesics may be necessary for some women.

Less frequent breast-feeding problems include an impaired let-down reflex and a poor milk supply. Virtually any woman can produce milk, but, if she cannot release it, production will not continue. The let-down reflex depends on the pituitary release of oxytocin. Signs and symptoms of let-down include sensations ranging from a sense of tightening or pressure to a pronounced pins-and-needles feeling in the nipple. The most powerful trigger for this surge of oxytocin is the infant suckling. Like most reflexes mediated by the hypothalamus, the let-down reflex is inhibited most commonly by psychologic factors. The treatment of impaired let-down includes increased maternal rest, comfort, privacy, and removal of distractions. If this is unsuccessful, a trial of synthetic oxytocin (Syntocinon, available as a nasal spray) has proved useful for some women.

Milk supply is determined by a simple supply-and-demand feedback loop. Problems of insufficient milk production are primarily related to inadequate frequency or length of feedings, provided that nutrition is adequate. Once again, the availability of a support person is of critical importance for mothers who are breast-feeding, should problems arise.

The question of contraception during lactation is important. The contraceptive effect of breast-feeding alone has been observed in third-world settings. A mother who is breast-feeding exclusively has only a one in 1,250 chance of ovulating during the first 9 weeks postpartum. After this time, however, ovulation occurs more often and is unpredictable, prompting the need for reliable contraception. Barrier contraception has no contraindications, and the intrauterine device is acceptable for the multigravid, breast-feeding mother who is aware of the risks involved. Steroidal contraceptives appear to have little or no effect on milk composition, but the combined oral contraceptive may have an adverse effect on breast milk production. The degree to which lactation is suppressed relates to the dosage and timing of therapy. The minidose progestin-only pill and injectable progestin do not adversely affect breast milk production.

As a general rule, it should be assumed that any drug ingested by a nursing mother may be present in breast milk at 1%–2% of the maternal dosage. The excretion of a drug in breast milk is increased for the pharmacologic agents with any of the following properties: low molecular weight, high lipid solubility, low protein binding, small volumes of distribution, and a long half-life. Metabolism of the drug by the neonate depends on the infant's stage of development. The current literature should be reviewed before administering any drug to breast-feeding patients. Relative contraindications must be considered in light of the risk-benefit relationship. Pharmacologic measures to suppress lactation were attempted as early as 1940. The first medications used were chlorotrianisene (TACE), a progestin with weak estrogenic properties, and a combination of testosterone enanthate and estradiol valerate (Deladumone OB). Limitations of hormone therapy include questionable efficacy, risk of puerperal thromboembolism, and high incidence of rebound lactation. These medications were not prescribed after 1980, when the Food and Drug Administration (FDA) approved the nonsteroidal bromocriptine mesylate (Parlodel) for physiologic postpartum lactation suppression. The mechanism for action of this ergot derivative, a dopamine receptor agonist, is inhibition of the release of prolactin. Secondary to case reports of cardiovascular and cerebrovascular complications, in 1990 the FDA requested voluntary sales of Parlodel as a lactation suppressant to be halted. Successful clinical trials with long-acting dopamine agonists such as Capergoline are reported in Europe, but are not approved for this indication in the United States.

Although no drug is currently marketed to suppress postpartum lactation, patients should be reassured that stopping milk production is rarely problematic. Suppression of lactation can be achieved in approximately 60% of patients by mechanical compression and avoidance of nipple stimulation. Relief of modest symptoms can be achieved with ice packs and oral analgesics such as Ibuprofen, 600 mg t.i.d.

General
1. Ogle KS, Alfano MA. Common problems of initiating breast-feeding. *Postgrad Med* 1987;82:159.
   A thoughtful review of the management of common problems encountered in breast-feeding.
2. Shingleton WW, McCarty KS Jr. What you should know about breast pathology. *Contemp Obstet Gynecol* 1987;29:90.
   A practical look at breast pathology, containing a nice section on the major hormonal influences on the breast as well as the clinical correlates of histologic changes in the breast that may occur during or before pregnancy.
3. Whitehead RG. Nutritional aspects of human lactation. *Lancet* 1983;1:167.
   An excellent comprehensive report, although brief, in which the dietary role of breast milk is detailed.

Etiology
4. Yen SC, Jaffe RB. *Reproductive endocrinology*, 2nd ed. Philadelphia: Saunders, 1986.
   The composition of breast milk is detailed in this superlative report.
5. Darr MS, Taylor RB. A practical guide to drugs in breast milk. *Female Patient* 1988;13:42.
   A simple but comprehensive guide for the clinician and patient regarding the effects of drugs on breast milk.
6. Neifert MR, Seacat JM. How to help patients breastfeed successfully. *Contemp Obstet Gynecol* 1987;4:85.
   Using excellent visual aids, details how to assist patients in breast-feeding.
7. Bauchner J, Leventhal JM, Shapiro ED. Studies of breast-feeding and infections. How good is the evidence? *JAMA* 1986;256:887.
   An excellent compilation of 20 studies, meeting stringent methodologic standards, that examined the association between breast-feeding and infections in the neonate. The authors found that breast-feeding conferred minimal protection in nursing mothers from industrialized countries.

Diagnosis
8. Feller WF. Steps in evaluation of a breast mass. *Contemp Obstet Gynecol* 1988; 32:11.
   How to evaluate a breast mass and how to diagnose breast masses in pregnancy are discussed.
9. Scialli AR, Fabro S. What drugs are safe during nursing? *Contemp Obstet Gynecol* 1984;22:211.

This excellent article details how to determine which drugs are safe for mothers who are nursing.

10. Bergevin U, Doughtery C, Kramer MS. Do infant formula samples shorten the duration of breast-feeding? *Lancet* 1983;1:1148.
    The results from this large and elegant study indicate that, when babies are fed infant formula, this may shorten the duration of breast-feeding and may indeed hasten the age when they are given solid food.

Treatment

11. Ford K, Labbok M. Contraceptive usage during lactation in the United States: an update. *Am J Public Health* 1987;77:79.
    Barrier method contraception was found to be preferred in a survey of breast-feeding women conducted in the United States.

12. West CP. The acceptability of a progestin-only contraceptive during breastfeeding. *Contraception* 1983;27:563.
    Use of the progestin-only pill did not adversely affect either breast milk production or the infant.

13. Shapiro AG, Thomas L. Efficacy of bromocriptine versus binders as inhibitors of postpartum lactation. *South Med J* 1984;77:719.
    The use of breast binders was compared to bromocriptine therapy in 50 postpartum patients. Bromocriptine was more successful in suppressing breast problems but the side effects were higher; thus, the dosage was reduced from 2.5 to 1.25 mg twice a day, which is the currently recommended clinical dosage.

14. Defoort P, et al. Bromocriptine in an injectable form for puerperal lactation suppression: comparison with estrandron prolongatum. *Obstet Gynecol* 1987;70:866.
    Bromocriptine (injectable) was compared to estrandron. Both appeared to suppress lactation adequately.

15. Kremer J. Lactation inhibition by a single injection of a new depot-bromocriptine. *Br J Obstet Gynaecol* 1990;97:527.
    Encouraging results from the depot administration of Parlodel are reported.

16. Koetswang S. The effects of contraceptive methods on the quality and quantity of breast milk. *Int J Gynecol Obstet* 1987;25:115.
    An excellent review of the Third World experience with contraceptive agents in the postpartum period.

17. Dunson TR, et al. A multicenter clinical trial of progestin-only oral contraceptive in lactating women. *Contraception* 1993;47:23.
    Progestin-only oral contraceptive pills were effective for postpartum breast-feeding women.

Complications

18. Katz M, et al. Puerperal hypertension, stroke, and seizures after suppression of lactation with bromocriptine. *Obstet Gynecol* 1985;66:822.
    Two cases of cerebrovascular events that occurred after the use of bromocriptine are presented.

19. Yaffe SJ. Drugs and the nursing mother. *Female Patient* 1984;9:19.
    In this well-detailed report, a compendium of drugs is presented that are contraindicated in the breast-feeding mother. It also depicts nicely the pharmacologic principles at work in the secretion of drugs in breast milk.

20. Tchabo JG, Stay EJ. Gravidic macromastia: case report. *Am J Obstet Gynecol* 1989;160:88.
    The authors describe a rare condition called gravidic macromastia, in which the breasts become engorged as a result of marked hormonal influence. Medical therapy with dihydroprogesterone is recommended first, followed by surgical intervention if the former proves unsuccessful.

21. Kulig K. Bromocriptine-associated headache: possible life-threatening sympathomimetic interaction. *Obstet Gynecol* 1991;78:941.
    Cases involving a sympathomimetic interaction with Parlodel are reported.

22. Deutinger M, Deutinger J. Breast feeding after aesthetic mammary operations and cardiac operations through horizontal submammary skin incision. *Surg Gynecol Obstet* 1993;176:267.
Postpartum women who had undergone an aesthetic mammary operation were able to breast-feed their infants.

---

39. POSTPARTUM HEMORRHAGE

Baha M. Sibai, Farid Mattar, and Dorel Abramovici

Postpartum hemorrhage (PPH) is a serious complication of pregnancy and the puerperium that may result in serious maternal morbidity, and is a leading cause of maternal mortality in several countries, accounting for 28% of maternal deaths in the developing world. Defined as a blood loss exceeding 500 ml, the exact incidence is difficult to determine because the clinical estimation of blood loss during delivery is inaccurate by as much as 50%, compared to the actual loss that can be determined after delivery. When measured correctly, the mean blood loss during vaginal delivery and postpartum in one large series was found to be 500 ml, with 39% of the patients losing more than this. About 4% of the patients lose more than 1,000 ml, although the actual incidence of PPH severe enough to cause hemorrhagic shock is less than 1%. The bleeding is usually continuous but may be slow or brisk, depending on the cause. PPH is considered early if it occurs during the first 24 hours postpartum and late if it develops after this time.

Uterine atony is the cause of early PPH in approximately 90% of the cases; genital tract lacerations, including uterine, cervical, vaginal, and perineal lacerations account for 6%; and retained placental fragments are responsible in 3%–4% of the cases. The last accounts for most cases of late PPH, but routine exploration of the uterus after delivery can eliminate 90% of these. Other infrequent causes include uterine inversion and blood dyscrasia, such as von Willebrand's disease, factor VII deficiency, thrombotic thrombocytopenic purpura, and acquired coagulation problems associated with amniotic fluid embolism or abruptio placentae after fetal demise. The risk of PPH is increased if any of the following factors are present: (1) overdistention of the uterus owing to hydramnios, multiple pregnancy, or a macrosomic fetus; (2) high parity; (3) prolonged difficult labor, especially after oxytocin induction; (4) history of previous PPH; (5) preeclampsia; or (6) precipitous labor. Other correlates include general anesthesia, abnormal placentation such as placenta previa or accreta, abruptio placentae, and a succinate placental lobe, as well as operative delivery using either instrumentation or version and extraction.

Steps to be taken in the management of PPH include early recognition, aggressive correction of hypovolemia, and control of the specific bleeding sites. Patients with predisposing factors should be monitored closely, and blood should be available at the time of delivery. Universal therapy for all patients should include prompt blood and volume replacement, maintenance of good urinary output, and serial monitoring of the patient's vital signs, hematocrit, and central venous pressure. After the initial steps have been implemented, the patient should be examined under general anesthesia, with systematic exploration of the genital tract to identify the cause of bleeding.

The classic management of uterine atony consists of the mechanical stimulation of uterine contractions by means of firm (but not vigorous) massage of the uterus through the abdomen and concomitant bimanual compression of the elevated anteverted uterus. These measures should be performed in conjunction with the simultaneous administration of oxytocic agents in amounts sufficient to initiate and maintain uterine contractility. Mechanical maneuvers to stop the attendant bleeding include digital compression of the uterine arteries in the paracervical area and compression of the descending aorta against the maternal spine.

Oxytocin should be given by continuous intravenous administration in a dosage as high as 20–30 units per 500 ml of Ringer's lactate solution. It should never be given as a bolus because hypotension, myocardial arrhythmias, and cardiac arrest may occur. The simultaneous intramuscular administration of 0.2 mg of methylergonovine may be used in those who are normotensive if the uterus fails to respond to oxytocin. One large series found that oxytocin was as effective as a combination of oxytocin and ergometrine in the prevention of PPH, and that either was more effective when administered immediately after head delivery.

If the aforementioned measures fail to control the bleeding resulting from uterine atony within 15 minutes, other potent ecbolic agents such as prostaglandins may be used. The intramuscular administration of 0.25 mg of 15-methyl PGF_2 (a prostaglandin F_2 analogue) has been shown in several studies to be very effective in controlling PPH secondary to uterine atony when it is unresponsive to conventional methods. The drug can be injected directly into the myometrium or can be given intramuscularly. Some of the side effects reported include nausea, vomiting, diarrhea, pyrexia, and acute hypertension, with the last usually seen in preeclamptic patients. Prostaglandin E_2 has also been used, both intravenously and as vaginal suppositories, to treat severe cases of PPH even in preeclamptic patients. The use of tranexamic acid, a synthetic fibrinolytic inhibitor, was described to successfully control intractable PPH not responding to conventional medical therapy. Misoprostol, a PGE_1 analogue, was also found to be effective in the prevention of PPH. Misoprostol has the additional advantages of being an oral agent, not requiring special storage conditions, and having a shelf life of several years.

If all the aforementioned measures fail to control the bleeding resulting from uterine atony, other recommended methods of treatment include the instillation of heated solutions into the uterus, intrauterine packing, or surgical intervention, although the efficacy of intrauterine packing remains controversial. Some consider it a valuable procedure for uterine atony, whereas other believe it is unphysiologic and ineffective, contributes to further bleeding, predisposes to infection, and may delay definitive treatment by obscuring the amount of blood loss. Most agree, however, that intrauterine packing can be used as a temporary measure in preparation for surgical management, and occasionally, it may be a lifesaving or uterus-preserving measure. Surgical intervention may include laparotomy with these options: ligation of the uterine arteries, ovarian blood supply, or hypogastric arteries, or total or subtotal hysterectomy, depending on the condition of the parturient as well as the desire to preserve fertility. The selective arterial infusion of antidiuretic hormone (Pitressin), embolization, or both, may be used to control life-threatening PPH in some cases when laparotomy is not possible.

Recently, two novel surgical approaches were described: (1) stepwise uterine devascularization of the uterine and ovarian arteries, and (2) the B-Lynch uterine brace or compression suture. Both have been proposed as effective alternatives to hysterectomy for the management of intractable PPH.

Retained fragments of the placenta can be removed digitally once the proper cleavage plane is found by means of manual exploration just after delivery. This can be facilitated by the use of placental forceps to grasp fragments and a piece of gauze spread out over the gloved fingers to remove small fragments and adherent placental membranes. Occasionally, curettage of the uterus may be necessary using a large blunt curette. The diagnosis of placenta accreta should be suspected in the absence of a cleavage plane and inability to remove placental fragments. Treatment usually requires hysterectomy, although intrauterine packing has been used successfully in some cases.

Vaginal and cervical lacerations are usually the result of the use of instruments at delivery, but may also result from precipitous spontaneous delivery. The most common sites for cervical lacerations are at the three and nine o'clock positions. Control of bleeding is usually achieved by simple suture repair after large vessels are isolated and tied individually. Deep lacerations should be closed in layers to avoid hematoma formation, and the repair should start above the apex of the laceration. Vaginal packing may be helpful in preventing venous oozing or bleeding from varicosities. Laceration of the lower uterine segment or rupture of the uterus should be suspected following difficult midforceps operations, internal uterine manipulation, and hyperstimulation (oxytocin), as well as in the setting of vaginal delivery after previous cesarean section. Bleeding resulting from uterine rupture may be internal, and the diagnosis can be confirmed by digital exploration of the uterus. Treatment of uterine rupture includes laparotomy, with the options comprising repair of the laceration, as well as total or subtotal hysterectomy, depending on the type, extent, and site of laceration, as well as the patient's condition and the desire to preserve the uterus.

Acute puerperal inversion of the uterus is a rare cause of PPH and one that is usually associated with excessive fundal pressure, strong traction on the umbilical cord, grand multiparity, placenta accreta, and uterine atony. Classic symptoms include shock, hemorrhage, and pain. If the diagnosis is made early and general anesthesia is available, manual replacement is possible in most cases. Applying constant slow pressure, Trendelenburg positioning, and filling the vagina with warm sterile saline solution may also be helpful in restoring the organ to its correct position.

The incidence of late PPH is about one in 1,000 deliveries, with most cases occurring between day 6 and 10 after delivery. Frequent causes are subinvolution of the uterus and retained placental fragments. Other causes include endometritis and withdrawal bleeding from estrogens. Many of these patients can be managed conservatively with uterotonic agents, especially if placental inspection and uterine exploration are done routinely at the time of delivery. The use of curettage along with the simultaneous administration of oxytocin is necessary in about 65% of the patients, but may be associated with potential complications, such as uterine perforation and an increased incidence of Asherman's syndrome.

The potential complications of PPH include postpartum infection, anemia, transfusion hepatitis, Sheehan's syndrome, and Asherman's syndrome, especially if curettage was part of the management. Sheehan's syndrome, or acute pituitary necrosis, occurs in a small number of patients after severe PPH, and is associated most commonly with prolonged shock and secondary ischemic necrosis of the anterior pituitary gland. Prolactin-secreting cells are the first to be affected by anterior pituitary ischemia; hence, the diagnosis should be suspected early in the absence of lactation. Treatment consists of hormonal replacement.

In summary, the best management of PPH is prevention, but, when it occurs, good clinical acumen in combination with treatment is called for.

General
1. Hayashi R. Obstetric hemorrhage and hypovolemic shock. In: Clark SL, et al. eds. *Critical care in obstetrics*. Philadelphia: Blackwell Scientific, 1991.
   The pathophysiologic causes of hemorrhagic shock are listed, and a step-by-step approach to the management of obstetric hemorrhage is discussed.
2. Harris BA. Acute puerperal inversion of the uterus. *Clin Obstet Gynecol* 1984; 27:134.
   The etiology, incidence, classification, clinical course, and treatment of postpartum uterine inversion are summarized.

Etiology
3. Benedetti TJ. Obstetric hemorrhage. In: Gabbe SG, Niebyl JR, Simpson JL, eds. *Obstetrics, normal and problem pregnancies*. New York: Churchill Livingstone, 1999;499–532.
   The various causes of postpartum hemorrhage are listed, and a step-by-step approach to management of obstetric hemorrhage is discussed.
4. Hayashi RH. Heading off disaster in postpartum hemorrhage. *Contemp Obstet Gynecol* 1982;20:91.
   Definition, incidence, and the various factors associated with postpartum hemorrhage (PPH) are reviewed. The author also describes a step-by-step approach for managing patients with PPH stemming from uterine atony.

5. Brar HS, et al. Acute puerperal uterine inversion. New approaches to management. *J Reprod Med* 1989;34:173.
A retrospective review of 56 patients with uterine inversion is presented in this article. Patients who received oxytocin were at high risk for inversion. Magnesium sulfate or the beta mimetics were acceptable alternatives to general anesthesia in relaxing the uterus.

Diagnosis
6. Herbert WNP, Cefalo RC. Management of postpartum hemorrhage. *Clin Obstet Gynecol* 1984;27:139.
The etiology, predisposing factors, and management of postpartum hemorrhage are summarized.
7. Watson P, Besch N, Bowes WA. Management of acute and subacute puerperal inversion of the uterus. *Obstet Gynecol* 1980;55:12.
Eighteen cases of puerperal inversion of the uterus were studied. The most common signs were hemorrhage (94%) and shock (39%). Treatment regimens are summarized.

Treatment
8. Soriano D, et al. A prospective cohort study of oxytocin plus ergometrine compared with oxytocin alone for prevention of postpartum haemorrhage. *Br J Obstet Gynaecol* 1996;103:1068.
A total of 2,189 women were included. Oxytocin-ergometrine IM was comparable in efficacy to oxytocin IV alone, but had higher adverse effects. Either drug was associated with a significantly lower rate of PPH when administered at the second stage as opposed to the end of the third stage.
9. Alok K, Hagen P, Webb JB. Tranexamic acid in the management of postpartum haemorrhage. *Br J Obstet Gynaecol* 1996;103:1250.
A case report describing the successful use of tranexamic acid for the treatment of severe PPH following a cesarean section delivery for placenta previa/accreta, and after failure of conventional medical therapy.
10. El-Refaey H, et al. Use of oral misoprostol in the prevention of postpartum haemorrhage. *Br J Obstet Gynaecol* 1997;104:336.
A total of 2,347 consecutive patients were given 600 μg of oral misoprostol upon clamping of the umbilical cord. The rates of PPH (6%), need for further therapeutic oxytocics (5%), and the length of the third stage of labor (5 minutes) were lower than those reported without oxytocics, and comparable to Syntometrine (a combination of oxytocin and ergometrine).
11. AbdRabbo SA. Stepwise uterine devascularization: a novel technique for management of uncontrollable postpartum hemorrhage with preservation of the uterus. *Am J Obstet Gynecol* 1994;171:694.
This approach was used on 103 patients who failed the classic treatment of PPH, with a 100% success rate in avoiding hysterectomy and no complications.
12. B-Lynch C, et al. The B-Lynch surgical technique for the control of massive postpartum hemorrhage: an alternative to hysterectomy? Five cases reported. *Br J Obstet Gynaecol* 1997;104:372.
Reports a series of five cases of intractable PPH treated with a novel uterine brace or compression suture.
13. Drife J. Management of primary postpartum haemorrhage. Commentary. *Br J Obstet Gynaecol* 1997;104:275.
A broad description of the definition and management of PPH, with particular reference to medical treatment with ecbolic agents, uterine packing, and surgical intervention.
14. Magil B. PGF$_2$ for postpartum hemorrhage—how well does it work? *Contemp Obstet Gynecol* 1984;23:111.
Physicians who have participated in clinical trials of PGF$_2$ report their findings. The dosage and number of doses needed, the clinical efficacy, and the side effects are detailed. Definitions and the factors associated with postpartum hemorrhage are also discussed.

15. Garite TJ, Buttino L Jr. The use of 15-methyl F_2 alpha prostaglandin (prostin 15M) for the control of postpartum hemorrhage. *Am J Perinatol* 1986;3:241.
    Describes the use of prostin 15M in 26 patients with postpartum hemorrhage who did not respond to conventional treatment, including fundal massage plus oxytocin, and methylergonovine. All patients had uterine atony. The success rate was 84.6% (22 patients responded). Two patients underwent hysterectomy because of placenta accreta, one patient required dilatation and curettage, and one patient underwent bilateral uterine artery ligation. The mean number of doses given was 2.2 (range, one to seven doses).
16. Hayashi RH, Castillo MS, Noah ML. Management of severe postpartum hemorrhage with an F_2 analogue. *Obstet Gynecol* 1984;63:806.
    Fifty-one patients with postpartum hemorrhage unresponsive to conventional therapy were studied. The use of an intramuscular PGF_2 analogue in the management of these patients is detailed.
17. Gaye H, Gough JD, Gillmer MDG. Control of persistent primary postpartum haemorrhage due to uterine atony with intravenous prostaglandin E_2. Case report. *Br J Obstet Gynaecol* 1983;90:280.
    Describes the successful use of PGE_2, given intravenously, in a patient with intractable primary postpartum hemorrhage stemming from uterine atony.
18. Gunning JE. For controlling intractable hemorrhage: the gravity suit. *Contemp Obstet Gynecol* 1983;22:23.
    The gravity suit can be a lifesaving measure in some patients with severe postpartum hemorrhagic shock. A detailed description of how and when to use the suit is presented.
19. Hestler JD. Postpartum hemorrhage and reevaluation of uterine packing. *Obstet Gynecol* 1975;45:501.
    Reports on 153 patients with postpartum hemorrhage. Uterine packing, surgical intervention, and conservative management are compared.
20. Malviya VK, Deppe G. Control of intraoperative hemorrhage in gynecology with the use of fibrin glue. *Obstet Gynecol* 1989;73:284.
    The authors describe the use of fibrin glue in three patients. They believe that, if used in conjunction with good surgical technique, it would decrease the need for blood transfusions.
21. Gilbert WM, et al. Angiographic embolization in the management of hemorrhagic complications of pregnancy. *Aust J Obstet Gynecol* 1992;166:493.
    This procedure is described in managing 109 women with pregnancy-related hemorrhage, including three due to postcesarean bleeding, four because of vaginal wall hematomas, two due to cervical pregnancies, and one due to postpartum bleeding. The procedure was successful in all cases and the average length of time for the procedure was 167 minutes. The authors conclude that angiographic embolization is effective for controlling postpartum hemorrhage in hemodynamically stable patients.
22. Altabef KM, et al. Intravenous nitroglycerin for uterine relaxation of an inverted uterus. *Am J Obstet Gynecol* 1992;166:1237.
    Nitroglycerin (50–100 mg IV) was used for uterine relaxation to permit replacement of a tightly contracted, inverted uterus. Relaxation with this drug was rapid, effective, and without adverse side effects.

Complications
23. Visscher JC, Visscher RD. Early and late postpartum hemorrhage. In: Sciarra JJ, ed. *Gynecology and obstetrics. Vol. 2.* Maryland: Harper and Row, 1980;1–5.
    A most complete reference to the causes of both early and late postpartum hemorrhage. The steps taken to prevent this complication are discussed.
24. Feinberg BB, et al. Angiographic embolization in the management of late postpartum hemorrhage. A case report. *J Reprod Med* 1987;32:929.
    Bilateral selective embolization of the internal iliac arteries was used to control late recurrent postpartum hemorrhage. The authors recommend using this procedure as a means of preserving fertility.

25. Weckstein LH, Masserman JSH, Garite TJ. Placenta accreta: a problem of increasing clinical significance. *Obstet Gynecol* 1987;69:480.
   The case of a woman with placenta previa and accreta is described. The risk factors, incidence, and recommendations for management are discussed.
26. DeSimone CA, et al. Intravenous nitroglycerin aids manual extraction of a retained placenta. *Anesthesiology* 1990;73:787.
   The authors describe the use of intravenous nitroglycerin in 22 patients who required uterine relaxation for manual removal of the placenta. The method was successful in all cases, and there were no maternal side effects.
27. Duggan PM, et al. Intractable postpartum hemorrhage managed by angiographic embolization: case report and review. *Aust NZ J Obstet Gynaecol* 1991;31:229.
   A comprehensive review of using this technique to control intractable postpartum hemorrhage. The technique and risks from angiographic embolization are detailed.
28. Khan GQ, et al. Controlled cord traction versus minimal intervention techniques in delivery of the placenta: a randomized controlled trial. *Am J Obstet Gynecol* 1997;177:770.
   In this large, prospective study, the authors found that cord traction for delivery of the placenta results in a significantly lower incidence of postpartum hemorrhage and retained placenta, as well as less need for uterogenic agents, compared with minimal intervention.

40. PUERPERAL INFECTIONS

Marian H. Ascarelli

Puerperal infection is a general term that describes any postpartum infection of the genital tract. Puerperal fever is defined as an oral temperature of 38.0°C (100.4°F) or higher that is noted to occur on two occasions on any two of the first 10 days postpartum, exclusive of the first 24 hours when taken by standard oral technique four times a day. Most puerperal fever is due to infection in the genital tract; however, other sources of febrile morbidity must be excluded. Although death from infection is rare in developed nations, pelvic infections are among the most serious complications that can occur during the postpartum period. The primary determinant of the risk for genital tract infection is route of delivery. Patients delivered vaginally have approximately a 2% incidence of endometritis, which increases to 6% in high-risk patients. In patients delivered by cesarean section, the incidence is 15%–35% if prophylactic antibiotics are given and can be as high as 90% in patients not receiving prophylactic antibiotics, especially in an indigent population. The principal risk factors for post-cesarean endomyometritis are young age, low socioeconomic status, extended duration of labor with ruptured membranes, multiple vaginal exams, and delivery for cephalopelvic disproportion. The placental implantation site is primarily involved in the infectious process, and the collection of serosanguinous material within the uterine and pelvic cavities provides an excellent medium for organism proliferation with subsequent tissue invasion in the presence of surgical trauma, suture material, and devitalized tissue. Clinical manifestations of endomyometritis include fever, tachycardia, lower abdominal or uterine tenderness, malaise, and purulent or foul-smelling lochia. Infection is usually polymicrobial in nature and caused by bacteria that normally colonize the female lower genital tract. The most frequently isolated pathogens are *Escherichia coli, Klebsiella pneumoniae,* and Proteus species. Anaerobes such as Bacteroides species, Peptococcus, and Peptostreptococcus are frequently present, while group B and group D (Enterococcus) Streptococcus are also important pathogens. Several antibiotic regimens have proven to be efficacious in the treatment of postcesarean endomyometritis. Clindamycin plus an aminoglycoside, a broad-spectrum cephalosporin such as cefoxitin, cefotetan, or moxalactam, or an extended-spectrum penicillin such as mezlocillin can be utilized for antibiotic therapy. Mezlocillin alone or clindamycin plus an aminoglycoside are the most cost-effective treatment regimens. Most patients demonstrate a response within 72 hours of initiation of treatment, and antibiotics should be continued until the patient has been completely afebrile for 24–48 hours. There is no evidence that continued oral antibiotic therapy after discharge from the hospital offers any additional benefit. Treatment failure is usually due to a resistant organism or a concurrent wound infection. Other less common complications of endomyometritis that are associated with poor treatment response are necrotizing fasciitis, peritonitis, parametrial phlegmon, pelvic abscess, and septic pelvic thrombophlebitis.

Wound infections occur in 3%–15% of patients who undergo cesarean section and occur more commonly in patients with diabetes, obesity, anemia, poor hemostasis, immunosuppression or corticosteroid use, chorioamnionitis, and emergency cesarean delivery. Wound infection often does not become manifest until 4–7 days postsurgery and is often preceded by symptomatic endomyometritis. Persistent fever may be the only symptom, or infection may be accompanied by skin erythema surrounding the incision and a serous, serosanguinous, or purulent drainage from the operative site. Surgical drainage of the wound is the treatment of choice; however, when associated skin cellulitis is present, adjunctive therapy with antimicrobials is indicated. Packing of the wound with sterile gauze dressing twice or three times daily usually results in the formation of good granulation tissue, at which time the wound can often be successfully closed using steristrips, sutures, or staples. In some cases, healing by secondary intention may be more prudent. In all cases where a wound infection is diagnosed, the physician must ensure that the fascial closure is intact and that a dehiscence has not occurred. Episiotomy infections are rare due to the increased vascularity of the perineal tissues that develops during pregnancy. When infection develops at the episiotomy site, pain in excess of predicted intensity is common. Treatment includes opening of the infected site with subsequent debridement, and healing is allowed to occur by the process of granulation. Patients with diabetes are at increased risk for such infections, and progression to necrotizing fasciitis can occur. Early diagnosis and aggressive treatment including surgical debridement and intravenous antibiotic therapy is crucial in order to avoid the excessively high morbidity and mortality that accompanies this complication.

Septic pelvic thrombophlebitis is a rare complication of delivery and is more common in patients who have experienced operative vaginal delivery or cesarean section. It often presents following treatment for endomyometritis whereby continued fever spikes without other clinical symptomatology occur despite antibiotic therapy. It is most often a diagnosis of exclusion, and blood cultures may be positive in up to 35% of cases. Treatment with therapeutic doses of heparin can be utilized as both a diagnostic and therapeutic treatment modality. In many cases there will be prompt defervescence within 48–72 hours after heparin has been initiated and confirms the diagnosis. Most authorities recommend that 7–10 days of full anticoagulation be given, maintaining the partial thromboplastin time (PTT) levels at two times the pretreatment control value. The need for continued anticoagulation as an outpatient after discharge from the hospital is controversial.

Respiratory infections occur almost exclusively in patients who have been delivered by cesarean section. Obesity, underlying pulmonary disease, smoking, and general anesthesia are risk factors for the development of a postoperative pulmonary infection. Prophylactic pulmonary treatments that facilitate alveolar distention and sputum expectoration may be useful in high-risk patients for the prevention of atelectasis and bacterial pneumonia, while careful anesthetic technique is the most important factor in preventing aspiration. Clinical signs and symptoms of pneumonitis may include fever, cough, purulent sputum, chest pain, tachycardia, dyspnea, tachypnea, and hypoxemia. Appropriate clinical evaluation as well as laboratory studies including arterial blood gas measurements, chest x-ray, gram stain, and culture of the sputum are required to make an accurate diagnosis. Antibiotic therapy for pneumonic infections should be targeted to include coverage for community-acquired as well as nosocomial infection.

Urinary tract infections are relatively common and generally present with the onset of lower abdominal or back pain, dysuria, frequency, urgency, and low-grade fever. Pyelonephritis should be suspected if the temperature elevation is marked, costovertebral angle tenderness is present, and there is elevation of the white blood count. A clean catch midstream urinary specimen should be obtained for urinalysis and culture, and the former is usually diagnostic of infection. In most cases the offending organism will be *E. coli*, but other gram-negative organisms as well as enterococcus may also cause infection. Due to the widespread resistance of *E. coli* to ampicillin in many patient populations, the treatment of choice is usually a cephalosporin, which is given for 7–10 days. Gentamycin is often added in cases of pyelonephritis where a resistant organism is suspected or the patient appears toxic. Specific antibiotic sensitivities of the organism can be further utilized to direct therapy when needed.

Breast engorgement may cause a brief temperature elevation that rarely exceeds 39°C in 15% of postpartum patients. This usually lasts less than 24 hours and occurs 48–72 hours postpartum. It is critical to exclude other causes of fever, especially infection. Ice packs, breast support, binders, and analgesics are usually all that are required in patients who wish to bottle feed, while regular emptying of the breast will cause resolution of symptoms in breast-feeding women. Conversely, approximately 10% of lactating patients experience mastitis or breast infection that usually has its onset 10–14 days postpartum. Predisposing factors to mastitis are primarily inadequate emptying of the breast which is more likely to occur when the infant is improperly positioned for feeding. The infectious source is the mouth flora of the infant that enters the breast through a cracked or fissured nipple which predisposes to infection when incomplete emptying of the breast occurs. Breast engorgement in the early stage of infection further impedes emptying due to ineffective suckling, thereby permitting more bacteria to enter the duct, exacerbating the problem. Pain, temperature elevation, and V-shaped area of breast erythema are the most common presenting symptoms. *Staphylococcus aureus* is usually the offending organism; however, group A and group B beta-hemolytic Streptococcus, *E. coli*, and Bacteroides species can also be causative agents. Uncomplicated mastitis can be successfully treated with an oral antibiotic for 7–10 days, generally a penicillinase-resistant penicillin such as dicloxacillin and continued breast-feeding is recommended. Alternatively, a cephalosporin or erythromycin can also be utilized. Analgesics, ice packs, and breast support can be used adjunctively. This treatment usually results in prompt resolution of symptoms, and the best maternal response occurs in patients who receive antibiotics within the first 24 hours of symptoms and continue to breast-feed. In cases where clinical improvement does not occur or exacerbation of symptoms occurs, abscess formation should be suspected. This complication is seen in 5%–10% of women treated for puerperal mastitis, most commonly when there is a delay in diagnosis and treatment. Definitive treatment that utilizes open drainage, wound packing, and intravenous antibiotics should be employed in these circumstances. Proper breast care to reduce nipple fissuring can also reduce the risk of mastitis. Vitamin E capsules expressed directly onto the nipple may be helpful in maintaining the nipples in optimal condition for breast-feeding. Lanolin should be avoided due to the increased fissuring that occurs with its use.

General

1. Soper DE. Postpartum endometritis: pathophysiology and prevention. *J Reprod Med* 1988;33:97.
   Endometritis may spread to the adnexa, broad ligaments, peritoneal cavity, and pelvic veins, causing pelvic abscesses, peritonitis, or septic pelvic thrombophlebitis.
2. Fortunato SJ, Dodson MG. Therapeutic considerations in postpartum endometritis. *J Reprod Med* 1988;33:101.
   Early and more severe patterns of onset, especially with evidence of septic shock, suggest less-common infections, particularly Streptococcus pyogenes, Escherichia coli, *and* Clostridium welchii.

Etiology
3. Hohnson SR, et al. Maternal obesity and pregnancy. *Surg Gynecol Obstet* 1987; 164:431.

   In obese women undergoing cesarean section, there was an increased incidence of blood loss of more than 1 liter, operating time longer than 2 hours, and postoperative wound infection.
4. Hoyme UB, Kiviat N, Eschenbach DA. Microbiology and treatment of late postpartum endometritis. *Obstet Gynecol* 1986;68:226.

   Endometritis occurring 7–42 days after delivery may be related to retained products of conception and to infections with Chlamydia or genital mycoplasmas. Erythromycin therapy was successful in 10 of the 13 women followed in this study.
5. Walmer D, Walmer KR, Gibbs RS. Enterococci in post-cesarean endometritis. *Obstet Gynecol* 1988;71:159.

   In the National Nosocomial Infection System report on obstetric bacteremias, staphylococci were the most common (20.4%), anaerobes were next (12.2%), then Escherichia coli (8.2%); thereafter, the "breakthrough" organism enterococci was the most common (6.1%).
6. Newton ER, Prihoda TJ, Gibbs RS. A clinical and microbiologic analysis of risk factors for puerperal endometritis. *Obstet Gynecol* 1990;75:402.

   Cesarean delivery and certain organisms, such as bacterial vaginosis or high-virulence organisms, predict endometritis. Clinical variables may be facilitators rather than predictors of endometritis.
7. Seo K, et al. Preterm birth is associated with increased risk of maternal and neonatal infection. *Obstet Gynecol* 1992;79:75.

   Among the women delivered by cesarean, the incidence of postpartum endometritis was higher in those with preterm rupture of membranes than in those with term rupture of membranes.
8. Olsen CG, Gordon RE Jr. Breast disorders in nursing mothers. *Am Fam Physician* 1990;41:1509.

   Mastitis develops in approximately 2.5% of nursing women, usually between 2 and 5 weeks after delivery.

Diagnosis
9. Awadalla SG, Perkins RP, Mercer LJ. Significance of endometrial cultures performed at cesarean section. *Obstet Gynecol* 1986;68:220.

   Staphylococcus aureus is occasionally found, usually in diabetics or with cervical lacerations, episiotomy, or other trauma. The infection is clinically similar to that caused by anaerobes.
10. Duff P, et al. Endometrial culture techniques in puerperal patients. *Obstet Gynecol* 1983;61:217.

    The most satisfactory culture procedure was brush biopsy or lavage through a double-lumen catheter.
11. Lev-Toaff AS, et al. Diagnostic imaging in puerperal febrile morbidity. *Obstet Gynecol* 1991;78:50.

    Only two of 31 patients with refractory puerperal febrile morbidity had negative imaging studies. Sonography is the usual initial modality, with computed tomography the usual back-up and magnetic resonance imaging used only occasionally.

Treatment
12. Soper DE, Brockwell NJ, Dalton HP. The importance of wound infection in antibiotic failures in the therapy of postpartum endometritis. *Surg Gynecol Obstet* 1992;174:265.

    Close correlation between endometritis and wound cultures suggests a frequent relationship. Wound infection should be suspected if still febrile for 48 hours or more after antibiotics commenced.
13. Faro S, et al. Comparative efficacy and safety of mezlocillin, cefoxitin, and clindamycin plus gentamycin in postpartum endometritis. *Obstet Gynecol* 1987; 69:760.

Single-agent therapy using the newer broad-spectrum beta-lactam drugs (e.g., semisynthetic penicillins, cefotaxime, moxalactam, timentin) appears to be clinically as effective as "gold-standard" therapy.

14. Pastorek JG II, Ragan FA Jr, Phelan M. Tobramycin dosing in the puerperal patient. *J Reprod Med* 1987;32:343.
Puerperal patients require much higher aminoglycoside dosages than usual, so that serum levels must be monitored for therapeutic reasons rather than for toxicity. The authors suggest replacing the aminoglycoside with one of the new monobactams (aztreonam) that has a wide range, minimal toxicity, and similar efficacy.

15. Dinsmoor MJ, Newton ER, Gibbs RS. A randomized, double-blind, placebo-controlled trial of oral antibiotic therapy following intravenous antibiotic therapy for postpartum endometritis. *Obstet Gynecol* 1991;77:60.
Oral antibiotic therapy is unnecessary after successful intravenous antibiotic therapy for endometritis.

16. Karstrup S, et al. Ultrasonically guided percutaneous drainage of breast abscesses. *Acta Radiol* 1990;31:157.
Avoiding surgical drainage, three of the four patients continued nursing during and after the period of treatment.

17. Calhoun BC, Brost B. Emergency management of sudden puerperal fever. *Obstet Gynecol Clin North Am* 1995;22:357.
Discusses the differential diagnosis of puerperal fever and its evaluation and treatment.

18. Hager WD. Puerperal mastitis. *Contemp Obstet Gynecol* 1989;33:27.
Discusses the differential diagnosis of puerperal inflammatory disorders of the breast and delineates management protocols.

19. Duff P. Review: Pathophysiology and management of postcesarean endomyometritis. *Obstet Gynecol* 1986;67:269.
Extensive review article discussing pathophysiology, clinical presentation, diagnosis, and treatment regimens.

20. Del Priore G, et al. Comparison of once-daily and 8-hour gentamycin dosing in the treatment of postpartum endometritis. *Obstet Gynecol* 1996;87:994.
Clinical trial demonstrated similar efficacy in the treatment of endometritis for both dosing regimens.

Complications
21. Cruse PE, Ford R. Epidemiology of wound infection: a 10-year prospective study of 62,930 wounds. *Surg Clin North Am* 1980;60:27.
Infection rate of clean wounds, 1.7%; of clean-contaminated wounds, 8.8%; of contaminated wounds, 17.5%; and of dirty wounds, 30%.

22. Dodson MK, Magann EF, Meeks GR. A randomized comparison of secondary closure and secondary intention in patients with superficial wound dehiscence. *Obstet Gynecol* 1992;80:321.
Secondary closure of superficial wound dehiscence is superior to healing by secondary intention.

23. Ramin SM, et al. Early repair of episiotomy dehiscence associated with infection. *Am J Obstet Gynecol* 1992;167:1104.
Successful early repairs were accomplished in 32 of 34 patients.

24. Ammari NN, et al. Postpartum necrotizing fasciitis: case report. *Br J Obstet Gynaecol* 1986;93:82.
The pathognomonic feature is subcutaneous necrosis. Moderate-to-severe systemic toxic reaction is usually associated. It is essential to make an early diagnosis followed almost immediately by surgical debridement to healthy margins.

25. Rivlin ME, Hunt JA. Surgical management of diffuse peritonitis complicating obstetric/gynecologic infections. *Obstet Gynecol* 1986;67:652.
Severe infections resistant to medical therapy are rare but require timely surgery to avoid serious morbidity and even mortality.

26. Cohen MB, et al. Septic pelvic thrombophlebitis: an update. *Obstet Gynecol* 1983;62:83.

A clinical response following the addition of heparin to the antibiotic regimen provides presumptive evidence of the diagnosis. Operative ligation of the ovarian veins is rarely necessary.

27. Rosenberg JM, et al. *Clostridium difficile* colitis in surgical patients. *Am J Surg* 1984;147:486.
   Features of significant antibiotic-associated pseudomembranous colitis include watery diarrhea, cramps, fever, leukocytosis, and rectal bleeding.
28. Pearlman M, Faro S. Obstetric septic shock: a pathophysiologic basis for management. *Clin Obstet Gynecol* 1990;33:482.
   Life-threatening complications of uncontrolled sepsis include septicemia, septic shock, adult respiratory distress syndrome, and multiple organ failure.
29. Witlin AG, Sibai BM. When fever persists in the postpartum patient. *Contemp Obstet Gynecol* 1996;41:39.
   Reviews the diagnoses that should be considered in the puerperal patient with refractory postpartum febrile morbidity.
30. Dunnihoo DR, et al. Postpartum ovarian vein thrombophlebitis: a review. *Obstet Gynecol Surv* 1991;46:415.
   Extensive review on postpartum pelvic and ovarian vein thrombosis with recommended strategies for diagnosis and management.

41. DEEP VEIN THROMBOSIS AND PULMONARY EMBOLISM

Baha M. Sibai

Deep venous thrombosis (DVT) is an uncommon but serious complication of pregnancy because of the ultimate risk of pulmonary embolism (PE) and potential fatal outcome. The incidence of DVT during pregnancy ranges from 0.5 to 3 per 1,000 (a fivefold increase from the nonpregnant state). It appears that the frequency of venous thromboembolism increases with advancing gestation, with an equal occurrence between the antepartum and postpartum periods. If untreated, there is a 16%–24% mortality rate. If adequately treated, however, PE occurs in less than 5%, with a mortality rate of less than 1%.

Pregnancy is considered a state of hypercoagulopathy owing to the progressive increase in the levels of all plasma coagulation factors (except XI and XIII). There is also a decrease in the fibrinolytic activity because of a reduction in the level of the circulating plasminogen activator. At the same time, there is progressive venous stasis because of venous dilation and elevated capacitance, as well as increased pressure on the pelvic vessels. Recently, reduced levels of coagulation inhibitors antithrombin III, protein C, and protein S have been implicated in the mechanism of DVT. Antithrombin III, protein C, and protein S are naturally occurring coagulation inhibitors. Levels of protein S decrease throughout pregnancy, whereas protein C and antithrombin III levels remain normal. In the presence of protein S, activated protein C selectively degrades the coagulation factors Va and VIIIa. A single-point mutation in the factor V gene, known as the factor V Leiden, leads to an activated protein C resistance, a condition associated with a three- to sevenfold increased risk of venous thromboembolism in nonpregnant subjects. This risk is further accentuated by the following individual factors: (1) cesarean birth, (2) instrumental vaginal delivery, (3) increased maternal age, (4) suppression of lactation by estrogens, (5) sickle-cell disease, (6) prior history of thrombophlebitis, (7) maternal cardiac disease, (8) prolonged immobilization, (9) obesity, (10) maternal infection, and (11) chronic venous insufficiency.

During pregnancy, deep venous thrombosis most frequently begins in the calf veins or the iliofemoral veins, and has a propensity to the left leg. The diagnosis of DVT during the antepartum period is usually made on the basis of certain clinical signs and symptoms, identified by nonspecific, noninvasive techniques. Diagnostic x-ray and radioisotopic studies are potentially harmful to the fetus and are not performed. Symptoms include swelling, muscle pain, and tenderness, as well as a positive Homans' sign and Lowenberg's test. Unfortunately, reliance on these findings alone will result in an incorrect diagnosis (false-positive or false-negative) in 50% of the cases. Moreover, it is important that DVT be differentiated from superficial inflammation of the vein, as the treatment and prognosis of this problem are radically different.

Investigations using venography have revealed that about half of the patients with DVT exhibit no clinical signs, whereas the venographic findings are normal in 45% of those with clinical signs. Clinical diagnosis is most reliable in the presence of significant thrombosis in a tense, swollen extremity, with attendant pain and tenderness that extends to the thigh. Noninvasive techniques such as the Doppler ultrasonic velocity flow detector and impedance plethysmography can be helpful in detecting major venous obstruction (mainstream occlusive thrombi from the popliteal vein to the vena cava and large clots below the knee), but are unreliable for identifying minor venous thrombosis in the calf muscle area (sural and tibial veins). Overall accuracy of these tests is about 80%–85%. The special advantages of these techniques are that they can be used as screening techniques, performed serially, and potentially used for day-to-day follow-up studies. Thermography is another noninvasive technique that is potentially useful for detecting calf vein and femoral vein thrombosis. This technique has an accuracy rate of 90% when compared to that of contrast-enhanced phlebography. Ascending contrast-enhanced phlebography can also be used in the evaluation of the patient with suspected DVT, and is the most sensitive and reliable of all tests for its detection. It can be used during pregnancy, but its disadvantages are that it is invasive and carries a moderate degree of risk. Hence, it should not be used as a screening procedure. The fibrinogen uptake test (using ^{125}I-labeled fibrinogen) is of value in diagnosing lower extremity venous thrombosis and is most valuable in screening patients with risk factors during the postpartum period. This test should not be used in patients who are breast-feeding or pregnant.

The diagnosis of pulmonary embolism depends on the clinical history, physical findings, appropriate laboratory tests, and results of specific procedures. The signs, symptoms, and laboratory data are often nonspecific, however, as nearly 50% of the cases arise without a prior diagnosis of thrombophlebitis having been made. The most common findings are dyspnea, tachypnea, chest pain, hemoptysis, and tachycardia. An arterial oxygen tension (P_aO_2) of less than 80 mm Hg at room air in conjunction with a positive lung scan is a useful finding in confirming the diagnosis. Both anteroposterior and lateral scans should be obtained to reduce the likelihood of false-negative results. If positive, the scan reveals a lung perfusion defect but does not delineate the cause. Pulmonary arteriography remains the most specific and reliable diagnostic procedure for the definitive diagnosis of pulmonary embolism. These techniques are used during gestation because of the serious nature of a pulmonary embolism, but they do have significant risks for both the fetus and the mother.

Symptomatic treatment in the form of bed rest, elevation of the affected extremity, the application of moist heat, and the wearing of elastic stockings may be helpful in managing DVT. Anticoagulant therapy consisting of either heparin or warfarin is the definitive mode of treatment for DVT, with or without pulmonary embolism. Heparin is the drug of choice in the antepartum period because it does not cross the placenta owing to its large molecular size and negative charge. Heparin is administered as a loading bolus followed by a continuous intravenous maintenance dose. For uncomplicated DVT, the loading dose is 80–100 IU/kg, with a minimum of 5,000 IU. Following the loading dose, the infusion rate is started at 15–25 IU/kg/hour, or a minimum of 1,000 IU/hour. Heparin therapy should be monitored and the maintenance dose adjusted accordingly to achieve an aPTT of 1.5–2.0 times the control value, or a blood heparin level in the range of 0.2–0.4 IU/ml. It is important to achieve therapeutic levels early to prevent extension of the clot. Intravenous heparin therapy should be continued for a minimum of 5 days, or until symptoms have resolved and there is no evidence of recurrence. Following this regimen, therapy is maintained using adjusted low-dose heparin, 5,000–10,000 IU subcutaneously every 12 hours to keep the aPTT in the desired range. Treatment should be continued for the duration of pregnancy and 6–12 weeks postpartum, with at least 3 months of therapy.

Heparin may be discontinued at the time of labor and resumed 6 hours after delivery, but its use may be continued throughout labor and delivery without an increase in blood loss. Patients with PE or iliofemoral thrombosis in the current pregnancy should continue to receive heparin IV during delivery. The decision to use regional anesthesia should be made on an individual basis. Regional anesthesia is not contraindicated if the aPTT is normal and heparin has not been administered within 4–6 hours of the procedure.

The major risk of heparin therapy is hemorrhage. Protamine sulfate binds with heparin and irreversibly inhibits its anticoagulant activity. It can be given in a dose of 1 mg per 100 IU heparin to decrease the bleeding complications. Another major complication is osteoporosis, with radiologically documented bone demineralization, and a risk (2%) of symptomatic spinal fractures. Osteoporosis can be minimized by the administration of calcium and vitamin D and may be reversible following cessation of therapy. Other rare side effects include hypotension, alopecia, allergic reactions, pain at the injection site, and thrombocytopenia. There are two types of thrombocytopenia: (1) an early, self-limiting, nonimmune type, occurring within the first week of treatment, and (2) a late, severe, IgG-mediated condition occurring after the first week of initiation of therapy. Extreme cases may result in arterial and venous thrombosis. Hence, a platelet count should be obtained periodically for the first 3 weeks of therapy, regardless of the heparin dose and regimen used.

Low molecular weight heparin (LMWH) has been reported to be safe and efficacious. Single daily dosing, absence of monitoring of activity, and less incidences of bleeding are all appealing advantages. But, at this point in time, it remains much more expensive than unfractionated heparin.

Oral warfarin can be used in the postpartum period, but is difficult to regulate and requires following with frequent prothrombin time assessment. Warfarin is a small molecule that readily crosses the placenta and can produce multiple congenital anomalies if given in the first trimester (namely, epiphyseal stippling and nasal and limb hypoplasia). If used later in pregnancy, it can cause fetal anticoagulation, leading to fetal or neonatal hemorrhage with subsequent central nervous system abnormalities, as well as placental abruption. Because of these major drawbacks, heparin is the drug of choice throughout pregnancy, and warfarin use should be limited to the postpartum period only. Both agents are safe during breast-feeding.

Prophylactic anticoagulation with heparin (minidose heparin) has been recommended in patients who are at a high risk of thromboembolism during pregnancy. These include women with a history of estrogen-related thromboembolism (oral contraceptive use, or prior pregnancy), antiphospholipid antibody syndrome, and prosthetic heart valves. Minidose heparin employs 5,000 IU heparin subcutaneously every 12 hours, increasing the dose to 7,500 IU and 10,000 IU in the second and third trimesters, respectively. This dose doesn't affect the aPTT, and there is no need to monitor dosage since there is no increase in hemorrhagic complications. The prophylactic minidose heparin is given throughout pregnancy and continued 6–12 weeks' postpartum. Therapeutic anticoagulation regimen in the manner described earlier is administered to patients with recurrent thromboembolic events, and abnormalities in antithrombin III, protein C, and protein S.

Pulmonary embolism constitutes a life-threatening situation that requires immediate aggressive management. Medical management consists of intravenous heparin therapy (the same as that for DVT), and intravenous treatment should be maintained for a minimum of 2 weeks. After this regimen, intermittent heparin is given or oral warfarin is used (as outlined previously). Supportive therapy in the form of oxygen therapy to keep the maternal PaO_2 above 70 mm Hg, bronchodilators, maternal sedation, and the immediate management of shock or congestive heart failure are of equal importance. If an embolism develops postpartum, anticoagulation should be continued for 3–6 months following initial therapy.

Embolectomy should be reserved for patients with massive embolization. Indications for vena caval interruption or insertion of an intracaval device include recurrent PE despite adequate anticoagulation, iliofemoral thrombosis in a patient with an absolute contraindication to anticoagulation, and the development of hemorrhagic complications with anticoagulation.

Septic pelvic thrombophlebitis is usually a complication of postpartum, postabortal, or postoperative pelvic infections. The clinical picture includes persistent spiking fever (with or without chills), and tachycardia—all in spite of adequate antibiotic therapy. The pelvic examination findings may be normal, and the diagnosis is made on the basis of the clinical response to a trial of heparin therapy after a computed tomography scan is performed to rule out a pelvic abscess. The treatment of choice is intravenous heparin and antibiotics maintained for a minimum of 5 days.

General
1. Toglia MR, Nolan TE. Venous thromboembolism during pregnancy: a current view of diagnosis and management. *Obstet Gynecol Surv* 1997;52:60.

   Provides a review of the recent diagnostic and therapeutic strategies for the evaluation of acute deep venous thrombosis and pulmonary embolism, including a stepwise approach to the treatment of these conditions in pregnancy.

2. Toglia MR, Weg JG. Venous thromboembolism during pregnancy. *N Engl J Med* 1996;335:108.

   A summary of the current knowledge on venous thromboembolism in pregnancy, including a rational approach to management.

3. Macklon NS, Greer IA. The deep venous system in the puerperium: an ultrasound study. *Br J Obstet Gynaecol* 1997;104:198.

   Describes the pathophysiological changes that may be responsible for the increased risk of deep venous thrombosis in the puerperium.

4. Witlin AG, Sibai BM. Postpartum ovarian vein thrombosis after vaginal delivery: a report of 11 cases. *Obstet Gynecol* 1995;85:775.

   A report of 11 patients with ovarian vein thrombosis following vaginal delivery, including detailed diagnostic criteria and therapy.

5. Sipes SL, Weiner CP. Venous thromboembolic disease in pregnancy. *Semin Perinatol* 1990;14:103.

   This comprehensive article details the pathogenesis, risk factors, prophylaxis, and management of thromboembolic disease.

6. Thromboembolic Risk Factors (THRIFT) Consensus Group. Risk of and prophylaxis for venous thromboembolism in hospital patients. *BMJ* 1992;305:567.

   Reports the results of a Consensus Conference in Great Britain. It describes the risk groups for venous thromboembolism, the incidence and outcome according to a classification that identifies a patient as low-risk, moderate-risk, or high-risk. Recommendations for prophylaxis are made for patients requiring gynecologic surgery, during pregnancy, or in the puerperium.

Etiology
7. Hellgren M, Svensson PJ, Dahlback B. Resistance to activated protein C as a basis for venous thromboembolism associated with pregnancy and oral contraceptives. *Am J Obstet Gynecol* 1995;73:210.

   The authors note a high prevalence of activated protein C resistance (60%) in women with a history of thromboembolism during pregnancy, and a lesser increase (30%) among women with thromboembolism during oral contraceptive use. They raise the question of whether general screening for the defect should be done early in pregnancy or prior to prescribing oral contraceptives.

8. Dizon-Townson DS, et al. The incidence of the factor V Leiden mutation in an obstetric population and its relationship to deep vein thrombosis. *Am J Obstet Gynecol* 1997;176:883.

   The authors report a 3% carrier state prevalence of factor V Leiden mutation with an associated 28 times increase in deep venous thrombosis among carriers.

9. Esmon CT. The regulation of natural anticoagulant pathways. *Science* 1987; 235:1348.

   An excellent and up-to-date summary of the natural anticoagulant pathways.

10. Tengborn L, et al. Recurrent thromboembolism in pregnancy and puerperium. Is there a need for thromboprophylaxis? *Am J Obstet Gynecol* 1989;160:90.
    The authors compared the effects of heparin prophylaxis versus no prophylaxis in patients during a pregnancy that followed a thromboembolic episode. The frequency of recurrent thrombosis was approximately half that seen in those who did not receive treatment.

Diagnosis

11. Didolkar SM, Koontz C, Schimberg PI. Phleborheography in pregnancy. *Obstet Gynecol* 1983;61:363.
    The authors compared the phleborheographic findings in 48 asymptomatic pregnant patients studied during the second or third trimesters or immediately postpartum to the normal phleborheographic findings in nonpregnant patients. This study indicated that both chronic and acute venous obstruction are absent during normal pregnancy.
12. Sandler DA, et al. Diagnosis of deep-vein thrombosis: comparison of clinical evaluation, ultrasound, plethysmography, and venoscan with x-ray venogram. *Lancet* 1984;2:716.
    Of multiple devices available for the diagnosis of deep venous thrombosis, only the x-ray venogram proved suitable for definitive diagnosis, while the venoscan (fibrinogen scintigraphy) was found to be suitable only as a screening device.
13. White RH, et al. Diagnosis of deep-vein thrombosis using duplex ultrasound. *Ann Intern Med* 1989;3:297.
    The authors reviewed all published studies comparing duplex ultrasound with venography for diagnosing deep-vein thrombosis. The sensitivity of duplex ultrasound in detecting proximal thrombosis ranged from 92% to 95% (average 93%), and the specificity ranged from 97% to 100% (average 94.8%).

Treatment

14. Sturridge F, de Swiet M, Letaky E. The use of low molecular weight heparin for thromboprophylaxis in pregnancy. *Br J Obstet Gynaecol* 1994;101:69.
    In a retrospective study of 16 patients treated with low molecular weight heparin, the authors found it to be a safe and effective alternative to standard heparin for the prophylaxis and treatment of thromboembolism in pregnancy. They recommend a higher prophylactic dose (40 mg instead of 20 mg daily) to achieve the same therapeutic level of heparin late in pregnancy.
15. Hahn CLA. Pulsatile heparin administration in pregnancy: a new approach. *Am J Obstet Gynecol* 1986;155:283.
    Fifteen women used a portable infusion pump to administer heparin, either subcutaneously or intravenously, for up to 25 weeks. Patient acceptability of the pump was excellent, and there were no untoward events.
16. Turpie AGG, et al. Randomized comparison of two intensities of oral anticoagulant therapy after tissue heart valve replacement. *Lancet* 1988;1:1242.
    Two intensities of treatment were used in patients receiving oral anticoagulants; the hemorrhagic complications associated with the standard regimen were more than twice as frequent as those seen for the treatment consisting of smaller doses of anticoagulants.
17. Dahlman TC, et al. Thrombosis prophylaxis in pregnancy with use of subcutaneous heparin adjusted by monitoring heparin concentration in plasma. *Am J Obstet Gynecol* 1989;161:420.
    Twenty-six pregnant women were given heparin prophylactically because of previous thromboembolic complications. The amount of heparin was adjusted to keep plasma levels about 0.1 IU/ml, measured as antifactor Xa activity. The average dose of heparin used was 16,400 IU/24 hours or 225 IU/kg of body weight. This method was not associated with adverse effects on either platelet count or on the amount of blood loss at delivery. None of the patients had fractures of the spine caused by osteoporosis. The authors concluded that a heparin dose of about 240 IU/kg body weight per 24 hours, divided into two doses (7,500–10,000 IU twice daily) is appropriate in most pregnant patients.

18. Porreco RP, McDuffie RS Jr, Peck SD. Fixed mini-dose warfarin for prophylaxis of thromboembolic disease in pregnancy: a safe alternative for the fetus? *Obstet Gynecol* 1993;81:806.

Warfarin, 1 mg daily, was given in the third trimester of pregnancy. Fetal cord blood samples were obtained at 33, 36, and 38 weeks. No fetal coagulation abnormalities were detected.

Complications

19. DeSwiet M, et al. Prolonged heparin therapy in pregnancy causes bone demineralization. *Br J Obstet Gynaecol* 1983;90:1129.

Prophylactic heparin therapy in pregnancy is associated with bone demineralization that is dose related.

20. Landefeld CS, et al. Identification and preliminary validation of predictors of major bleeding in hospitalized patients starting anticoagulant therapy. *Am J Med* 1987;82:703.

In this large study involving 617 patients on long-term anticoagulant therapy, the most common site of bleeding was in the gastrointestinal tract. A prediction profile of the risks of bleeding complications was detailed by the authors and included old age, a very elevated prothrombin time or partial thromboplastin time, liver dysfunction, and multiorgan disease.

21. Dahlman TC. Osteoporotic fractures and the recurrence of thromboembolism during pregnancy and the puerperium in 184 women undergoing thromboprophylaxis with heparin. *Am J Gynecol* 1993;168:1265.

A total of 184 women received prophylactic heparin treatment during pregnancy. Vertebral fractures occurred in 2.2%, and 2.7% of the women had recurrent thromboembolic problems.

---

42. POSTPARTUM DEPRESSION

Cheryl A. Glass and Joseph P. Bruner

Recent changes in health care delivery, shorter hospital stays, and the industry growth of a new mix of providers, from primary care physicians to nurse practitioners, bring the need to review the scope of postpartum depressive disorders. Research has elucidated that only a small portion of postpartum depression is recognized by health care providers. The short length of hospital stay after delivery and the traditional 6-week check-up examinations are not adequate observation periods to detect most cases of postpartum depression.

The incidence of depression in the general population is 15%–25% and is more common in women (a twofold increase over men). Depression in women also peaks during the childbearing period from 25 to 45 years of age. Research has linked depression to reproductive changes including those in the premenstrual, perimenopausal, and postpartum periods. Notably, childbirth has been recognized as a major risk factor in the development of depression. It has been estimated that approximately 40% of births are noted to have some degree of a postpartum mood disorder. Psychologic disorders noted in the postpartum period range from the "blues," commonly thought of as a "normal process," to postpartum psychosis and obsessive-compulsive disorders.

The mildest form of postpartum mood disorders is called the "postpartum" or "maternity blues." Approximately 40%–85% of women experience some degree of the "blues." Most authors describe each state with a descriptive set of symptoms, but in reality the symptoms may overlap and change over time with the expected adaptive changes that occur with their newborn. Symptoms include episodes of crying, sleep disturbances/insomnia, loss of appetite, confusion, anxiety, and mood swings from happiness to depression. The "blues" are generally experienced within the first week after delivery (days 3–7) and diminish by the second week (days 10–14). In general, most clinicians do not prescribe any medications or psychotherapy for the "blues," since they are generally self-limiting. However, a short course of a mild sedative to treat the insomnia is noted to be therapeutic by several authors.

On the other extreme, postpartum psychosis is rare. Only a very small portion (0.1%–0.2%) of women develop postpartum psychosis. Symptoms include severe depression, mania, and psychotic harmful thoughts. Postpartum psychosis generally is noted between weeks 2 and 4 postpartum, with greater than half of all cases seen within the first 14 days. All authors agree that inpatient hospitalization is required secondary to the significant risk of infanticide. Medications (antidepressants, neuroleptics, and lithium), and electroconvulsive therapy are utilized in the treatment of postpartum psychosis. Early diagnosis and therapy have produced a 95% improvement within 3 months of treatment. However, postpartum psychosis has a notable recurrence risk of between 14% and 25% in subsequent pregnancies.

Information on postpartum obsessive-compulsive disorder is minimal. The literature notes that the onset is usually premenstrual (luteal phase), antepartum (time period not specified), and postpartum (onset from 2 to 6 weeks from delivery). Postpartum obsessive-compulsive disorder may be linked to recognized (panic attacks or anxiety disorders) and unrecognized pathology prior to pregnancy. Symptoms include overwhelming thoughts of fear, or overprotection of the infant, or avoidance secondary to obsessive thoughts of hurting the baby. Patients with postpartum obsessive-compulsive disorder also have up to a 50% increased risk of postpartum depression. Pharmacotherapy is the mainstay of treatment.

Pregnancy and childbirth are generally considered a happy period for women and yet can be overshadowed with severe depression. The overall incidence of postpartum depression (PPD) ranges from 10% to 15% of all deliveries. Symptoms include a progression/extension of the "blues" to a debilitating depression that interferes with the care of the infant. Loss of interest/pleasure in activities, depressed mood, and the presence of at least five other symptoms (weight gain/weight loss, insomnia/hypersomnia, psychomotor agitation/retardation, fatigue or loss of energy, inability to think, suicide ideations, guilt or worthless feelings) must be present for at least 2 weeks to meet the Diagnostic and Statistical Manual of Mental Disorders 4th edition (DSM-IV) criteria for major depression.

There are several psychosocial risk factors for postpartum depression noted in the literature: (1) previous postpartum depression (recurrence in up to 30% of subsequent pregnancies); (2) family history of depression; (3) preterm delivery; (4) twin delivery; (5) marital problems (single, abusive relationship, lack of emotional and social support); (6) financial problems (housing, medical, loss of work); and (7) stressful events, such as death, moving, fetal loss, illegitimate birth (26%–32% of teens experience postpartum depression).

Drastic changes in hormonal markers (thyroid, progesterone, estrogen, and prolactin) and biochemical markers (brain norepinephrine, calcium, tryptophan, cyclic adenosine monophosphate [cAMP]) at the time of parturition have been hypothesized as the cause for postpartum depression. However, research has not reached any consensus that hormonal withdrawal or biochemical changes cause postpartum depression.

The insidious onset of symptoms may not become apparent until 6 months postpartum. There is also a social stigma surrounding depression because negative emotions are not considered acceptable. Women may need to be given "permission" to speak about their true feelings after delivery to overcome the fear and embarrassment. Statements such as "It is common for women to feel down after delivery and overwhelmed about caring for the baby. Did you experience any problems?" gives the woman an opportunity to discuss her feelings. Depression tools such as the Postpartum Depression Checklist (PDC), Kennerley Blues Questionnaire, and the Edinburgh Postnatal Depression Scales (EPDS) have all been utilized as screening tools for the recognition of postpartum depression.

Psychotherapy is the primary therapeutic treatment for postpartum depression. Antidepressant therapy is also a mainstay of treatment. Women prescribed tricyclic antidepressants (TCAs) must be aware that it often takes 2–3 weeks for a therapeutic response to be noted. The selective serotonin reuptake inhibitors (SSRIs) are becoming the most widely prescribed medication for depression since they have less anticholinergic side effects, less lag-time in therapeutic response, and the convenience of daily dosing. The information available related to compatibility with breast-feeding states that antidepressants are excreted in milk, few have known infant effects, and the American Academy of Pediatrics states that this may be of concern. Mothers should be counseled about continued breast-feeding, take their dose after feeding, and not breast-feed again at the peak level of the drug. Most authors concur that the recovery and treatment period for the diagnosis of postpartum depression is 1 year.

Depression is not isolated to the mother but involves the entire family secondary to the disruption of sleep and daily activities as well as isolation and withdrawal from society. One study on the male partner concluded that the partner assumes similar symptoms that require support, education, and possibly medication. The effects on the child include delayed cognitive and language development secondary to the loss of interaction with the mother.

Depending on the severity of depressive symptoms, referral to a support group, family counselor, or psychiatric care may be necessary. A prompt referral to a mental health facility is mandatory when there is any ideation about harming either the infant/children or herself.

A discharge telephone call within 1 week of delivery is recommended to evaluate the woman/family psychological adjustment and discuss any symptoms of depression. A woman with a previous history of depression should be evaluated in the office 1 week after discharge and again after her support systems have diminished (e.g., husband returned to work, mother returned to home).

Other providers such as pediatric staff should also be aware of and screen for postpartum depression during routine office visits. American Academy of Pediatrics guidelines emphasize an assessment within 48 hours after a short-stay hospitalization, which would be an ideal time to evaluate the family as a unit as well as performing the neonatal physical examination. Lastly, the yearly gynecological examination provides another opportunity for recognition and discussion of depressive symptoms that may have been felt after the 6-week postpartum examination.

General
1. Beck CT. Teetering on the edge: a substantive theory of postpartum depression. *Nurs Res* 1993;42:42.
   Using the grounded theory method, a substantive theory of postpartum depression was developed. The four-stage process of teetering on the edge includes (a) encountering terror, (b) dying of self, (c) struggling to survive, and (d) regaining control.
2. Bright DA. Postpartum mental disorders. *Am Fam Physician* 1994;50:595.
   General discussion of postpartum "blues," postpartum depression, and postpartum psychosis.
3. Stover AM., Marnejon JA. Postpartum care. *Am Fam Physician* 1995;52:1465.
   General review of postpartum issues with practical questions for the family physician to review in the postpartum period.
4. Susman JL. Postpartum depressive disorders. *J Fam Pract* 1996;43:S17.
   Review of postpartum "blues," depression, psychosis, risk factors, and family impact, with guidelines on pharmacotherapy.
5. Walther VN. Postpartum depression: a review for perinatal social workers. *Soc Work Health Care* 1997;24:99.
   Review of family impact, psychosocial contributing factors, and treatment.

Etiology
6. Handley SL, et al. Tryptophan, cortisol and puerperal mood. *Br J Psychiatry* 1980;136:498.
   This article suggests that tryptophan, a neurotransmitter precursor, is implicated in the psychologic changes that take place postpartum.
7. Lazarus JH, et al. Clinical aspects of recurrent postpartum thyroiditis. *Br J Gen Pract* 1997;47:305.
   The recurrence of postpartum depression was not related to thyroid function.

8. O'Hara MW, et al. Prospective study of postpartum blues: biologic and psychosocial factors. *Arch Gen Psychiatry* 1991;48:801.
   Predictors of postpartum "blues" were personal and family history of depression, social adjustment, stressful life events, and levels of free and total estriol.
9. Smith R, et al. Mood changes, obstetric experience and alteration in plasma cortisol, beta-endorphin and corticotrophin releasing hormone during pregnancy and the puerperium. *J Psychiatr Res* 1990;34:53.
   The findings from this prospective study of 97 primiparous Australian women suggest that, although antenatal mood states were primarily determined by obstetric events, a significant association exists between maternal postnatal mood states and serum level of beta-endorphin.
10. Nemeroff CB, et al. Antithyroid antibodies in depressed patients. *Am J Psychiatry* 1990;142:840.
    Elevated levels of antimicrosomal and antithyroglobulin antithyroid antibodies were detected in a sample of nonpregnant euthyroid psychiatric inpatients with prominent depressive symptoms.

Screening
11. Beck CT. A checklist to identify women at risk for developing postpartum depression. *J Obstet Gynecol Neonatal Nurs* 1998;27:39.
    A must read. Succinct, straight to the point.
12. Beck CT. A meta-analysis of predictors of postpartum depression. *Nurs Res* 1996; 45:297.
    Meta-analysis of 44 studies to determine the magnitude of postpartum depression to predictor variables: prenatal depression, previous depression, social support, life stress, child care stress, postpartum "blues," marital satisfaction, and prenatal anxiety.
13. Beck CT. Screening methods for postpartum depression. *J Obstet Gynecol Neonatal Nurs* 1995;24:308.
    Introduces the 11-symptom Postpartum Depression Checklist (PDC) as a screening tool.
14. Cox JL, et al. Detection of postnatal depression: development of the 10-item Edinburgh Postnatal Depression Scale. *Br J Psychiatry* 1987;150:782.
    Introduces the 10-item self-report scale (EPDS) to screen for postpartum depression.
15. Horowitz JA, et al. Identification of symptoms of postpartum depression: linking research to practice. *J Perinatol* 1996;16:360.
    Research on identification of postpartum depression with the use of a self-administered questionnaire composed of The Mother's Information Tool for demographics, Depression Adjective Check Lists and Brief Symptoms Inventory for birth and postpartum symptoms.
16. Posner NA, et al. Screening for postpartum depression: an antepartum questionnaire. *J Reprod Med* 1997;42:207.
    Discusses the development and design of an antepartum questionnaire (APQ) for screening and evaluation of postpartum depression.
17. Richman JA, et al. Gender roles, social support, and postpartum depressive symptomatology. *J Nerv Ment Dis* 1991;179:139.
    Study explores the phenomenon of male postpartum depressive symptoms.
18. Stowe ZN, Nemeroff CB. Women at risk for postpartum-onset major depression. *Am J Obstet Gynecol* 1995;173:639.
    Recommendations for early identification and treatment of postpartum depression are drawn from the review of prospective, cross-sectional, retrospective studies and clinical experience.

Diagnosis / Clinical Assessment
19. Busch P, Perrin K. Postpartum depression: assessing risk, restoring balance. *RN* 1989;52:46.
    Assessing the new mother's emotional status is essential, but the full range of care begins months before the birth. Education and support from nurses can help new mothers beat the postpartum "blues."

20. Beck CT, et al. Maternity blues and postpartum depression. *J Obstet Gynecol Neonatal Nurs* 1992;21:287.
    Investigation of the relationship between maternity "blues" and postpartum depression, with early discharge versus customary hospital length.
21. Gruen DS. Postpartum depression: a debilitating yet often unassessed problem. *Health Soc Work* 1990;15:261.
    Discusses the implication for social work practice in the identification, referral, and treatment of women with postpartum depression.
22. Horowitz JA, et al. Postpartum depression: issues in clinical assessment. *J Perinatol* 1995;15:268.
    Presents assessment approaches derived from research and clinical practice. The conclusion is that systematic assessment for postpartum depression should become the norm for clinical practice.

IX. ADVANCES IN OBSTETRICS

43. ANTEPARTUM DIAGNOSIS OF FETAL ANOMALIES

L. Wayne Hess, Darla B. Hess, Randall C. Floyd, and Robert F. Fraser II

Three to five percent of all liveborn infants have a significant congenital anomaly at birth. Most such infants are delivered of mothers with no known risk factors for a fetal malformation. The general public believes that most birth defects occur because of exposure during pregnancy to teratogenic drugs, chemicals, x-rays, or viruses. However, contrary to public assumption, the available scientific data reveal that, of all birth defects, only 2% are due to exposure to these teratogens; 98% occur secondary to random mutations, the expression of lethal genes in the parents, autosomal or multifactorial genetic expression, aneuploidy, and so on. This tremendous public confusion has substantially increased the difficult challenge obstetricians face when a malformed infant is delivered. Therefore, the obstetrician has an increased responsibility to detect fetal anomalies in those gravidas at risk.

The prevention of fetal anomalies has been increasingly emphasized by the American College of Obstetricians and Gynecologists (ACOG). All women of childbearing age are encouraged to undergo preconceptional evaluation and counseling. A careful past medical, family, and genetic history should be taken from all women of childbearing age. Other information, such as maternal and paternal age, ethnic background, type of employment, occupational exposures, and family pets, as well as cigarette, alcohol, and drug use, should be obtained. In addition, immunity to rubella should be ascertained. These preconception measures should allow the health-care provider to determine which obstetric patients are at risk for fetal anomalies, and therefore provide appropriate therapy, counseling, and fetal evaluation. Additionally, preconceptional folic acid supplementation may be considered to minimize the risk of a fetal neural tube defect (NTD) developing.

In most European countries, sonographic screening is recommended for all pregnancies. In this country, ultrasonography is routinely utilized only for selected indications during pregnancy. The availability of real-time ultrasonography in the office practice of obstetrics, on the other hand, has led to an increase in the frequency with which antepartal fetal anomalies are detected in the low-risk gravida. ACOG, however, has advised physicians who do not have special expertise in prenatal diagnosis to limit the office sonographic evaluation in these selected gravidas to a basic examination, which should include (1) the fetal number, (2) fetal presentation, (3) documentation of fetal life, (4) placental localization, (5) amniotic fluid volume, (6) gestational dating, (7) detection and evaluation of pelvic masses, and (8) survey of fetal anatomy for gross malformations. If this basic examination reveals a suspected fetal abnormality, the patient should be referred to a center where a physician with expertise in prenatal diagnosis can perform a targeted fetal ultrasonographic examination.

Historic screening of all gravidas for risk factors for congenital anomalies is now a standard part of practice in the United States. In addition, serum alpha-fetoprotein (AFP) or triple test screening should be offered to all patients between 15 and 17 weeks' gestation. For those patients with any positive test finding for anomalies, testing by means of a targeted sonographic examination, midtrimester amniocentesis, fetal echocardiography, cordocentesis, and so on is carried out, in addition to definitive counseling. These tests must be completed in time (usually by 22 weeks' gestation) to allow the patient the option of pregnancy termination if she desires. These tests should be performed by individuals and laboratories experienced in prenatal diagnosis.

The antenatal diagnosis of NTDs has received increasing public attention. The background risk for NTDs in the United States is one to two per 1,000 live births. Most NTDs occur in patients with no known predisposing risk factors. The recurrence risk for these defects follows the typical polygenic pattern, with a risk of 3%–5% if one primary relative has the disease, 5%–7% if two primary relatives have the disease, and so on. In those women with no risk factors but who have two verified serum AFP values greater than 2.5 multiples of the median, there is a 10% risk for NTDs. These patients are offered targeted fetal ultrasonographic evaluation and genetic amniocentesis. The targeted sonographic evaluation in these patients includes measurement of the inner and outer orbital diameter; evaluation of the ventricular atrium; measurement of the cerebellar dimensions; longitudinal, sagittal, and transverse evaluation of the fetal spinal column; exclusion of the lemon and banana signs, and so on. Amniotic fluid obtained during midtrimester amniocentesis in these women is generally evaluated, and this includes determination of the AFP content and fetal karyotype. If the amniotic AFP content is evaluated, the fluid is also tested for acetylcholinesterase to confirm an NTD. If an NTD is detected, the option of pregnancy termination should be available to the patient.

At 18–20 weeks' gestation, gravidas at risk for fetal anomalies should undergo a targeted fetal sonographic evaluation. This examination should be performed by a physician with special training and experience in targeted sonography. Careful fetal biometry with measurement of the appropriate fetal organs and biometric ratios should allow the detection of 60%–70% of all fetuses with anomalies. Targeted sonography is 90%–95% accurate in identifying the nature of lesions that are specifically assessed.

Gravidas at risk for fetal cardiac anomalies should undergo fetal echocardiography. This examination is generally performed jointly by a maternal-fetal medicine specialist and a cardiologist. The two-dimensional examination of the fetal heart should include four-chamber, left ventricular outflow tract, right ventricular outflow tract, and aortic and ductal arch views of the fetal heart. Color-flow mapping of the fetal heart allows the detection of unusual turbulence patterns. These areas can then be evaluated by either pulsed or continuous-wave Doppler. The doppler velocities across the valves will allow diagnosis of stenotic and regurgitant lesions.

M-mode fetal echocardiography should permit the accurate diagnosis of most fetal cardiac dysrhythmias. At times Doppler may be a helpful adjunct. If an anatomic anomaly of the fetal heart is detected, determination of the fetal karyotype is indicated, as aneuploidy exists in 30% of these fetuses. A fetus with a dysrhythmia has the following risks for a structural anomaly of the heart: supraventricular tachycardia, 10%; ventricular dysrhythmia, 1%–2%; and complete heart block, 50%–60%. Fetal supraventricular tachycardia (with no other fetal anomalies) is usually treated with maternal digoxin (with the goal of achieving a maternal serum level of 2 ng/ml) or verapamil (80 mg orally three times a day). If the digoxin fails to convert the dysrhythmia and verapamil is added as a second agent, the digoxin dose is reduced by 50% to prevent toxicity. A maternal 12-lead electrocardiogram should be obtained and the mother's electrolyte pattern assessed to confirm that these are normal before therapy is begun. Fetal ventricular dysrhythmias rarely require therapy. The finding of congenital heart block should prompt an evaluation for systemic lupis erythematosus or other connective tissue disease in the mother (antinuclear antibody and Rho antibody, also known as anti-SSA antibody). Infants with complete heart block frequently require transvenous cardiac pacing after delivery.

Other techniques for prenatal diagnosis that are available at selected centers in the United States include embryoscopy, chorionic villus sampling (vaginal and abdominal), genetic amniocentesis, fetal organ biopsy, and cordocentesis (percutaneous umbilical blood sampling). Cordocentesis appears to be the most promising of these techniques. Since its introduction by Daffos in 1985, it has enjoyed a rapid gain in popularity worldwide. This technique is capable of such diverse applications as fetal blood karyotyping, measurement of immunoglobulin M titers (to detect congenital infections), enzyme analysis, ABO grouping, determination of the Rh and other antigen status, hematocrit measurement, and assessment of the acid-base status. This technique carries a 1%–2% risk of causing fetal loss. It may be used for second- or third-trimester diagnosis.

The advent of the polymerase chain reaction (PCR), DNA probes, and other exciting molecular genetic techniques has substantially increased the prenatal diagnostic ability. Mitochondrial and nontraditional genetics (uniparental disomy) are also expanding the prenatal diagnostic horizons. Analysis of fetal cells in the maternal circulation may also soon allow prenatal diagnosis by noninvasive means.

In summary, all gravidas at risk should be screened for anomalies prior to 22 weeks' gestation. If an anomaly is detected before this time, the options of either pregnancy termination or informed continuation of the pregnancy are available to the patient. Those gravidas with anomalies first detected in the late second or third trimesters should be referred to a physician with expertise in prenatal diagnosis. Prenatal diagnosis in these fetuses will permit optimal planning for the timing, method, and place of delivery.

General
1. Simpson JL, Golbus MS. *Genetics in obstetrics and gynecology.* Philadelphia: Saunders, 1996.
   A basic text of genetics for obstetrics and gynecology.
2. Jones KL. *Smith's recognizable patterns of human malformations.* Philadelphia: Saunders, 1996.
   This excellent text is the most up-to-date and complete reference on all fetal anomalies. All aspects of each of the fetal malformations diagnosed after birth are listed in separate categories.
3. Satish J. Prenatal genetics in laboratory medicine. A cytogeneticist's perspective. *Clin Lab Med* 1992;12:493.
   Importance of laboratory findings to prenatal diagnosis.
4. Anderson RH. Simplifying the understanding of congenital malformations of the heart. *Int J Cardiol* 1991;32:131.
   A comprehensive review of fetal cardiac malformations.

Diagnostic Techniques
5. Lescale KB, Eddleman KA, Chervenak FA. Prenatal diagnosis of structural anomalies. *Curr Opin Obstet Gynecol* 1992;4:249.
   A comprehensive review of the various aspects of prenatal diagnosis.
6. Wilson GN. Human congenital anomalies: application of new genetic tools and concepts. *Semin Perinatol* 1992;16:385.
   An excellent review of the application of new genetic tools.
7. Neilson JP. Prenatal diagnosis in multiple pregnancies. *Curr Opin Obstet Gynecol* 1992;4:280.
   A comprehensive review of the aspects of prenatal diagnosis.
8. Cooper DN, Schmidtke J. Molecular genetic approaches to the analysis and diagnosis of human inherited disease: an overview. *Ann Med* 1992;24:29.
   The field of molecular genetics in review.
9. Larsen JW Jr. Diagnosis of abnormalities of the human fetus during the first, second, and third trimesters. *Teratology* 1992;46:23.
   A comprehensive review of all prenatal diagnostic techniques.
10. Canick JA, Knight GJ. Multiple-marker screening for fetal Down syndrome. *Contemp Obstet Gynecol* 1992;36:3.
    The accuracy and limitations of triple-screen prenatal testing are described.
11. Wald NJ, Kennard A. Prenatal biochemical screening for Down's syndrome and neural tube defects. *Curr Opin Obstet Gynecol* 1992;4:302.
    A comprehensive review of the biochemical screening done to detect fetal anomalies.
12. Chervenak FA, Isaacson G, Campbell S. *Ultrasound in obstetrics and gynecology.* Boston: Little, Brown, 1993.
    A comprehensive test of prenatal diagnosis via ultrasonography.
13. Hill LM. New ultrasound observations of fetal anomalies in the second trimester. *Curr Opin Radiol* 1992;4:93.
    A review of recent developments in ultrasound diagnosis.
14. Hess DB, Hess LW. *Fetal echocardiography.* New York: Appleton & Lange, 1998.
    Comprehensive textbook of fetal echocardiography.
15. Lippman A, et al. Canadian multicentre randomized clinical trial of chorion villus sampling and amniocentesis. Final report. *Prenat Diagn* 1992;12:385.
    The Canadian chorionic villus sampling trial.
16. Pergament E, et al. The risk and efficacy of chorionic villus sampling in multiple gestations. *Prenat Diagn* 1992;12:377.
    First-trimester prenatal diagnosis in twins.

17. Ruitenbeek W, et al. The use of chorionic villi in prenatal diagnosis of mitochondriopathies. *J Inherit Metab Dis* 1992;15:303.
    A new diagnostic technique in the field of nontraditional genetics.
18. Reece EA. Embryoscopy: new developments in prenatal medicine. *Curr Opin Obstet Gynecol* 1992;4:447.
    A review of the applications of embryoscopy for making a prenatal diagnosis.
19. Cutting GR, Antonarakis SE. Prenatal diagnosis and carrier detection by DNA analysis. *Pediatr Rev* 1992;13:138.
    DNA analysis for prenatal diagnosis.
20. Chueh J, Golbus MS. The search for fetal cells in the maternal circulation. *J Perinat Med* 1992;19:411.
    An exciting potential future diagnostic technique.

Prognosis and Therapy
21. Stoll C, et al. Evaluation of prenatal diagnosis by a registry of congenital anomalies. *Prenat Diagn* 1992;12:263.
    A critical assessment of the accuracy of prenatal diagnostic techniques.
22. Northern Regional Survey Steering Group. Fetal abnormality: an audit of its recognition and management. *Arch Dis Child* 1992;67:770.
    A general review of the management involved.
23. Chambers HM. The perinatal autopsy: a contemporary approach. *Pathology* 1992; 24:45.
    A contemporary approach to the fetal or neonatal autopsy.
24. Simpson JL, et al. Vitamins, folic acid and neural tube defects: comments on investigations in the United States. *Prenat Diagn* 1991;11:641.
    A possible method to prevent neural tube defects is described.
25. Smythe JF, Copel JA, Kleinman CS. Outcome of prenatally detected cardiac malformations. *Am J Cardiol* 1992;69:1471.
    A multicenter review of the various aspects of the prenatal detection of cardiac malformations.
26. Karson EM, Polvino W, Anderson WF. Prospects for human gene therapy. *J Reprod Med* 1992;37:508.
    Practical recommendations for gene therapy are offered.
27. Mateau TM, et al. The psychological effects of false-positive results in prenatal screening for fetal abnormality: a prospective study. *Prenat Diagn* 1992;12:205.
    This describes the maternal stress incurred as the result of incorrect prenatal diagnosis.

---

44. GENETIC COUNSELING

Joseph P. Bruner and Cheryl A. Glass

The 2%–3% incidence of serious birth defects found at delivery in the general population has remained unchanged for decades. Of all malformations 15%–20% are thought to be genetic, 8%–10% are a result of environmental factors or maternal disease (i.e., diabetes), and the remaining 65% are of unknown etiology. As advances are made in the treatment of other obstetric and newborn complications, genetics will play a proportionately larger role in neonatal morbidity and mortality. As the paradigm shifts toward prevention and primary care, knowledge and understanding of preconceptional and genetic counseling are paramount. All health care providers for women must understand the basics of such counseling. This chapter's emphasis is on genetic counseling.

Genetic counseling addresses two major areas: hereditary and environmental disorders. The hereditary category includes those mendelian disorders inherited in an autosomal dominant, autosomal recessive, or X-linked recessive fashion, as well as polygenic or multifactorial and chromosomal aberrations (Table 44-1). Environmental factors encompass exposure to viruses, radiation, and drugs, including alcohol and tobacco.

TABLE 44-1. Overview of disorders

Chromosomal aberrations
  Monosomy—absence of a chromosome (MAY be fatal)
    Example: Sex chromosome monosomy XO (Turner syndrome)
  Trisomy—presence of an extra chromosome (MAY be fatal—mental and physical anomalies)
    Example: Trisomy 13 (Patau syndrome)
    Trisomy 19 (Edward's syndrome)
    Trisomy 21 (Down syndrome)
    Female sex chromosome trisomy XXX
    Male sex chromosome trisomy XXY (Klinefelter syndrome) and XYY
Structural abnormalities
  Arises from a deficiency, duplication, or rearrangement/exchange of genetic information.
    Example: Translocation (chromosomal breakage and exchange)
    Mosaicism (accident at cell division during mitosis)
Autosomal dominant
  Appear in every generation because the mutation is a homozygous state. The parent with the autosomal dominant gene can transmit either their abnormal or normal gene—random meiosis process. Each pregnancy has a 50/50 chance of inheriting the disorder.
    Example: Achondroplasia (dwarfism, short-limbed)
Autosomal recessive
  Appear when both parents carry the heterozygotic mutation. Each pregnancy has a 1 in 4 chance of inheriting the disorder, and a 1 in 2 chance of being a carrier of the disorder.
    Example: Cystic fibrosis
    Phenylketonuria
    Tay-Sachs disease
    Oculocutaneous albinism
    Infantile polycystic kidney disease
    Sickle cell anemia
X-linked recessive
  The dominant and recessive mutations only apply to the female partner. The females with 2 X chromosomes will be affected if they are heterozygous for the X-linked dominant trait. The males, having only one X chromosome, will always be affected if they inherit the X-linked mutation.
    Example: Color blindness
    Hemophilia A and B
    Duchenne's muscular dystrophy
    Lesch-Nyhan syndrome
    Glucose-6-phosphate dehydrogenase deficiency
Multifactorial inheritance
  Arises secondary to the interaction of environmental and genetic factors. The following have a 2–5% incidence of recurrence in blood relatives.
    Example: Congenital heart disease
    Club foot
    Neural tube defects
    Pyloric stenosis
    Cleft lip/palate
    Congenital hip dysplasia

General counseling begins with the performance of screening procedures to identify those individuals at greater risk of producing offspring with genetic abnormalities than the population at large. This identification process requires a thorough family and reproductive history, as well as information regarding possible exposure to various environmental factors. Counseling is best carried out when both parents are involved and when the needs of both parents are identified. The timing of the counseling session is of critical importance, because some interventions, such as folate administration or glycemic control, should be carried out before conception occurs, whereas others, such as maternal serum alpha-fetoprotein (MSAFP) determinations or triple screening, must be timed for 15–18 weeks' gestation.

Counseling is the process that opens the lines of communication between the health-care provider and the patient for the purpose of disseminating accurate and reliable information, thereby allowing the patient and her partner to make fundamental decisions about conception, abortion, antenatal procedures, and tests. The objectives of genetic counseling are to provide information, assist in the decision-making process and adjustment to the problem at hand, and ultimately to decrease the incidence of genetic defects at birth.

Adequate genetic counseling requires that the abnormality of concern be clearly defined and that the information presented to the parents be accurate, understandable, and timely. A thorough family history (pedigree) and physical examination, combined with serum screens (i.e., Sickledex^R and/or electrophoresis) and various investigative procedures, are necessary to establish an accurate diagnosis. The risks, benefits, and failures of each diagnostic procedure, such as amniocentesis and ultrasound, should be explained in an honest and noncoercive manner (informed consent versus directional persuasion). Accurate data dissemination and a description of the full range of alternatives must be presented to the couple. Confidentiality is of the utmost importance, as is the development of a trusting relationship between the health-care provider and patient. It is essential to follow up on each couple that receives counseling.

Women delivering after the age of 35 years constitute one of the largest categories of patients requiring counseling during the prenatal period. The risk of delivering an infant with trisomy 21, or Down syndrome, increases in direct proportion to maternal age, reaching one in 385 pregnancies at age 35 years and one in 11 pregnancies at age 49. Therefore, the American College of Obstetricians and Gynecologists (ACOG) recommends that "standard medical practice is to offer prenatal diagnosis to women who will be 35 or older when their infant is born" (based on EDC, not delivery date). There is increasing information in the literature concerning advanced *paternal* age (increased risk has exponential rise, rather than a linear increase) in regards to the increased risk of chromosomal abnormalities. At the present, ACOG suggests that "counseling on an individual basis is recommended for couples to address their specific concerns if advancing paternal age is an issue." Besides this age-related risk, couples that have had a previous infant with Down syndrome face a recurrence risk in future pregnancies of approximately 1%, regardless of maternal age. Couples in whom one parent has a known chromosomal rearrangement, such as a balanced translocation, are also at risk for giving birth to a child with a chromosomal aberration, and are candidates for counseling, prenatal diagnosis, or both.

One of the most common methods of genetic screening is high-resolution ultrasound imaging of the fetus using transvaginal or, more commonly, transabdominal transducers. A fetal femur length less than 91% of that expected for the gestational age, a nuchal skin fold thickness greater than 5 mm, or other findings, noted between 15 and 20 weeks' gestation, are associated with Down syndrome; the finding of a posterior nuchal cystic hygroma has been linked to Turner's syndrome; and cardiac defects and overlapping digits in the hand reportedly occur in 100% of fetuses with trisomy 13 or 18. These findings, however, are considered too nonspecific for making a reliable diagnosis of fetal aneuploidy, and invasive testing after appropriate counseling is required to establish the diagnosis.

Another common indication for genetic counseling is the patient at risk for delivering a child with a neural tube defect (NTD). NTDs are among the most common birth defects in humans. These anomalies, which include spina bifida, anencephaly, and encephalocele, occur in approximately six per 1,000 live births. The incidence varies by geographic location, seasonal influence, and use of anticonvulsants (maternal and paternal). In general, delivery of one child with an NTD is associated with a 4%–5% recurrence risk and delivery of two children with an NTD is associated with a 10% recurrence in a future pregnancy.

MSAFP testing is offered/performed at 15–18 weeks' gestation. Table 44-2 lists complications associated with unexplained elevated and low MSAFP values. It is imperative that the test be corrected for maternal age, race, and the presence of diabetes mellitus. Universal screening with the measurement of MSAFP levels in pregnancy may detect up to 20% of the cases of trisomies in women younger than 35 years at delivery. Abnormal values should prompt further investigation by means of ultrasound imaging to date and evaluate the pregnancy. Approximately 90% of the structural fetal anomalies can be detected by an experienced ultrasonographer. Although ultrasound scanning should identify all cases of anencephaly, amniotic fluid assays for alpha-fetoprotein and acetylcholinesterase may identify an additional 5% of small NTDs undetectable by current high-resolution imaging techniques. Use of the triple screen to detect abnormally low values of serum estriol and abnormally elevated levels of human chorionic gonadotropin, in addition to the MSAFP measurement, may identify up to 60% of the cases of Down syndrome in this low-risk population.

In 1991, the Medical Research Council Vitamin Study Group reported that the daily intake of 4 mg of folic acid periconceptually prevented 71% of the NTDs in women with one affected offspring. On January 1, 1998, a population-based prevention strategy was put into effect by the U.S. Food and Drug Administration (FDA). The FDA now requires enriched flour to have 140 mcg of folic acid per 100 gms of flour. This public health strategy will increase the folic acid intake of most childbearing-aged females.

Women at risk for delivering an infant with NTDs because of the previous delivery of such an infant should be placed on 4 mg/day of folic acid for at least 4 weeks prior

TABLE 44-2. Associations noted with abnormal MSAFP testing

Abnormally elevated MSAFP
1. Elevated presumably due to fetomaternal hemorrhage secondary to abnormal placentation.
   A. Threatened abortion/demise
   B. Fetal hydrops and ascites
2. Elevated with structural anomalies
   A. Ventral wall defects: omphalocele and gastroschisis
   B. Cystic hygroma (usually with Turner's)
   C. Esophageal and duodenal atresia
   D. Urinary tract disease, congenital nephrosis, polycystic kidneys, bladder neck obstruction
3. Associated with other pregnancy complications (unknown etiology):
   A. Preterm labor
   B. Intrauterine growth retardation
   C. Stillbirth
Abnormally low MSAFP
1. Missed abortion
2. Fetal trisomy
3. Hydatidiform mole

The maternal serum alpha-fetoprotein (MSAFP) must be corrected for maternal weight, race, singleton/twin gestation, history of insulin-dependent diabetes, and history of neural tube defects.
MSAFP is reported in multiples of the median (MOM): <0.5 MOM is abnormally low; >2.5 MOM is abnormally high; >4.5 MOM is abnormal in twins.

to conception and should remain on it through the first trimester. Yet we should caution against achieving 4 mg/day of folic acid by ingesting several prenatal vitamins, as this practice may expose women to toxic levels of other vitamins (e.g., vitamin A). Since folic acid supplementation cannot be expected to prevent all NTDs, prophylaxis does not preclude MSAFP or ultrasound testing later in pregnancy.

Since 1952, an increasing number of diseases, known as *inborn errors of metabolism,* have been determined to be secondary to an abnormality in a fetal metabolic process. Most of these disorders are inherited in an autosomal recessive or X-linked fashion. Detection of the approximately 100 inborn errors currently amenable to prenatal diagnosis is generally performed by enzyme activity assay of cultured amniotic fluid cells or of placental villi obtained by chorionic villus sampling (CVS). One notable exception is phenylketonuria (PKU), which is diagnosed with newer molecular techniques.

Although several mendelian disorders can also be diagnosed by enzymatic determination, DNA analysis for diagnosis can now be performed on any nucleated cell. Table 44-3 lists a few of the disorders detectable in utero by recently developed molecular techniques. This list is by no means exhaustive, but serves as a guide.

Invasive testing is now possible throughout gestation through the use of transcervical or transabdominal CVS, early amniocentesis, midtrimester amniocentesis, and cordocentesis. Couples should be informed that genetic amniocentesis performed at 15–16 weeks' gestation is associated with an approximately 0.5% incidence of spontaneous abortion. The risk may be slightly higher in the setting of early amniocentesis, performed between 12 and 14 weeks. Amniocentesis should be performed under ultrasonic guidance to minimize the risk of maternal and fetal injury. Thorough screening with ultrasound is necessary before the procedure to rule out the presence of fetal anomalies, twins, and fetal death, and to accurately ascertain the gestational age. Those women who are Rh negative with Rh-positive partners should receive Rh immunoglobulin after any invasive procedure to prevent maternal sensitization.

Although amniocentesis has provided the means for the early detection of many chromosomal and metabolic disorders, one drawback has been the need to wait until the second trimester before performing it. Long-term culture of retrieved amniocytes

TABLE 44-3. DNA analysis availability

21-hydroxylase deficiency
Adult-onset polycystic kidney disease
Alpha 1 antitrypsin deficiency
Becker's muscular dystrophy
Chronic granulomatous disease
Congenital adrenal hyperplasia
Cystic fibrosis
Duchenne's muscular dystrophy
Familial hypercholesterolemia
Fragile X mental retardation
Glucose-6-phosphate deficiency
Hemophilia A and B
Huntington's chorea
Lesch-Nyhan disease
Myotonic dystrophy
Neurofibromatosis (NF)
Norrie's disease
Ornithine transcarbamylase deficiency
Phenylketonuria (PKU)
Retinoblastoma
Sickle cell anemia
Tay-Sachs disease
Thalassemia
von Willebrand's disease

may require an additional 2–3 weeks before the results are available. This long waiting period contributes to mounting patient anxiety. However, rapid prenatal diagnosis using fluorescence in situ hybridization (FISH) protocol on amniotic fluid may gain popularity. Rapid aneuploidy detection by the FISH method can be used as an adjunct in cases of increased risk for a fetal trisomy (based on family history of multiple marker/MSAFP). Therefore, if a fetal abnormality is detected, the option of pregnancy termination may be offered earlier than the traditional amniocentesis time frame of 2–3 weeks.

Finally, effective fetal therapy may depend on early diagnosis followed by the prompt initiation of treatment. For these reasons, interest in the first-trimester diagnosis of fetal anomalies has increased markedly over the past several years. CVS is one method that makes this possible. It consists of a placental biopsy performed under ultrasound guidance at 10–12 weeks' to 6 days' gestation. Because the chorionic material obtained in the procedure is genetically identical to that of the fetus, it can be subjected to the same chromosomal, metabolic, and DNA analyses possible with amniocentesis, except for alpha-fetoprotein testing. However, the studies are performed directly on fetal derived tissue, which permits results to be available within a few days, rather than the weeks necessary for amniotic fluid studies. Although the risk involved depends to some degree on operator experience, CVS compares favorably to amniocentesis in terms of safety. A large multicenter trial revealed the procedure loss rate of CVS to be slightly greater than that seen for amniocentesis, but the difference did not reach statistical significance. Reports of fetal limb malformations following CVS have caused concern about developmental risks, but the procedure has been shown to be a comparably safe alternative to genetic amniocentesis. Appropriate counseling, an expert operator, and an experienced laboratory are mandatory components of a CVS program.

Cordocentesis is an invasive technique that allows the in utero diagnosis of a wide range of fetal disorders. Also known as *percutaneous umbilical blood sampling* (PUBS), cordocentesis consists of the fine-needle aspiration of fetal blood using high-resolution ultrasound guidance. Because the most common aspiration site is a blood vessel in the umbilical cord, cordocentesis is technically feasible only after about 18–20 weeks' gestation. In a review of more than 5,000 cases, the National PUBS Registry has determined the fetal loss rate to be only 1.15% per procedure.

The cytogenetic analysis of lymphocytes obtained from fetal blood yields a fetal karyotype in 2 days or less. Use of cordocentesis for rapid karyotyping enables the physician and patient to work together to quickly formulate optimal management strategies.

Armed with basic knowledge of genetic screening and counseling and with appropriate information concerning the risk factors, health-care providers can play a crucial role in the overall management of reproductive-aged women at genetic risk. Although it is not necessary that each provider be expert in genetic counseling, each clinician does have the responsibility to recognize the potential for genetic disorders and to provide the means of obtaining accurate counseling and testing for his or her patients.

General
1. Antenatal diagnosis of genetic disorders. *ACOG Tech Bull* no. 108, September 1987.
   Succinct discussion on genetic history, indications for testing, screening tools, neural tube defects, amniocentesis, chorionic villus sampling, brief ultrasound and fetoscopic topics.
2. Boss JA. First trimester prenatal diagnosis: earlier is not necessarily better. *J Med Ethics* 1994;20:3.
   Must read. The emotional case of chorionic villus sampling (CVS) in terms of the greater number of both spontaneous and selective abortions following CVS, the use of CVS for sex selection, and, because of the greater social acceptability of first-trimester abortion, the possibility of increased pressure on women to undergo prenatal diagnosis by health insurance companies, medical professionals, and government agencies all need to be weighed against the advantages of early prenatal diagnosis.

3. Forsman I. Evolution of the nursing role in genetics. *J Obstet Gynecol Neonatal Nurs* 1994;23:6.
   General discussion of the evolution of counseling by nurses working in a multidisciplinary team.

4. Gore D. Parental adjustment to a child with genetic disease: one parent's reflections. *J Obstet Gynecol Neonatal Nurs* 1994;23:6.
   A mother of two children with cystic fibrosis discusses feelings of guilt, marital stress, communication, coping strategies, and family planning.

5. Larrabee K, Cowan M. Clinical nursing management of sickle cell disease and trait during pregnancy. *J Perinatal Neonatal Nurs* 1995;9:2.
   Strategies for the synthesis of knowledge pertaining to pathophysiology, genetic counseling, life events that may have affected the patient's health history, treatment modalities, and psychosocial need may improve obstetrical and neonatal outcomes. Clinical management strategies for the prenatal, intrapartum, and postpartum courses are provided.

6. May KA, Mahlmeister LR, eds. The genetic code and fetal development. In: *Maternal and neonatal nursing: family-centered care 3rd ed.* Philadelphia: Lippincott, 1994;251–274.
   Nursing textbook that provides basic, understandable information on counseling and patient care.

7. Penticuff J. Ethical issues in genetic therapy. *J Obstet Gynecol Neonatal Nurs* 1994;23:6.
   Basic thought-provoking discussion on the ethical issues in genetic therapy including confidentiality, prevention of harm, discrimination in the allocation of beneficial genetic therapies, and "neo-eugenics."

8. Raff BS, Eunpu D. The genome project. *J Obstet Gynecol Neonatal Nurs* 1994; 23:6.
   Basic overview of the National Center for Human Genome Research.

9. Riding H, Cadle R. Primary care genetics: evaluation and counseling. *Physician Assist* July 1993.
   General discussion of amniocentesis, chorionic villus sampling, ultrasound, maternal serum alpha-fetoprotein, percutaneous umbilical blood sampling, DNA analysis, genetic counseling, and multifactorial genetic disease.

10. Ross LJ. Developmental disabilities: genetic implications. *J Obstet Gynecol Neonatal Nurs* 1994;23:6.
    Thought-provoking discussion about knowledge and new techniques in genetics that can aid in a better understanding of developmental disabilities.

11. Tinkle M. Folic acid and food fortification: implications for the primary care practitioner. *Nurse Pract* 1997;22:3.
    This article reviews the key concepts related to folic acid and provides an overview of the implications of the fortification program.

12. Vitamin A supplementation during pregnancy. *ACOG Comm Opin* no. 112, August 1992.
    Supplementation with 5,000 IU of vitamin A per day should be considered the maximum intake prior to and during pregnancy. Women using retinol and retinyl esters should be cautioned about the potential teratogenicity.

13. Williams JK, Lea DH. Applying new genetic technologies: assessment and ethical considerations. *Nurse Pract* 1995;20:7.
    Ethical considerations in the use of genetic testing include protection of privacy, protection from coercion, and assuring client understanding of implications of test results. Practitioner responsibilities also include educating clients regarding benefits and limitation of testing, collaborating with genetic counseling resources, and monitoring the client for potential adverse outcomes of testing.

14. Wright L. Prenatal diagnosis in the 1990s. *J Obstet Gynecol Neonatal Nurs* 1994;23:6.
    Great review, simple and easy to understand article covering family history, maternal serum alpha-fetoprotein / multiple marker screening, ultrasound, chorionic villus sampling, amniocentesis, percutaneous umbilical blood sampling, and laboratory analysis, including fluorescence in situ hybridization technique.

Counseling
15. Advanced paternal age: risks to the fetus. *ACOG Comm Opin* no. 189, October 1997.
    Recommendation for genetic counseling on an individual basis for couples to address specific concerns if advanced paternal age is an issue.
16. Cohen-Overbeek TE, et al. Spontaneous abortion rate and advanced maternal age: consequences for prenatal diagnosis. *Lancet* 1990;336(8706):27.
    Research suggests the justification of late first-trimester chorionic villus sampling in women of advanced maternal age because the spontaneous abortion rate and the procedure-related abortion risk do not exceed the risk of fetal chromosomal abnormality.
17. Dailey JV, et al. Role of the genetic counselor: An overview. *J Perinat Neonat Nurs* 1995;9:3.
    Highlights concepts inherent in the process of genetic counseling, as well as touching upon some of the ethical concerns faced by counselors.
18. Perry LE. Preconceptional care: a health promotion opportunity. *Nurse Pract* 1996;21:11.
    Succinct overview of preventive care. Teaching and assessment tools included.
19. Phillips OP, Elias S. Prenatal genetic counseling issues in women of advanced reproductive age. *J Women's Health* 1993;2:1.
    Among healthy women of advanced maternal age (AMA), the major risks associated with pregnancy relate primarily to increased risk of spontaneous abortion and abnormal offspring due to chromosome abnormalities. A table is included on age-related risk and total risk for chromosome abnormalities associated with AMA.
20. Preconceptional care. *ACOG Tech Bull* no. 205, September 1995.
    Good review of the components of preconceptional care.
21. Summers L, Price RA. Preconception care: an opportunity to maximize health in pregnancy. *J Nurse-Midwifery* 1993;38:4.
    Good overview of the components of preconception care: (1) appropriate and ongoing risk assessment, (2) health promotion, and (3) medical and psychological interventions and follow-up.

Genetic Diagnosis
22. Genetic screening for hemoglobinopathies. *ACOG Comm Opin* no. 168, February 1996.
    Initiation of screening for hemoglobinopathies depends on the ethnic background of the patient, medical history, RBC indices, and purposes of the testing procedure.
23. Screening for Tay-Sachs disease. *ACOG Comm Opin* no. 162, 1995.
    Serum screening for Tay-Sachs disease (TSD) should be offered before pregnancy if both partners are Ashkenazi Jews, French-Canadian, or of Cajun descent, or have a family history of TSD. If only one partner is high risk, only that partner needs to be tested. If the high-risk partner is determined to be a carrier, the other partner should also be screened. If both partners are carriers of TSD, genetic counseling and prenatal diagnosis should be offered. Women on oral contraception pills (OCDs) need leukocyte testing in conjunction with TSD screen.
24. Spence WC, et al. Molecular fragile X screening in normal populations. *Am J Med Genet* 1996;64:181.
    Ongoing analysis indicates that screening of pregnant or preconceptual populations for fraX carrier status is accepted by many patients and is an important addition to current medical practice.
25. Ward K. Prenatal diagnosis and genetics. In: Scott JR, et al., eds. *Danforth's obstetrics and gynecology*, 8th ed. Philadelphia: Lippincott, 1999.
    Excellent textbook chapter that provides understandable information on genetics and an overview of testing.

Ultrasound
26. Fleischer AC, Jeanty P. Obstetric sonography. In: Eden RD, Boehm FH, eds. *Assessment and care of the fetus: physiological, clinical, and medicolegal principles.* Norwalk, CT: Appleton & Lange, 1990;247–258.
    Excellent textbook chapter that provides basic, understandable information on the use of ultrasound in obstetrics.

27. Reinsch RC. Choroid plexus cysts—association with trisomy: prospective review of 16,059 patients. *Am J Obstet Gynecol* 1997;176:6.

When a choroid plexus cyst was associated with an additional risk factor (advanced maternal age, other abnormalities on ultrasound, past obstetric history, or family history), 10.5% of the patients had an abnormality. Amniocentesis is recommended when a choroid plexus cyst is found in association with additional risk factors.

28. Shields LE, et al. Isolated fetal choroid plexus cysts and karyotype analysis: is it necessary? *J Ultrasound Med* 1996;15:389.

Research suggests that the risk of finding an abnormal fetal karyotype in the presence of isolated choroid plexus cysts is up to 2.4%. On the basis of the data, genetic counseling and prenatal diagnosis should be offered to these patients.

29. Crandall BF. Alpha fetoprotein. In: Eden RD, Boehm FH, eds. *Assessment and care of the fetus: physiological, clinical, and medicolegal principles.* Norwalk, CT: Appleton & Lange, 1990;267–281.

Excellent textbook chapter that provides basic, understandable information on alpha-fetoprotein.

30. Hershey DW, et al. Maternal serum alpha-fetoprotein screening of fetal trisomies. *Am J Obstet Gynecol* 1985;153:2.

Short review of 32 trisomy pregnancies in light of reports concerning the association of low maternal serum alpha-fetoprotein with fetal chromosomal trisomies.

31. Folic acid for the prevention of recurrent neural tube defects. *ACOG Comm Opin* no. 120, March 1993.

Unless contraindicated, women who have had a fetus with a neural tube defect in a previous pregnancy should be offered treatment with 4 mg of folic acid daily, preferably starting 1 month prior to the time that the patient plans to become pregnant and continuing throughout the first 3 months of pregnancy.

32. Tinkle MB, Sterling BS. Neural tube defects: a primary prevention role for nurses. *J Obstet Gynecol Neonatal Nurs* 1997;26:5.

Great review of neural tube defect research including etiology, folic acid, and genetic/environmental factors. Primary prevention is the emphasis.

33. Wald N, et al. Amniotic fluid acetylcholinesterase measurement in the prenatal diagnosis of open neural tube defects: second report of the collaborative acetylcholinesterase study. *Prenat Diagn* 1989;9:2.

In a study of 32,642 women, the acetylcholinesterase (AChE) test yielded a detection rate for open spina bifida of 99%, 98% for anencephaly, and a false-positive rate of 0.34% excluding miscarriages, intrauterine fetal demise (IUFD), and serious fetal abnormalities. The best result was obtained by a combination of elevated maternal serum alpha-fetoprotein (>2.0 multiples of the median [MOM]) and AChE. Using this policy, open spina bifida detection rate was 96% and the false-positive rate was 0.14%.

34. Ward BE, et al. Rapid prenatal diagnosis of chromosomal aneuploidies by fluorescence in situ hybridization: clinical experience with 4,500 specimens. *Am J Hum Genet* 1993;52:4.

Review of the prenatal fluorescence in situ hybridization (FISH) protocol experience. FISH can provide a rapid and accurate clinical method for prenatal identification of chromosome trisomies.

Amniocentesis

35. French BN, et al. Evaluation of the Health Belief Model and decision making regarding amniocentesis in women of advanced maternal age. *Health Ed Q* 1992;19:2.

The Health Belief Model was developed as an attempt to explain an individual's decision regarding obtaining preventive health care. It is not necessarily the lack of knowledge that prevents women who are at risk because of advanced maternal age from having an amniocentesis, but their perceptions regarding amniocentesis.

36. Johnson MP, et al. Amniocentesis. In: Eden RD, Boehm FH, eds. *Assessment and care of the fetus: physiological, clinical, and medicolegal principles.* Norwalk, CT: Appleton & Lange, 1990;283–290.

Excellent textbook chapter that provides basic, understandable information on amniocentesis.

Chorionic Villus Sampling
37. Burton BK, et al. Limb anomalies associated with chorionic villus sampling. *Obstet Gynecol* 1992;79(5):726.
   Overview of reported limb deformities associated with chorionic villus sampling. A vascular etiology, related to either decreased fetal perfusion or thrombosis of the sampling site with subsequent embolization, is suggested.
38. Chorionic villus sampling. *ACOG Comm Opin* no. 160, October 1995.
   Chorionic villus sampling (CVS) should not be performed before 10 weeks' gestation. Transcervical and transabdominal CVS when performed between 10–12 weeks' gestation are relatively safe and accurate. CVS requires appropriate genetic counseling before the procedure. Counseling should include comparing and contrasting the risks and benefits of amniocentesis and CVS.
39. Elias S, Simpson JL. Sampling the chorionic villi. *Contemp Obstet Gynecol* 1991;36(Technology issue):11.
   Review of chorionic villus sampling (CVS; should be considered historical since discussion of performance at 9 weeks' gestation). Discusses the team approach to CVS, including training, counseling, technical, performance, interpretation of studies, and postprocedure counseling.
40. Jauniaux E. Fetal testing in the first trimester of pregnancy. *Female Patient* 1997;22:10.
   First-trimester ultrasound has changed the perception of human development and conception. The author makes good points for discussion on defects and testing availability.
41. Golbus MS, et al. Chorionic villus sampling. In: Eden RD, Boehm FH, eds. *Assessment and care of the fetus: physiological, clinical, and medicolegal principles.* Norwalk, CT: Appleton & Lange, 1990;259–265.
   Excellent textbook chapter that provides basic, understandable information on chorionic villus sampling.

Cordocentesis
42. Nicolaides KH, et al. Cordocentesis. In: Eden RD, Boehm FH, eds. *Assessment and care of the fetus: physiological, clinical, and medicolegal principles.* Norwalk, CT: Appleton & Lange, 1990;291–306.
   Excellent textbook chapter that provides basic, understandable information on percutaneous umbilical blood sampling.

45. ANTEPARTUM ASSESSMENT OF FETAL WELL-BEING

Christy Michelle Isler

The average perinatal mortality rate in the United States is approximately 13 per 1,000 live births. In certain high-risk populations, this number may increase to 30–40 per 1,000 live births. There are now several tests available that may substantially reduce perinatal mortality. Not all physicians agree on which method of testing is best nor which patients should be tested; however, indications for antepartum fetal testing would include hypertension, insulin-requiring diabetes mellitus, oligohydramnios, intrauterine growth restriction, and postdatism. Other conditions include multiple gestation, isoimmunization, maternal renal disease, maternal collagen vascular disease, maternal heart disorders, a previous unexplained fetal demise, or decreased fetal movement. Although various chemical tests, such as estriol and human placental lactogen, have been utilized in the past to evaluate fetal well-being, monitoring of fetal heart rate and other biophysical parameters give a more immediate result and have proven to be more reliable.

Maternal awareness of fetal activity is a simple, inexpensive, and effective screening method of fetal well-being. Two major techniques have been described. In the first method, described by Sadovsky, fetal movements perceived by the mother are recorded for 30–60 minutes two to three times each day. More sensitive testing, such as a nonstress test (NST), should be performed if the mother does not feel three fetal movements in one hour or if no movements are perceived for 12 hours. The second method, described by Pearson and Weaver, is the Cardiff Count-to-Ten chart. Each day fetal movements are noted from the time of waking. When ten fetal movements have been perceived, the time of day is recorded. If the patient does not perceive 10 movements in 12 hours or if it takes longer each day to perceive ten movements, then follow-up testing should be instituted. Of these two methods the Cardiff Count-to-Ten method has been shown to be most reliable in predicting fetal well-being.

Because accelerations of the fetal heart rate with fetal movement are associated with a favorable fetal outcome, the NST was developed. The NST involves fetal heart rate observation for a period of 20 minutes by external fetal monitor. The tracing is interpreted as reactive if two accelerations of at least 15 beats per minute, which each last at least 15 seconds, are noted. Should the tracing be nonreactive, there is an an additional 20 minutes of observation to allow for fetal sleep-wake cycle variations. The presence of mild variable decelerations are not necessarily associated with an adverse perinatal outcome; however, they may indicate the need for an ultrasound exam to detect oligohydramnios. In the uncompromised fetus, only 50% of NSTs will be reactive at 24–28 weeks' gestation; however, by 32 weeks' gestation, the incidence of nonreactive tests should be comparable to that seen at term. In order to shorten the time required to obtain a reactive NST, vibroacoustic stimulation using an artificial larynx has been employed. The incidence of nonreactive tests can be decreased by 50% in this manner. The reactive NST in association with vibroacoustic stimulation appears to be as good a predictor of fetal well-being as the nonstimulated NST. In most conditions requiring antepartum fetal assessment, an NST can be performed on a weekly basis. However, the testing interval may need to be increased to twice weekly in conditions such as intrauterine growth restriction, diabetes, and prolonged gestation. With a reactive NST the perinatal mortality rate in the following week is five per 1,000, most of which are due to acute accidents. Nonreassuring NST testing should be further evaluated with a more sensitive test of fetal well-being such as a contraction stress test (CST) or biophysical profile.

The knowledge that fetal heart rate decelerations in association with uterine contractions predicted fetal morbidity allowed investigators to develop the oxytocin challenge test in the 1970s. A baseline fetal heart rate tracing is obtained for 15–20 minutes with an ultrasound transducer, and uterine activity is measured with a tocodynamometer. At least three contractions within a 10-minute period are required. These contractions may be spontaneous or may be induced with oxytocin given via an intravenous infusion. More recently, nipple stimulation has been used to induce uterine contractions. The introduction of nipple stimulation has reduced the time required to perform a CST as well as the expense of the test. It is important to monitor maternal blood pressure during the CST to insure that a positive test is not a result of maternal supine hypotension.

The CST may be interpreted in one of five ways. The CST is interpreted as negative if no late decelerations occur with three contractions in a 10-minute interval, as positive if late decelerations follow more than half the contractions, as suspicious if inconsistent late decelerations occur with fewer than half of the contractions, as unsatisfactory if fewer than three contractions within ten minutes are noted or if the tracing is of poor quality, and as hyperstimulation if there are decelerations but uterine contractions occurred with a frequency of every two minutes or less. Most physicians avoid the CST when the patient is at risk for preterm labor, has preterm premature rupture of membranes, or there is a contraindication to uterine contractions, such as with placenta previa or prior classical cesarean section. Perinatal death rate has been estimated at one per 1,000 within 1 week of a negative CST. A suspicious CST should be investigated further, most often with the test repeated within 24 hours.

The fetal biophysical profile (BPP) can be used to reduce the number of false-positive NST tests obtained. The BPP consists of an NST combined with a 30-minute ultrasound observation period. Two points are given for each component of the BPP as follows: (1) reactive NST, (2) one or more episodes of sustained fetal breathing of 30 seconds or more, (3) three or more discrete body or limb movements, (4) one or more episodes of extension of an extremity with return to flexion, indicating normal fetal tone, and (5) a quantitative amniotic fluid volume assessment with a pocket measuring 2 cm or greater in two perpendicular planes. A score of eight or 10 is considered normal and scores below four are considered abnormal. A score of six to 10 is equivocal and should be further evaluated. The BPP may be used as early as 26–28 weeks' gestation. Once again, the vibroacoustic stimulator can be used to decrease the false-positive rate of this test.

Doppler velocimetry takes advantage of the frequency shift that occurs when a sound wave strikes a moving object. This has been helpful in looking at various measures of volumetric flow. Either continuous or pulse Doppler velocimetry has been utilized to evaluate the fetal condition. There are methodologic problems, but measurement of the systolic to diastolic (S/D) ratio is most widely used. Higher values, indicative of a greater resistance to flow, reflect placental pathology, not asphyxial change. This method has been of particular use with the evaluation of conditions predisposing to intrauterine growth restriction, such as chronic hypertension, pregnancy-induced hypertension, and collagen vascular disease. By 30 weeks' gestation, the S/D ratio in the umbilical artery should be less than three. The S/D ratio falls with increasing gestational age.

There are many unanswered questions concerning the topic of antepartum fetal surveillance. In general, fetal testing should begin once viability has been reached, and the physician ordering such tests should be prepared to act on the results. Most would begin weekly fetal testing at approximately 32 weeks' gestation in high-risk pregnancies; however, in certain conditions, testing could begin much earlier or be performed more frequently. Antepartum fetal testing is used to predict compromise from uteroplacental insufficiency in chronic conditions. It is unable to predict acute compromise due to cord accidents or acute abruption. After correcting for congenital anomalies, the risk of stillbirth occurring within 1 week of a reassuring test is low no matter which test is employed.

General
1 Druzin ML, et al. Antepartum fetal evaluation. In: Gabbe SG, Niebyl JR, Simpson JL, eds. *Obstetrics: normal and problem pregnancies*. New York: Churchill Livingstone, 1996;327–367.
   Methods of antepartum fetal evaluation are reviewed, as is the associated issue of perinatal mortality.
2. Shalev E, et al. A comparison of the nonstress test, oxytocin challenge test, Doppler velocimetry and biophysical profile in predicting umbilical vein pH in growth-retarded fetuses. *Int J Gynaecol Obstet* 1993;43:15.
   The nonstress test and contraction stress test are the best indirect methods of evaluating fetal well-being in growth-restricted fetuses.
3. Nageotte MP, et al. The value of a negative antepartum test: contraction stress test and modified biophysical profile. *Obstet Gynecol* 1994;84:231.
   The frequency of adverse perinatal outcome after a negative modified biophysical profile and a negative contraction stress test is comparable.
4. Rouse DJ, et al. Determinants of the optimal time in gestation to initiate antenatal fetal testing: a decision-analytic approach. *Am J Obstet Gynecol* 1995;173:1357.
   A discussion of factors that determine when in gestation the antepartum fetal testing should be undertaken.
5. Antepartum fetal surveillance. *ACOG Tech Bull* no. 188, January 1994.
   Currently accepted methods of fetal evaluation are presented including procedures for performing the individual tests.
6. Rayburn WF. Fetal movement monitoring. *Clin Obstet Gynecol* 1995;38:59.
   Daily fetal movement charting by the compliant patient is a worthwhile adjunct in antenatal surveillance.

Nonstress Test and Contraction Stress Test
7. Paul RH, et al. Nonstress test. *Clin Obstet Gynecol* 1995;38:3.
   A review of the nonstress test in antepartum surveillance.

8. Ware DJ, et al. The nonstress test: reassessment of the gold standard. *Clin Perinatol* 1994;21:779.
   The physiologic basis, clinical applications, and current role of the nonstress test are discussed.
9. Smith CV. Vibroacoustic stimulation for risk assessment. *Clin Perinatol* 1994; 21:797.
   Vibroacoustic stimulation appears to be a reasonable and safe clinical technique when used in conjunction with other fetal surveillance methods.
10. Tongsong T. Comparison of the acoustic stimulation test with nonstress test: a randomized, controlled clinical trial. *J Reprod Med* 1994;39:17.
    Clinical trial demonstrating the ability of vibroacoustic stimulation to lower the incidence of nonreactive nonstress tests.
11. Lagrew DC. The contraction stress test. *Clin Obstet Gynecol* 1995;38:11.
    A review of the contraction stress test and its uses in antepartum surveillance.

Ultrasound and Doppler

12. Manning FA. Dynamic ultrasound-based fetal assessment: the fetal biophysical profile score. *Clin Obstet Gynecol* 1995;38:26.
    Interpretation of biophysical profile use and scoring.
13. Inglis SR, et al. The use of vibroacoustic stimulation during the abnormal or equivocal biophysical profile. *Obstet Gynecol* 1993;82:371.
    Vibroacoustic stimulation can improve biophysical profile scores without increasing the false-negative rate of the test.
14. Manning FA. Fetal biophysical profile: a critical appraisal. *Fetal Matern Med Rev* 1997;9:103.
    A discussion of the biophysical profile and its ability to predict perinatal morbidity.
15. Maulik D. Doppler ultrasound velocimetry for fetal surveillance. *Clin Obstet Gynecol* 1995;38:91.
    The rationale behind Doppler velocimetry testing along with its efficacy in predicting perinatal outcome are discussed.
16. Farmakides G, et al. Doppler velocimetry: where does it belong in evaluation of fetal status? *Clin Perinatol* 1994;21:849.
    Appropriate use of Doppler velocimetry to decrease perinatal morbidity and mortality is reviewed.

---

46. LABORATORY TESTS OF FETAL LUNG MATURITY

Neil S. Whitworth

During weeks 25–26 of gestation, the fetal pulmonary alveolar epithelium begins to differentiate into type I and type II pneumocytes. The type II pneumocytes synthesize a surface active material (surfactant), which is both stored and then secreted in the form of lamellar bodies. There is a modest but progressive increase in surfactant production beginning at week 26. This is followed by a striking increase at week 34, which continues until delivery of the fetus. Pulmonary surfactant consists largely of phospholipids (80%–90%), with phosphatidylcholine the major active component (60%–70%), together with lesser quantities of phosphatidylglycerol (PG; 5%–10%) and other phospholipids.

The primary function of pulmonary surfactant is to maintain a low, stable surface tension (<10 dyn/cm^2) at the alveolar air-liquid interface. This action lowers the pressure needed to inflate the lungs and decreases the likelihood of alveolar collapse. A deficiency of surfactant at the time of birth is usually a result of preterm delivery before the surfactant production pathways are fully developed. It is also thought to be associated with certain maternal-fetal disorders that interfere with surfactant synthesis, even in the term infant. In either case, surfactant deficiency is the principal etiologic factor responsible for the neonatal respiratory distress syndrome (RDS). RDS affects 10%–15% of infants weighing less than 2,500 g at birth, and it remains the leading cause of morbidity and mortality in preterm neonates. For this reason, developing laboratory tests for determining the status of fetal lung maturity (FLM) has been the object of considerable research, and these tests continue to play an important role in the management of pregnancy.

Virtually all laboratory tests for FLM are based on the analysis of various constituents and characteristics of amniotic fluid. This is thought to be an accurate and practical approach to estimating the status of pulmonary surfactant, as (1) lamellar bodies are carried into amniotic fluid by fetal respiratory movements, and (2) amniotic fluid specimens are relatively accessible to amniocentesis or vaginal collection in the case of ruptured membranes. Although numerous tests for FLM have been developed, the analytic principles underlying these tests fall into one of two general categories: (1) those based on the biochemical analysis of amniotic fluid phospholipids, e.g., the lecithin-sphingomyelin (L/S) ratio and PG concentration, and (2) those based on measurement of the biophysical characteristics of amniotic fluid, such as the optical density and surfactant activity.

Recommendations for the appropriate clinical use of FLM tests have been derived from the literally hundreds of published studies that have evaluated and compared the predictive accuracy of these tests. There are, however, several methodologic features of these studies (particularly the earlier investigations) that render these comparisons less than ideal. RDS, the ultimate end point when it comes to evaluating test performance, has not always been clearly defined, and RDS criteria may vary from study to study. At times, important variables that can affect the incidence of RDS have not been well controlled, for example, gestational age, fetal sex, and mode of delivery. Amniotic fluid specimens contaminated with blood or meconium are frequently excluded from the analysis. However, because these contaminants can occur in up to 20% of the specimens, this exclusion likely introduces substantial patient sample bias. Patient demographics and obstetric risk factors are often insufficiently considered. In particular, evidence indicates that the results yielded by FLM test validation studies conducted in relatively normal term pregnancies do not generalize well to the high-risk obstetric populations encountered at tertiary-care facilities. Studies of new methods to predict FLM generally suffer from verification bias. This is because the new test is usually compared to the L/S ratio, and elective delivery will rarely be allowed if the ratio indicates pulmonary immaturity. Test results that show immaturity are therefore less likely to be verified than those that show maturity.

Before reviewing characteristics of the various FLM tests it is important to realize that the accuracy of test results is highly dependent on the quality of the amniotic fluid specimen submitted to the laboratory for analysis. Specimens collected by transabdominal amniocentesis are thought to yield the most reliable test results. While vaginal amniotic fluid samples are often collected in the case of ruptured membranes, the test results of these specimens may be altered by vaginal secretions and other factors. Samples that are to be analyzed the day of collection may be stored at 4°C. Specimens that will be stored or transported for longer periods of time should be frozen. Do not centrifuge the sample since this can remove substantial amounts of surfactant from amniotic fluid. Contamination with blood may lower the test result of mature specimens and raise the test result of immature samples. Contamination with significant amounts of meconium can completely invalidate FLM test results. While these factors may limit the application of FLM tests, several aspects of FLM test performance are well established, and these tests can aid the obstetrician in situations requiring an estimate of RDS risk for the neonate.

Although introduced more than 25 years ago, the L/S ratio is still a widely used test of FLM, and it is the standard to which newer tests of FLM are compared. The test uses thin-layer chromatography (TLC) to isolate the amniotic fluid phospholipids, and the analytes are then quantified by densitometry or planimetry. The test takes about 3 hours to perform, is technically difficult, and requires a well-trained, experienced test operator. For this reason, the means for determining the L/S ratio are rarely available on an around-the-clock basis. Because of test difficulty and many procedural variations, L/S ratio results are highly variable between laboratories. In recent surveys of L/S ratio proficiency testing conducted by the College of American Pathologists, the percent coefficient of variation between laboratories was found to be as high as 40%. As a result, it has been recommended that each laboratory establish its own L/S ratio reference values for FLM, rather than relying on the widely published textbook value of 2.0:1. Despite these drawbacks, the L/S ratio is one of the most accurate FLM tests available. If the L/S ratio shows maturity, the probability of RDS occurring in an infant delivered at that time is very low (1%–3%). Earlier studies had suggested that the mature predictive value ([PV_{Mat}], or the percentage of mature test results that correctly predict lung maturity) of the L/S ratio was less accurate in certain classes of diabetic pregnancies. However, the findings from more recent investigations indicate that the customary FLM reference values are valid for diabetic populations. The immature predictive value ([PV_{Imm}], or the percentage of immature test results that correctly predict RDS) of the L/S ratio is considerably lower than the PV_{Mat} and is usually reported to be about 50%. Although most concern has been focused on minimizing the falsely mature FLM test result, to avoid the consequences of a neonate with RDS, the high rate of falsely immature results seen for the L/S ratio is not inconsequential. This is particularly true for those high-risk obstetric situations in which it may be desirable to deliver the fetus as soon as possible.

The other amniotic fluid phospholipid frequently measured as a test of FLM is PG. Originally, the test methodology used two-dimensional TLC, which is even more laborious than the L/S ratio procedure. This test has largely been replaced by a commercially available immunoagglutination test for PG (AmnioStat-FLM, Irvine Sci., Santa Ana, CA). The results of this newer test correlate highly with the TLC procedure, and 0.5 μg/ml is set as the PG concentration indicative of FLM. The test turnaround time is relatively fast (less than 30 minutes) and the procedure is simple to perform. However, the manufacturer does caution that the test results may be unreliable if there is more than moderate blood or meconium contamination. The presence of PG in amniotic fluid is a very accurate marker for FLM, and the PV_{Mat} for this test is often reported to range from 98% to 100%. The absence of PG, however, is not an accurate predictor of RDS, as the PV_{Imm} is only about 30%. This is due to the fact that substantial amounts of PG do not appear in amniotic fluid until 36–37 weeks' gestation, and up to 25% of term mature amniotic fluid specimens do not exhibit PG. Other amniotic fluid phospholipids, combinations of phospholipids, and even hormones have been measured to serve as tests for FLM, but none has achieved the widespread use of the L/S ratio and PG measurement.

Many of the other rapid tests of FLM rely on the biophysical characteristics of amniotic fluid rather than on its chemical makeup. One of the best-known of these tests is the surfactant foam test (shake test). The shake test depends on the capacity of fetal pulmonary surfactant to produce stable foam in the presence of a graded series of ethanol dilutions. A commercial form of the test is available, the Lumadex Foam Stability Index, or FSI (Beckman Instruments, Brea, CA), which simplifies measurement and provides semiquantitative results. A Lumadex FSI of 0.47 or greater is considered to indicate lung maturity. In addition to its foaming properties, mature amniotic fluid exhibits a characteristic opalescence, which is due in part to the increasing concentration of surfactant-containing lamellar bodies. This property can be quantified by measuring the optical density (OD) of the sample at a wavelength of 650 nm, and is the basis for the OD_{650} test of FLM. Both of these tests take less than 30 minutes to perform and do not require great technical expertise. The reliability of the shake and OD_{650} tests is subject to the effects of blood and meconium contamination and also the potential dilutional effects associated with oligohydramnios or polyhydramnios. When the results of either of these tests indicate lung maturity, the incidence of RDS is low (1%–3%). Like the PG test, however, an immature test result is unreliable, with the PV_{Imm} reported to be as low as 10% and usually not much higher than 30%.

Of the newer tests of FLM, two have received particular attention. The lamellar body density test is a variant of the OD_{650} test and uses the platelet channel of an electronic cell counter to directly determine the concentration of amniotic fluid lamellar bodies. The pulmonary maturity cut-off point for this test is not well standardized and has reportedly ranged from 10,000 to 50,000 cell counts/μl. The assay must also be calibrated for each model of cell counter. The second procedure, the TDx FLM test (Abbott Lab, Abbott Park, IL), is a modification of the older microviscosity test. This test is now widely used and employs a fluorescence polarization method to measure the amniotic fluid surfactant phospholipid-to-albumin ratio. Recent reports indicate that normative values for this test need not be adjusted when dealing with diabetic pregnancies. The automated equipment required for these procedures is available in most, if not all, hospital laboratories and is simple to operate. These tests can be performed rapidly with a degree of precision higher than that of the L/S ratio and the results appear to correlate well with the results of other tests of FLM. The PV_{Mat} of these procedures has been uniformly reported to be comparable to that of other FLM tests (97%–99%). The PV_{Imn} is not as well documented, as studies of these newer tests inherently suffer from verification bias. The results of some investigations suggest that the PV_{Imn} is at least as accurate as the L/S ratio (~50%), while other evidence indicates that the value may be considerably lower.

Several factors should be considered when adopting a strategy of FLM testing. The utility of FLM testing is dependent on gestational age. There is little benefit in terms of patient management to testing beyond 37 weeks' gestation because the incidence of RDS is very low at this time (<1%). Furthermore, a test result showing immaturity at this stage of gestation is likely to be false, and may cause the obstetrician to delay an otherwise appropriate delivery. Similarly, FLM testing at week 30 or less is generally not useful because the likelihood of RDS is so high (≥60%) that it is often just as effective to assume that RDS will occur if delivery takes place at this time. As a result, FLM testing is most useful during intermediate stages (weeks 32–35), when conditions prevail that may threaten either the mother or the fetus, for example, preterm labor, premature rupture of membranes, situations necessitating labor induction or cesarean section, and poorly documented gestational age. The clinician should also keep in mind that, although the PV_{Mat} of all FLM tests is highly accurate (97%–99%), a price is paid for this accuracy in the form of a high falsely immature rate. The PV_{Imm} for the L/S ratio is only 50% and is even lower for many other tests (≤30%). A final consideration is the logistics of test performance. The L/S ratio, although the most accurate measure of FLM, is a lengthy test and may not be available during evenings or weekends, making it probable that the physician will wait several hours or longer for a test result. As an alternative, the rapid tests of FLM at least offer an accurate PV_{Mat} and the test turn-around time can be less than 30 minutes.

Given these considerations, a sequential protocol can provide an efficient scheme for FLM testing. Begin FLM testing with any of the simple, rapid tests (e.g., AmnioStat-FLM or TDx FLM). The result will be quickly available and, if it shows maturity, the result is highly reliable and can be acted on. If the test shows immaturity, the result is not reliable and testing must therefore proceed to the more accurate, but difficult, L/S ratio. If the L/S ratio shows immaturity, the risk for RDS is approximately 50%.

The extent to which new developments, such as fetal ultrasound assessment or RDS therapy with exogenous surfactant, may alter the nature of obstetric management and FLM testing is not yet established. The protocol just described can, however, provide the clinician with a rapid and cost-effective means of evaluating FLM.

General
1. Amenta JS, Brocher SC, Serenko-Aber AL. Comparing different statistical methods for evaluating diagnostic effectiveness of clinical tests: respiratory distress syndrome as a model. *Clin Chem* 1988;34:273.
   Discusses the appropriate statistical procedures for evaluating fetal lung maturity (FLM) tests and establishing FLM reference values.
2. Bourbon JR, Farrell PM. Fetal lung development in the diabetic pregnancy. *Pediatr Res* 1985;19:253.

Reviews the influence of maternal diabetes on fetal lung development and the incidence of respiratory distress syndrome.

3. Dubin SB. The laboratory assessment of fetal lung maturity. *Am J Clin Pathol* 1992;97:836.
   A comprehensive review of the utility of several laboratory tests in predicting fetal lung maturity.
4. Scarpelli EM. *Pulmonary physiology: fetus, newborn, child, and adolescent*, 2nd ed. Philadelphia: Lea & Febiger, 1990.
   Comprehensive presentation of the topic of fetal pulmonary physiology.
5. Schreiner RL, Bradburn NC. Newborns with acute respiratory distress: diagnosis and management. *Pediatr Rev* 1988;9:279.
   Reviews the etiology, diagnosis, and management of neonatal respiratory distress syndrome.

Laboratory Analysis
6. Amenta JS, Brocher SC, Serenko-Aber AL. Evaluating the clinical effectiveness of amniotic fluid assays in predicting respiratory distress syndrome in the neonate. *Clin Chem* 1987;33:647.
   Uses stepwise discriminant function analysis to evaluate the clinical effectiveness of phospholipid tests of fetal lung maturity.
7. Ashwood ER, et al. Lamellar body counts for rapid fetal lung maturity testing. *Obstet Gynecol* 1993;81:619.
   The results from this 3-year prospective study indicate that the lamellar body density test is a useful and rapid screening test for fetal lung maturity.
8. Ashwood ER, Palmer SE, Lenke RR. Rapid fetal lung maturity testing: commercial versus NBD-phosphatidylcholine assay. *Obstet Gynecol* 1992;80:1048.
   The rapid TDx fetal lung maturity test performance correlates highly with that of the more laborious L/S ratio.
9. Dubin SB. Characterization of amniotic fluid lamellar bodies by resistive-pulse counting: relationship to measures of fetal lung maturity. *Clin Chem* 1989;35:612.
   First description of the use of resistive-pulse counting of amniotic fluid lamellar body concentration as a fetal lung maturity test.
10. Gluck L, et al. Diagnosis of the respiratory distress syndrome by amniocentesis. *Am J Obstet Gynecol* 1971;109:440.
    The original paper describing the clinical utility of the L/S ratio in predicting respiratory distress syndrome.
11. Kjos SL, et al. Prevalence and etiology of respiratory distress in infants of diabetic mothers: predictive value of fetal lung maturation tests. *Am J Obstet Gynecol* 1990;163:898.
    The L/S ratio, phosphatidylglycerol, and OD_{650} tests were used to predict fetal lung maturity in a population of 526 diabetic mothers. The results suggest that the conventional test cutoff values are valid for diabetic patients.
12. Livingston EG, et al. Use of the TDx-FLM assay in evaluating fetal lung maturity in an insulin-dependent diabetic population. *Obstet Gynecol* 1995;86:826.
    This multicenter investigation demonstrates that the standard normative values for the TDx test are appropriate for use with diabetic pregnancies.
13. Oulton M, Fraser M, Robinson S. Correlation of absorbance at 650 nm with the presence of phosphatidylglycerol in amniotic fluid. *J Reprod Med* 1990;35:402.
    The OD_{650} test is a useful rapid screening test for the initial evaluation of fetal lung maturity.
14. Ragosch V, et al. Prediction of respiratory distress syndrome by amniotic fluid analysis: a comparison of the prognostic value of traditional and recent methods. *J Perinat Med* 1992;20:351.
    Compares test performance of the L/S ratio, AmnioStat-FM phosphatidylglycerol test, and TDx fetal lung maturity test. The PV_{Mat} for all tests was high and the falsely immature rate was lowest for the L/S ratio.
15. Richardson DK, et al. Diagnostic tests in obstetrics: a method for improved evaluation. *Am J Obstet Gynecol* 1985;152:613.

Uses receiver operating characteristics curve analysis to suggest that the L/S ratio is a more accurate predictor of respiratory distress syndrome than the Lumadex FSI or OD_{650} test.

16. Sher G, Statland BE. Assessment of fetal pulmonary maturity by the Lumadex foam stability index test. *Obstet Gynecol* 1983;61:444.
    The authors present their observations from the initial validation study of the Lumadex-FSI test of fetal lung maturity.
17. Steinfeld JD, et al. The utility of the TDx test in the assessment of fetal lung maturity. *Obstet Gynecol* 1992;79:460.
    TDx fetal lung maturity (FLM) test performance was improved by the adoption of less conservative FLM reference values.
18. Towers CV, Garite TJ. Evaluation of the new Amniostat-FLM test for the detection of phosphatidylglycerol in contaminated fluids. *Am J Obstet Gynecol* 1989;160:298.
    Evaluates the performance of the second-generation ultrasensitive AmnioStat-FLM test for phosphatidylglycerol. The results indicate good concordance with the chromatographic phosphatidylglycerol procedure.
19. Wong SS, Schenkel O, Qutishat A. Strategic utilization of fetal lung maturity tests. *Scand J Clin Lab Invest* 1996;56:525.
    Uses a literature review containing 1,759 patients to compare performance of the L/S ratio, TDx, and phosphatidylglycerol tests of fetal lung maturity.

Strategies for Using Fetal Lung Maturity Tests
20. Committee on Educational Bulletins of the American College of Obstetricians and Gynecologists. Assessment of fetal lung maturity. *Int J Gynaecol Obstet* 1997;56:191.
    This educational bulletin from the American College of Obstetricians and Gynecologists details recommendations for the use of fetal lung maturity tests.
21. Garite TJ, Freeman RK, Nageotte MP. Fetal maturity cascade: a rapid and cost-effective method for fetal lung maturity testing. *Obstet Gynecol* 1986;67:619.
    Shows that a sequential test protocol combining rapid fetal lung maturity tests with the L/S ratio can provide timely test results with a cost savings of 30%.
22. Hagen E, Link JC, Arias F. A comparison of the accuracy of TDx-FLM assay, lecithin-sphingomyelin ratio, and phosphatidylglycerol in the prediction of neonatal respiratory distress syndrome. *Obstet Gynecol* 1993;82:1004.
    Shows that the accuracy of fetal lung maturity test performance varies greatly as a function of gestational age.
23. Lee IS, et al. Lamellar body count in amniotic fluid as a rapid screening test for fetal lung maturity. *J Perinatol* 1996;16:176.
    Test specificity and the PV_{Imm} were improved when the lamellar body density test was used as a screening procedure preceding the L/S ratio.
24. Myers ER, et al. Cost-effectiveness of fetal lung maturity testing in preterm labor. *Obstet Gynecol* 1997;90:824.
    The decision to use tocolysis and corticosteroids in the management of preterm labor (34–36 weeks) is more cost-effective when the decision is based on the results of fetal lung maturity testing.

GYNECOLOGY

X. GENERAL GYNECOLOGY

47. UTERINE FIBROIDS

Abraham Rubin

Fibroids (myomas, fibromyomas, leiomyomas) are the most common benign tumors of the female genital tract. They usually occur in the uterus, but can also be found in the round ligament, the ovary, and rarely in the labia majora. These growths are solid tumors but may undergo degeneration, and even liquefaction, sometimes producing softening of the tumors. Degenerations, which may be hyaline, cystic, carneous, or fatty, are usually due to diminished blood supply when the tumor becomes large. Red degeneration (or necrobiosis) may occur during pregnancy or postpartum, and it has been encountered in menopause. It is due to venous obstruction producing intense congestion and necrosis. Malignant (sarcomatous) change is a rare complication in the menopausal woman.

Uterine fibroids may be either submucous (growing into the cavity), intramural, or subserous (bulging into the peritoneal cavity). This last type may develop a pedicle, become attached to other structures (usually the omentum), and obtain extra blood supply from these areas. Knowing the anatomic site of the myomas is important with regard to their symptomatology, complications, and management. Little has been documented regarding their etiology. It has been established that they are more common, grow more extensively, and occur at a younger age in the black population. They are somehow associated with infertility (either as a possible cause or effect), and appear to be related to hormonal influences. They may get larger during pregnancy and with estrogen administration. However, the prolonged use of oral contraceptives effectively reduces the risk of developing fibroids by 30% after 10 years. Use of birth control pills does not lead to an increased risk of developing fibroids. These tumors diminish in size postmenopausally and may regrow or recur after surgical removal. They can be extremely large, irregular, and multiple, yet remain benign tumors. They have been found in patients as young as 11 years of age.

The etiology of myomata remains obscure. Estrogen and progesterone appear to be essential for their growth (hence the shrinkage and degeneration in the postmenopausal woman). Both hormones contribute through gene regulation in opposing ways. There is a potential role for cytokines in the pathogenesis of leiomyomata. Pathologically, fibroids are distinguished by their pseudocapsule and whorled macroscopic appearance on cross section. Leiomyoma is the correct term for these tumors, because they arise from a single smooth muscle cell. Deposits of calcium, after longstanding degeneration, account for the tumor's gritty texture on cutting and the typical stippled appearance seen on x-ray films.

The most frequent presenting feature is menorrhagia (75% of the patients), and it is the resultant anemia that may cause the patient to seek medical attention. Infertility, dysmenorrhea (usually of the congestive type), and the presence of an abdominal mass account for most of the other symptoms. Acute episodes, such as retention of urine owing to sudden enlargement and impaction in the cul-de-sac, are occasionally encountered. A large number of patients harbor symptomless fibroids that are identified only during routine vaginal or general medical examinations. Autopsy shows that 20% of women older than 30 years have symptomless fibroids; 50% of the patients with symptoms present before age 35 years.

The majority of signs and symptoms that occur in women with fibroids are due to the submucous fibroids, and include dysmenorrhea, menorrhagia (resulting from an increased bleeding surface area), metrorrhagia, and intermittent pain. The submucous fibroid can become pedunculated and can be delivered through the cervix. The surface of the exposed tumor can become eroded and septic and can produce marked metrorrhagia, which will bring the patient to the hospital. Submucous fibroids may also induce abortion, stemming from interference with placentation, or postpartum hemorrhage, resulting from incomplete placental separation. However, the spontaneous abortion rate associated with fibroids is overall not greater than that for the general population. Patients with large fibroids are at increased risk for premature delivery. The size, number, and location of the fibroids do not influence pregnancy outcome, and the overall mode of delivery does not differ from that of patients who have no fibroids. The incidence of fibroids in pregnancy is 0.3–2.5 per 100 live births.

Intramural fibroids cause the least problems, only producing symptoms because of their size. The mechanism whereby they affect fertility has not yet been elucidated. They are most likely the result, rather than the cause, of sterility. Subserous fibroids are also asymptomatic unless they are very large or become pedunculated. The latter group may cause some peritoneal irritation or rarely, if very mobile, undergo torsion. Even extremely large fibroid uteri seldom produce more than slight mechanical obstruction or anatomical obstruction of the ureters. Edema of the legs and increased varicosities may also be noted with large tumors. In the postmenopausal woman, sudden enlargement (with or without pain) could indicate either cystic degeneration or sarcomatous degeneration. The latter occurs in less than 0.5% of patients.

Leiomyosarcomas occur postmenopausally—the average age is 55—and with greater frequency in the black population. Incidence is unrelated to parity. The most common presenting symptom is vaginal bleeding. The tumor is nonencapsulated with a bulging, homogeneous, grayish-white, soft pultaceous mass in which the whorled appearance has disappeared. This malignancy must not be confused with cellular leiomyoma. The latter are fibroid tumors that have increased cellularity and closely opposed nuclei microscopically. They have a low mitotic count compared to sarcomas, with little or no anaplasia. They have a propensity to enlarge rapidly during pregnancy.

The benign metastasizing leiomyoma is a condition in which uterine myomata are found together with pulmonary nodules of well-differentiated benign smooth muscle. It is probably related to dissemination of intravenous leiomyomatas; this refers to the presence of well-differentiated smooth muscle in the lumina of uterine and pelvic veins. Microscopically, wormlike cords of tumor can be seen extending from the myometrium into veins of the broad ligament. There is no inclination toward extravascular invasion. Clinical symptoms are vaginal bleeding and, infrequently, abdominal enlargement.

Leiomyomatosis peritonealis disseminata is a rare pathological entity. Multiple, 1–2-cm, raised white nodules are seen on the peritoneal surface, including the liver and bowel. These are often associated with large uterine leiomyomas. They are grossly indistinguishable from a disseminated malignant tumor but are benign, both microscopically and in their clinical behavior. The condition is metaplastic rather than metastatic in its pathogenesis.

The diagnosis of myomata is usually clinical. Bimanual pelvic examination reveals a characteristically firm to hard, irregularly shaped, enlarged uterus. Abdominal x-rays may show the soft tissue tumor and the presence of calcification, which, if present, will appear as concentric white rings. Ultrasound may also be helpful, as it will confirm that the tumors are not extrauterine masses. Intravenous pyelography may show evidence of pressure effects on the ureters, and should be included in the workup. Differential diagnosis includes ovarian tumors, chronic tuboovarian abscess, hydro-salpinx, uterine sarcoma, and adenomyosis.

The management of myomata will depend essentially on the patient's age, parity, and symptoms. It will also be influenced by her desire for future pregnancies. As a rule, a total abdominal hysterectomy (vaginal hysterectomy may be performed if feasible) is the procedure of choice in the older patient in whom fertility is not a factor. The treatment of leiomyosarcoma is total abdominal hysterectomy and bilateral salpingo-oophorectomy. The 5-year survival rate is only 20.7%. Pelvic recurrence is the most common initial indication of treatment failure. Metastases to peritoneum and lung are next in frequency.

In the younger patient, small submucous fibroids may be removed by curettage after cervical dilatation (Laminaria is an effective dilator) or with polyp-forceps under hysteroscopic vision. When the fibroid has become pedunculated and presents through the cervix, the tumor may be twisted off or the pedicle cut at the base. This is followed by immediate curettage or hysteroscopic review, if the cervix is not dilated more than 1 cm, to make sure that there are no small residual fibroid polyps.

Hysterosalpingography may reveal whether submucous fibroids are present and establish the patency, or otherwise, of the fallopian tubes. Laparoscopy may be done before definitive surgical intervention to determine whether myomectomy or hysterectomy is indicated. The final decision usually depends on the condition of the tubes. Myomectomy is performed when there is tubal patency or when tuboplasty is possible, when the uterus is not too large (not more than 20 weeks' gestational size), and when the fibroids are not too numerous. Small subserous or pedunculated subserous fibroids may be evaporated by laser performed via laparoscopy. Destruction of the tumor may also be performed using high-voltage electric probes. This procedure (myolysis) should only be performed on patients who have no desire for future fertility because uterine rupture has been reported in patients who have become pregnant.

The administration of long-acting gonadotropin-releasing hormone (GnRH) agonists by injection given monthly or in three monthly injections may reduce the tumor's size by 40%–60% after 2–6 months of therapy. Three months is probably sufficient before surgical removal. Rapid regrowth occurs when treatment ceases. Side effects of the agonist treatment include hot flashes, dry vagina, acne, seborrhea, and, rarely, hoarseness and loss of libido. GnRH analogues have potent antiestrogenic and anti- progestogenic properties. GnRH injection causes the uterine volume and tumor size to decrease, thereby sometimes making laparoscopic or vaginal hysterectomy feasible. It also promotes restoration of blood volume in anemic patients. Mifepristone (RU-486), a synthetic steroid with antiprogesterone activity, has been shown in a small study to reduce the size of leiomyomata by 87%. There were fewer side effects than with GnRH agonists.

The main complications of myomectomy are hemorrhage at operation and postoperative sepsis. Prophylactic antibiotics should be administered in all patients undergoing myomectomies. The disadvantage of resecting the fibroids only is that there is a 10% recurrence rate. With young patients, 50% will conceive in the first 2 years after myomectomy if there are no other infertility factors. The pregnancy rates in women older than 35 years are only 5%–10%. Interventional radiology to embolize the uterine arteries is being used in selected clinics with promising results using Ivalo (polyvinyl alcohol) particles. The vessels are approached via femoral artery catheterization. This can be done under sedation. Pelvic pain can be a problem after the pro cedure because of ischemia. Long-term follow-up is still awaited.

Asymptomatic myomas, when the uterus is less than 12 weeks' gestational size and not palpable suprapubically, may be treated expectantly. Two or three examinations annually will indicate whether they are dormant or enlarging. The rare acute red degeneration that occurs in pregnancy responds to pain relief and antipyretic treatment. Obstructed labor due to fibroids is extremely rare and requires cesarean section for delivery. The fibroids shrink rapidly postpartum, and surgical treatment should be delayed for at least 6 weeks after delivery.

Review

1. Buttram VC Jr, Reiter RC. Uterine leiomyomata. Etiology, symptomatology and management. *Fertil Steril* 1981;36:433.
   A good overview of various aspects of leiomyomata and their possible etiologies.
2. Howkins J, Stallworthy J. Abdominal myomectomy. In: *Bonney's gynecological surgery,* 8th ed. London: Balliere-Tindall, 1974;410–448.
   A clear, concise, well-illustrated, step-by-step approach to myomectomy. It remains the standard text for the abdominal approach to fibroids.
3. Glavind K, et al. Uterine myoma in pregnancy. *Acta Obstet Gynecol Scand* 1990; 69:617.
   Good review of the effects of pregnancy on fibroids.
4. Fedele L, et al. Diffuse uterine leiomyomatosis. *Acta Eur Fertil* 1982;13:125.
   A detailed review.

Etiology

5. Soules MR, McCarty KS Jr. Leiomyomas. Steroid receptor content. Variations within normal menstrual cycles. *Am J Obstet Gynecol* 1982;143:6.
   The number of estrogen receptors is significantly greater in fibroids than in normal myometrium.

6. Chandrasekhar Y, et al. Insulin-like growth factor I and II binding in human myometrium and leiomyomas. *Am J Obstet Gynecol* 1992;166:64.
   The number of insulin-like growth factor receptors is increased in leiomyomata compared to myometrium. This may therefore play a role in the generation and growth of the tumor.
7. Rein MS, Barbieri RL, Friedman AJ. Progesterone: a critical role in the pathogenesis of uterine myomas. *Am J Obstet Gynecol* 1995;172:14.
   Detailed evaluation of progesterone's role in the etiology of myomas.
8. Andersen J. Growth factors and cytokinase in uterine leiomyomas. *Semin Reprod Endocrinol* 1996;14:269.
   Cytokinase may play an important role in the etiology of fibroids.

Diagnosis
9. Weinstein D, Aviad Y, Polishuk WZ. Hysterography before and after myomectomy. *Am J Roentgenol* 1977;129:899.
   The value of preoperative hysterography in confirming the diagnosis and localization of myomas is stressed.
10. Samuelson S, Ovall SJ. The value of laparoscopy in the differential diagnosis between uterine fibromyomata and adnexal tumors. *Acta Obstet Gynecol Scand* 1970;49:175.
    Laparoscopy may be indicated for the evaluation of subserous fibroids.
11. Gross BH, et al. Sonographic features of leiomyomas. Analysis of 41 problem cases. *J Ultrasound Med* 1983;2:401.
    A detailed picture of the sonographic appearances of fibroids.
12. Tada S, et al. Computed tomographic features of uterine myoma. *J Comput Assist Tomogr* 1981;5:866.
    Appearance of fibroids on computed tomographic scan.
13. Mark AS, et al. Adenomyosis and leiomyoma: differential diagnosis with MR imaging. *Radiology* 1987;163:527.
    Assesses capability of making the distinction.
14. La Sela GB, et al. Panoramic diagnostic microhysteroscopy. Analysis of results obtained from 976 outpatients. *Acta Obstet Gynecol Scand* 1987;141:91.
    Excellent review of the use of hysteroscopy for the diagnosis of submucous fibroids.
15. Treissman DA, Bate JT, Randall PT. Epidural use of morphine in managing the pain of carneous degeneration of a uterine leiomyoma during pregnancy. *Can Med Assoc J* 1982;126:505.
    Novel therapy for this painful condition.
16. Davis JL, et al. Uterine leiomyomas in pregnancy. A prospective study. *Obstet Gynecol* 1990;75:41.
    The size of fibroids had no influence on pregnancy status.
17. Rubin A, Ford JA. Uterine fibromyomata in urban blacks. A preliminary survey of the relationship between symptomatology, blood pressure and haemoglobin levels. *South Afr Med J* 1974;48:2060.
    An association between fibroids and hypertension has been sought, because the two conditions frequently coexist. This relationship is probably only statistical, however, as both disorders are very common in black patients.
18. Burton CA, et al. Surgical management of leiomyomata during pregnancy. *Obstet Gynecol* 1989;74:707.
    Leiomyomata may require surgical treatment because of symptoms or an uncertain diagnosis. Surgical treatment is safe in selected cases.

Management
19. Hutchins FZ Jr. Myomectomy after selective preoperative treatment with a gonadotropin releasing hormone analog. *J Reprod Med* 1992;37:699.
    This article describes the effective and safe preoperative management to reduce the size of a tumor and thus decrease the morbidity associated with the procedure.
20. Schlaff WD, et al. A placebo-controlled trial of depot gonadotropin-releasing hormone analogue (leuprolide) in the treatment of uterine leiomyomata. *Obstet Gynecol* 1989;74:856.
    Long-acting preparations allow for three-monthly, rather than monthly, dosing.

21. Dubiuisson JB, et al. Myomectomy by laparoscopy: a preliminary report of 43 cases. *Fertil Steril* 1991;56:827.
    A report on 43 patients who underwent removal of 92 myomata. No patients required laparotomy or transfusions.
22. Berkeley AS, DeCherney AH, Polan ML. Abdominal myomectomy and subsequent fertility. *Surg Gynecol Obstet* 1983;156:319.
    A reminder of the positive effects of myomectomy.
23. Neuwirth RS. Hysteroscopic management of symptomatic submucous fibroids. *Obstet Gynecol* 1983;62:509.
    A relatively easy and effective way of removing small submucous fibroids under direct visualization per vaginam.
24. Indman PD. Hysteroscopic treatment of menorrhagia associated with uterine leiomyomas. *Obstet Gynecol* 1993;81:716.
    Of 51 women treated, three subsequently required hysterectomy.
25. Reyniak JV, et al. Microsurgical laser technique for abdominal myomectomy. *Microsurgery* 1987;8:92.
    Laser treatment can effectively vaporize small fibroids.
26. Friedman AJ, Haas ST. Should uterine size be an indication for surgical intervention in women with myomas? *Am J Obstet Gynecol* 1993;168:751.
    The authors argue against the routine removal of asymptomatic fibroid uteri based on the size of the uterus exceeding the size of a 12-week gestation.
27. Arcangell S, Pasquerette MM. Gravid uterine rupture after myolysis. *Obstet Gynecol* 1997;5:857.
    Rupture of a gravid uterus at 25 weeks is discussed.
28. Davis KM, Schaff MD. Medical management of uterine fibromyomata. *Obstet Gynecol Clin North Am* 1995;22:727.
    A review of many different medical managements that are in use for the treatment of fibroids.
29. Ravina JH, et al. Arterial embolization to treat uterine myomata. *Lancet* 1995; 346:8976.
    The technique and usefulness for treatment of symptomatic fibroids is described. This may be the future therapy for many patients unsuitable for surgery.

48. PROLAPSE

Michel E. Rivlin

Weakness of the pelvic supporting structures may allow the pelvic organs to descend into the vagina. This process is termed *genital prolapse*. Descent of the anterior vaginal wall with protrusion of the bladder is called a *cystocele*. If the urethra sags as well, this is called a *cystourethrocele*. A protrusion of the rectum through the posterior vaginal wall is termed a *rectocele*; it is frequently found in association with a herniation of the intestine through the cul-de-sac, termed an *enterocele*. The degree of descent of the uterus varies and is deemed grade I if there is descent between the normal position and the ischial spines, grade II for descent between the spines and the hymen, grade III for descent within the hymen, and grade IV if through the hymen. One or more forms of uterovaginal prolapse usually exist in an individual patient.

The fixed, unyielding support of the pelvic organs is derived from the pelvic bones, while the major soft tissue support is afforded by the muscular pelvic floor. This latter is formed by the levator muscles (pubococcygeus, iliococcygeus, and ischiococcygeus). The more superficial perineal muscles and the urogenital diaphragm also provide some limited muscular support, although they are much less important than the levators in this regard. In addition to the pelvic floor muscles, certain connective tissues, called the *endopelvic fascia,* play a vital role in pelvic organ support. These include the paired uterosacral ligaments, passing from the cervix to the sacrum, and lateral thickenings in the base of the broad ligament, called *transverse cervical, cardinal,* or *Mackenrodt's ligaments,* which suspend the cervix and upper vagina from the pelvic side walls. The anterior and posterior vaginal walls are also supported by the pubocervical and rectovaginal fascia, respectively.

Prolapse is almost always a result of traumatic neuromuscular damage to the pelvic supporting structures incurred during childbirth and tends to be progressive with increasing parity. Lack of estrogen after the menopause frequently aggravates the condition. As in any other hernial condition, obesity, chronic cough, constipation, and occupations involving much standing and lifting may be contributory factors. Under normal conditions and in the erect position, the levator plate (central tendon of the levator muscles) lies in the horizontal plane; the uterus, vagina, and rectum all lie parallel to the plate, with the latter two structures lying in the hollow of the sacrum. When intraabdominal pressure increases, all three structures are forced against the levator plate, which contracts to support them. In addition, contraction of the levator, particularly the crura (i.e., the puborectalis and pubococcygeus), narrows the urogenital and anal hiatus. If structural or functional impairment of the levator occurs, the crura fail to narrow the pelvic hiatus, and the levator sags, assuming a position that is inclined from the horizontal. Increased intraabdominal pressure results in a widened and elongated pelvic hiatus.

Mild to moderate pelvic relaxation is often associated with stress urinary incontinence (SUI). Poor transmission of abdominal pressure to the urethra is the main pathophysiologic reason for SUI. With the loss of anatomic support to the bladder base, the urethrovesical junction descends with the Valsalva maneuver and is no longer in the intraabdominal pressure domain. With the anatomic displacement of the urethrovesical junction and proximal urethra outside of its normal intrapelvic location above the urogenital diaphragm, any abdominal pressure increase is well transmitted to the bladder but is poorly transmitted to the urethra, and this results in the formation of a pressure gradient across the urethrovesical junction and an involuntary loss of urine. Substantial SUI is usually associated with demonstrable defects in anterior vaginal wall support, most often with concurrent defects in uterine and posterior vaginal wall support. Other symptoms of prolapse include a feeling of bulging in the vagina or a dragging feeling. Rarely, when prolapse is marked, it may be necessary to apply digital pressure to allow micturition or defecation. Residual urine, owing to incomplete emptying of a cystocele, may be a source of urinary tract infections (UTIs). There may be dyspareunia owing to the vaginal bulge, or the patient may complain of feeling too large. Backache that is most painful on arising and abates during the day is likely to be orthopedic in origin. If it is absent on arising, worsens during the day, and is relieved by lying down, the traction caused by genital prolapse may be the problem. In major degrees of prolapse, the protruding cervix and vagina may ulcerate, with consequent bleeding and discharge.

Prolapse is diagnosed on the basis of findings revealed by pelvic examination, which should be carried out in both the lithotomy and standing positions. The anterior and posterior vaginal walls are examined separately for the presence of descent with straining, as is the cervix. When primary damage involves the upper suspensory system, the cervix or vaginal vault will appear first, followed by any cystocele and rectocele. In cases of primary damage to the lower supportive system, the order is reversed. SUI is assessed if present. The size and position of the uterus are outlined on bimanual examination; the uterus is usually axial or retroverted with prolapse. It is not uncommon for the cervix to be well supported and for vaginal wall prolapse to result in elongation of the supravaginal cervix. Particular care must be taken to assess levator muscle tone and to determine whether there is an enterocele. A urine culture should be performed for every patient. Many patients with no urinary complaints may become incontinent when the prolapse is reduced, and this must be taken into account when planning surgical correction. Uroflowmetry and measurement of residual urine may help identify the patients at risk. The cystometrogram also identifies underlying detrusor instability or a hypotonic bladder. Multichannel pressure testing and fluoroscopy can comprehensively define the function of the lower urinary tract, but are not universally available. If third-degree descensus is present, an intravenous pyelogram is required, because ureteric obstruction is common in major instances of prolapse.

Medical treatment of prolapse is confined to patients with mild forms, especially young women in the first few months after childbirth. Conservative therapy includes pelvic floor exercises, weight loss, control of cough, and management of constipation. In older women, estrogen therapy may improve the condition of the vaginal mucosa and relieve minor symptoms. All these measures are also useful in preparing patients for surgical repair.

Vaginal pessaries have a place as a temporary measure after childbirth, during pregnancy, or in patients for whom surgical treatment is contraindicated. This last group includes aged and medically debilitated women for whom the operative risk appears too great, as well as those who refuse the procedure. Pessaries are usually made of plastic in the shape of a ring and are placed in a fashion similar to that of the contraceptive diaphragm. Pessaries should be cleaned and reinserted every few months because, if neglected, they may cause vaginal ulceration. A modern pessary should cause less trouble than a dental plate.

Conservative measures are usually insufficient in all but the mildest cases of prolapse. Surgical correction is usually required as the definitive therapy, but, because prolapse is seldom a health hazard, surgical repair should not be recommended unless the symptoms warrant the operative risk. Urinary and local vaginal infections or ulcerations must be cleared up before the operation. In planning the procedure, the patient's attitude toward future pregnancy, the presence or absence of SUI, and the importance of coital activity to the individual must be considered in detail.

The favored procedure for the treatment of uterine descent is a vaginal hysterectomy with support of the vaginal vault by the transverse cervical and uterosacral ligaments. When these tissues are inadequate, the vaginal apex may be suspended from the sacrospinous ligaments or the iliococcygeus fascia. If an enterocele is present, the peritoneal sac is excised and closed, and the uterosacral ligaments are approximated in the midline to prevent further herniation. In most cases, this procedure is followed by anterior vaginal wall repair (colporrhaphy), with particular attention to support of the urethrovesical angle if SUI is a problem. If there is a rectocele and a deficient perineum, posterior vaginal wall repair and restoration of the perineal body (colpoperineorrhaphy) complete the procedure.

Surgical procedures for prolapse may be carried out by the abdominal route with the exception of the posterior compartment repairs. These procedures include operations for anterior compartment defects, including cystocele with or without SUI, such as retropubic urethrocystopexy or paravaginal repairs. For central descent, a sacral colpopexy may be performed with suspension of the vaginal apex to the sacrum using a graft. Enterocele is prevented by permanent sutures obliterating the cul-de-sac in a Moschcowitz or Halban fashion. In summary, all defects encountered in the individual patient should be corrected by appropriate techniques through either an abdominal, or a vaginal, or a combined approach.

For those women who desire further pregnancies, surgical treatment can be delayed. If this is not possible, modified repairs can be performed, although these are much less likely to be successful. If these patients become pregnant, delivery should be by cesarean section; otherwise, the repair is likely to break down at the time of delivery. In older women in whom intercourse is no longer a factor, a stronger repair is possible, as less attention needs to be given to maintaining a functional vagina.

Postoperative care is chiefly directed at urinary function and the relief of pain associated with the posterior repair. Hemorrhage and infection are the major postoperative complications, but the incidence of infection is much reduced by the administration of perioperative prophylactic antibiotics, especially in premenopausal patients.

Long-term postoperative complications include dyspareunia and vault prolapse. Dyspareunia may be relieved by vaginal dilatation and estrogen therapy. Vault prolapse is usually due to failure of the enterocele repair. Several operative procedures, by both abdominal and vaginal routes, have been used to alleviate this difficult surgical problem, but no completely satisfactory method has yet been developed.

Reviews
1. American College of Obstetricians and Gynecologists. Pelvic organ prolapse. *ACOG Tech Bull* no. 214, 1995.
   Prolapse may involve damage to the cardinal and uterosacral ligament complex, the urogenital diaphragm, including its pubourethral components, the pelvic diaphragm, and the perineal body. A basic surgical rule is to overrepair the primary site of damage to reduce the chance of recurrence.
2. Nichols DH. Surgery for pelvic floor disorders. *Surg Clin North Am* 1991;71: 927.
   Important goals of reconstructive surgical treatment include upward relocation of the vesicourethral junction to a point where it is once again under the influence of intraabdominal pressure, as well as restoration of normal vaginal depth and axis.

Anatomy
3. DeLancey JO. Anatomy and biomechanics of genital prolapse. *Clin Obstet Gynecol* 1993;36:897.
   The levator ani muscles form an occlusive layer on which the pelvic organs rest. The endopelvic fascia suspends the organs from the pelvic side walls.
4. Wall LL. The muscles of the pelvic floor. *Clin Obstet Gynecol* 1993;36:910.
   Fibers of the pubovisceral muscle pass behind the rectum, forming a sling that pulls it toward the pubic bones.
5. Norton PA. Pelvic floor disorders: the role of fascia and ligaments. *Clin Obstet Gynecol* 1993;36:926.
   Reviews the possibility that an underlying abnormality of connective tissue in pelvic floor ligaments and fascia is a cause of pelvic support disorders.

Etiology
6. Smith ARB, Hosker GL, Warrell DW. The role of partial denervation of the pelvic floor in the aetiology of genitourinary prolapse and stress incontinence of urine. A neurophysiological study. *Br J Obstet Gynaecol* 1989;96:24.
   Deleterious effect of childbirth on the integrity of pelvic floor innervation and muscle strength.
7. Olsen AL, et al. Epidemiology of surgically managed pelvic organ prolapse and urinary incontinence. *Obstet Gynecol* 1997;89:501.
   The lifetime risk of undergoing an operation for prolapse or incontinence was 11.1%. Most patients were older, postmenopausal, parous, and overweight. Nearly half were smokers. Reoperation was common (29%).
8. Strohbehn K, Jakary JA, Delancey JO. Pelvic organ prolapse in young women. *Obstet Gynecol* 1997;90:33.
   A higher than expected prevalence of congenital anomalies was found in this study of young women, as well as rheumatologic and neurologic diseases.
9. Wiskind AK, Creighton SM, Stanton SL. The incidence of genital prolapse after the Burch colposuspension. *Am J Obstet Gynecol* 1992;167:399.
   Thirty-five percent of 131 patients required surgical treatment for prolapse after the Burch procedure. Repair of one vaginal compartment may predispose another compartment to prolapse.

Diagnosis
10. Bump RC, et al. The standardization of terminology of female pelvic organ prolapse and pelvic floor dysfunction. *Am J Obstet Gynecol* 1996;175:10.
    Standardized nomenclature providing an objective site-specific system for describing, quantitating, and staging pelvic support in women.
11. Jackson SL, et al. Fecal incontinence in women with urinary incontinence and pelvic organ prolapse. *Obstet Gynecol* 1997;89:423.
    There is a high rate of fecal incontinence in women with urinary incontinence and pelvic organ prolapse. Clinicians should inquire routinely and specifically about fecal incontinence.
12. Mouritsen L. Techniques for imaging bladder support. *Acta Obstet Gynecol Scand [Suppl]* 1997;166:48.

Literature about imaging techniques, especially voiding cystourethrography, ultrasonography, and magnetic resonance imaging, were studied and their diagnostic value evaluated. Dynamic ultrasonography is the first-line imaging method for studying bladder support.

13. Healy JC, et al. Patterns of prolapse in women with symptoms of pelvic floor weakness: assessment with MR imaging. *Radiology* 1997;203:77.

Magnetic resonance imaging clearly shows pelvic visceral prolapse and pelvic floor configuration on straining.

Medical Therapy

14. Wu V, et al. A simplified protocol for pessary management. *Obstet Gynecol* 1997;90:990.

A plastic ring, a rubber doughnut, or an inflatable pessary may be used in the elderly patient. To retain a pessary comfortably, the patient must have some strength in the pelvic diaphragm measured at the levator sling—the hiatus at which the levator ani crosses the sides of the vagina.

15. Taskin O, et al. The effects of episiotomy and Kegel exercises on postpartum pelvic relaxation: a prospective controlled study. *J Gynecol Surg* 1996;12:23.

The Kegel exercise program involves isometric contractions of the muscle of the pelvic diaphragm. An effective regimen consists of 15 consecutive strong contractions lasting 3 seconds each and performed six times daily.

Surgical Procedures

16. Lee RA. Vaginal hysterectomy with repair of enterocele, cystocele, and rectocele. *Clin Obstet Gynecol* 1993;36:967.

This article reviews correction of the defective pelvic structures and restoration of them to a normal functional and anatomical position.

17. Kohli N. Incidence of recurrent cystocele after anterior colporrhaphy with and without concomitant transvaginal needle suspension. *Am J Obstet Gynecol* 1996; 175:1476.

The incidence of recurrent cystocele is significantly higher after anterior colporrhaphy with concomitant needle bladder neck suspension compared with anterior colporrhaphy alone.

18. Youngblood JP. Paravaginal repair for cystourethrocele. *Clin Obstet Gynecol* 1993;36:960.

This describes a technique intended specifically for the repair of lateral detachment of the vagina with resultant cystocele and stress urinary incontinence.

19. Kahn MA, Stanton SSL. Posterior colporrhaphy: its effects on bowel and sexual function. *Br J Obstet Gynaecol* 1997;104:82.

Correction of pelvic anatomic defects without appropriate preoperative evaluation is likely to result in unacceptably high failure rates.

20. O'Leary JA, O'Leary JL. The extended Manchester operation. *Am J Obstet Gynecol* 1970;107:546.

The Fothergill or Manchester procedure, consisting of anterior repair with cervical amputation, has been largely replaced by vaginal hysterectomy with repair.

21. Grody MHT, Chatwani A, Nyirjesy P. Bilateral cervical uterosacral suspension and cardinal cervical fixation for uterovaginal prolapse in young women. *J Pelvic Surg* 1997;3:11.

There are several treatments from which to choose for the repair of symptomatic prolapse in the patient who wishes to retain fertility.

22. Allahbadia GN. Obstetric performance following conservative surgery for pelvic relaxation. *Int J Gynaecol Obstet* 1992;38:293.

Less than 2% of the cases of prolapse occur in nulliparous women.

23. Ahranjani M, et al. Neugebauer-Le Fort operation for vaginal prolapse. *J Reprod Med* 1992;37:959.

This operation obliterates the central portion of the vagina, leaving lateral channels for drainage. It can be performed under local anesthesia in very debilitated patients, but is seldom required in modern practice.

24. Langmade CJ, Oliver JA Jr. Partial colpocleisis. *Am J Obstet Gynecol* 1986; 154:1200.
    For older, debilitated patients not requiring a functional vagina, avoiding scarring between the anterior and posterior walls prevents the stress urinary incontinence often reported after complete colpocleisis.
25. Nichols DH. Types of enterocele and principles underlying choice of operation for repair. *Obstet Gynecol* 1972;40:257.
    The types of enteroceles covered include congenital (persistent sac), pulsion (plus eversion of the vaginal wall), traction (plus cystocele and rectocele pulling the vault into eversion), and iatrogenic (anterior or posterior to the vagina).
26. Given FT Jr. Posterior culdoplasty: revisited. *Am J Obstet Gynecol* 1985;153:135.
    Culdoplasty, consisting of the narrowing or obliteration of the cul-de-sac of Douglas, can be performed by either a vaginal or an abdominal approach for the prophylaxis or therapy of enterocele. Commonly used procedures, are, in general, modifications of the techniques introduced by Moschcowitz, Halban, and McCall.

Vaginal Inversion
27. De Vries MJ, et al. Short-term results and long-term patients' appraisal of abdominal colposacropexy for treatment of genital and vaginal vault prolapse. *Eur J Obstet Gynecol Reprod Biol* 1995;59:35.
    The procedure consisted of retroperitoneal interposition of a Mersilene mesh between a prolapsed vaginal vault or uterus and the anterior surface of the sacrum. There was a favorable result on prolapse-related complaints. Functional complaints and pain are not substantially relieved.
28. Paraiso MFR, et al. Pelvic support defects and visceral and sexual function in women treated with sacrospinous ligament suspension and pelvic reconstruction. *Am J Obstet Gynecol* 1996;175:1423.
    The coccygeus muscle and sacrospinous ligament are the same fibromuscular structure. In suspending the prolapsed vagina from the ligament, great care must be taken to avoid injury to the pudendal nerve and vessels laterally and the sciatic nerve and inferior gluteal vessels superiorly.
29. Ross JW. Techniques of laparoscopic repair of total vault eversion after hysterectomy. *J Am Assoc Gynecol Laparosc* 1997;4:173.
    Initial results of laparoscopic repair of total pelvic vault eversion are comparable to those of other surgical approaches. Careful anatomic evaluation of the different defects, together with urodynamic studies, are necessary in treating this difficult disorder.

49. STRESS INCONTINENCE

Mendley A. Wulfsohn

Stress urinary incontinence (SUI) can be defined as an involuntary loss of urine from an intact urethra that occurs without any conscious desire to void and as the result of a rise in intraabdominal pressure. It is by far the most common cause of urinary incontinence in the female. Minor degrees of SUI may occur in at least 50% of nulliparous women, though only 1% of all patients requiring surgical correction are nulliparous. Pregnancy and childbirth undoubtedly play roles in the causation of SUI in susceptible subjects by damaging the supports of the bladder neck and urethra. SUI is four times as common in white as in African-American women, but the reason for this is uncertain.

The following are the five mechanisms responsible for continence: (1) The bladder neck, or internal sphincter, consists of smooth muscle derived from the detrusor muscle fibers. (2) The distal sphincter, which is a smooth muscle sphincter that surrounds the middle and lower portion of the urethra, is relatively weak in the female; both smooth muscle sphincters are innervated by alpha-adrenergic receptors. (3) The external sphincter is a striated muscle that surrounds the middle third of the urethra and acts together with the pelvic floor musculature; reflex contractions of these muscles, occurring with sudden rises in abdominal pressure, tend to prevent SUI; damage to this external sphincter mechanism is therefore important in the pathogenesis of SUI. (4) The resilience and elasticity of the epithelium lining the urethra play a small additional role in continence; this is important in elderly patients with a lack of estrogen and atrophic changes in the distal urethral epithelium. (5) The upper third of the urethra lies above the pelvic diaphragm, and thus is intraabdominal; this ensures that any rise in intraabdominal pressure is transmitted to both the bladder and the upper urethra simultaneously; prolapse of the upper urethra below the pelvic floor therefore eliminates this mechanism.

Patients with grade I SUI complain of a transient leaking of urine with sudden increases of intraabdominal pressure, such as during coughing, sneezing, or exertion during sporting activities. Incontinence does not occur while at rest in bed. In grade II SUI, the symptoms are more severe, with incontinence occurring with lesser degrees of exertion, such as walking, standing up from a sitting position, or even sitting up in bed. Grade III SUI is so severe that there is almost continuous leaking while the person is erect or with virtually any movement while lying down. About 5%–10% of patients also have incidental urinary tract infection (UTI) that requires control.

The general physical examination should be directed toward the detection of neurologic disease, chronic respiratory conditions, large bowel disorders, and the presence of a pelvic mass. Signs of senile atrophy should be observed, and the appearance and size of the urethral meatus should be noted. The presence and extent of descent of the anterior vaginal wall are noted when the patient coughs or strains. At the same time, cystocele, rectocele, and uterine prolapse are sought. The patient should be examined when the bladder is comfortably full. SUI can be demonstrated when the patient is coughing. Failing this, the table may be tilted downward 45 degrees. If this technique fails, she can be tested while in the erect position with a receiver between the thighs.

The Marshall (Bonney) test consists of the digital elevation of the vagina on either side of the bladder neck, which prevents demonstrable stress incontinence. This is an unreliable test, however, because only the slightest compression of the urethra itself will prevent all forms of incontinence. The Q-tip test is performed by inserting a lubricated Q-tip into the urethra. Anterior rotation of the Q-tip with straining indicates prolapse of the bladder base. Cystoscopy and urethroscopy should be performed to rule out any other bladder disorder. Motility of the bladder neck can be observed during cystoscopy by getting the patient to cough or strain. Renal ultrasound imaging should be done before any surgical procedure.

SUI must be distinguished from other forms of incontinence. Urinary fistulas in the vagina usually produce a constant dribbling incontinence, but a small fistula may cause leakage only during stress. Rarely, an ectopic ureteral opening into the female genital tract presents with pseudostress incontinence. Chronic urinary retention may also present with stress as well as overflow incontinence. Urgency incontinence is usually readily distinguishable by taking a careful history. However, there are some patients with bladder instability whose symptoms and signs are difficult to distinguish from those of SUI. Pure urgency incontinence must be confirmed by urodynamic evaluation. Surgical treatment in this type of patient is likely to have a poor outcome. Giggle incontinence is an inborn abnormality in which a detrusor contraction is initiated by laughter.

The anatomy of the bladder outlet can be demonstrated radiologically by filling the bladder with contrast material via a catheter. Fluoroscopy is then performed, and x-ray studies are taken with the patient in the erect position. Observations are made with the patient at rest, while coughing and straining, and during voiding. In type 0 and I SUI the base of the bladder is situated at or above the upper border of the pubic symphysis at rest, and the vesical neck is closed. During stress, the bladder neck opens and descends less than 2 cm. In type 0, actual leakage cannot be demonstrated, although normally it is present. In type I, the incontinence is visualized. The bladder base has a similar appearance at rest in type IIA, but, when the patient strains, the vesical neck opens and descends below the lower border of the symphysis. Because the distal urethra is fixed, descent of the bladder base results in flattening of the posterior vesicourethral angle. With progressive prolapse, the urethra comes to lie horizontally and the angle may exceed 180 degrees. However, the loss of the posterior vesicourethral angle is not the cause of SUI, but reflects the anatomic deformity, which is a cystourethrocele. In type II B SUI, the bladder base is below the lower border of the pubic symphysis at rest. During stress, further descent may or may not take place, but the urethra opens and incontinence ensues. Type III is the most severe variety of SUI and often occurs after previous failed surgery. The position of the bladder base varies, but, universally, the bladder neck and proximal urethra are open at rest, and leaking occurs with minimal stress (e.g., by gravity).

It is important to carry out urodynamic studies on most patients with SUI. A filling cystometrogram is first performed. While the bladder is being filled with water at a fixed rate, simultaneous rectal (intraabdominal) and intravesical pressures are measured. By measuring both pressures, it is possible by subtraction to determine the true detrusor pressure and to record uninhibited bladder contractions. Detrusor instability is defined as any reflex contraction of 15 cm of water or more that cannot be inhibited by the patient. In rare cases, unstable contractions may be initiated by coughing or by changing to the erect posture (postural hyperreflexia). When a significant bladder contraction occurs immediately after coughing the symptoms may closely resemble those of genuine SUI. A considerable number of women with SUI also complain of urinary urgency, and about 16% have urodynamically demonstrable detrusor instability. This condition is not a contraindication to the surgical correction of proven true SUI, as instability will resolve 80% of the time after operation. Bladder instability may develop in a small number of patients de novo postoperatively.

The measurement of leak-point pressure (LPP) is the second important parameter which requires evaluation during urodynamics. There are two types of LPP. (1) Valsalva LPP (VLPP) is measured when the bladder is filled with approximately 300 cc of fluid. At this point the patient is asked to strain. The total vesical pressure is measured at the moment that leakage is observed. VLPP of less than 100 cm of water is strongly suggestive of intrinsic sphincter deficiency (ISD), also called type III SUI. (2) Detrusor LPP (DLPP) is not an important measurement in the evaluation of SUI. DLPP is the detrusor pressure which is recorded at the time that the patient leaks during a detrusor contraction.

Conservative therapy can be tried in mild cases of SUI. Pelvic floor exercises and faradic stimulation of the perineal muscles are occasionally successful. Better results can be expected if this is combined with biofeedback. Alpha-adrenergic receptor stimulants may be tried to increase tone in the bladder neck and urethral smooth muscle. Oral or vaginal doses of conjugated estrogen may be helpful in elderly patients with atrophic vaginitis. Incontinence associated with detrusor instability requires treatment with anticholinergic agents or detrusor relaxants. UTI must be cleared. In the elderly, vaginal pessaries may adequately control SUI. Disposable urethral inserts represent one of the newer nonsurgical treatment modalities. Several different designs are currently undergoing clinical trials. Generally they consist of a gel-like material which when activated swells in the bladder and urethra and result in occlusion of the urethral lumen. These plugs require removal and replacement each time the patient voids. Transurethral submucosal injection of collagen into the submucosal tissues of the proximal urethra have been successful in 70%–80% of cases. This procedure should be reserved for patients with ISD with little or no mobility of the bladder neck. Between 2.5 and 7.5 cc of collagen are injected under local anesthesia in an attempt to occlude the urethral lumen. Two or three repeat injections are not uncommonly required before a successful result is obtained. Surgical treatment should be offered to patients who have significant SUI.

Numerous operations have been designed for the cure of SUI, but controversy exists as to which type of operation is best suited for which type and grade of defect. Undoubtedly, the first operation should be the best operation, because subsequent repairs become progressively more difficult and achieve a lower success rate. There are four main groups of operations in common use today, all of which are aimed at the restoration of normal anatomy, elongation of the urethra, and fixation of the bladder neck: (1) Anterior vaginal repairs are aimed at correcting the defective pelvic floor and buttressing the bladder neck with sutures apposing the pubocervical fascia (Kelly plication); the low success rates associated with this procedure have been largely responsible for eliminating its use. (2) Retropubic vesicourethropexy procedures (Marshall-Marchetti and Burch) entail the placement of sutures between the paraurethral and paravesical tissues and the pubic bones, or Cooper's ligament, thereby elevating and fixating the bladder neck. (3) In endoscopic vesical neck suspension operations (Stamey and Raz), the area of the bladder neck is elevated by the placement of heavy polypropylene sutures in the pubocervical fascia. These sutures are passed suprapubically using specially designed needles. They may be tied down to the rectus fascia or tied to bone anchors which are placed in the pubic bones on both sides. During the operation, cystoscopy is performed to confirm the correct position of the suspension sutures and to assure that the bladder is not perforated. Retropubic suspension operations and needle suspension procedures have an initial high success rate but in recent times it is becoming increasingly evident that there is a high long-term failure rate. (4) Sling operations are usually required for treatment of type III SUI. Many authorities now believe that a sling procedure should be performed as the first procedure on young women with SUI. Materials that can be used for pubovaginal slings include autologous fascia, allogenic fascia, synthetic materials, and vaginal mucosa. Sling procedures are reported to have a success rate of 95%. Rarely, it becomes necessary to insert an artificial urinary sphincter, although the complication rate is high if there have been multiple previous operations. When all else has failed, urinary diversion may be the last resort for managing intractable incontinence. When indicated, needle suspension and pubovaginal sling procedures should be combined with vaginal hysterectomy and cystocele and rectocele repairs. In repairing a large cystocele, even when no preoperative stress incontinence has been demonstrated, serious consideration should be given to supporting the bladder neck since stress incontinence may ensue once the urethrovesical angle has been straightened.

Reviews

1. Varner RE, Sparks JM. Surgery for stress urinary incontinence. *Surg Clin North Am* 1991;71:1111.
   Updated review of pathogenesis and management. Conservative and surgical approaches to management are reviewed.
2. Dupont MC, Albo ME, Raz S. Diagnosis of stress urinary incontinence. An overview. *Urol Clin North Am* 1996;23:407.
   An overview of the evaluation and diagnosis of stress incontinence. The relevance of the distinction between anatomic incontinence and intrinsic sphincter deficiency is discussed.
3. Morley R, Cumming J, Weller R. Morphology and neuropathology of the pelvic floor in patients with stress incontinence. *Int Urogynecol J Pelvic Floor Dysfunct* 1996;7:3.
   Stress incontinence is associated with neurological and collagenous changes in the pelvic floor.
4. Thind P, Lose G, Colstrup H. Initial urethral pressure increased during stress episodes in genuine stress incontinent women. *Br J Urol* 1992;69:137.
   Bladder and urethral pressures are measured simultaneously with a double-microtip transducer catheter. Findings suggest the presence of a defective active closure mechanism in urinary bladder incontinence.
5. Mushkat Y, Bukovsky I, Langer R. Female urinary stress incontinence—does it have familial prevalence? *Am J Obstet Gynecol* 1996;174:617.
   There is a threefold prevalence among first-degree relatives of patients with stress incontinence. There may be a genetic factor.

Diagnostic Studies

6. Viktrup L, et al. The symptoms of stress incontinence caused by pregnancy or delivery in primiparas. *Obstet Gynecol* 1992;79:945.
    Stress incontinence occurs as a natural consequence of pregnancy in 32% of primiparas. Persistent stress urinary incontinence occurs in only 1%. The importance of obstetric factors as an etiologic agent is unclear.
7. Demirci F, Fine PM. Ultrasonography in stress urinary incontinence. *Int J Pelvic Floor Dysfunct* 1996;7:125.
    Ultrasonography is an inexpensive, reliable, and noninvasive modality for evaluating the urethrovesical junction.
8. Gordon D, et al. Comparison of ultrasound and lateral chain urethrocystography in the determination of bladder neck descent. *Am J Obstet Gynecol* 1989;160:182.
    Diagnostic procedures include urethroscopy, urodynamics, cystometry, urethral closure pressure profiles, uroflowmetry, electromyography of the pelvic floor, radiologic procedures, and ultrasound.
9. Migliorini GD, Glenning PP. Bonney's test—fact or fiction? *Br J Obstet Gynaecol* 1987;94:157.
    This study invalidates the Bonney test by objectively demonstrating that the test restores continence by directly obstructing the urethra and urethrovesical junction.
10. Bhatia NN, Bergman A. Pessary tests in women with urinary incontinence. *Obstet Gynecol* 1985;65:220.
    The authors found that use of a pessary differentiated patients with bladder instability from those with stress urinary incontinence caused by correctable anatomic defects.
11. Cummings JM, et al. Leak point pressures in women with urinary stress incontinence: correlation with patient history. *J Urol* 1997;157:811.
    Low valsalva leak point pressure can be expected in women who have had previous surgery and have severe leakage. In addition, 47% of patients without predisposing factors have a low leak point pressure. This could account for many failures of routine suspension procedures.
12. Faerber GJ, Vashi AR. Variations in leak point pressure with increasing vesical volume. *J Urol* 1998;159:1909.
    The ideal volume required to fill the bladder for testing for leak point pressure is 250–300 cc.
13. Blavias JG, Olsson CA. Stress incontinence: classification and surgical approach. *J Urol* 1988;139:727.
    A videourodynamic study led to the formulation of a modified classification for stress urinary incontinence based on the nature of vesical neck descent and the integrity of the intrinsic sphincteric mechanisms.

Therapy

14. Marshall VF, Marchetti AA, Krantz KE. The correction of stress incontinence by simple vesicourethral suspension. *Surg Gynecol Obstet* 1949;88:509.
    In this procedure, sutures appose paraurethral tissues and the bladder neck to the back of the pubis.
15. Barnett RM. The modern Kelly plication. *Obstet Gynecol* 1969;34:667.
    In this anterior vaginal approach, plicating sutures are placed at the bladder neck.
16. Karram MM, Bhatia NN. Management of coexistent stress and urge urinary incontinence. *Obstet Gynecol* 1989;73:4.
    The authors recommend initial medical management with various combinations of oxybutynin, imipramine, and estrogen.
17. Wilson PD, et al. An objective assessment of physiotherapy for female genuine stress incontinence. *Br J Obstet Gynaecol* 1987;94:575.
    Successful treatment with pelvic floor exercises with or without faradic stimulation is more likely in younger patients and in those with lesser degrees of stress urinary incontinence.
18. Bhatia NN, Bergman A, Karram MM. Effects of estrogen on urethral function in women with urinary incontinence. *Am J Obstet Gynecol* 1989;160:176.
    Improvement in half the cases was associated with increased urethral closure pressure and improved abdominal pressure transmission to the proximal urethra.

19. Bartholomew B, Grimaldi T. Collagen injection therapy for type III stress urinary incontinence. *AORN J* 1996;64:74.
    This article discusses a viable alternative to surgery for the treatment of intrinsic sphincter deficiency.
20. McGuire EJ. Abdominal procedures for stress incontinence. *Urol Clin North Am* 1985;12:285.
    The author prefers the Burch colposuspension to the classic Marshall-Marchetti procedure, because the latter is more likely to cause urethral compression. A rectus fascia sling is used for the nonfunctioning urethral sphincter mechanism resulting from multiple failed operations, scarring, and some types of neurologic disease.
21. Trockman BA, Leach GE. Needle suspension procedures: past, present, and future. *J Endourol* 1996;10:217.
    A review of the evolution and future of transvaginal needle suspension procedures.
22. Webster GD, et al. Management of type III stress urinary incontinence using artificial urinary sphincter. *Urology* 1992;39:499.
    The artificial sphincter is an excellent first option for treating type III stress incontinence due to intrinsic urethral weakness resulting from various causes.
23. Radomski SB, Harshorn S. Laparoscopic Burch bladder neck suspension: early results. *J Urol* 1996;155:515.
    Short-term results indicate an 85% success rate.
24. Cross CA, et al. Transvaginal urethrolysis for urethral obstruction after anti-incontinence surgery. *J Urol* 1988;159:1199.
    Urethrolysis is an acceptable procedure for urethral obstruction resulting from previous incontinence surgery. Operative techniques are described.
25. Staskin D, et al. Effectiveness of a urinary control insert in the management of stress urinary incontinence: early results of a multicenter study. *Urology* 1996; 47:629.
    Preliminary results indicate that a urethral insert may be a safe, effective, and well-tolerated alternative to other methods of treatment.
26. Cross CA, Cespedes RD, McGuire EJ. Our experience with pubovaginal slings in patients with stress urinary incontinence. *J Urol* 1998;159:1195.
    Describes only one of several sling techniques available today. Pubovaginal slings are effective and durable. Voiding dysfunction is uncommon and is temporary in most patients.
27. Blavias JG. Editorial: female urology. *J Urol* 1998;159:1202.
    Needle bladder neck suspensions have a 50% failure rate at 5 years. A sling made of fascia or other biocompatible material is strongly favored.

50. DYSMENORRHEA AND PELVIC PAIN

Michel E. Rivlin

Dysmenorrhea, the occurrence of painful uterine cramps during menstruation, may be either *primary* and due to no discernible organic cause, or *secondary* and due to a demonstrable pelvic lesion. It is estimated that more than 50% of menstruating women experience dysmenorrhea, and, in about 10%, the symptoms are incapacitating for several days each month. Primary dysmenorrhea usually begins at menarche or shortly thereafter. The pain appears either several hours before or immediately after the start of menses and is most severe on the first and second days. The pain is spasmodic, occurs over the lower abdomen, and may radiate to the back and thighs. Systemic symptoms, such as nausea, vomiting, and diarrhea, may accompany the pain. The relationship between premenstrual syndrome (PMS) and dysmenorrhea is obscured by the traditional definitions—PMS is regarded as a constellation of variable symptoms and dysmenorrhea is restricted to pain. However, PMS has been shown to more commonly afflict women with dysmenorrhea, and menstrual pain may precede the onset of bleeding. Furthermore, PMS symptoms may persist into the menstrual period, and dysmenorrhea sufferers often have symptoms like those in PMS (e.g., nausea, breast discomfort, and depression). It is therefore an artificial distinction to separate the premenstrual stage from the menstrual period, and appropriate management must be based on this perspective.

Primary dysmenorrhea and its frequently associated symptoms appear to be related to the increased production and release of endometrial prostaglandins (PGE$_{2a}$ and PGE$_2$) during menstruation, which triggers increased and abnormal uterine activity. The condition is limited to ovulatory cycles because the estrogen-primed endometrium requires luteal-phase progesterone levels to enhance the production and concentration of prostaglandins. The abolition of ovulation by oral contraceptives is therefore highly effective in relieving dysmenorrhea.

The myometrial contractions brought about by the particularly high prostaglandin levels reduce uterine blood flow, resulting in uterine ischemia and hypersensitization of pelvic nerve terminals to prostaglandins and endoperoxides, thereby reducing the threshold for the physical and chemical stimuli of pain. Nonsteroidal antiinflammatory drugs (NSAIDs) inhibit prostaglandin production and thus represent another means of managing dysmenorrhea. They are successful in relieving the dysmenorrhea in about 80% of sufferers. Arachidonic acid is metabolized by two important enzyme systems: cyclooxygenase, leading to prostaglandin formation, and 5-lipoxygenase, leading to leukotriene production. The NSAIDs readily suppress menstrual prostaglandin release by inhibiting cyclooxygenase. It is possible that nonresponse to NSAIDs may be related to the continued production of leukotrienes, which also stimulate uterine contractions. Lipoxygenase inhibitor therapy may therefore prove useful in this event.

The causes of *secondary dysmenorrhea* include endometriosis, intrauterine devices (IUDs), pelvic inflammatory disease, adenomyosis, congenital müllerian system malfusions, cervical stenosis, ovarian cysts, and, arguably, pelvic congestion and Allen-Master syndrome. The diagnosis is based on the patient's history, physical examination findings, and response to NSAIDs. These drugs are usually ineffective in relieving secondary dysmenorrhea, so a failure of response may help identify those patients who need to undergo diagnostic laparoscopy. NSAIDs can effectively suppress IUD-induced dysmenorrhea and menorrhagia.

The treatment of primary dysmenorrhea depends on the patient's choice of contraception, if any. If oral contraception is not requested, NSAIDs are prescribed for patients not suffering from a gastric ulcer or NSAID hypersensitivity. If patients do not respond to this treatment after 3 to 4 months, an alternative NSAID is prescribed or oral contraception is added. If there is still no response, laparoscopy is performed, and, if an organic cause is found, further therapy is directed at the underlying disease. Surgical interruption of the uterine nerves is occasionally performed for the treatment of severe intractable cases.

Chronic pelvic pain (which, by definition, persists for more than 6 months) is one of the most common complaints of gynecologic patients. Even after a thorough evaluation, including diagnostic laparoscopy, the cause may remain obscure. Furthermore, the relationship between certain types of pathologic conditions and the pain response may be inconsistent and often inexplicable. For instance, the incidence and severity of pain that occurs in endometriosis do not correlate with the amount of disease present, nor do the site, density, or number of adhesions (postinfective or postoperative) in those with a complaint of pelvic pain differ from those in patients without pain. Many of these women are presumed to suffer from chronic pelvic inflammatory disease and are given repeated courses of antibiotics, which may result in chronic vaginal candidiasis. Many others undergo a variety of surgical procedures, including dilatation and curettage, cyst aspiration, lysis of adhesions, hysterectomy, and oophorectomy. Some sufferers see physicians 20 times a year. Thus, the outcome of traditional management has often led to loss of hormonal and reproductive function, continued pain, and frustration for both the patient and physician.

Nerves carrying pain impulses from the pelvic organs are numerous. Sympathetic fibers from T10 to L1, which are contained within the inferior hypogastric nerve, course along the vena cava and sacrum to enter the uterus through the uterosacral ligaments. Parasympathetic fibers from S1 to S4 travel within the nervi erigentes, emerging in the lateral pelvis and forming ganglia lateral to the cervix (Frankenhauser's ganglion). Autonomic nerves from the outer two thirds of the tubes and from the ovaries enter the cord at the T9–T10 level and are carried via the aortic and mesenteric ganglia and plexuses. Somatic pain is readily perceived and well localized, whereas visceral pain is poorly localized, and the patient's description is usually vague. The most effective triggers of visceral pain are stretch, inflammation, and ischemia.

Characteristically, women who suffer from chronic pelvic pain are 25 to 35 years of age and also complain of dysmenorrhea and dyspareunia. The pain is continuous and poorly localized to the lower abdomen. There is an insistent belief that the pain has an organic cause, and there is a desire for surgical therapy. There is a history of menorrhagia, but the hematocrit is generally normal. Careful questioning often reveals a history of sexual or physical abuse (36%), with an attendant lack of self-esteem and a negative attitude toward sex. The patient usually has a poor relationship with her partner and family. Previous pelvic procedures, especially tubal ligation, are common. Invariably these patients resent suggestions that their problem has a psychiatric or psychosomatic basis.

The initial evaluation, once the history is taken, includes a physical and pelvic examination. Pelvic ultrasonography may be helpful in confirming the normalcy of the pelvic structures. Other causes of pelvic pain may be ruled out with further studies, including barium enema, proctoscopy, and pyelography. Consultation with a gastroenterologist, urologist, orthopedist, or neurologist may be indicated. Laparoscopy is the major tool for guiding diagnosis and management in these women. About a third of each will be found to have endometriosis, adhesions, or a normal pelvis. The finding of minor pelvic pathology may prove difficult to interpret; however, endometriosis should, of course, be treated with standard therapy. The role of pelvic adhesions in causing pain is controversial, and although adhesiolysis has been found to relieve pain in some patients, surgical measures to achieve lysis might produce more adhesions, and patients should be made aware of this fact. When pelvic findings are normal, such patients may be helped by understanding the emotional origins of their problem. Referral to a pain clinic for management, together with psychologic or psychiatric treatment, is frequently necessary because these patients need to understand the connection between stress and pain. Psychologic evaluation provides information about the patient's treatment responses and prognosis. Women accept this when they are reassured that it is a routine measure and not performed to ascertain whether the pain is psychogenic. Psychologic treatment may include behavior therapy and either marital or sexual therapy, or both, plus psychotherapy, as necessary. At the outset, the patient must understand not to expect a cure. Instead, she will be seen regularly by interested therapists, with the goal of achieving a reduction in the level of pain sufficient to permit her return to normal activities.

Pelvic congestion has been proposed as an entity causing pelvic pain. Congestion of the uterus and broad ligament has been noted on radiographic studies and at laparoscopy. A constellation of findings, including secondary dysmenorrhea, low back pain, dysuria, menorrhagia, dyspareunia, and, frequently, retroflexion of the uterus, are thought to stem from this syndrome. Various approaches to therapy, including psychiatric consultation, vasoconstrictor drugs, and hysterectomy, have been tried, with differing results. Traumatic laceration of uterine supporting tissues, the *Allen-Master syndrome,* also has been explored as a cause of pelvic pain. Similar complaints and findings have been associated with repair of the lacerations or hysterectomy.

In patients with recalcitrant pain who still wish to have children, especially those with associated dysmenorrhea, a presacral neurectomy may be performed. The presacral nerve (superior hypogastric plexus) fibers also may be interrupted in the uterosacral ligaments via the laparoscope. Resection does not interfere with bladder or bowel function because the innervation of these organs is predominantly parasympathetic. The procedure is commonly performed in association with conservative surgical treatment for endometriosis, with results that are better than those when surgical treatment is performed for the chronic midline pelvic pain alone. Patients who respond to uterosacral block appear to be suitable candidates for the procedure. In the worst cases, the patient undergoes extremes of treatment, including castration with hysterectomy, in futile efforts to relieve her pain. An operation may bring tremendous relief and even euphoria. However, this elation lasts only until suspicion falls on another body part. Unconscious feelings of guilt or unworthiness return, and the patient repeats the process.

Experience with the multidisciplinary management of pelvic pain at specialized pain clinics suggests that many of these patients have coexisting problems that are both somatic and nonsomatic in nature. Conditions such as the irritable bowel syndrome, urethral syndrome, interstitial cystitis, and myofascial syndrome are important somatic disorders that must be considered in the differential diagnosis of such patients; concurrent psychopathology includes the somatoform pain disorder, somatization, posttraumatic stress disorder, and depression. Advocates of a multidisciplinary approach, including both organic and psychologic interventions, suggest that the frequency with which hysterectomy is performed for this disorder can be markedly reduced.

Dysmenorrhea

1. Osathanondh R. Dysmenorrhea. *Curr Ther Endocrinol Metab* 1997;6:246.
   Risk factors for primary dysmenorrhea include nulliparity and a positive family history; the results of a physical examination should be normal.
2. Jamieson DJ, Steege JF. The prevalence of dysmenorrhea, dyspareunia, pelvic pain, and irritable bowel syndrome in primary care practices. *Obstet Gynecol* 1996;87:55.
   The reported prevalence rates were 90%, 46%, 39%, and 12%, respectively.
3. Mehlisch DR, Fulmer RI. A crossover comparison of bromfenac sodium, naproxen sodium, and placebo for relief of pain from primary dysmenorrhea. *J Womens Health* 1997;6:83.
   Uterine activity in dysmenorrheic patients is characterized by high resting pressure, high frequency, and high active pressure. If NSAIDs are unsuccessful, additional analgesics should not be added because this may potentiate gastrointestinal and other side effects.
4. Ekstrom P, et al. Stimulation of vasopressin release in women with primary dysmenorrhea and after oral contraceptive treatment—effect on uterine contractility. *Br J Obstet Gynaecol* 1992;99:680.
   Oral contraceptives reduce the sensitivity of the uterus to PGF_{2a} and vasopressin.
5. Creatsas G, et al. Prostaglandins: PGF_{2a}, PGE_2, 6-keto-PGF_{1a}, and TXB_2 serum levels in dysmenorrheic adolescents before, during, and after treatment with oral contraceptives. *Eur J Obstet Gynecol Reprod Biol* 1990;36:292.
   The role of prostacyclin in relation to other prostanoids such as thromboxane, PGF_{2a}, and PGE_2 needs to be considered. Some patients have reduced prostacyclin (prostacyclin relaxes the uterus, induces vasodilatation, and is platelet antiaggregatory) levels as the source of their dysmenorrhea. NSAIDs block production of all these prostanoids.
6. Rees MCP, et al. Leukotriene release by endometrium and myometrium throughout the menstrual cycle in dysmenorrhea and menorrhagia. *J Endocrinol* 1987; 113:291.
   The pattern of leukotriene release is similar to that of the prostaglandins: the endometrial concentrations varied throughout the menstrual cycle and were always higher than the myometrial values.
7. Transdermal nitroglycerine in the management of pain associated with primary dysmenorrhea: a multinational pilot study. The Transdermal Nitroglycerine/ Dysmenorrhea Study Group. *J Intern Med Res* 1997;25:41.
   Endogenous nitric oxide mediates smooth-muscle relaxation with subsequent vasodilatation in the vascular, pulmonary, gastrointestinal, and genitourinary tissues. Transdermal nitroglycerin (a nitric oxide donor) has been found effective in inhibiting uterine contractility.

8. Milson I, Hedner N, Mannheimer C. A comparative study of the effect of high-intensity transcutaneous nerve stimulation and oral naproxen on intrauterine pressure and menstrual pain in patients with primary dysmenorrhea. *Am J Obstet Gynecol* 1994;170:123.
   Transcutaneous electrical nerve stimulation is effective in the treatment of dysmenorrhea, possibly due to the gate-control mechanism postulated for stimulation-produced analgesia. This involves the bombardment of the thalamic receptors with impulses traveling on myelinated A fibers, which prevents slower-transmitting A-delta and C fibers from passing their information through the gate to the central nervous system pathways and receptors.
9. Chen FP, et al. Comparison of laparoscopic presacral neurectomy and laparoscopic uterine nerve ablation for primary dysmenorrhea. *J Reprod Med* 1996; 41:463.
   Presacral neurectomy was better than uterosacral resection at 12 months follow-up (81% versus 51%).

Pelvic Pain
10. ACOG Technical Bulletin. Chronic pelvic pain. American College of Obstetricians and Gynecologists. *Int J Gynaecol Obstet* 1996;54:59.
    The bulletin lists 53 causes of chronic pelvic pain.
11. Ryder RM. Chronic pelvic pain. *Am Fam Physician* 1996;54:2225.
    Equal attention to both organic and other causative factors from the outset is more likely to be successful than a standard approach; some believe that laparoscopy is seldom helpful.
12. Savidge CJ, Slade P. Psychological aspects of chronic pelvic pain. *J Psychosom Res* 1997;42:433.
    Evidence that women with pelvic pain without discernible pathology differ in personality, psychological state, or life experiences from women with an identifiable cause for the pain, or those without chronic pelvic pain, is inconclusive.
13. Stewart DE. Chronic gynecologic pain. *Gen Hosp Psychiatry* 1996;18:230.
    The specific psychiatric diagnoses of major depressive disorder, somatoform disorders, borderline personality disorder, and posttraumatic stress disorder have been found to occur more frequently in the chronic pelvic pain population than in the general population.
14. Kamm MA. Chronic pelvic pain in women—gastroenterological, gynaecological or psychological? *Int J Colorectal Dis* 1997;12:57.
    It is critically important to rule out occult nongynecologic diagnoses such as myofascial syndrome, irritable bowel syndrome, urethral syndrome, interstitial cystitis, and psychogenic problems, including somatization, depression, stress disorders, and hypochondriacal or hysterical neuroses.
15. Badura AS, et al. Dissociation, somatization, substance abuse, and coping in women with chronic pelvic pain. *Obstet Gynecol* 1997;90:405.
    Association between a positive abuse history and high levels of dissociation, somatization, and substance abuse is often noted in the chronic pelvic pain population. These psychological variables may be addressed as part of a biopsychosocial model of treatment for chronic pelvic pain patients.
16. Thornton JG, et al. The relationship between laparoscopic disease, pelvic pain and infertility; an unbiased assessment. *Eur J Obstet Gynecol Reprod Biol* 1997; 74:57.
    There is little or no association between minimal endometriosis, pelvic adhesions, or dilated pelvic veins and pain.
17. Stenchever MA. Symptomatic retrodisplacement, pelvic congestion, universal joint, and peritoneal defects: fact or fiction? *Clin Obstet Gynecol* 1990;33:161.
    An objective appraisal is presented of several time-honored but poorly documented diagnoses, including Allen-Masters syndrome (universal joint), retrodisplacement, and pelvic congestion, that have been implicated in the causation of pelvic pain.
18. Slocumb JC. Chronic somatic, myofascial, and neurogenic abdominal pelvic pain. *Clin Obstet Gynecol* 1990;33:145.

The author suggests that many patients suffer from abdominal wall or myofascial pain, or both, rather than from pelvic visceral pain. Hyperpathic trigger points can be identified and treated with local anesthetic blocks, followed by long-lasting improvement.

19. Peters AA, et al. A randomized clinical trial on the benefit of adhesiolysis in patients with intraperitoneal adhesions and chronic pelvic pain. *Br J Obstet Gynaecol* 1992;99:59.
   Adhesiolysis is not useful for alleviating moderate adhesions, but may be beneficial in patients with severe adhesions involving the intestinal tract.
20. Capasso P, et al. Treatment of symptomatic pelvic varices by ovarian vein embolization. *Cardiovasc Intervent Radiol* 1997;20:107.
   Pelvic vascular congestion as a cause of pelvic pain is conjectural and difficult to justify.
21. Hills SD, Marchbanks PA, Peterson HB. The effectiveness of hysterectomy for chronic pelvic pain. *Obstet Gynecol* 1995;86:941.
   Cure rates were less than 50% in women with no abnormal physical findings.
22. Flor H, Fydrich T, Turk DC. Efficacy of multidisciplinary pain treatment centers: a meta-analytic review. *Pain* 1992;49:221.
   Multiple services were directed to the needs of the individual patient.

---

51. ENDOMETRIOSIS

Randall S. Hines

Endometriosis is the condition in which endometrial tissue occurs aberrantly in various locations. It is not a neoplasm despite the fact that it can grow into the bowel or bladder. On rare occasions, it may be the site for the development of a malignant growth. Endometriosis is diagnosed by the presence of endometrial glands and stroma outside the uterus, usually on other pelvic or abdominal organs, although it can occur almost anywhere in the body.

The etiology of endometriosis is not known, but there are multiple theories. The most commonly held theory is that of retrograde menstruation with local implantation. To explain endometriosis in sites such as the ureter, urethra, or umbilicus, another theory suggests that the coelomic epithelium, which forms the müllerian ducts, from which the endometrium arises, can, at any time in adult life, be restimulated by some unknown mechanism and be transformed once again into endometrial tissue. Endometriosis in pelvic lymph nodes or distant sites, such as the lungs or limbs, can be explained by the theory of lymphatic or vascular embolization. Genetics may play a role in the etiology of endometriosis. Two studies have shown a 6% to 7% incidence of endometriosis in first-degree relatives. This is consistent with a multifactorial mode of inheritance. Related to genetics, aberrations in the immune system are thought to occur in some women. A decreased clearance of endometrial cells and abnormal production of cytokines by white cells in the peritoneal fluid of women with endometriosis may be evidence of changes in these patients.

The incidence of endometriosis has been reported to range from 7% to 10% of menstruating women in different studies, and in 30% to 50% of patients presenting with infertility. The true incidence is unknown. Endometriosis may be found in teenagers and rarely after menopause. It occurs most commonly in women between the ages of 30 and 40 who have delayed marriage and childbearing. The incidence of infertility is approximately 30% to 40% in patients with the disease, and the remaining sufferers are usually of low parity.

Half of the patients with endometriosis are asymptomatic. For this reason, it must always be considered in infertile women. Other symptoms of endometriosis depend more on the site of involvement and its nerve supply than the size of individual endometriomata or the extent of the involvement. The ovary is the most common site, occurring in approximately 40% of cases. Involvement of the cul-de-sac and uterosacral ligaments, the next most common site, causes a fixed retroversion and is associated with deep dyspareunia. Progressively worsening dysmenorrhea is another common secondary symptom. Painful defecation due to bowel involvement or hematuria due to bladder involvement are symptoms more rarely encountered. The diagnosis must always be considered in cases of vague, chronic abdominal pain. Rupture of an endometriomatous cyst may cause acute abdominal pain accompanied by all the signs of an "acute abdomen." Although the majority of patients have negative pelvic examination results, extensive pathology may produce tender, nodular swellings along the uterosacral ligaments, or a tender, fixed retroverted uterus, and tender, fixed ovarian tumors with surrounding fibrosis. These patients are often incorrectly diagnosed as suffering from pelvic inflammatory disease.

The correct diagnosis of endometriosis depends on confirmation by laparoscopy. There is tremendous variety in the appearance of the lesions from red vesicular to brown, powder burn, black, or white lesions. There is often an excessive amount of peritoneal fluid containing large amounts of prostaglandin. This has been postulated as the possible cause for the associated infertility (perhaps by affecting tubal transport) in those patients with minimal lesions. Numerous other theories have also been postulated as to the mechanisms by which endometriosis may cause infertility. In severe cases (stage III or IV), physical factors such as scarring and adhesions interfering with tubal mobility, obstructing tubes, or interfering with ovulation and ovum transport are self-explanatory. In mild cases, these factors do not apply. Other explanations include luteinized unruptured follicle syndrome, luteal phase defects, a cytotoxic effect of peritoneal fluid and peritoneal macrophages phagocytosing and degrading sperm, and many more. However, none of these theories have been conclusively demonstrated to explain endometriosis-associated infertility.

Laparoscopic visualization of a classic lesion is considered sufficiently diagnostic to allow treatment to begin, even in the absence of a histologic diagnosis. Atypical lesions require biopsy. Histologic specimens may not always supply a pathologic diagnosis because there may have been so much pressure or scarring that the endometriomatous tissue (e.g., in the case of a "chocolate" cyst of the ovary) can no longer be seen. The best therapeutic regimen for the treatment of endometriosis depends on the age of the patient, the severity of the symptoms, and the symptomatic presentation (pain versus infertility). Laparoscopy and surgical management are recommended for any patient with enough symptomatology to warrant surgery. A variety of surgical techniques provide similar efficacy, from excision to cautery to laser. Although pregnancy may not cure endometriosis, it usually causes considerable involution of the lesions. For patients with pain who have not had surgery or are in need of suppressive therapy, oral contraceptives are given continuously for a period of 6 to 9 months. This therapy is indicated in patients with recurrent disease after a previous conservative operation.

Pain may be treated with danocrine (Danazol), a synthetic derivative of testosterone that may act via suppression of gonadotropin-releasing hormone (GnRH) or gonadotropin secretion, or both. Side effects include menopausal symptoms, weight gain, edema, and mild virilization when used at high dosages. However, mild to moderate cases can be managed effectively with fewer side effects at lower dosage levels. These cases require nonhormonal contraception, however, because ovulation may occur and virilization of female fetuses may follow. Danazol therapy also may be used for 6 to 8 weeks prior to conservative surgery to make dissection of lesions simpler and more complete. Five percent to 20% of patients will experience a recurrence each year. Recognition of adequacy of therapy or recurrence may be obtained after completion of medical therapy by second-look laparoscopy or by testing for the cell surface antigen CA-125, which has been noted to be elevated in patients with endometriosis and correlated with the amount of disease present. It should be remembered, however, that elevation of the CA-125 antigen is nonspecific and has been noted in many other conditions. A more common aggressive medical therapy would use GnRH analogs in the form of a nasal spray, nafarelin, daily injections of leuprolide acetate, or monthly injections of leuprolide acetate depot 3.75 mg intramuscularly, or 11.25 mg used every 3 months. The menopausal-like side effects are better tolerated than the androgenic side effects of danocrine. The use of GnRH analogs has become the most popular form of medical treatment for endometriosis, due to the lack of side effects. In the majority of patients whose major complaint is infertility, conservative surgery produces the best results. The surgery should be completed at laparoscopy with laparotomy for large adnexal masses or failed conservative surgery. Destruction of the lesion can be done through electrocoagulation or vaporization with the CO_2 or KTP laser. In older patients in whom pregnancy is not a consideration and relief of pain is the main objective, laparotomy with total hysterectomy and bilateral salpingo-oophorectomy with excision of any other visible endometriomatous lesions and lysis of adhesions are the treatments of choice. These women may be placed on maintenance estrogen therapy postoperatively because exacerbation of the endometriosis is uncommon.

Rarely, surgery is indicated for obstruction of the rectosigmoid at the level of the cul-de-sac due to an endometrioma, or for small bowel obstruction of the distal ileum or at the ileocecal junction. In the latter case, obstruction is most likely due to adhesions between loops of bowel with subsequent kinking. Surgery also may be indicated for endometriomatous involvement of the ureter. Malignant change is rare, occurring in less than 1% of patients; the lesion is an endometrioid adenocarcinoma. The prognosis for 5-year survival is good, averaging more than 70%. Stromal endometriosis is a rare myometrial tumor, composed of endometrial stroma. It often spreads locally, but true malignant change with remote metastases due to sarcomatous transformation is extremely uncommon.

Adenomyosis is a related condition in which endometrial glands and stroma extend diffusely through tissue spaces in the myometrium and are by convention located more than one high-power field from normal surface endometrium on microscopic examination. Adenomyosis is thought to represent a downgrowth from the basal endometrium, but it may be due to venous or lymphatic embolization. Because it is composed of basal-type endometrium, which is normally insensitive to hormonal stimulus, secretory activity occurs in less than 30% of cases. On gross examination, the lesion is not encapsulated and has a honeycomb appearance. Clinically, the condition is usually found in older, multiparous women. Menorrhagia is the most common symptom, and the large, boggy uterus also may cause pelvic discomfort, bladder and bowel pressure, deep dyspareunia, and even a noticeable abdominal mass. However, it is rare for the uterus to be larger than a 12 to 14 weeks' gestation. Magnetic resonance imaging under certain conditions may be used for diagnosis. Treatment for symptomatic adenomyosis is hysterectomy. Rarely, in the young woman still desirous of having children, local excision with metroplasty may be attempted.

Review
1. Barbieri RL. Endometriosis. A comprehensive review. *Curr Prob Obstet Gynecol Fertil* 1989;11:1.
   Staging each patient according to the American Fertility Association classification provides a point from which to measure disease regression, stability, or progression.
2. Olive DL, Haney AF. Endometriosis-associated infertility; a critical review of therapeutic approaches. *Obstet Gynecol Surv* 1986;41:538.
   Despite extensive literature on the treatment of endometriosis-associated infertility, there are very few answers which can be called definitive.
3. Speroff L, Adamson GD, eds. Endometriosis. *Semin Reprod Endocrinol* 1997;15:199.
   The authors provide a comprehensive discussion on endometriosis.

Etiology
4. Ridley JH. The histogenesis of endometriosis. *Obstet Gynecol Surv* 1968;23:1.
   None of the theories explain why all women do not get the disease.

5. Scott RB, TeLinde RW, Wharton LR Jr. Further studies on experimental endometriosis. *Am J Obstet Gynecol* 1953;62:1082.
   *Six in 10 monkeys with experimentally induced retrograde menses developed
   endometriosis.*
6. DiZerega GS, Barber DL, Hodgen GD. Endometriosis, role of ovarian steroids in
   initiation, maintenance, and suppression. *Fertil Steril* 1980;33:649.
   Estrogen is essential for the development of endometriosis and its continued activity.

Clinical Presentation
7. Simpson JL, et al. Heritable aspects of endometriosis: I. Genetic studies. *Am J
   Obstet Gynecol* 1980;137:327.
   *An apparently unaffected patient with an affected first-degree relative has a 7%
   risk of developing endometriosis. A polygenic, multifactorial form of inheritance
   seems most likely.*
8. Metzger DA, et al. Association of endometriosis and spontaneous abortion: effect
   of control group selection. *Fertil Steril* 1986;45:18.
   *These results suggest that the spontaneous abortion rate in untreated endo-
   metriosis may not be as high as previously reported. Well-defined control groups
   are also stressed.*
9. Mostoufizadeh M, Scully RE. Malignant tumors arising in endometriosis. *Clin
   Obstet Gynecol* 1980;23:951.
   *Rare, but true incidence is not known. Endometrioid carcinoma, clear cell car-
   cinoma, stromal sarcoma, and mixed mesodermal adenosarcoma have been
   described.*
10. Wheeler JM. Epidemiology of endometriosis-associated infertility. *J Reprod Med*
    1989;34:41.
    *Population-based epidemiologic methods using accepted criteria for causality applied
    to the endometriosis literature failed to demonstrate an association between
    endometriosis and infertility.*

Diagnosis
11. Buttram VC Jr. Evolution of the revised American Fertility Society classification
    of endometriosis. *Fertil Steril* 1985;43:347.
    *Endometriosis is classified as stage I through IV (mild, moderate, severe, or extreme)
    depending on the extent of the disease.*
12. Martin DC, et al. Laparoscopic appearances of peritoneal endometriosis. *Fertil
    Steril* 1989;51:63.
    *An increased awareness and histologic confirmation of the protean presenta-
    tion of endometriosis is associated with a significant increase in the diagnosis
    of endometriosis at laparoscopy.*

Medical Management
13. Management of endometriosis. ACOG Tech Bull No. 85, March 1985.
    It is important to emphasize that the management should be strictly individualized.
14. Barbieri RL. CA-125 in patients with endometriosis. *Fertil Steril* 1986;45:767.
    *The development of the CA-125 antigen is reviewed. Its value in following the
    course of treated endometriosis is discussed.*
15. Buttram VC Jr, Reiter RC, Ward S. Treatment of endometriosis with Danazol:
    report of a 6-year prospective study. *Fertil Steril* 1985;43:353.
    This is a summary of modern concepts and management.
16. Henzl MD, et al. Administration of nasal nafarelin as compared with oral Danazol
    for endometriosis. *N Engl J Med* 1988;318:485.
    Nafarelin is equally effective and is better tolerated than Danazol.
17. Waller KG, Shaw RW. Gonadotropin-releasing hormone analogues for the treat-
    ment of endometriosis: long-term follow-up. *Fertil Steril* 1993;59:511.
    *The women were highly likely to suffer a recurrence, particularly if their disease
    was severe at the outset.*

18. Taylor PJ, Kredenster JV. Nonsurgical management of minimal and moderate endometriosis to enhance fertility. *Int J Fertil* 1992;37:138.
    A rational clinical approach is described that is aimed at discouraging too-rapid recourse to the apparent panacea of the highly technological new reproductive approaches.
19. Malinak LR. Surgical therapy and adjunct therapy of endometriosis. *Int J Gynecol Obstet* 1993;40[Suppl]:43.
    Combined surgery and pre- or postoperative medical therapy is recommended in young non-infertile women and those with extensive or severe disease.

Surgical Management
20. Adamson GD, et al. Comparison of CO_2 laser laparoscopy with laparotomy for treatment of endometriomata. *Fertil Steril* 1992;57:965.
    This is the first controlled study using prospectively tabulated data that confirms that CO_2 laser laparoscopy is safe and effective treatment for endometriomata.
21. Meyers WC, Kelvin FM, Jones RS. Diagnosis and surgical treatment of colonic endometriosis. *Arch Surg* 1979;114:169.
    Radiographic findings are nonspecific.
22. Moore JG, et al. Urinary tract endometriosis: enigmas in diagnosis and management. *Am J Obstet Gynecol* 1979;134:162.
    If the ureter is involved, danger to renal function is great and castration is nearly always indicated, as is freeing the ureter.
23. Marcoux S, et al. Laparoscopic surgery in infertile women with minimal or mild endometriosis. *N Engl J Med* 1997;337:217.
    A randomized trial demonstrated the efficacy of surgery for infertility.

52. PEDIATRIC GYNECOLOGY

Michel E. Rivlin

Most children are seen regularly by pediatricians and are referred to gynecologists only for specific problems. In obtaining the history and performing the physical examination, great care and sensitivity must be exercised, in view of the physical and emotional immaturity of the patient. Inspection of the external genitalia is part of the neonatal and well-child examination, whereas complete gynecologic examination is reserved for the child with symptoms or signs of a genital disorder. Specially designed equipment may be necessary (e.g., a vaginoscope and virginal speculum) or adapted (e.g., nasal speculum, otoscope, or laparoscope). Sonographic evaluation is helpful in more complex situations and on occasion, examination under anesthesia may be necessary.

Newborn infants demonstrate the effects of maternal hormones, with breast budding, prominent external genitalia, and vaginal discharge. The ratio between the cervix and the corpus is 3:1, and the ovaries are abdominal organs. In early childhood (2 months to 7 years), an estrogen-poor phase, the uterus regresses and only regains the size present at birth by age 6. The breasts are undeveloped, and the diameter of the hymenal orifice is 0.5 cm. During late childhood (7 to 10 years), the onset of ovarian estrogen production results in the appearance of the breast bud, but external genital effects are not yet apparent. In the premenarche period (11 to 12 years), the hymenal orifice increases from 0.7 to 1.0 cm and the ratio of the cervix to the corpus alters from 1:1 toward the adult ratio. Puberty is the early stage of adolescence culminating in menarche. The changes and problems of puberty are discussed in Chapter 82.

Congenital anomalies of the genitalia may be related to intersex problems with sexual ambiguity in which the true gender cannot be immediately determined. These include genetic abnormalities and are discussed in the endocrinology section of this manual. A newborn with ambiguous genitalia requires immediate investigation, not only because of parental anxiety but because one of the causes, salt-losing congenital adrenal hyperplasia, may be rapidly fatal in the first week of life if the serum electrolyte levels are not closely monitored and corrected. Congenital anomalies of the genital tract in chromosomally normal females can result from agenesis or abnormalities of tissue fusion and canalization. Because the wolffian and müllerian ducts develop in close proximity, urinary tract anomalies are commonly associated, occurring in up to 20% of the cases. Persistence of the urogenital membrane results in an imperforate hymen, which may be found at birth as a mucocolpos. However, it may not be diagnosed until adolescence, when primary amenorrhea with recurrent pelvic pain leads to the discovery of a hematocolpos. A portion of the membrane should be removed for drainage.

The upper two thirds of the vagina are formed by the canalization of müllerian tissue, and the lower one third from the urogenital sinus. Varying degrees of failure of canalization may occur, including longitudinal and transverse vaginal septa and the absence of the vagina. Asymptomatic longitudinal septa require no treatment, but transverse septa usually require excision, and vaginal agenesis requires the construction of an artificial vagina, generally when sexual maturity is achieved.

Uterine anomalies range from the minor arcuate deformity (subseptate uterus) to a double uterus (didelphia) with one (unicollis) or two (bicollis) cervices. These anomalies are seldom discovered until pregnancy occurs, with the exception of a rudimentary uterine horn that does not communicate with the other uterine cavity or the vagina, resulting in a hematometra or pyometra and necessitating surgical intervention. If pregnancy occurs in such a horn, it may result in rupture with hemoperitoneum. Ideally, a horn should be removed before pregnancy occurs.

Vulvar pruritus may be due to any of several vulvar or perineal dermatologic disorders. *Lichen sclerosus,* a hypotrophic disorder usually affecting postmenopausal women, is occasionally seen in young girls. Treatment is symptomatic, and steroid creams also may be helpful. The lesion may abate or resolve during puberty. A *labial adhesion* is quite common in prepubertal children, probably related to the thin skin covering the labia becoming denuded by local irritation and scratching, resulting in adherence in the midline. No therapy is required unless it becomes symptomatic with dysuria and recurrent vulvar and vaginal irritation. Treatment consists of twice-daily local application of estrogen cream for 7 to 10 days and proper instruction with regard to perineal hygiene. Surgical separation is rarely required. Recurrence is common until puberty.

Vulvovaginitis is probably the most common gynecologic disorder in children because the estrogen-poor atrophic mucosa is susceptible to infection and because perineal hygiene is often inadequate, resulting in contamination by stool. Symptoms include a mucopurulent discharge, perineal pruritus, and dysuria. Nonspecific infections are usually polymicrobial. Specific infections include *Neisseria gonorrhoeae,* chlamydia trachomatis, and candidiasis. Inoculation may occur secondary to upper respiratory or urinary tract infections. Allergic and chemical reactions are common, and careful inquiry into the kinds of soaps and detergents the patient is exposed to may suggest the cause. Panties made of synthetic material and tight clothing may aggravate the situation; loose cotton clothing should be recommended. If the predominant symptom is pruritus, a pinworm (*Enterobius vermicularis*) infestation is likely; diagnosis is based on identifying the eggs on a sticky tape placed on the perianal area overnight. A foreign body is suspected if the discharge is bloody and malodorous. In first infections, inspection of the external genitalia with microscopic examination and culture of the discharge is sufficient. Rectal examination should be performed to evaluate the pelvic organs. In the event of recurrence or nonresponse, vaginoscopy is necessary to rule out the presence of a foreign body or tumor. Therapy is directed toward the specific cause, and proper hygienic instructions are given to the mother and child. Recurrence with foreign bodies is common, and removal may require general anesthesia.

Injuries to the genitalia during childhood are usually accidental. Most are minor, but a few require major surgical treatment. It is important to determine how the injury was sustained because the child will require protection if she is a victim of physical or sexual abuse. General anesthesia is frequently necessary in order to perform an adequate examination. Contusions and hematomas of the vulva may be relieved by ice packs and analgesics, but if they are large or increasing in size, surgical incision and control of bleeding points or packing may be necessary. Vaginal wounds generally involve the lateral walls but may involve the peritoneal cavity, necessitating laparotomy. Thus, if the hymen is torn, an intravaginal examination should be performed and the bladder and rectum checked for trauma.

Genital tumors, although rare, must be considered in girls with a chronic genital ulcer, nontraumatic genital swelling, fetid or bloody discharge, abdominal pain or enlargement, or premature sexual maturation. Almost every tumor of the adult also has been encountered in children, but about half of the genital tumors in the pediatric group are premalignant or malignant. Vulvar tumors are generally benign and include hymenal cysts of the newborn, which usually disappear within a few weeks. Condyloma acuminatum, viral warts similar to those in the adult, teratomas, and hemangiomas also occur. Most benign vaginal tumors are cystic remnants of the mesonephric duct (Gartner's duct cyst) and require surgical excision or marsupialization if they become large enough to cause symptoms. Sarcoma botryoides is the most common neoplasm of the lower genital tract in girls younger than 16 years of age. The tumor usually involves the vagina, but the cervix also may be affected. In this condition, the vaginal mucosa bulges into a series of polypoid growths. Diagnosis is made on the basis of biopsy findings that usually indicate the presence of rhabdomyoblasts. Prognosis has improved with the advent of combination chemotherapy together with conservative surgical treatment, with or without irradiation. Clear cell adenocarcinoma of müllerian origin, often associated with antenatal exposure to synthetic estrogens, is now primarily seen in postmenarcheal females.

Ovarian tumors are the most frequent genital neoplasm encountered in children and adolescents. Non-neoplastic ovarian cysts occasionally occur in children or infants and are generally follicular or corpus luteal in origin. Unless acute complications occur, conservative management is preferable. The incidence of malignant degeneration of neoplasms is higher in children than in adolescents or adults, and ovarian neoplasms in children have a malignancy rate of 35% overall. The tumors in about 65% are of germ cell origin (e.g., teratoma, dysgerminoma, endodermal sinus tumor, gonadoblastoma, and choriocarcinoma); 12% are derived from specialized stroma (e.g., granulosa-theca cells or Sertoli-Leydig cells). The remaining tumors are chiefly epithelial in origin, as in the adult. The most common symptoms are abdominal pain and an abdominal mass. Stromal tumors and germ cell tumors may cause isosexual precocious puberty. At least a fourth of all childhood ovarian tumors are diagnosed only at the time of exploratory laparotomy. Conservative surgical treatment (unilateral adnexectomy) is justified for most premenarcheal patients with stage I cancer, once localization to the ovary has been established by surgical staging. If extension has occurred, a more radical operation (removal of the uterus with adnexa) is indicated. Adjunctive chemotherapy, with or without radiotherapy, also may be indicated, especially in the event of advanced disease or for those lesions with greater malignant potential, such as the papillary serous epithelial tumor.

General
1. Hairston L. Physical examination of the prepubertal girl. *Clin Obstet Gynecol* 1997;40:127.
   External genitalia are most easily examined with the child in a frog-legged position. Allowing the mother to hold the child on her lap also may be helpful.
2. Arbel-DeRowe Y. The contribution of pelvic ultrasonography to the diagnostic process in pediatric and adolescent gynecology. *J Pediatr Adolesc Gynecol* 1997;10:3.
   Sonography may obviate the need for an unpleasant and uninformative examination or the need for general anesthesia.
3. Bond GR. Unintentional perineal injury in prepubescent girls: a multicenter, prospective report of 56 girls. *Pediatrics* 1995;95:628.
   Hymenal injuries are rarely the result of unintentional injury—the presence of a hymenal injury should suggest sexual abuse.

Vulvovaginitis
4. Dodds ML. Vulvar disorders of the infant and young child. *Clin Obstet Gynecol* 1997;40:141.
   Topics explored include diaper rash, labial adhesions, vitiligo, dermatitis, lichen sclerosis, lichen simplex, and Behçet syndrome.
5. Koumantakis EE. Vulvovaginitis during childhood and adolescence. *J Pediatr Adolesc Gynecol* 1997;10:39.
   Candida (23%), beta-hemolytic streptococci group B (15%), and enterococci (10%) were the most frequent pathogens involved in this study of 1,778 cases.
6. Pokorny SF. Prepubertal vulvovaginopathies. *Obstet Gynecol Clin North Am* 1992;19:39.
   Most (95%–98%) prepubertal gynecologic problems involve the vulva or the vagina. These consist of bleeding problems, which are the most serious, abnormal appearance, which is the most worrisome, and pruritus / discharge, which is the most annoying.
7. Paradise JE, Willis ED. Probability of vaginal foreign body in girls with genital complaints. *Am J Dis Child* 1985;139:472.
   Vaginal bleeding is the most reliable clue to a vaginal foreign object in premenarcheal girls.
8. Berkowitz CD, Elvik SL, Logan MK. Labial fusion in prepubescent girls: a marker for sexual abuse? *Am J Obstet Gynecol* 1987;156:16.
   This article considers 10 cases of labial fusion in 500 girls evaluated for sexual abuse. The patient's history or physical findings, or both, were consistent with abuse in six of the 10. It is suggested that the fusion may have resulted from trauma, particularly vulvar coitus.
9. Trotman MDW, Brewster EM. Prolapse of the urethral mucosa in prepubertal West Indian girls. *Br J Urol* 1993;72:503.
   Surgical treatment is seldom necessary because most patients respond to a short course of locally applied estrogen cream.

Congenital Anomalies of the Genital Tract
10. The American Fertility Society classification of mullerian anomalies. *Fertil Steril* 1988;49:944.
    The American Fertility Society classification is discussed: class I, hypoplasia / agenesis; class II, unicornuate; class III, didelphus; class IV, bicornuate; class V, septate; class VI, arcuate; class VII, diethylstilbestrol-related.
11. Doyle MB. Magnetic resonance imaging in mullerian fusion defects. *J Reprod Med* 1992;37:33.
    Sonography, computed tomography, and magnetic resonance imaging have largely replaced purely diagnostic surgery.
12. Lindenman E, Shepard MK, Pescovitz OH. Mullerian agenesis: an update. *Obstet Gynecol* 1997;90:307.
    These patients have normal ovaries and XX chromosomes, but an absent or rudimentary uterus, tubes, and the upper two thirds of the vagina.
13. Candiani GB, Fedele L, Candiani M. Double uterus, blind hemivagina, and ipsilateral renal agenesis: 36 cases and long-term follow-up. *Obstet Gynecol* 1997; 90:26.
    Endometriosis is a common associated finding when congenital anomalies obstruct normal menstruation.

Tumors
14. Parker Jones K. Gynecologic issues in pediatric oncology. *Clin Obstet Gynecol* 1997;40:200.
    Potential ovarian failure from chemotherapy and radiation treatment of childhood cancers.
15. Farghaly SA. Gynecologic cancer in the young female: clinical presentation and management. *Adolesc Pediatr Gynecol* 1992;5:163.
    Unfortunately, the rarity of these tumors and the nonspecificity of their symptomatology result in delays in diagnosis past the point of potential cure.

16. Muram D, et al. Ovarian cancer in children and adolescents. *Adolesc Pediatr Gynecol* 1992;5:21.

Ovarian tumors are the most common genital neoplasm in children and adolescents, accounting for 1% of all cancers in this age group.

17. Millar DM, et al. Prepubertal ovarian cyst formation: 5 years experience. *Obstet Gynecol* 1993;81:434.

Cysts larger than 5 cm are at risk for torsion; ultrasound-guided aspiration has been suggested for the eradication of these larger cysts.

18. Shulman LP, et al. Marker chromosomes in gonadal dysgenesis: avoiding unnecessary surgery. *Adolesc Pediatr Gynecol* 1992;5:39.

Gonadoblastoma, dysgerminoma, and other germ cell malignancies occur in 15% to 30% of females possessing Y chromosomal material in their karyotype. Accurate identification is essential because early bilateral gonadectomy is recommended.

19. Hicks ML, Piver MS. Conservative surgery plus adjuvant therapy for vulvovaginal rhabdomyosarcoma, diethylstilbestrol clear cell adenocarcinoma of the vagina, and unilateral germ cell tumors of the ovary. *Obstet Gynecol Clin North Am* 1992;19:219.

Early stage disease (I or II) for these three groups of childhood cancers may be treated with high cure rates and retention of childbearing capacity.

20. Waggoner SE, et al. Influence of in utero diethylstilbestrol exposure on the prognosis and biologic behavior of vaginal clear-cell adenocarcinoma. *Gynecol Oncol* 1994;55:238.

Prognosis was worse in cases not associated with diethylstilbestrol exposure.

53. LAPAROSCOPY AND HYSTEROSCOPY

Michel E. Rivlin

Inspection of the internal pelvic organs with an illuminated telescope through a small incision in the gas-distended abdominal cavity is termed *laparoscopy* (less commonly, *celioscopy* or *peritoneoscopy*). The major diagnostic application of the procedure is in the evaluation of female infertility, with particular regard to tubal patency and ovarian evidence of ovulation. The other major diagnostic application lies in the elucidation of the cause of pelvic pain. The presence of endometriosis, pelvic inflammatory disease, or ectopic pregnancy explains the symptoms; the absence of organic pathology may provide reassurance to both the patient and physician. Diagnostic laparoscopy also may be helpful in the staging and follow-up of patients with pelvic cancer.

The most common indication for performing therapeutic laparoscopy is tubal sterilization, with the fallopian tubes either fulgurated with electrocautery or closed by clips or bands. Many other surgical procedures have been performed with the laparoscope, including the removal of intraabdominal foreign bodies (particularly perforated intrauterine devices [IUDs]), ovarian biopsy in patients with endocrine disorders such as suspected ovarian failure, or the fulguration of endometriotic implants. Skilled laparoscopists can aspirate ovarian cysts, capture intact ova for in vitro fertilization, drain pelvic abscesses, remove ectopic pregnancies, ventrosuspend the uterus, lyse tubal adhesions, and perform fimbriolysis and salpingostomy. In recent years, advances in instrumentation have greatly increased the applications of this minimally invasive surgical approach, allowing the performance of myomectomy, appendectomy, adnexectomy, bladder suspension, lymphadenectomy, presacral neurectomy, and, most significantly, hysterectomy. The adaptation of the carbon dioxide laser to the operating laparoscope has introduced a new format for the performance of a variety of operative procedures, such as the fulguration of endometrial implants and the dissolution of pelvic adhesions. The distinction between diagnostic and therapeutic laparoscopy is no longer clear-cut because it has become common practice to deal with abnormalities found at laparoscopy at the time of diagnosis, as many such problems can be managed through the laparoscope.

Laparoscopy is contraindicated in patients with severe cardiorespiratory disease, diffuse peritonitis, or ileus. The presence of hiatal herniation or an ostomy is also a contraindication. The procedure is relatively contraindicated, dependent to a large degree on the laparoscopist's skill or experience, in obese patients and in those with abdominal scars from previous operations.

Peritoneoscopy may be regarded as a minor surgical but a major anesthetic procedure. This is because general anesthesia with endotracheal intubation and muscle relaxation is the usual anesthesia used. Regional or local anesthesia is also satisfactory, however, particularly when the operation is performed on an outpatient basis.

Celioscopy is performed with the patient supine, her legs supported by stirrups angled 15 degrees downward, and her buttocks protruding over the edge of the table. This position is essential because manipulative instruments are introduced through the uterine cervix to enhance visualization by moving the pelvic organs during the procedure. Furthermore, these instruments are canalized so that colored dyes (indigo carmine or methylene blue) may be injected for the assessment of tubal patency (chromopertubation).

The first step in the procedure is creating the pneumoperitoneum. The gas used is either carbon dioxide or nitrous oxide and it is introduced through a spring-loaded needle (Veress or Palmer), generally inserted subumbilically. Gas is insufflated at 1 L/minute and the gas pressure should not exceed 20 mm Hg. The usual amount of gas required varies from 2 to 5 L. When liver dullness in response to percussion is lost, the patient is placed in the Trendelenburg position and the needle is withdrawn.

Next, the telescope is introduced. To do this, a 1-cm subumbilical incision is made through the skin and fascia. A trocar and valve sleeve are introduced at an angle of 45 degrees toward the pelvis. The trocar is removed, and the telescope is passed through the sheath. (Some surgeons prefer to introduce the trocar and valve sleeve directly and before the creation of the pneumoperitoneum.) The gas insufflator is attached on automatic flow to maintain the pneumoperitoneum. The fiberoptic light source is attached to the telescope, and viewing commences. Telescope diameters vary from 4 to 10 mm, and their objectives are usually angled 180 degrees forward. If a double-channeled operating laparoscope is used, this may obviate the need for placement of ancillary instruments through a further incision.

Additional instruments, if required, are passed through further incisions, generally placed in the iliac fossae through a smaller trocar and cannula. These incisions are made under direct laparoscopic vision. A wide variety of ancillary instruments are available. These include tubal clip or band applicators; ovarian biopsy forceps; apparatuses for suction or aspiration; electrocautery or laser instruments capable of coagulation, vaporization, or cutting; forceps; graduated probes; scissors; loops; and needles for the placement of intraabdominal sutures. In addition, there are clip applicators such that individual titanium clips can be applied or two lines of staples may be placed simultaneously with an inbuilt knife to cut the tissue between the staples.

The mortality rate associated with diagnostic laparoscopy is 11 per 100,000, and the incidence of laparotomy performed for intraabdominal complications is 8.5 per 1000. Complications may occur owing to the anesthesia, improper gas insufflation, and perforation of viscera or vessels, as well as the operative procedure itself, including hemorrhage or burns.

Anesthetic complications are related to increases in intraabdominal pressure over 20 mm Hg, particularly when carbon dioxide is the insufflating gas. Reduced pulmonary excursion and carbon dioxide absorption result in hypercapnia, causing cardiac arrhythmias and cardiac arrest (one in 5,000 procedures). Careful technique that includes close cardiac and abdominal pressure monitoring, as well as active ventilation, minimizes the incidence of this problem. The alternative use of nitrous oxide, which does not cause hypercapnia and is nonirritant, is not entirely without problems because it is an ignitable gas and is only slowly absorbed. This must be kept in mind, particularly when electrocautery is used.

Almost every conceivable viscus or vessel has been injured by the Veress or other cannulas. Most of these injuries are minor and require no special attention other than close observation. Of course, immediate laparotomy is necessary to manage major bleeding or visceral injury.

When operative procedures are performed, bleeding is the most common complication encountered. Hemostasis can generally be achieved by electrocoagulation, although laparotomy may be required. The more serious complications are due to electrical burns. These result from accidentally touching adjacent tissues or from sparking of the current to these structures. Bowel burns are commonly involved and, if recognized and superficial, may be treated conservatively because most resolve when managed in this way. In those cases in which unrecognized bowel burns become progressive, a clinical picture similar to that of pelvic inflammatory disease or appendicitis develops. Laparotomy with bowel resection, together with antibiotic therapy, is then necessary. The hazards of electrical burns are lessened by the use of bipolar rather than unipolar electrodes, whereas regular inspection and testing of equipment with particular attention to insulation is mandatory. Many surgeons prevent these problems by using clips or bands rather than electrosurgical techniques when performing tubal sterilization.

The introduction of minimally invasive surgical techniques into the practice of operative gynecology has had a revolutionary impact, such that, within a few years, the discipline may become almost exclusively endoscopic. The downside of the situation is that much expensive equipment is required and operating times may be prolonged ("foreveroscopy"). Extensive retraining and study are also required so that gynecologic endoscopic surgery, with its advantages of a shortened hospital stay and postoperative convalescent time, can be effective, safe, and free of unnecessary complications.

Hysteroscopy is the direct visualization of the endometrial cavity using an endoscope. It may be performed under local or general anesthesia. Women with recurrent abnormal bleeding, repetitive abortion, uterine synechiae, abnormal hysterosalpingograms, and infertility are all candidates for diagnostic hysteroscopy. Operative procedures that can be performed under hysteroscopic guidance with video monitoring include removal of IUDs, resection of submucous myomas, lysis of synechiae, incision of uterine septa, removal of endometrial polyps, electrosurgical or laser ablation of the endometrium, falloposcopy and balloon tuboplasty for obstructed fallopian tubes, and the placement of silicone plugs into the tubes for sterilization. The cavity of the uterus must be distended for the procedure, and the mediums used for this purpose include 32% dextran, 5% dextrose and water, 1.5% glycine, and carbon dioxide gas. Dextran is preferred by many clinicians for its good optic qualities and immiscibility with blood. However, it is antigenic, which may lead to anaphylaxis; instruments also must be cleaned shortly after the procedure because it is sticky. The flow of carbon dioxide must be limited to less than 100 ml/minute, and the volume of 5% dextrose and water or 1.5% glycine must be carefully monitored to prevent fluid overload. A variant instrument, the contact hysteroscope, does not require a distending medium. The interpretation of findings is similar to that for colposcopy, relying on the color, contour, and vascular pattern. A microhysteroscope may be used to examine the endocervical canal after vital staining.

Contraindications to hysteroscopy include acute pelvic infection and pregnancy. Active bleeding and uterine cancer are relative contraindications. Complications occur in fewer than 2% of the procedures and include uterine perforation, pelvic infection, and hemorrhage.

Complications due to the distending media include the potential for gas embolism with carbon dioxide. Fluid media may cause dilutional hyponatremia with acute pulmonary edema if fluid overload occurs.

Light amplification by the stimulated emission of radiation (*laser*) is a technique that is widely used in medicine. It involves the use of energized light to vaporize tissue. Lasers generate an intense narrow beam of light in waves that must all be of one wavelength (monochromatic), exactly in phase (coherent), and parallel (collimated), so that the peaks and valleys of the waves line up and amplify each other until they are absorbed by a target. In an atomic laser, the lasing medium emits only a single, predominant wavelength of light when its atoms have been excited and then allowed to return to the resting state. This wavelength is determined by the medium, which may be solid, liquid, or gas. Three types of lasers are commonly used in gynecology: the argon laser, the neodymium: yttrium-aluminum-garnet (Nd:YAG) laser, and the carbon dioxide laser. Each of these lasers is used for specific purposes, as dictated by its wavelength and tissue-absorption qualities. The carbon dioxide laser has been evaluated most extensively for pelvic procedures and may be handheld or used through an endoscope. It destroys tissue by instantaneously boiling intracellular water. Adjusting the spot size helps control the power density, which ranges from warming to incisional vaporization. The depth of laser action is precisely controlled by the power density, exposure time, and the use of energy-absorbing "backstop" probes or fluids. Nd:YAG lasers have been favored for use in hysteroscopy procedures because they can penetrate deep into tissue, producing an excellent coagulative effect. Protective goggles must be worn while this laser is in operation. As with electrocautery, great care must be taken to prevent injury to vessels and viscera.

Reviews
1. Nezhat C, Nezhat F, Nezhat C. Operative laparoscopy (minimally invasive surgery); state of the art. *J Gynecol Surg* 1992;8:111.

   The average postoperative stay is 0.5 to 2 days for operative laparoscopy versus 5 to 5.7 days for laparotomy. Women can return to full activity in 7 to 10 days.

2. Garry R. Laparoscopic alternatives to laparotomy: a new approach to gynaecological surgery. *Br J Obstet Gynaecol* 1992;99:629.

   Incorporating a laparoscopy-mounted videocamera, a videorecorder, and a video monitor allows the surgeon to operate in an upright position directly from the video monitor. Magnification of the pelvic organs by the monitor simplifies the procedure.

Technique
3. Philipsen T, Hansen BB. Comparative study of hysterosalpingography and laparoscopy in infertile patients. *Acta Obstet Gynecol Scand* 1981;60:149.

   For a conclusive evaluation of the tubal factor, hysterosalpingography should be replaced by laparoscopy, according to the findings in this series of 168 patients investigated by both techniques.

4. Penfield AJ. How to prevent complications of open laparoscopy. *J Reprod Med* 1985;30:660.

   For the procedure of open laparoscopy, a special cannula is inserted through a small laparotomy incision; sutures ensure a gas-tight seal. This is an especially useful approach in the obese or when adhesions are suspected.

Anesthesia
5. Tan PL, Lee TL, Tweed WA. Carbon dioxide absorption and gas exchange during pelvic laparoscopy. *Can J Anaesth* 1992;39:677.

   A sharp increase in the arterial carbon dioxide tension and a decrease in pH was noted with carbon dioxide, but there were no changes with nitrous oxide.

6. Versichelen L, et al. Physiopathologic changes during anesthesia administration for gynecologic laparoscopy. *J Reprod Med* 1984;29:697.

   Large changes in total lung compliance and venous pressures yielded only marginal general effects, probably because of volume-controlled mechanical respiration and the limitation of insufflation pressures.

7. Sniadach MS, Alberts MS. A comparison of the prophylactic antiemetic effect of ondansetron and droperidol on patients undergoing gynecologic laparoscopy. *Anesth Analg* 1997;85:797.

   Equivalent effectiveness and significant cost savings may be obtained by using droperidol prophylactically for laparoscopic surgery.

Applications
8. Lipscomb GH, Ling FW. Development of a program teaching laparoscopic sterilization using local anesthesia. *Obstet Gynecol* 1995;86:609.

Electrical methods are preferable in women with adhesions and tubal pathology. Clips (Hulka and Filshie) and rings (Yoon) are preferable in women who may later request sterilization reversal.

 9. Daniell JF, Lalonde CJ. Advanced laparoscopic procedures for pelvic pain and dysmenorrhea. *Baillieres Clin Obstet Gynaecol* 1995;9:795.
    Laparoscopy is necessary to establish a diagnosis in women with chronic pelvic pain. Pain may be relieved by laparoscopic procedures including adhesiolysis, uterine suspension, uterosacral transection, and presacral neurectomy.
10. Alexander JM, et al. Treatment of the small unruptured ectopic pregnancy: a cost analysis of methotrexate versus laparoscopy. *Obstet Gynecol* 1996;88:123.
    In a surgically stable patient, especially with an unruptured accessible tube, both conservative and radical procedures are possible using electrocautery, endocoagulation, laser, or intraabdominal sutures.
11. Eschenbach DA, et al. Acute pelvic inflammatory disease: associations of clinical and laboratory findings with laparoscopic findings. *Obstet Gynecol* 1997;89:184.
    Laparoscopy provides accurate diagnosis, possible identification of bacteria, and the potential for adjunctive surgical intervention.
12. Dubrisson JB, et al. Laparoscopic myomectomy and myolysis. *Curr Opin Obstet Gynecol* 1997;9:233.
    Laparoscopy is recommended for myomas under 8 cm in diameter and under 3 in number.
13. Parker WH. The case for laparoscopic management of the adnexal mass. *Clin Obstet Gynecol* 1995;38:362.
    If cancer is unexpectedly found, the surgeon should be prepared to proceed with staging laparotomy.
14. Redwine DB, Sharpe DR. Laparoscopic surgery for intestinal and urinary endometriosis. *Baillieres Clin Obstet Gynaecol* 1995;9:775.
    Laparoscopic surgery is suitable for many, but not all, patients with endometriosis.
15. Tulandi T. Reconstructive tubal surgery by laparoscopy. *Obstet Gynecol Surv* 1987;42:193.
    Laparoscopic salpingostomy, fimbrioplasty, and adhesiolysis may yield results equivalent to those of surgical procedures performed through a laparotomy. However, for tubal anastomosis, the superior results of microsurgical procedures are unlikely to be accomplished by laparoscopic techniques.
16. Lyons TL. Minimally invasive treatment of urinary stress incontinence and laparoscopically directed repair of pelvic floor defects. *Clin Obstet Gynecol* 1995;38:380.
    Promising early experience with laparoscopic pelvic reconstruction and treatment of urinary incontinence are described.
17. Munro MG, Deprest J. Laparoscopic hysterectomy: does it work? A bicontinental review of the literature and clinical commentary. *Clin Obstet Gynecol* 1995;38:401.
    Ambulatory laparoscopic supracervical hysterectomy may be the standard operation in the future.

Complications
18. Harkki-Siren P, Kurki T. A nationwide analysis of laparoscopic complications. *Obstet Gynecol* 1997;89:108.
    Diagnostic and sterilization laparoscopies appear to be safe, but operative laparoscopies are associated with serious complications.
19. Hulka JF, et al. Laparoscopic-assisted vaginal hysterectomy: American Association of Gynecologic Laparoscopists 1995 membership survey. *J Am Assoc Gynecol Laparosc* 1997;4:167.
    Complication rates appeared to be in the same range as those reported for vaginal hysterectomy and total abdominal hysterectomy. Inferior epigastric injury was the most common complication.
20. Saidi MH, et al. Diagnosis and management of serious urinary complications after major operative laparoscopy. *Obstet Gynecol* 1996;87:272.
    Serious urinary complications occurred in 1% to 6% of major operative laparoscopy cases.

21. Levy BS, Soderstrom RM, Dail DH. Bowel injuries during laparoscopy. Gross anatomy and histology. *J Reprod Med* 1985;30:168.
    Bowel injuries ascribed to electrical damage actually may have resulted from trauma. The authors suggest that unipolar techniques with appropriate low-voltage generators should be reconsidered in view of the increased failure rate associated with bipolar methods.

Hysteroscopy

22. Istre O. Fluid balance during hysteroscopic surgery. *Curr Opin Obstet Gynecol* 1997;9:219.
    Careful perioperative monitoring of the deficit of collected irrigating medium is mandatory to prevent dilutional hyponatremia. Monitoring the serum sodium and osmolality also may be helpful.
23. Perino A, et al. Role of leuprolide acetate depot in hysteroscopic surgery: a controlled study. *Fertil Steril* 1993;59:507.
    Preoperative agonist therapy led to a significant reduction in operating time, blood loss, and the amount of distention medium required.
24. Perrot N, et al. Sonohysterography: a new study method of the uterine cavity: evaluation of 84 cases and comparison to hysteroscopy. *Contracept Fertil Sex* 1997;25:325.
    Pelvic ultrasonography after saline distension of the uterine cavity is a useful noninvasive diagnostic aid for lesions projecting into the uterine cavity such as fibroids or polyps.
25. Hamou J, et al. Can microcolpohysteroscopy be used to screen cervical lesions? *Contracept Fertil Sex* 1997;25:358.
    There are three types of hysteroscopes: rigid panoramic, rigid contact, and flexible panoramic.
26. Torrejon R, et al. The value of hysteroscopic exploration for abnormal uterine bleeding. *J Am Assoc Gynecol Laparosc* 1997;4:453.
    Dilatation and curettage and hysteroscopy are similar in terms of specificity, but hysteroscopy is significantly more sensitive (98% versus 65%). In particular, dilatation and curettage may miss fibroids and polyps.
27. Balmaceda JP, Ciuffardi I. Hysteroscopy and assisted reproductive technology. *Obstet Gynecol Clin North Am* 1995;22:507.
    The infertility investigation includes hysterosalpingogram as a vital screening procedure; when an intrauterine abnormality is detected, hysteroscopic identification of the lesion is necessary.
28. Bacsko G. Uterine surgery by operative hysteroscopy. *Eur J Obstet Gynecol Reprod Biol* 1997;71:219.
    Bleeding, infection, and uterine perforation were attributed to the procedure. Allergic reactions and a symptom complex consisting of acute noncardiogenic pulmonary edema and disseminated intravascular coagulation, related to the distending medium, are the major, albeit rare, complications.
29. Goldrath MH. Hysteroscopic endometrial ablation. *Obstet Gynecol Clin North Am* 1995;22:559.
    The iatrogenic Asherman syndrome may obviate the need for hysterectomy in many women with uterine bleeding problems. This is particularly valuable in patients for whom a major surgical procedure is contraindicated. The most common technique is the use of a resectoscope with either a cutting loop or rollerball electrode.
30. March CM. Intrauterine adhesions. *Obstet Gynecol Clin North Am* 1995;22:491.
    An operative hysteroscopy for the treatment of Asherman syndrome is often followed by the placement of an IUD and the institution of cyclic hormone therapy to prevent the reformation of adhesions and to encourage endometrial regeneration. However, the necessity for this adjunctive therapy has not been demonstrated.
31. Jacobsen LJ, DeCherney A. Results of conventional and hysteroscopic surgery. *Hum Reprod* 1997;12:1376.
    Hysteroscopic metroplasty with either scissors, resectoscope, or laser is superior to the Strassman, Jones, and Tompkins procedures for most septate uteri, including the avoidance of pelvic adhesions and the need for cesarean section.

54. HYSTERECTOMY

Michel E. Rivlin

The uterus may be removed through an incision in the abdominal wall. A total abdominal hysterectomy is the removal of both the corpus and cervix. The cervix may be left in situ; this is a subtotal hysterectomy. An alternative method, vaginal hysterectomy, consists of removal of the uterus through the vagina. At the time of hysterectomy, one or both tubes or ovaries also may be removed, a procedure termed a *unilateral* or *bilateral salpingo-oophorectomy.*

Hysterectomy is the second most common surgical procedure performed in the United States. Annually, more than 600,000 women undergo the procedure. Recent advances in operative techniques, the development of alternative therapies, the reevaluation of indications, and the reassessment of health-care expenditures and cost-benefit analyses are likely to lead to changes in the thinking regarding the procedure. Hysterectomy in the treatment of cancer is discussed in relevant chapters in Section XVI, Gynecologic Oncology.

Leiomyomas, dysfunctional uterine bleeding, and pelvic relaxation account for more than half of the procedures performed. Other indications include adnexal diseases, such as endometriosis or pelvic inflammatory disease (PID), and, in this event, the uterus is removed together with the abnormal adnexa. Obstetric emergencies may necessitate the procedure, although in the absence of preexisting gynecologic abnormalities, hysterectomy during pregnancy should be discouraged because of the increased risk of hemorrhage and urinary tract injury. Hysterectomy for sterilization should generally be performed only when preexisting gynecologic disease or other circumstances warrant the increased risk over alternative procedures. Quality-of-life considerations, including menstrual problems, contraceptive difficulties, and cancer fears, may play important roles in a woman's decision to undergo the operation.

A preoperative workup to rule out the existence of preinvasive or invasive cancer is necessary, including colposcopy, curettage, or cone biopsy, if indicated by the results of Papanicolaou (Pap) smears or endometrial biopsy. In nonurgent cases, anemia and local infections should be treated preoperatively. Many surgeons require that an intravenous pyelogram and barium enema be obtained before the operation. Adequate counseling, especially regarding menstrual, reproductive, and sexual function, is essential because the procedure carries profound physical and psychological implications.

The vaginal approach is used in 30% to 35% of hysterectomies. The usual indication for this is pelvic relaxation, although the method is suitable for any hysterectomy in skilled hands, provided no contraindications exist. These contraindications include the presence of intraabdominal or pelvic abnormalities that necessitate abdominal exploration, a uterus too large to remove vaginally, or a narrow subpubic angle that would limit access. The vaginal route is associated with a shorter and more comfortable recovery but a higher incidence of febrile morbidity than the abdominal procedure.

Abdominal hysterectomy is performed through a transverse or vertical abdominal incision. No clear consensus exists regarding the age at which normal ovaries should be removed as prophylaxis against cancer. In view of the adverse effects of castration in terms of menopausal symptoms, osteoporosis, and vascular disease, many gynecologists remove these organs only in perimenopausal or postmenopausal patients. The total procedure is currently preferred because the retained cervical stump may cause problems later, including cancer (0.3%). Subtotal procedures are favored by a few who feel that Pap smears limit the risk of cancer and the operation is faster, easier, and safer. The safety of total hysterectomy is increased by the use of an intrafascial technique, although this is not suitable for patients with cervical precancer; in these women, an extrafascial approach is indicated.

In performing both vaginal and abdominal hysterectomy, it is important to support the vaginal vault (cuff) with the transverse cervical and uterosacral ligaments as prophylaxis against vault prolapse, an uncommon late complication of hysterectomy. Most gynecologists close the cuff routinely, although many leave it open to provide pelvic drainage if infection is present.

In recent years, a variety of hysterectomy procedures involving laparoscopy have been introduced. These range from diagnostic laparoscopy before vaginal hysterectomy, through laparoscopy-assisted vaginal hysterectomy, in which variable portions of the procedure are begun through the laparoscope with completion of the operation per vaginam, all the way to complete laparoscopic hysterectomy. Advantages include faster postoperative recovery and avoidance of large abdominal incisions. Disadvantages include longer operating times and higher costs. As more surgeons learn the techniques, laparoscopic methods are gaining in popularity.

Occasionally, postoperative bleeding may occur early or late and may be manifested by frank bleeding or a pelvic hematoma. Vaginal or abdominal resuturing is necessary in most instances, although late hemorrhage from the cuff usually responds to vaginal packing. Postoperative infections are not uncommon and may affect the urinary tract, abdominal or vaginal incisions, adnexa, or lungs. In severe cases, pelvic abscess, peritonitis, wound dehiscence, septicemia, and septic pelvic thrombophlebitis can occur. Febrile morbidity is most common in premenopausal patients undergoing vaginal hysterectomy. The administration of prophylactic antibiotics in high-risk patients has markedly lessened the incidence of all these infectious complications, although their routine use remains controversial. Thromboembolism is a major source of postoperative mortality. The use of low-dose prophylactic heparin may lessen the incidence, especially in patients at high risk, such as the markedly overweight.

Injuries to the bladder, ureters, or bowel are uncommon, but if not recognized and repaired at the time of operation, they may lead to serious infections and the formation of urinary or fecal fistulas. Complications common to major abdominal or pelvic procedures, such as anesthetic and blood transfusion problems, drug reaction, and ileus or intestinal obstruction, also may occur.

The emotional and psychosexual sequelae of hysterectomy are of great significance. The incidence of depression after the procedure has been estimated to be two to three times that after other operations. Hormone replacement in premenopausal patients undergoing surgical castration and adequate preoperative and postoperative counseling and support are both important elements of care.

From this review of the complications, although the more serious are uncommon, it is clear that the added risks do not warrant hysterectomy purely for sterilization or as cancer prophylaxis. Nevertheless, it remains one of the safest major procedures, with a death-to-case ratio of 1:1,000 to 2:1,000. The average patient may expect to be discharged from 3 to 5 days after the operation, and few procedures improve the quality of life more than an indicated hysterectomy in a well-informed patient.

Incidence
1. Lepine LA, et al. Hysterectomy surveillance United States, 1980–1993. *MMWR CDC Surveill Summ* 1997;46:1.
   Regional differences are highest in the South, lowest in the Northeast. The cost of the 600,000 annual procedures is in excess of $5 billion.
2. Kramer MG, Reiter RC. Hysterectomy: indications, alternatives, and predictors. *Am Fam Physician* 1997;55:827.
   One in three American women has the procedure by age 60, a higher percentage than in any other country.
3. Marks NF, Shinberg DS. Socioeconomic differences in hysterectomy: the Wisconsin Longitudinal Study. *Am J Public Health* 1997;87:1507.
   The higher the educational status, the lower the hysterectomy rate, and vice versa.
4. Hillis SD, et al. Tubal sterilization and long-term risk of hysterectomy: findings from the United States collaborative review of sterilization: The U.S. Collaborative Review of Sterilization Working Group. *Obstet Gynecol* 1997; 89:609.
   The cumulative probability of undergoing hysterectomy 14 years after sterilization was 17%. The incidence was higher in women with previous gynecologic disorders.

Management
5. Kovac SR. Which route for hysterectomy? Evidence-based outcomes guide selection. *Postgrad Med* 1997;102:153.
   The ratio of abdominal to vaginal operations is 3:1, probably reflecting surgeons' experience. The indications and contraindications require critical evidence-based reevaluation.
6. Munro MG, Parker WH. A classification system for laparoscopic hysterectomy. *Obstet Gynecol* 1993;82:624.
   The term laparoscopic hysterectomy has been applied to a variety of procedures, ranging from adhesiolysis only to total hysterectomy under endoscopic direction. This paper recommends a classification system.
7. Munro MG. Supracervical hysterectomy: a time for reappraisal. *Obstet Gynecol* 1997;89:133.
   Some have argued that supracervical hysterectomy better preserves bladder and sexual function and may be associated with reduced surgical and postoperative morbidity.
8. Davies A, Magos AL. Indications and alternatives to hysterectomy. *Baillieres Clin Obstet Gynaecol* 1997;11:61.
   The only valid alternatives to hysterectomy, if medical therapy fails, are endometrial ablation and myomectomy.
9. Crosignani PG, et al. Endometrial resection versus vaginal hysterectomy for menorrhagia: long-term clinical and quality-of-life outcomes. *Am J Obstet Gynecol* 1997;177:95.
   Endometrial ablation may be considered as an alternative to hysterectomy for abnormal uterine bleeding in selected patients.
10. Stevermer JJ, Chambliss ML. Pap smear of the vaginal cuff. *J Fam Pract* 1997; 44:250.
    Although it is probably not necessary as a routine, follow-up is nevertheless important because vaginal cancer may follow hysterectomy for either dysplasia or for an unrelated disease.
11. Williams TJ, Johnson TR, Pratt JH. Time interval between cervical conization and hysterectomy. *Am J Obstet Gynecol* 1970;107:790.
    Unless hysterectomy is done within 48 hours of conization, 6 weeks should elapse before proceeding; otherwise, an increase in morbidity is likely.
12. Lu PY, et al. Elective versus emergency cesarean hysterectomy on a teaching service 1981 to 1991. *South Med J* 1997;90:50.
    The indications for emergency obstetric hysterectomy generally include uterine rupture, placental disorders, and extension of the incision during cesarean section.

The Ovaries
13. Hefni MA, Davies AE. Vaginal endoscopic oophorectomy with vaginal hysterectomy: a simple minimal access surgery technique. *Br J Obstet Gynaecol* 1997; 104:621.
    Technical advances have resulted in a threefold increase in the removal of ovaries with vaginal hysterectomy.
14. Parazzini F, et al. Hysterectomy, oophorectomy in premenopause, and risk of breast cancer. *Obstet Gynecol* 1997;90:453.
    Risk is lower and the protection increases with time from surgery.
15. Kritz-Silverstein D, Barrett-Cooper E, Wingard DL. Hysterectomy, oophorectomy, and heart disease risk factors in older women. *Am J Public Health* 1997;87:676.
    Women who had ovaries removed prior to menopause and who did not receive estrogen have double the risk of coronary heart disease.
16. Dean S. Hysterectomy and bone mineral density. *Br J Hosp Med* 1997;57:207.
    Hysterectomy adversely affects the ovaries, leading to premature ovarian failure in 34% of cases. The effect of premenopausal hysterectomy on osteoporosis has not been established.
17. Zalel Y, et al. Is it necessary to perform a prophylactic oophorectomy during hysterectomy? *Eur J Obstet Gynecol Reprod Biol* 1997;73:67.

Prophylactic removal of healthy ovaries for cancer prophylaxis is not universally accepted, even in older women.

18. Parazzini F, et al. Hysterectomy, oophorectomy, and subsequent ovarian cancer risk. *Obstet Gynecol* 1993;81:363.

Hysterectomy halves the risk of ovarian cancer, possibly because it permits the opportunity to examine the ovaries or because it leads to altered ovarian blood flow.

19. Bukovsky L, et al. Ovarian residual syndrome. *Surg Gynecol Obstet* 1988;167:132.

In 1% to 3% of cases in which one or both ovaries are retained at the time of hysterectomy, subsequent symptoms of lower abdominal and back pain, deep dyspareunia, and urinary complaints may necessitate removal of the residual adnexa.

20. Pettit PD, Lee RA. Ovarian remnant syndrome: diagnostic dilemma and surgical challenge. *Obstet Gynecol* 1988;71:580.

The patient who has pain after undergoing bilateral oophorectomy (usually for endometriosis) may harbor remnants of ovarian tissue, whether or not a mass is present. Surgical correction requires mobilization of the ureter throughout its entire pelvic course to facilitate resection of the mass.

Complications

21. Hill DJ. Complications of hysterectomy. *Baillieres Clin Obstet Gynaecol* 1997; 11:181.

A delayed complication of a subclinical hemorrhage is hematoma. Most are self-limiting and resolve. Drainage is unnecessary, unless there is infection or the location relative to the vaginal cuff allows easy access.

22. Ryan MM. Hysterectomy: social and psychosexual aspects. *Baillieres Clin Obstet Gynaecol* 1997;11:23.

The rate of psychological disorder is higher than normal both before and after hysterectomy.

23. Harris WJ. Early complications of abdominal and vaginal hysterectomy. *Obstet Gynecol Surv* 1995;50:795.

Many vesicovaginal fistulas develop from an unsuspected bladder injury. It is recommended that, after a difficult dissection, the bladder be distended with fluid or a dye solution to rule out such an injury.

24. Meikle SF, Nugent EW, Orleans M. Complications and recovery from laparoscopy-assisted vaginal hysterectomy compared with abdominal and vaginal hysterectomy. *Obstet Gynecol* 1997;89:304.

Laparoscopic cases had a shorter hospital stay and speedier postoperative recovery, but surgery was lengthier and the rate of bladder injury was higher.

25. Thakar R, et al. Bladder, bowel, and sexual function after hysterectomy for benign conditions. *Br J Obstet Gynaecol* 1997;104:983.

A literature review did not demonstrate any consistent alterations in bladder, bowel, and sexual function.

26. Hemsell DL. Prophylactic antibiotics in gynecologic and obstetric surgery. *Rev Infect Dis* 1991;13:821.

Antimicrobial prophylaxis for vaginal hysterectomy is generally indicated, whereas for abdominal hysterectomy, it should be reserved for patients at high risk for infection. A single dose, given relatively soon before the operation, of an antibiotic active against either aerobic or anaerobic flora is recommended. The pharmacokinetics and antimicrobial spectrum of an agent, although paramount in determining the efficacy for established infection, have little impact in terms of prophylactic efficacy.

27. Eason E, Aldis A, Seymour RJ. Pelvic fluid collections by sonography and febrile morbidity after abdominal hysterectomy. *Obstet Gynecol* 1997;90:58.

Fever during the first 24 to 48 hours is usually pulmonary in origin, requiring treatment of atelectasis. A pelvic abscess or cuff abscess, on the other hand, causes fever at about 72 hours. Wound infections become evident at about the third day, with the exception of clostridial or streptococcal infections, which present earlier.

28. Shaikh N, Saveranamuthu J, Williams G. Ureteric injury unrecognized during gynaecological operations. *J Obstet Gynaecol* 1992;12:133.

Bleeding is a common problem that attends pelvic procedures, and can lead to ureteral injury. Direct pressure can control most bleeding. The ureter and the bleeding point are positively identified before suturing or cauterizing, to ensure hemostasis without ureteral damage.

29. Bakri YN, Linjawi T. Angiographic embolization for control of pelvic genital tract hemorrhage: report of 14 cases. *Acta Obstet Gynecol Scand* 1992;71:17.

    Approximately 30% of the blood volume is lost before a significant decrease in blood pressure occurs. In the event of postoperative hypovolemic shock, an immediate return to the operating room is mandated. In less acute cases, restoration of the blood volume in conjunction with angiographic embolization of the bleeding vessel is possible.

30. Kvist-Poulsen H, Borel J. Iatrogenic femoral neuropathy subsequent to abdominal hysterectomy: incidence and prevention. *Obstet Gynecol* 1982;60:516.

    Femoral neuropathy with thigh numbness, paresthesia, and weakness may result from improper positioning in the stirrups with marked thigh flexing or nerve stretching, or from retractor pressure on the psoas muscles through which the nerve runs. Perineal or sciatic nerve damage may occur in the lithotomy position resulting from compression along the leg or buttock.

31. Kim YB, DuBeshter B, Niloff JM. Continuous single-layer closure of midline abdominal incisions in high-risk gynecologic patients. *J Gynecol Surg* 1992;8:15.

    The incidence of disruption of a suture line (dehiscence) ranges from 0.28% to 0.51% for abdominal hysterectomy. Obesity, anemia, vertical incision, and medical disorders (diabetes and renal) are all risk factors. Closure of a vertical incision should utilize the Smead-Jones technique with a nonabsorbable suture.

32. Greer IA. Epidemiology, risk factors and prophylaxis of venous thromboembolism in obstetrics and gynaecology. *Baillieres Clin Obstet Gynaecol* 1997; 11:403.

    Pharmacologic methods with heparin, warfarin, and dextrose, and mechanical methods with pneumatic calf compression and graduated elastic compression stockings are all effective prophylactic agents.

XI. INFECTIOUS AND VENEREAL DISEASES

55. GONORRHEA

Michel E. Rivlin

Neisseria gonorrhoeae is the causative agent of gonorrhea (GC), an infection that primarily involves the mucous membranes of the genitourinary tract, pharynx, and anus. The organism is a gram-negative diplococcus found in polymorphonuclear leukocytes. The virulence of the organism is associated with specific colony types. Only those that contain pili are capable of producing infection. Pili are proteinaceous surface appendages and are the primary mediators of attachment. Pilated gonococci have been shown to adhere to sperm and a variety of human epithelial cells. Colonies isolated from uncomplicated infection and from the endocervix in women are opaque, whereas colonies isolated in the setting of disseminated infection and the endocervix during menstruation are transparent. Gonococcal typing is essential to conduct an effective epidemiologic study. Auxotyping entails identifying the specific nutritional requirements of the organism; the most common is the wild type (requiring no additives). Auxotypes correlate well with patterns of infection and antibiotic sensitivity. Thus, arginine, hypoxanthine, and uracil-requiring AHU strains are associated with disseminated infection and are very sensitive to antibiotics. A less useful typing method is plasmid analysis. In 1976, strains of gonococci were found to contain an extrachromosomal deoxyribonucleic acid (DNA), a plasmid that produces beta-lactamase, and this in turn inactivates penicillin. Similar strains of penicillinase-producing *N. gonorrhoeae* (PPNG) have since appeared worldwide. Another resistant strain that has appeared is beta-lactamase negative. Chromosomally mediated resistant *N. gonorrhoeae* (CMRNG) has intranuclear DNA that renders the cell membrane impermeable to penicillin. Both PPNG and CMRNG respond to therapy with either spectinomycin, quinolones, or a third-generation cephalosporin. CMRNG strains resistant to tetracycline and spectinomycin have been found. Quinolone-resistant strains (QRNG) have appeared in recent years. Finally, serology is used to type the organism, often in conjunction with auxotyping, and this yields information on the auxotype/serovar classes.

In the United States, an estimated 600,000 new GC infections occur each year. Rates have decreased gradually and reached a 30-year low in 1995 of 149 per 100,000. The male:female ratio is 1.5:1. Risk factors include young age (15 to 24 years), an increased number of sex partners, and nonuse of barrier contraception. Cases occur primarily in the southern states, and the male:female ratio is reversed in young teenagers. Transmission is almost entirely accomplished by sexual contact. A male has a 20% to 25% risk, and a female has an 80% to 90% risk of transmission per single sexual contact. There is a short incubation time of 3 to 5 days, but this can range from 1 to 14 days. In adults, transmission can take place after fellatio and genital-rectal exposure in addition to genital intercourse. In children, besides sexual exposure, nonsexual contact with the infectious discharge may lead to vaginal or ocular infection.

Uncomplicated urogenital or anal infection is frequently asymptomatic. There is a much higher prevalence of signs and symptoms in women who seek care, including dysuria, suprapubic discomfort, purulent cervical discharge, intermenstrual spotting and bleeding, or menorrhagia. The cervix or urethra, or both, may be red and edematous, and there may be a purulent discharge. Pharyngitis may be present with edema, erythema, and complaints of sore throat, or it may be asymptomatic. Proctitis may be associated with blood and pus in stools and diffuse erythema or it may be asymptomatic. Ophthalmia neonatorum arises between 2 and 3 days after delivery, and symptoms consist of bilateral conjunctivitis and a profuse purulent discharge. If left untreated, corneal ulceration and scarring occur. In 15% to 20% of women with uncomplicated anogenital GC, upper genital tract infection (pelvic inflammatory disease [PID]) occurs, usually at the end of or just after menstruation (see Chapter 63). Gonococcal vaginitis is rare, although it may be seen in prepubertal and postmenopausal females. Perihepatitis (Fitz-Hugh-Curtis syndrome) may be found in conjunction with PID and results from either direct or contiguous spread of the infection. Disseminated gonococcal infection (DGI) affects 1% to 3% of infected patients, but predominates in women, showing a female:male ratio of approximately 4:1. This usually appears during pregnancy, especially in the third trimester or within 7 days of the onset of menses. DGI manifests an early bacteremic stage consisting of chills, fever, and a dermatitis that includes a variety of skin lesions of gonococcal emboli that are asymmetrically distributed. These start as macules, which become vesicular, pustular, and then purpuric, and are mostly seen on the hands, fingers, feet, and toes. Blood cultures are positive in half of the patients during this stage. Joint symptoms are frequently present and are then characteristic of the later septic arthritis stage, in which purulent synovial effusions occur commonly in the knees, ankles, and wrists. Tenosynovitis, involving the extensor and flexor tendons of the hands and feet, is also a common finding. Patients also experience erythema, swelling, tenderness, and pain on motion along the tendon sheath.

The diagnosis may be made by GC culture. To obtain material for culture, a dry, sterile cotton-tipped swab is inserted into the endocervical canal; this is moved from side to side, and after 15 to 30 seconds, organisms should have absorbed to the swab. Ideally, the specimen is cultured directly onto selective medium (Thayer-Martin) and incubated immediately at 36°C in 5% to 7% carbon dioxide (a candle jar provides an adequate concentration of carbon dioxide). Fermentation reactions differentiate *N. gonorrhoeae* from *N. meningitidis*. The former ferments glucose, the latter maltose. A single endocervical swab will miss approximately 10% of GC infections. Microscopic examination of a gram-stained specimen from the infected site is diagnostic of GC in only 40% to 50% of women compared with 95% of men. The Gonozyme test is a solid-phase enzyme immunoassay (ELISA) for detecting gonococcal antigens and is more sensitive than gram staining (78%–100%), but the specificity is variable (70%–100%). The number of false-positive results that this would produce, particularly in low-prevalence populations, has consequently limited use of the test. Polymerase chain reaction (PCR) and *ligase chain reaction* (LCR) are expensive but more sensitive than culture or ELISA. Furthermore, these tests are accurate using self-obtained first-voided samples and vaginal swabs, obviating the need for cervical sampling. Depending on the history, samples may be taken from the urethra, pharynx, and rectum in addition to the endocervical sample. Furthermore, blood testing for syphilis is indicated if GC is diagnosed. The differential diagnosis includes trichomoniasis, candidiasis, anaerobic vaginosis, herpes, and chlamydial cervicitis.

The Centers for Disease Control and Prevention (CDC) recommended regimens for treatment of uncomplicated anogenital GC (1998), including concomitant therapy for coexisting chlamydia since that organism is found in 20% to 40% of GC cases. A single-dose regimen for GC is given, followed by a tetracycline or doxycycline regimen for chlamydia. Ceftriaxone 125 mg intramuscularly followed by doxycycline 100 mg twice daily for 7 days orally are given. Alternatively, azithromycin may be prescribed as a single 1-g dose for chlamydial infection. If tetracyclines are contraindicated (during pregnancy or in children) or not tolerated, erythromycin ethylsuccinate 800 mg four times daily may be substituted. Alternatives to ceftriaxone include the quinolones (ciprofloxacin 500 mg or ofloxacin 400 mg orally), cefixime 400 mg orally, cefotaxime 500 mg intramuscularly, ceftizoxime 500 mg intramuscularly, and cefotetan 1 g intramuscularly and cefoxitin 2 g intramuscularly with probenicid 1 g orally. Spectinomycin 2 g intramuscularly is useful for patients who are intolerant of other agents. Other effective quinolones include norfloxacin 800 mg orally, enoxacin 400 mg orally, and lomefloxacin 400 mg orally. Pharyngeal infections should be treated with ceftriaxone; patients who cannot receive ceftriaxone should be treated with ciprofloxacin. Patients with incubating syphilis are likely to be cured by all the aforementioned regimens other than spectinomycin and the quinolones.

The disease is notifiable, and contacts should be identified, examined, cultured, and treated presumptively. Follow-up culture (test of cure) following ceftriaxone/doxycycline therapy is not essential because failure is rare. Reculture 1 to 2 months later (rescreening) detects both failures and reinfections. Those with persistent symptoms or treated with alternative regimens should have a culture 4 to 7 days after therapy. If

GC persists after treatment, antibiotic sensitivities are indicated, although reinfection is more common than resistance. Additional therapy with ceftriaxone/doxycycline should be given. Pregnant women should have endocervical GC culture at first visit and, in high-risk cases, repeated in late pregnancy. Treatment regimens are the same except for tetracycline and doxycycline, which are contraindicated in pregnancy. Therapy of PID is discussed in Chapter 63. Patients with DGI should be hospitalized for therapy, the details of which are beyond the scope of this chapter. All newborn infants should receive ophthalmic prophylaxis with erythromycin or tetracycline ointments or silver nitrate instillation. Infants born to mothers with untreated GC should be treated, and those with GC ophthalmia require parenteral therapy. Dosage schedules are included in the CDC recommendations.

The major long-term complications of GC include PID and the sequelae of PID, such as ectopic pregnancy, infertility, and chronic pelvic pain (see Chapter 63). An association between maternal gonorrhea and DGI, and perinatal complications such as premature ruptured membranes, chorioamnionitis, prematurity, intrauterine growth retardation, neonatal sepsis, and postpartum endometritis, has been recognized. The gonococcus is a highly adapted pathogen that has acquired or developed antibiotic resistance and has surface structures that can undergo phase and antigenic variation, ensuring the continuing high prevalence of the disease. The search for a vaccine continues; the ideal candidate would have conserved antigenic components common to all gonococci.

Review
1. Nicholas H. Sexually transmitted diseases. Gonorrhoea: symptoms and treatment. *Nurs Times* 1998;94:52.
   Widespread use and abuse of beta-lactam–producing agents, together with increasing global travel, have facilitated the dissemination of antibiotic-resistant gonococci.
2. Jephcott AE. Microbiological diagnosis of gonorrhoea. *Genitourin Med* 1997;73:245.
   When culture specimens are transported elsewhere for testing, instead of tested on-site, 16% fewer infections are detected.

Epidemiology
3. Sung L, MacDonald NE. Gonorrhea: a pediatric perspective. *Pediatr Rev* 1998;19:13.
   Because of the legal implications in children, standard cultures are required, and presumptive isolates should then be confirmed by at least two other modalities (e.g., serology, biochemistry, enzyme substrate). Isolates should be conserved for retesting or additional testing.
4. Mertz KJ, et al. Screening women for gonorrhea: demographic screening criteria for general clinical use. *Am J Public Health* 1997;87:1535.
   Age, marital status, and prevalence of infection at provider site are indicators of high-prevalence groups.
5. van Duynhoven YT, et al. Molecular epidemiology of infections with *Neisseria gonorrhoeae* among visitors to a sexually transmitted diseases clinic. *Sex Transm Dis* 1997;24:409.
   Beta-lactamase produced by the Gonococcus hydrolyzes the beta-lactam ring of the antibiotic's molecule. The ability to produce the enzyme is transmitted in a plasmid, a small extranuclear deoxyribonucleic acid (DNA) particle.
6. Belongia EA, et al. A population-based study of sexually transmitted disease incidence and risk factors in human immunodeficiency virus–infected people. *Sex Transm Dis* 1997;24:251.
   Patients infected with HIV should receive the same treatment regimens as those who are HIV-negative.

Genital Gonorrhea
7. Carne CA. Epidemiological treatment and tests of cure in gonococcal infection: evidence for value. *Genitourin Med* 1997;73:12.
   The author recommends a test of cure that includes a rectal swab.
8. Niruthisard S, et al. Use of nonoxynol-9 and reduction rate of gonococcal and chlamydial cervical infections. *Lancet* 1992;339:1371.

Spermicides together with diaphragm or condom appreciably decrease the risk of acquiring gonorrhea.

9. Oh MK, et al. Urine-based screening of adolescents in detention to guide treatment for gonococcal and chlamydial infections. Translating research into intervention. *Arch Pediatr Adolesc Med* 1998;152:52.

   The authors discuss an effective management tool for at-risk groups where cervical swab specimens may be difficult to obtain.

Extragenital Gonorrhea

10. van Bogaert LJ. Controversies in the approach to ophthalmia neonatorum. *S Afr Med J* 1997;87:79.

    Ophthalmic ointments or drops containing tetracycline or erythromycin should be instilled into the conjunctiva of all newborns to protect against gonococcal and chlamydial conjunctivitis.

11. Rompalo AM, et al. The acute arthritis-dermatitis syndrome. The changing importance of *Neisseria meningitidis. Arch Intern Med* 1987;147:281.

    Early (septicemic) phase of migratory polyarthritis with fever is followed by septic phase with inflammation and effusion in one joint. Blood culture is diagnostic in the early phase and joint culture in the later phase.

12. Suleiman SA, Grimes EM, Jones HS. Disseminated gonococcal infections. *Obstet Gynecol* 1983;61:48.

    Disseminated disease is more common with asymptomatic than with symptomatic infection.

Diagnosis

13. Barlow D. The diagnosis of oropharyngeal gonorrhoea. *Genitourin Med* 1997;73:16.

    Pharyngeal infections are more difficult to eradicate than genital infections. Ceftriaxone or ciprofloxacin or ofloxacin are recommended with azithromycin or doxycycline for possible chlamydial infection.

14. Stary A, et al. Comparison of ligase chain reaction and culture for detection of *Neisseria gonorrhoeae* in genital and extragenital specimens. *J Clin Microbiol* 1997;35:239.

    Ligase chain reaction testing with swabs or urine was better than culture for the diagnosis of genital or extragenital gonorrhea.

Treatment

15. Centers for Disease Control. 1998 Guidelines for treatment of sexually transmitted diseases. *MMWR* 1998;47(RR-1).

    This contains recommendations for the treatment of uncomplicated, complicated, and disseminated disease as well as resistant organisms in adults, children, neonates, and pregnant women.

16. Jones RB, et al. Randomized trial of trovafloxacin and ofloxacin for single-dose therapy of gonorrhea. Trovafloxacin Gonorrhea Study Group. *Am J Med* 1998; 104:28.

    Many antibiotics are effective against GC. These include the cephalosporins such as ceftazidime and cefoxitin; combinations of ampicillin or amoxicillin with beta-lactamase inhibitors such as clavulanic acid and sulbactam; aminoglycosides; and newer agents such as the monobactams and quinolones.

17. Knapp JS, et al. Fluoroquinolone resistance in *Neisseria gonorrhoeae. Infect Dis* 1997;3:584.

    Quinolones have a high tendency to induce resistance in N. gonorrhoeae organisms and are not considered safe for pregnant women or children.

18. Schwebke JR, et al. Positive screening tests for gonorrhea and chlamydial infection fail to lead consistently to treatment of patients attending a sexually transmitted disease clinic. *Sex Transm Dis* 1997;24:181.

    Methods must be sought to enhance patient compliance with follow-up of test results and treatment if indicated.

19. Cavenee MR, et al. Treatment of gonorrhea in pregnancy. *Obstet Gynecol* 1993;
    81:33.
    Repeat cultures during the third trimester are recommended for any patient
    treated for GC earlier in that pregnancy.

56. SYPHILIS

Michel E. Rivlin

Syphilis is a sexually transmitted disease caused by *Treponema pallidum,* a spirochete with a length of 6 to 15 mm and a width of only 0.15 mm, which is not easily
grown in vitro. On dark-field microscopic examination, the organism is observed to
exhibit a rotary motion. Serologic studies provide the usual means of diagnosis. In
1995, rates of primary and secondary syphilis were six and three per 100,000 population, respectively. Rates are much higher in certain groups. Like other STDs,
syphilis disproportionately affects poor, inner-city residents and minorities. Increased
rates are associated with drug use, drug-related sexual behavior, and prostitution.
Patients with concomitant human immunodeficiency virus (HIV) infection may be
subject to more aggressive syphilitic infections, and the response to therapy may
be less successful in these patients.
    The transmission of syphilis by sexual contact requires exposure to moist mucosal
or cutaneous lesions. The incubation period before the primary lesion develops at the
site of initial inoculation ranges from 10 to 90 days, with an average of 21 days. The
chancre (the initial lesion of primary syphilis) is usually solitary, although multiple
lesions can occur. It begins as a papule that erodes and ulcerates. It is usually painless, punched out, and clean with raised borders. The entire lesion is indurated, and
draining lymph nodes are enlarged, hard, and nontender. The lesions are usually genital. Extragenital sites include the lips, tongue, tonsils, fingers, nipples, and anus.
Diagnosis at this stage may be based on the findings from dark-field examination of
a direct scraping from the lesion or by direct fluorescent antibody tests of lesion exudate or tissue. The results of serologic tests are often negative initially. The differential diagnosis includes neoplasm, chancroid, lymphogranuloma venereum, granuloma
inguinale, herpes, and fungal infection. Untreated, the chancre heals in a few weeks.
    Within a few weeks or months, secondary syphilis may develop. This is a stage of
spirochetemia that can involve any cutaneous or mucosal surface as well as any organ.
Four major syndromes may be seen: rash, a generalized lymphadenopathy, a flulike
illness, and visceral involvement. The skin lesions are usually dry and symmetrical
and are most marked on the palms and soles. In warm, moist areas, such as the perineum, condylomata lata may form. Lesions may occur on mucosal surfaces and are
called mucous patches; these are found in about 30% of patients, generally in the
mouth, palate, and pharynx. Organs that may be involved include the liver (10%) and
long bones (rarely). The skin lesions must be differentiated from common skin eruptions, including drug reactions and acute exanthemata. Serology results are invariably positive and, like the chancre, the lesions are highly infective. In the latent stage
that follows, there are no clinical signs, and the diagnosis is based on positive serology in the absence of concurrent disease that may produce a false-positive reaction.
The early latent phase begins after the first attack of secondary syphilis has passed
and lasts for about 1 year. Late latent syphilis is rarely infectious, except that the
pregnant woman may transmit infection to the fetus regardless of the duration of the
illness. Tertiary syphilis is manifested by a diffuse vascular disease and the formation of lesions termed gummas that may occur throughout the body. It occurs many
years after secondary syphilis in about 30% of untreated patients. Most commonly,

the cardiovascular and central nervous systems are involved. Serology is usually reactive. The clinical spectrum of syphilis acquired in utero includes stillbirth, neonatal death, neonatal illness in the first months of life, and development of the stigmata of congenital syphilis in later life.

Two blood tests are commonly performed for syphilis: a nontreponemal reagin test, such as the rapid plasma reagin (RPR) or the Venereal Disease Research Laboratory (VDRL) test, and a treponemal test, such as the fluorescent treponemal antibody absorption (FTA ABS) test or the microhemagglution assay for antibody to *T. pallidum* (MHA TP). The preferred test for both screening and monitoring a patient's response to treatment is the VDRL test. The test result becomes positive 1 or 2 weeks after the appearance of the chancre. It is positive in about 66% of primary cases, 99% of secondary cases, and 70% of tertiary cases. Acute false-positive reactions occur in 1% to 2% of the general population and may occur transiently with acute febrile illnesses, immunizations, and pregnancy. Repeated false-positive results may be caused by other chronic infections (e.g., chronic active hepatitis), autoimmune diseases (e.g., systemic lupus erythematosus), or narcotic addiction. The false-positive VDRL titer is usually low (no more than 1:8). The FTA ABS test is used as a confirmatory test. Results are positive in 85% of primary and 100% of secondary cases, and may be the only positive test result in patients with tertiary syphilis. False-positive results may occur in patients with diseases associated with hypergammaglobulinemia, although the VDRL result is usually negative in these diseases. Treponemal tests are expensive and not quantitative. Once results are positive, they do not reverse. They are not, therefore, used for either screening or evaluating the response to treatment. Mothers with treated syphilis may passively transfer immunoglobulin G (IgG) to the fetus, resulting in positive serology findings in the newborn. Because maternal immunoglobulin M (IgM) is not passively transferred, an IgM FTA ABS assay is used to diagnose congenital infection. Unfortunately, a 35% false-negative rate and a 10% false-positive rate are associated with the test. Many physicians therefore choose to treat all VDRL-positive neonates. Cerebrospinal fluid (CSF) examination, consisting of serology plus a search for cells and determination of the protein content, is essential in all syphilitics with unexplained neurologic abnormalities. All patients with syphilis should be tested for HIV and retested 3 months later.

Penicillin is the drug of choice for treating all stages of syphilis, and resistance of the organism to the antibiotic has never been described. The CDC recommendations for primary, secondary, or latent (<1 year) infection are to administer a depot form of the drug (benzathine penicillin G 2.4 million units intramuscularly) as a single dose. In penicillin-allergic patients, doxycycline (100 mg twice daily for 14 days) is recommended; in those unable to tolerate that drug, erythromycin (500 mg four times daily for 14 days) is recommended. Ceftriaxone also has been recommended as an alternative therapy, 1 g intramuscularly daily for 10 days, but there is only limited experience with this regimen. For patients with late latent infection (>1 year), the penicillin regimen is extended to three injections administered at weekly intervals, and the duration of therapy with the alternative drugs is increased to 30 days. The therapy for neurosyphilis and congenital syphilis is beyond the scope of this manual. The therapy in pregnant women is the same, except that doxycycline is contraindicated; in addition, the fetal levels achieved with erythromycin are only 6% to 20% of the maternal levels. The CDC recommendations have therefore been modified for pregnancy in that penicillin is deemed the only acceptable therapy. If allergy to penicillin is documented by skin testing, reactive patients should be desensitized in consultation with an expert and penicillin given only where adequate emergency facilities are available.

After the initiation of antibiotic therapy, the Jarisch-Herxheimer reaction may occur. This is an acute flulike syndrome that peaks by 12 hours and resolves by 24 hours. Premature labor or fetal distress may be precipitated in the second half of pregnancy. Treatment is symptomatic and consists of antipyretics and fluids. Patients may resume sexual activity once lesions have healed, and from 7 to 10 days after a complete course of therapy. Follow-up is accomplished by repeat quantitative nontreponemal tests performed at 3, 6, and 12 months after treatment. Repeat treatment is indicated if the VDRL titer increases fourfold or fails to decrease fourfold within a year. The retreatment schedules are the same as those for syphilis of more than 1 year's duration. Careful follow-up is particularly important in patients treated with antibiotics other than penicillin. In the setting of late syphilis, the titers may not decrease, and if there are no other signs of disease activity, this is not an indication for retreatment. Cases of syphilis should be reported to the local or state health department within 48 hours of diagnosis, which usually offer referral and follow-up services. Sexual partners of the patient are notified without identification of the index case.

Review
1. Buckley HB. Syphilis: a review and update of the "new" infection of the '90s. *Nurse Pract* 1992;17:25.
   The stages of syphilis are used as a guide for therapy, as well as to indicate the duration of the disease and to identify the infectious individual.
2. Farnes SW, Setness PA. Serologic tests for syphilis. *Postgrad Med J* 1990;87:37.
   A fourfold change in titer (e.g., from 1:16 to 1:4, or 1:8 to 1:32) is necessary to demonstrate a clinically significant difference. A low titer persistence is termed a serofast reaction.

Epidemiology
3. Schramm M. Syphilis resurgent. *Aust N Z J Obstet Gynecol* 1997;37:377.
   All sexually transmitted diseases are inextricably linked—behaviorally, epidemiologically, biologically, clinically, economically, organizationally, and historically. Health professionals should build on the similarities and draw on their common skills in the prevention of sexually transmitted diseases.
4. Mushinski M. Sexually transmitted diseases: United States, 1995. *Stat Bull Metrop Insur Co* 1997;78:10.
   Rates of primary and secondary syphilis increased through the mid-1980s to a record high of 20.3 cases per 100,000 population in 1990. Since then, rates have dropped 69% to 6.3, the lowest rate in 35 years.
5. Dada AJ, et al. A serosurvey of *Haemophilus ducreyi*, syphilis, and herpes simplex virus type 2 and their association with human immunodeficiency virus among female sex workers in Lagos, Nigeria. *Sex Transm Dis* 1998;25:237.
   Genital ulcerative diseases facilitate HIV infections. Control of these diseases is an important factor in limiting the spread of HIV.
6. Peterman TA, et al. Partner notification for syphilis: a randomized, controlled trial of three approaches. *Sex Transm Dis* 1997;24:511.
   The trading of sex for drugs at crack houses encourages frequent sexual encounters with anonymous partners, rendering traditional methods of contact tracing less effective.

Diagnosis
7. Hira SK, et al. Clinical manifestations of secondary syphilis. *Int J Dermatol* 1987; 26:103.
   The author of this article does not believe that lumbar puncture for evidence of neurosyphilis is necessary in patients with secondary syphilis.
8. Feder HM Jr, Manthous C. The asymptomatic patient with a positive VDRL test. *Am Fam Physician* 1988;3:185.
   A patient with a low-titer VDRL or RPR may have active disease. Lumbar puncture is indicated (1) for patients with possible congenital syphilis or with signs or symptoms of neurosyphilis, (2) prior to nonpenicillin treatment of latent or tertiary syphilis, and (3) in cases of syphilis treatment failure.
9. Erbelding EJ, et al. Syphilis serology in human immunodeficiency virus infection: evidence for false-negative fluorescent treponemal testing. *J Infect Dis* 1997; 176:1397.
   HIV-infected patients can have abnormal test results, but in the majority, serologic tests are reliable for diagnosis and evaluation of treatment response.

10. Sanchez PJ, et al. Molecular analysis of the fetal IgM response to *Treponema pallidum* antigens: implications for improved serodiagnosis of congenital syphilis. *J Infect Dis* 1989;159:508.
    Immunoglobulin G (IgG) can be passively transferred from the mother, but IgM is not transferred. Fetal serum IgM reactivity can therefore be used as an important molecular marker for the diagnosis of congenital syphilis.
11. Sanchez PJ, Wendel GD. Syphilis in pregnancy. *Clin Perinatol* 1997;24:71.
    Maternal follow-up should include a monthly nontreponemal serologic test for syphilis for the remainder of pregnancy. Retreatment is necessary for women who exhibit a fourfold increase in the test titer or who do not show a fourfold decrease in the titer within 3 months of treatment.
12. Sison CG, et al. The resurgence of congenital syphilis: a cocaine-related problem. *J Pediatr* 1997;130:289.
    Maternal use of cocaine is significantly related to congenital syphilis.
13. Nathan L, et al. In utero infection with *Treponema pallidum* in early pregnancy. *Prenat Diagn* 1997;17:119.
    Amniocentesis samples were tested for syphilis, confirming that in utero infection in early pregnancy occurs and that the infection can be eradicated by maternal treatment.
14. Stoll BJ, et al. Clinical and serologic evaluation of neonates for congenital syphilis: a continuing diagnostic dilemma. *J Infect Dis* 1993;167:1093.
    A major problem is the inability to identify which asymptomatic but possibly infected neonate is really uninfected.
15. Barton JR, et al. Nonimmune hydrops fetalis associated with maternal infection with syphilis. *Am J Obstet Gynecol* 1992;167:56.
    Fetuses with hydrops as a result of maternal syphilis survived the perinatal period after penicillin therapy and preterm delivery.

Treatment
16. Centers for Disease Control. 1998 Guidelines for Treatment of Sexually Transmitted Diseases. *MMWR* 1998;47(RR-1).
    This represents the CDC treatment recommendations for the spectrum of syphilitic diseases. Approximately 50% of those treated for primary syphilis will experience the Jarisch-Herxheimer reaction.
17. Chisholm CA, et al. Penicillin desensitization in the treatment of syphilis during pregnancy. *Am J Perinatol* 1997;14:553.
    Oral desensitization is as effective as intravenous desensitization, and is easier and less expensive.

Perinatol
18. Rolfs RT, et al. A randomized trial of enhanced therapy for early syphilis in patients with and without human immunodeficiency virus infection. The syphilis and HIV study group. *N Engl J Med* 1997;31:307.
    Current recommendations for treating early syphilis appear adequate for most patients, whether or not they have HIV infection.
19. Schroeter AL, et al. Therapy for incubating syphilis: effectiveness of gonorrhea treatment. *JAMA* 1971;218:711.
    Standard gonorrhea therapy is successful in clearing incubating syphilis, but it will not clear established infection. The routine use of spectinomycin (which does not appear to cure incubating syphilis) in areas where a sizable proportion of gonorrhea infections are caused by beta-lactamase–producing organisms may partially explain the increase in infectious syphilis.
20. Guinan ME. Treatment of primary and secondary syphilis: defining failure at three- and six-month follow-up. *JAMA* 1987;257:359.
    In patients treated successfully, there was an approximate fourfold and eightfold drop in VDRL titers at 3 and 6 months, respectively. All should be followed until symptom-free and seronegative or, if positive at 2 years, until a stable low titer is reached.

57. GENITAL HERPES

Michel E. Rivlin

Herpes simplex virus (HSV) belongs to a large group of deoxyribonucleic acid (DNA) viruses that includes varicella zoster, cytomegalovirus, and the Epstein-Barr virus. The virus is fairly large and complex, measuring 150 to 200 μm in diameter. The DNA core of HSV is surrounded by a glycoprotein envelope derived from the host cell. After the virus penetrates the cell wall, the nucleocapsid is released and the DNA enters the nucleus. There are two subtypes of HSV, but clinical differentiation is not necessary. Fifty percent of DNA differs between HSV type 1 and type 2. Herpes infections that occur above the waist are generally caused by HSV type 1, and those below the waist are usually due to HSV type 2, although 20% to 25% of genital cases are due to type 1. In both HSV types, the dorsal spinal ganglia are thought to harbor latent viral infection. When this latent virus is activated, it migrates down the axons and produces lesions in the skin supplied by the sensory neurons. Type 2 infections have a recurrence rate of about 95%, versus about 50% for type 1 infections. The serologic prevalence of type 2 genital infection in the middle-class population of the United States ranges between 20% and 55%, but only about a third of these patients have a history of symptomatic genital infections. The prevalence in lower socioeconomic groups is between 40% and 60%. An estimated 300,000 to 500,000 new cases occur annually in the United States.

Transmission is known to result from genital or oral-genital sexual contact. The attack rate (percentage of those who contract it after exposure) for susceptible individuals is thought to be 75%. If intercourse is avoided during symptomatic periods, transmission to the partner does not appear to be inevitable. The incubation period tends to range from 2 to 10 days, although it may vary from 1 to more than 30 days.

The clinical manifestations depend on the immune status of the individual. There are three distinct clinical syndromes. First-episode primary infection occurs in patients who do not have circulating antibodies to either herpes viral type. The second syndrome occurs in women who already have antibody to HSV, and this is termed a first-episode nonprimary genital infection. The third group comprises those patients with recurrent disease who have previously had primary genital herpes infection and now have activation of latent herpes, or recurrent disease. The most severe forms of disease are confined to patients with first-episode primary infection or those whose immune system is compromised (e.g., resulting from corticosteroid therapy, pregnancy, malignancy, or immunosuppression). Both humoral and cell-mediated immune responses are important. Antibodies appear about 7 days after the primary infection and peak in 2 to 3 weeks. There is little rise in the antibody titer during recurrent episodes. When the cell-mediated immune response is suppressed, life-threatening infections may occur. Generally the area of outbreak is more limited and the symptoms are less severe in patients with antibodies from previous type 1 infections.

The characteristic signs of the first-episode primary infection include systemic symptoms in association with pain, dysuria, and the presence of multiple, painful vesicular or ulcerative genital lesions. More than 40% of the patients complain of systemic symptoms such as fever and malaise, 85% have multiple bilateral lesions, and 80% have tender lymphadenopathy. The mean duration of viral shedding is 11 days, and 87% of women shed virus from the cervix. Lesions first appear in the form of vesicles or pustules that ulcerate, crust, and finally heal in an average of 19 days. Local pain lasts for a mean of 12 days. Local and systemic symptoms have a mean duration of almost 3 weeks. Dysuria, which occurs in 83% of women, may be due to urine passing over the genital lesions or to a true urethritis, as the organism is also one of the causes of the urethral syndrome. Viral shedding takes place when the lesions are in the vesicular, pustular, and wet ulcer forms.

Extragenital infection occurs in about 26% of women with primary genital herpes. These lesions usually appear in the second week and are most commonly a result of autoinoculation from infected genital sites. They are usually located on the buttocks and fingers. Pharyngitis is noted in 10% of women with primary disease. Other complications, generally of the primary episode, include secondary urethral and bladder infections, urinary retention, and secondary bacterial invasion. Rectal herpes can cause significant pain and debilitation. Neurologic complications include inflammatory radiculomyelopathy, transverse myelitis, and aseptic meningitis. These are all uncommon but have been reported.

Recurrent infections have a periodicity of 1 to 3 months. Fifty percent of affected women experience a protracted remission after 7 years, and the duration of recurrences is considerably briefer than the initial episode. Many patients believe emotional stress, coitus, insomnia, and menstrual distress play major roles in initiating recurrent disease. Unique to recurrent infection is the prodrome, which affects 50% of the women and lasts just over a day. It is characterized by a tingling or itching sensation in the area where the eruption will occur. Viral shedding lasts up to a week, and healing is usually complete by 2 weeks. Urethritis is unusual, and typically there are only a few lesions that tend to recur in the same site. Local symptoms of pain or itching, if present, are generally mild.

Most cases are diagnosed clinically based on the appearance of typical herpetic lesions and the patient's history. The usual diagnostic laboratory procedure is viral culture. To perform this, the lesions are swabbed after the vesicles or pustules are broken with a sterile needle and the exudate sample is transferred immediately for viral culture. Cytologic examination of a Tzanck preparation or Papanicolaou (Pap) smear may demonstrate multinucleated giant cells. These preparations can be made using scrapings obtained from the bases of the vesicles or the cervix. Unfortunately, cytologic analysis positively identifies only about 30% to 50% of the patients with herpes, whereas culture results are positive in 80% of the same patients. Herpes antigen detection methods include direct immunofluorescence and enzyme-linked immunosorbent assays. The diagnostic sensitivities of these tests are intermediate between those of cytologic studies and viral culture. HSV DNA detection by the polymerase chain reaction (PCR) appears to be more sensitive than viral culture.

The differential diagnosis of HSV includes ulcerative lesions of the genital tract. In Western countries, HSV accounts for 20% to 50% of such lesions. *Treponema pallidum* is another important etiologic agent. In developing countries, chancroid (*Haemophilus ducreyi* infection) is the most common cause. Lymphogranuloma venereum strains of *Chlamydia trachomatis* are also associated with genital ulcers, often in conjunction with suppurative lymphadenopathy. Granuloma inguinale, or donovanosis, causes a chronic, slowly progressive genital ulceration that is spread by contiguity. The causative organism of this disease is *Calymmatobacterium granulomatis*. There is no adenopathy in this condition. In view of the multiple infectious causes of genital ulcers, clinical and laboratory confirmation of a diagnosis should be sought.

Noninfectious causes of genital ulcerations, such as the mucosal lesions associated with Behçet syndrome or inflammatory bowel disorders (Crohn's disease), also may be confused with genital herpes. A history of inflammatory bowel disease symptoms in a patient with Crohn's disease and the finding of oral, ocular, and central nervous system involvement in a patient with Behçet syndrome may help differentiate the conditions, although the differentiation between herpes and Behçet syndrome may be difficult if there is not a long history of either.

The treatment of choice for primary herpetic episodes is the antiviral nucleoside acyclovir. The drug's specificity for HSV-infected cells depends on its phosphorylation to its active form, acyclovir triphosphate, which is performed far more efficiently by HSV-specific thymidine kinase in infected cells than by cellular kinases in normal cells. The drug inhibits viral replication but does not eradicate latent infection. Therapy consisting of 200 mg orally five times daily for 7 to 10 days, initiated within 6 days of the onset of lesions, shortens the median duration of first-episode eruptions by 3 to 5 days and may reduce the number and intensity of systemic symptoms. Only about 2% of patients require hospitalization, and these may be treated intravenously. The topical application of acyclovir ointment confers only marginal benefit in decreasing viral shedding. Treatment for recurrent episodes should be limited to those patients who typically have severe symptoms and are able to begin therapy at the time of the prodrome or within 2 days of the onset of lesions. Acyclovir shortens the mean clinical course of recurrences by about 1 day. The safety of acyclovir in pregnancy and in neonates and children has not been established, and prophylactic administration to women with lesions at delivery or to their infants is not indicated.

Valacyclovir, a valine ester of acyclovir, and famciclovir, a prodrug of penciclovir, have enhanced oral bioavailability and therefore provide the advantage of less-frequent dosing. First-episode infections are treated with valacyclovir 1 g orally twice daily for 7-10 days or famciclovir 250 mg twice daily for 7 to 10 days. Dosage for episodic recurrences is valacyclovir 500 mg twice daily for 5 days or famciclovir 125 mg twice daily for 5 days. For daily suppressive therapy, dosages vary between 500 and 1,000 mg daily of valacyclovir and 250 mg twice daily of famciclovir. Immunocompromised patients may develop infections with acyclovir-resistant strains and may require parenteral therapy in higher dosage or, if nonresponsive, with systemic foscarnet.

The prevention of transmission depends on patient education. Patients should be advised to abstain from skin-to-skin contact when active oral or genital infections are present. The use of a condom may be helpful, although it is by no means always successful. Continuous oral acyclovir (200 mg orally two to five times daily) can reduce the frequency of recurrent episodes by at least 75%, but, when discontinued, the disease reverts to its natural course. Continuous treatment should be reserved for patients who suffer six or more recurrences annually, or those who either have severe symptoms or are immunocompromised. Many patients prefer suppressive to episodic treatment, and long-term therapy (up to 3 years) appears to be well tolerated. Acyclovir-resistant strains are associated with decreased or absent viral thymidine kinase enzyme activity. In immunocompromised patients, these strains may cause serious infections, and other antiviral agents may be indicated.

Psychological disability has been reported in up to 80% of patients surveyed. Nearly half of those infected avoid interpersonal relationships or abstain from sexual activity for varying periods. In one survey, 25% of patients reported that they had been rejected by partners because of the herpetic infection, and 18% felt that herpes contributed to the dissolution of a relationship. If the physician is not able to offer sufficient educational and psychologic support, these patients should be encouraged to seek out the services offered by national support groups and the assistance of trained psychological or psychiatric personnel.

Besides the fear of infecting a sexual partner, women are frequently concerned about transmission of the infection during pregnancy; this topic is addressed in Chapter 9. Furthermore, HSV infections have been associated with genital cancers. Women with HSV-2 antibodies exhibit a higher incidence of cervical dysplasia and cancer; however, when controlled for sexuality, these differences are not significant. In addition, HSV-2–specific DNA binding antigens have been found in the setting of cervical dysplasia and cancer. However, although an epidemiologic association exists, a causal link has not been established. Nevertheless, the epidemiologic associations do indicate that women with genital HSV infections should have a Pap smear at least once a year.

Reviews
1. Brugha R. Genital herpes infection: a review. *Int J Epidemiol* 1997;26:698.
   Silent spread of the infection is the rule, not the exception, with reactivation of previously unrecognized lesions.
2. Schmogyi M, Wald A, Corey L. Herpes virus type 2 infection: an emerging disease? *Infect Dis Clin North Am* 1998;12:47.
   A 30% increase in the prevalence of herpes virus type 2 over the past 13 years has been noted in the United States.

3. Fleming DT, et al. Herpes simplex virus type 2 in the United States, 1976 to 1994. *N Engl J Med* 1997;337:1105.
   Serologic assays used for epidemiologic studies accurately discriminate between type 1 and type 2 antibodies. These tests may become available for clinical use in the future.

Diagnosis
4. Boggess KA, et al. Herpes simplex virus type 2 detection by culture and polymerase chain reaction and relationship to genital symptoms and cervical antibody status during the third trimester of pregnancy. *Am J Obstet Gynecol* 1997;176:443.
   Polymerase chain reaction detected viral shedding in 14% versus 2% with viral culture. It is uncertain whether viral DNA is infectious.
5. Hensleigh PA, et al. Genital herpes during pregnancy: inability to distinguish primary and recurrent infections clinically. *Obstet Gynecol* 1997;89:891.
   Clinical assessment does not accurately discriminate primary and nonprimary genital infections.
6. Frankel RE, et al. High prevalence of gynecologic disease among hospitalized women with human immunodeficiency virus infection. *Clin Infect Dis* 1997; 25:706.
   Of 67 patients, 83% had gynecologic disease, 51% vaginitis, 45% dysplasia, 23% condyloma, 20% herpes, and 5% pelvic inflammatory disease.

Clinical Features
7. White C, Wardropper AG. Genital herpes simplex infection in women. *Clin Dermatol* 1997;15:81.
   Transmission occurred during periods of asymptomatic viral shedding in 70% of women infected.
8. Brown ZA, et al. The acquisition of herpes simplex virus during pregnancy. *N Engl J Med* 1997;337:509.
   Seroconversion during pregnancy occurred in 2% of susceptible women; if completed before labor, results were good; if not, perinatal morbidity was encountered.
9. Sucato G, et al. Evidence of latency and reactivation of both herpes simplex virus (HSV)-1 and HSV-2 in the genital region. *J Infect Dis* 1998;177:1069.
   Superinfection with a different herpes strain can occur; the frequency is not known.
10. Wald A, et al. Genital herpes in a primary care clinic. Demographic and sexual correlates of herpes simplex type 2 infections. *Sex Transm Dis* 1997;24:149.
    HSV-2 is present in one of five of the general population nationwide by serologic studies.
11. Keller ML, Jadack RA, Mims LF. Perceived stressors and coping responses in persons with recurrent genital herpes. *Res Nurs Health* 1991;14:421.
    The distress associated with the initial diagnosis may be similar to that of a grief reaction, with initial shock, numbness, and early denial. Thereafter, insomnia, depression, and rage are common.
12. Scott LL, Hollier LM, Dias K. Perinatal herpesvirus infections. Herpes simplex, varicella, and cytomegalovirus. *Infect Dis Clin North Am* 1997;11:27.
    Infection may occur in utero, by means of transplacental or ascending infection, or through exposure to genital lesions during delivery, or it may be acquired postnatally from relatives or attendants.

Therapy
13. Centers for Disease Control and Prevention. 1998 guidelines for treatment of sexually transmitted diseases. *MMWR* 1998;47(RR-1).
    Higher doses are usually recommended for the first episode of proctitis or stomatitis, although it is unclear whether these dosages are necessary.
14. Mertz GJ, et al. Oral famciclovir for suppression of recurrent genital herpes simplex virus infection in women. A multicenter, double-blind, placebo-controlled trial. *Arch Intern Med* 1997;157:343.

This drug neither eradicates latent virus nor affects the risk, frequency, or severity of recurrences after the drug is discontinued.

15. Tyring SK, et al. A randomized, placebo-controlled comparison of oral valacyclovir and acyclovir in immunocompetent patients with recurrent genital herpes infections. *Arch Dermatol* 1998;134:185.

    It is recommended that patients interrupt therapy after 1 year to reassess the frequency of recurrences because marked pattern changes may occur in up to 25% of the cases.

16. Brocklehurst P, et al. A randomised placebo controlled trial of suppressive acyclovir in late pregnancy in women with recurrent genital herpes infection. *Br J Obstet Gynaecol* 1998;105:275.

    Prophylactic acyclovir in late pregnancy lessened the number of recurrences but did not decrease the number of cesarean sections.

17. Safrin S, et al. A controlled trial comparing foscarnet with vidarabine for acyclovir-resistant mucocutaneous herpes simplex in the acquired immunodeficiency syndrome. The AIDS Clinical Trials Group. *N Engl J Med* 1991;325:551.

    Foscarnet was more effective and less toxic than vidarabine; however, there was a high frequency of relapse once treatment was stopped.

---

58. CHLAMYDIA

Michel E. Rivlin

Two species make up the genus *Chlamydia*. *Chlamydia psittaci* is the causative agent of psittacosis, whereas *Chlamydia trachomatis* is a specifically human pathogen. There are three major groups of infections caused by the 15 *C. trachomatis* serotypes recognized. L1, L2, and L3 cause lymphogranuloma venereum (LGV) and are more invasive with a broader tissue spectrum than the other strains. Serotypes A, B, and C are the agents responsible for endemic blinding trachoma. The remaining serotypes, D through K, are the sexually transmitted agents that cause urethritis, cervicitis, epididymitis, salpingitis, urethral syndrome, newborn conjunctivitis, and pneumonia. The chlamydial organism has a unique growth cycle existing in two forms. The infectious particle, the *elementary* body, is capable of entering uninfected cells where it reorganizes to produce an *initial* body. The initial body undergoes binary fission with coexisting initial and elementary bodies contained within an expanding lysosome, which appears as a rounded intracytoplasmic inclusion. Within 48 to 72 hours, the host cell bursts, releasing the highly infectious elementary bodies. Infection spreads from cell to cell along the epithelial surface in this manner. The elementary bodies have an affinity for columnar and pseudostratified epithelium. *C. trachomatis* is a bacterium containing DNA and RNA, possesses a cell wall, and is susceptible to antibiotics. However, it has similarities to viruses in that it is an obligate intracellular parasite.

Genitourinary chlamydial infections are the most common sexually transmitted diseases (STDs) in the United States, with an estimated 4 million cases annually. Infections are most prevalent in young, promiscuous, indigent, unmarried, inner-city women, especially with concomitant or prior history of other STDs. For instance, women with endocervical gonorrhea (GC) have a 25% to 50% rate of co-existing chlamydial infection. Male partners with nongonococcal urethritis (NGU) have a 29% to 68% rate of chlamydial infection. In the United States, approximately 4% to 5% of sexually active women carry chlamydia in their cervix, and this site appears to play a central role in transmission, with *horizontal* spread to male partners and *vertical* spread to neonates. The infection rate for an infant of an infected mother is 60% to 70%, with a 10% to 20% risk of pneumonia and a 25% to 55% risk of conjunctivitis. The incidence of *ascending* infection to the endometrium, fallopian tubes, and pelvic peritoneum is not known, but it is estimated that chlamydia is associated with 5% to 10% of acute pelvic inflammatory disease (PID) in the United States.

Seventy percent of women with genital chlamydial infections are asymptomatic. *Mucopurulent cervicitis* has been associated with a variable incidence of chlamydial infection. Diagnosis of mucopurulent cervicitis is established by the presence of yellow or green endocervical secretions on a white swab and by cervical friability (bleeds to touch). When compared with gonococcal or mixed aerobic/anaerobic salpingitis, women with chlamydial *salpingitis* are often less clinically ill, with minimal or no leukocytosis. However, paradoxically, sequelae may be even more severe, possibly due to delayed or absent treatment, resulting in tubal infertility and an increased risk of ectopic pregnancy and chronic pelvic pain. The *acute urethral syndrome* is characterized by frequency, dysuria, and pyuria, with a negative urinary culture. Chlamydia has been found in many of these cases studied. Acute *epididymitis* complicates NGU in 5% of men with the disease, and *Chlamydia* is the etiologic agent in 23% to 55% of men with NGU. Here again, the condition is clinically milder than the GC infection. Chlamydiae also have been associated with *proctitis* and *prostatitis*. Their role in *endometritis* and *bartholinitis* is unclear, but the organism has been found in both entities. Acute *perihepatitis* associated with salpingitis (Fitz-Hugh-Curtis syndrome) is probably usually chlamydial rather than gonococcal in origin. Chlamydial infection is the leading cause of *conjunctivitis* and afebrile interstitial *pneumonia* among infants younger than 6 months of age in the United States and also may cause *otitis media* in this group. The effect of maternal chlamydial infection on pregnancy outcome and perinatal complications, such as preterm delivery, premature rupture of membranes, and postpartum endometritis, remains controversial.

Chlamydia trachomatis may be isolated using tissue culture. To perform this, cycloheximide-treated McCoy cells are first incubated and then stained with iodine or Giemsa, or both, and examined microscopically for the presence of inclusions. Culture, however, is difficult, expensive, and slow. Two major rapid direct antigen tests are commercially available. They are faster but do require skilled personnel for interpretation. These tests react to chlamydial antigen in clinical specimens. They use either fluorescein-conjugated monoclonal antibodies to visualize the chlamydial elementary bodies in smears or enzyme immunoassay, which provides an objective colorimetric test. The most sensitive and specific tests, superior to culture and antigen assays, employ DNA amplification techniques. They are the polymerase chain reaction (PCR) and the ligase chain reaction (LCR) tests. The DNA tests may be used on urine and vulvar samples in addition to cervical samples. These tests do not require the maintenance of a cold chain to store specimens en route to the laboratory. Serologic testing is of little clinical value because neither seropositives nor seronegatives reliably correlate with infection or absence of infection.

Diagnosis and treatment of chlamydial infections are frequently based on the clinical syndrome. Uncomplicated urethral, endocervical, or rectal infections are best treated with a single 1-g dose of azithromycin, an azalide antibiotic, with observation of therapy. Alternatively, tetracycline (500 mg orally four times daily for 7 days) or doxycycline (100 mg orally twice daily for 7 days) may be used. Erythromycin is the obstetric treatment of choice. Erythromycin ethylsuccinate 400 to 800 mg four times daily for 7 days is preferred. Amoxicillin 500 mg three times daily for 7 days or azithromycin 1 g are alternative regimens. As discussed in Chapter 64, an antichlamydial agent is part of a combination therapy approach to the treatment of PID. Neonatal infections are best treated with systemic erythromycin. Additional drugs that have demonstrated activity against *Chlamydia* include ofloxacin, sulfamethoxazole-trimethoprim, rifampin, and clindamycin. Sex partners should be treated, and tests of cure should be performed in pregnant women. Cure rates of 95% are to be expected, and persistent positive testing suggests noncompliance or reinfection.

Empiric treatment is effective in an individual patient but does not address the larger issues of epidemiologic control. Three general approaches can be used. First, the reservoir can be reduced by the routine use of antichlamydial therapy when treating GC; by effective treatment of NGU, including the sexual contact; and by managing mucopurulent cervicitis as with NGU in men. Second, topical erythromycin should replace silver nitrate for ocular prophylaxis in the neonate. Third, the routine testing of pregnant women is probably warranted when the prevalence of the disease exceeds 6% to 12%.

Prevalence / Screening

1. Centers for Disease Control and Prevention. *Chlamydia trachomatis* genital infections—United States, 1995. *JAMA* 1997;277:952.
   Screening is indicated at the following types of clinics: STD, adolescent, family planning, abortion, detention center, prenatal.
2. Howell MR, et al. Screening women for *Chlamydia trachomatis* in family planning clinics: the cost effectiveness of DNA amplification assays. *Sex Transm Dis* 1998;25:108.
   There is a positive relationship between assay sensitivity and cost. DNA amplification techniques can provide cost savings in that urine tests on unexamined women are as reliable as cervical samples.
3. Lloyd F, et al. Screening for *Chlamydia trachomatis* in women referred for legal abortion. *J Obstet Gynaecol* 1991;11:224.
   Doxycycline prophylaxis can prevent C. trachomatis infection following legal abortion. Infected women tended to be younger and unmarried, and the prevalence of infection was 9.8%.
4. Todd CS, et al. *Chlamydia trachomatis* and febrile complications of postpartum tubal ligation. *Am J Obstet Gynecol* 1997;176(Pt 1):100.
   Women infected with Chlamydia *at delivery were more likely to experience febrile postoperative complications after tubal ligation.*

Diagnosis

5. Sellors J, et al. *Chlamydia* cervicitis: testing the practice guidelines for presumptive diagnosis. *CMAJ* 1998;13:41.
   Friability, ectopy, and polymorph count were poorly predictive of Chlamydia *or GC; screening of at-risk women is preferred.*
6. Dean D, Ferrero D, McCarthy M. Comparison of performance and cost-effectiveness of direct fluorescent-antibody, ligase chain reaction, and PCR assays for verification of chlamydial enzyme immunoassay results for populations with a low to moderate prevalence of *Chlamydia trachomatis* infections. *J Clin Microbiol* 1998;36:94.
   DNA amplification techniques using ligase chain reaction can be done on urine and are 95% accurate, superior to direct antigen assays or culture.
7. Hammerschlag MR, et al. Use of polymerase chain reaction for the detection of *Chlamydia trachomatis* in ocular and nasopharyngeal specimens from infants with conjunctivitis. *Pediatr Infect Dis J* 1997;16:293.
   Because neither silver nitrate nor antibiotics are effective in preventing neonatal chlamydial ophthalmia, the most effective control method may be by screening and treating pregnant women.
8. Kellock DJ, et al. Lymphogranuloma venereum: biopsy, serology, and molecular biology. *Genitourin Med* 1997;73:399.
   Rare in the United States, the diagnosis usually is made serologically and by exclusion of other causes of inguinal lymphadenopathy or genital ulcers.

Clinical Features

9. Davis A. Chlamydia: the most common sexually transmitted infection. *Nurs Times* 1998;94:56.
   More cases of chlamydia are documented than of gonorrhea, syphilis, and herpes combined. The annual cost of treating the infections and its complications exceeds $1.4 billion.
10. Tait IA, Duthie SJ, Taylor-Robinson D. Silent upper genital tract chlamydia infection and disease in women. *Int J STD AIDS* 1997;8:329.
    The majority of women are asymptomatic, and historical variables are typically not predictive of risk.

11. Brunham RC, et al. *Chlamydia trachomatis*–associated ectopic pregnancy: serologic and histologic correlates. *J Infect Dis* 1992;165:1076.
   Chlamydia trachomatis antibodies and tubal plasma cell infiltration were associated with ectopic pregnancy.
12. Jones RB, et al. *Chlamydia trachomatis* in the pharynx and rectum of heterosexual patients at risk for genital infection. *Ann Intern Med* 1985;102:757.
   Pharyngeal infection occurs in 3% to 5% of persons with genital Chlamydia *who participate in orogenital sex. It is not clear that* C. trachomatis *causes symptomatic pharyngitis.*
13. Sweet RL, et al. *Chlamydia trachomatis* infection and pregnancy outcome. *Am J Obstet Gynecol* 1987;156:824.
   Management strategy for chlamydial infection provides for treatment in the late third trimester in order to avoid perinatal transmission to the vaginally delivered neonate.
14. Mosure DJ, et al. Genital chlamydia infections in sexually active female adolescents: do we really need to screen everyone? *J Adolesc Health* 1997;20:6.
   Frequent recurrences with the same serovar suggest reinfection or relapse. Adolescents should be rescreened regularly.
15. Wasserheit JN. Epidemiological synergy: interrelationships between human immunodeficiency virus infection and other sexually transmitted diseases. *Sex Transm Dis* 1992;19:61.
   Chlamydial infections may facilitate HIV transmission.

Treatment
16. 1998 Guidelines for treatment of STD. *MMWR* 1998;47:RR-1.
   Treatment regimens and guidelines for the management of chlamydial infections from the Centers for Disease Control.
17. Hillis SD, et al. Doxycycline and azithromycin for prevention of chlamydial persistence or recurrence one month after treatment in women. A use-effectiveness study in public health settings. *Sex Transm Dis* 1998;25:5.
   Compliance with prolonged therapy is questionable and single-dose, directly observed therapy is preferable if financially feasible.
18. Kuhn GJ, et al. Diagnosis and follow-up of *Chlamydia trachomatis* infections in the ED. *Am J Emerg Med* 1998;16:157.
   The high cost of testing cannot be justified without proper follow-up. In this report, 105 of 181 women were inadequately treated at the initial visit.
19. Adair CD, et al. *Chlamydia* in pregnancy: a randomized trial of azithromycin and erythromycin. *Obstet Gynecol* 1998;91:165.
   Azithromycin was associated with significantly fewer gastrointestinal side effects, had similar efficacy, and was easy to administer.
20. Scholes D, et al. Prevention of pelvic inflammatory disease by screening for cervical chlamydial infection. *N Engl J Med* 1996;334:1362.
   Diagnosis and treatment of chlamydial cervicitis decreases the incidence of pelvic inflammatory disease.

---

59. HUMAN PAPILLOMAVIRUS

Michel E. Rivlin

The spectrum of disease resulting from infection with human papillomavirus (HPV) includes both the clinical (genital warts and condyloma acuminata) and subclinical involvement of the cervix, vagina, vulva, perineal body, and anus. Furthermore, there is an association with intraepithelial neoplasia of these areas and the male genitalia. It has also been shown that HPV deoxyribonucleic acid (DNA) is present in most squamous cancers of the female and male genital tracts. Although HPV is probably not the primary etiologic agent responsible for these cancers, it is probably a strong cocarcinogen. Finally, juvenile laryngeal papillomatosis is an uncommon, but important disorder caused by the virus.

The prevalence of HPV is linked to sexual activity, and HPV frequently coexists with other sexually transmitted diseases (STDs). Genital warts are the most common viral STD in the United States, and a minimum of 10% to 20% of sexually active adults are thought to be infected, with the predominant age 15 to 30 years. Approximately 2% to 3% of unselected Papanicolaou (Pap) smears are positive for the virus, and DNA testing indicates an additional 20%. Finding HPV in any area of the genital tract suggests that the virus is present in the remainder of the tract. HPV lesions are difficult to eradicate, with a very high recurrence rate that is possibly related to the existence of untreated lesions in sexual partners, but probably more often to persistent, latent virus in otherwise normal-appearing skin and squamous mucous membranes in other areas.

Human papillomavirus is classified as a subgroup of the papovaviruses because of the icosahedral virion capsids (i.e., the protein shell of a virus that acts as an antigen) and circular double-stranded DNA. Attempts to cultivate the virus have been unsuccessful, but advances in molecular biology, particularly nucleic acid hybridization (i.e., the formation of a complex between two single-stranded nucleic acid molecules), have led to the definition of more than 60 distinct types of HPV. The types are based on the viral DNA sequence (genotype) rather than on antigenic features (serotype). More than 30 virus types have been found to be associated with anogenital tract lesions. HPV types 16, 18, and 45 tend to be found in the presence of high-grade lesions and invasive cancers, whereas types 6 and 11 are usually associated with condyloma acuminata or low-grade lesions. However, cervical intraepithelial neoplasia (CIN) type I frequently contains types 16 and 18. In minor and early lesions, the DNA is circular and remains episomal (i.e., a foreign DNA molecule that is distinct from the host DNA and replicating autonomously). In more severe lesions, the virus is integrated into the host cell genome by opening its circular form, binding covalently to the host DNA, and then replicating with it (integrated DNA). In advanced lesions, abnormal host cell DNA replication results in a marked tendency toward aneuploidy, as demonstrated by flow cytometry. The lesions associated with HPV 6 and 11 usually have a diploid or polyploid DNA histogram.

The oncoproteins encoded by high-risk HPVs such as E6 and E7 inactivate tumor suppressor gene products such as p53 and RB. This disturbs cell cycle control, leading to genetic instability, enhancing the risk of mutations with tumor progression. This interplay of cellular and viral factors determines whether the outcome is active infection, viral latency, or ultimately genital cancer.

The carcinogenic potential of HPVs was first recognized when squamous cell cancers arose from Shope HPV-induced warts of domestic rabbits. The rate of malignant conversion depended on the viral strain, host species, and individual rabbit response. The frequency and speed of conversion were strongly increased by concomitant exposure to chemical carcinogens. Furthermore, the viral genome persisted in the cancer cells in a high copy number and continuously expressed viral gene products. The potential role of HPV was first substantiated in the setting of squamous cell cancers arising in epidermodysplasia verruciformis (a disease characterized by multiple flat warts of nongenital skin in patients with congenitally impaired cellular immunity). The importance of host immunity is further demonstrated by the rapid enlargement and spread of condylomata associated with the natural immunosuppression of pregnancy and the abnormal immunosuppression observed for some drugs and diseases (e.g., renal transplantation). Humoral immunity appears to protect against infection and spread, but cell-mediated immunity probably determines whether lesions regress, persist, or progress to become premalignant and malignant disease. Molecular cloning techniques of HPV DNA types from benign and malignant tumors of the oral, laryngeal, epidermal, and anogenital areas have provided probes (known DNA- or ribonucleic acid [RNA]-labeled to detect a given target DNA or RNA, respectively; the label is a radioactive or biotinylated nucleotide that is incorporated into the probe) to establish the consistent relationship between the HPV types of various pathologic conditions. Molecular probe technologies screening for virus infection by hybridization analysis are more accurate than cytologic smears. These techniques include in situ hybridization and the hybrid capture system. The tests vary in their sensitivity, the type of specimen needed (swabs or fixed tissues), level of difficulty, time required, and cost. Some of the tests incorporate the use of restriction endonucleases (enzymes that cut DNA at unique sites). Polymerase chain reaction (PCR) technology has further expanded the ability to recognize specific viral DNA using extremely small samples. The clinical application of this technology is unclear because the natural history of HPV infections is not known, so the use of routine HPV DNA typing may be indicated only in questionable situations.

Many HPV-infected women complain of fleshy warts on the external genitals, usually around the vulva, introitus, perineum, anus, or urethra. The cervix also may have fleshy fibroepithelial proliferations. The virus has a predilection for adolescents, probably because of their cervical biologic immaturity. Teenagers typically have larger areas of squamous cell metaplasia than do adults, and this affords the easy access to basal epithelium necessary for infection. Condylomata acuminata cause symptoms of itching, burning, pain, and tenderness. Cervical or vaginal infections are usually asymptomatic. Up to 50% of the patients with perineal warts also have them in the anal canal. The latent period from the time of exposure to the development of lesions averages about 3 months, but can be much longer. Warts may be difficult to control in pregnant women and may bleed or even necessitate abdominal delivery to prevent extensive vaginal damage. There is also a small but potentially serious risk of transmission to the infant, who may later manifest anogenital or laryngeal papillomata (HPV types 6 and 11). Possible modes of transmission include the transplacental and intrapartal routes, as well as postnatal contact, and there is usually a latent period of years before the lesions become clinically significant. Because the mode of transmission is unknown and the risk unclear, there is no consensus regarding the need for cesarean versus vaginal delivery. To avoid this dilemma, many advocate eradication of the warts during pregnancy and have reported success with various modes of therapy.

Human papillomavirus preferentially infects the basal cell layer, thereby inducing cellular proliferation. Exophytic warts are characterized by the marked proliferation of epithelial cells and upward papillomatous protrusion. Basal layers contain many mitoses; superficial layers exhibit marked koilocytosis, acanthosis, and parakeratosis. Flat warts, commonly seen on the cervix, display similar changes but are nonpapillomatous. Exfoliated cells exhibit koilocytosis (perinuclear cavitation), nuclear enlargement, and chromatin smudging. After the application of 5% acetic acid (vinegar), flat cervical warts were found to be blanched, white, flat, epithelial lesions on colposcopy. Blood vessels protruding through the epithelial surface may create an undulating or "spiked" appearance. CIN owing to HPV is similar but also may have an irregular vascular pattern with a punctate or mosaic appearance. Exophytic warts seldom require biopsy for diagnosis, although cervical flat warts usually rule out CIN. The differential diagnosis of anogenital warts includes molluscum contagiosum (poxvirus), verruca vulgaris (nongenital HPV infection), secondary syphilis (condylomata lata), squamous hyperplasia, and vulvar intraepithelial and invasive neoplasias. It is advised that the genitals and perianal area in the male partner also be inspected under magnification after the application of 5% acetic acid because the reported rate of condyloma transmission is 64%, the virus frequently being of the same type in both men and women.

Visible lesions can be eradicated by means of any of a wide variety of treatment alternatives, but all are associated with a high rate of symptomatic clinical recurrence. Therefore, both the patient and her partner must be counseled about the unpredictable natural history of the disease and possible increased risk of lower genital tract malignancy. A widely used treatment is topical podophyllin, a keratolytic agent that is then washed off thoroughly in 4 hours because it is toxic and otherwise absorbed. Recurrence is common, and if there is no response after four weekly applications, other treatments are indicated. Topically applied trichloroacetic or bichloroacetic acid, other keratolytics, is more efficacious, but repeated treatments may be required. Topically administered 5-fluorouracil may be the treatment of choice for vaginal, perianal, and urethral warts, but severe reactions are common. Cryotherapy and electrocautery reportedly achieve cure rates of 63% and 90%, respectively, and may be performed under local anesthesia in an ambulatory setting. Carbon dioxide laser ablation using colposcopic guidance can be expanded to include all HPV-related diseases; however, the time, cost, and morbidity rates of laser vaporization must be taken into account. There is also a possibility, although no conclusive documentation exists, that smoke from vaporized tissue may contain viral particles that could possibly induce respiratory tract lesions in treatment personnel. Intralesional alpha interferon therapy is modestly effective, with complete remission observed in about 50% of cases. However, dose-related side effects and high costs have limited the use of this treatment to refractory cases. Patient-applied treatments include podofilox 0.5% solution or gel and imiquimod 5% cream. Imiquimod is a topically active immune enhancer applied three times a week for up to 16 weeks.

The treatment of lesions in pregnant women is difficult, but good results have been reported with both cryotherapy and laser ablation. Trichloroacetic acid may be used, but imiquimod, podophyllin, 5-fluorouracil, and immunotherapy should be avoided during pregnancy. The male partner should be examined, and any visible lesions should be treated using the same therapeutic modalities as those used in the female. There is no vaccine against HPV, nor is there any specific antiviral drug or protocol. The only currently effective means of minimizing the risk of transmission is barrier contraception. Frequent anxiety-provoking follow-up visits and repeated treatments over the course of many years may be required. This is often difficult and frustrating for both the patient and the physician.

Reviews
1. Lorincz AT, Reid R. Human papillomavirus I. *Obstet Gynecol Clin North Am* 1996;23:3.
   Eight chapters review various aspects of the basic science and clinical aspects of HPV infection.
2. Lorincz AT, Reid R. Human papillomavirus II. *Obstet Gynecol Clin North Am* 1996;23:4.
   A further eight chapters conclude the review started in the previous volume. Reid's chapter on management is particularly informative.

Virology
3. Matsuura Y, et al. Low grade cervical intraepithelial neoplasia associated with human papillomavirus infection. Long-term follow-up. *Acta Cytol* 1998;42:625.
   The unpredictable clinical evolution of cervical dysplasia is linked to the diversity of genital types associated with the disease.
4. Autillo-Touati A, et al. HPV typing by in situ hybridization on cervical cytologic smears with ASCUS. *Acta Cytol* 1998;42:631.
   HPV DNA testing provides objective information that could be helpful in the follow-up of low-grade cytologic abnormalities.
5. Minkoff H, et al. A longitudinal study of human papillomavirus carriage in human immunodeficiency virus-infected and human immunodeficiency virus-uninfected women. *Am J Obstet Gynecol* 1998;178:982.
   Immunosuppressed persons may respond to therapy less well and have more frequent recurrences, and malignancy might occur more frequently.

HPV Infections
6. Ho GY, et al. Natural history of cervicovaginal papillomavirus infection in young women. *N Engl J Med* 1998;338:423.
   Differing disease patterns arise partly from the predilection of specific viral types for certain sites and through variations in host response. Disease expression may represent the focal breakdown of host surveillance within a field of latent infection.

7. Arends MJ, Buckley CH, Wells M. Aetiology, pathogenesis, and pathology of cervical neoplasia. *J Clin Pathol* 1998;51:96.
   Cervical dysplasia is a common and early manifestation of cervical HPV infection, particularly types 16 and 18.
8. Kruger-Kjaer S, et al. Different risk factor patterns for high-grade and low-grade intraepithelial lesions on the cervix among HPV-positive and HPV-negative young women. *Int J Cancer* 1998;76:613.
   Tobacco smoking is associated with sexual behavior; however, it seems likely that there is also a direct carcinogenic effect of cigarette smoking on the cervix.
9. Badaracco G, et al. Concurrent HPV infection in oral and genital mucosa. *J Oral Pathol Med* 1998;27:130.
   There is a high incidence of oral HPV lesions in patients with extensive genital condylomata.
10. Vernon SD, Unger ER, Reeves WC. Human papillomavirus and anogenital cancer. *N Engl J Med* 1998;338:921.
    Coexistence of anal intraepithelial neoplasia in women with high-grade cervical lesions is indicative of a multifocal disease process.
11. van Beurden M, et al. Human papillomavirus DNA in multicentric vulvar intraepithelial neoplasia. *Int J Gynecol Pathol* 1998;17:12.
    In contrast to the natural history of cervical lesions, the natural history of vulval, vaginal, and anal intraepithelial neoplasia is poorly understood.
12. Venturoli S, et al. Evaluation of immunoassays for the detection and typing of PCR amplified human papillomavirus DNA. *J Clin Pathol* 1998;51:143.
    Polymerase chain reaction techniques are highly efficient in detecting specific viral DNA.
13. Bergman A, Nalick R. Prevalence of human papillomavirus infection in men. Comparison of the partners of infected and uninfected women. *J Reprod Med* 1992;37:710.
    There were HPV-associated lesions in 69% of the men with infected partners and in 2% of the men with uninfected partners.

HPV and Pregnancy

14. Geijersstam V, et al. Trends in seroprevalence of human papillomavirus type 16 among pregnant women in Stockholm, Sweden, during 1969–1989. *Int J Cancer* 1998;76:341.
    The association of serum antibodies to HPV proteins with HPV-related disease is well established and useful for epidemiologic studies, but low sensitivity precludes diagnostic use.
15. Watts DH, et al. Low risk of perinatal transmission of human papillomavirus: results from a prospective cohort study. *Am J Obstet Gynecol* 1998;178:365.
    Whether adult-onset disease is due to latent virus or to later infection (e.g., by oral sex) is not known. Because genital infection is common and respiratory papillomatosis is rare (350 new cases in the United States annually), it is estimated that 80 cesarean deliveries would be needed to protect one baby at risk.
16. Ray R, et al. Pathological case of the month. Recurrent respiratory papillamatosis. *Arch Pediatr Adolesc Med* 1998;152:407.
    Laryngeal papillomas exhibit a bimodal age distribution, with the first peak in children 2 to 5 years of age and the second peak in adults. The clinical course is commonly characterized by multiple recurrences after surgical excision. They may produce respiratory obstruction. In most juvenile patients, they regress, generally at about the time of puberty.

Treatment

17. Centers for Disease Control. Guidelines for treatment of sexually transmitted diseases. *MMWR* 1998;47:RR1.
    Useful guide to details of available therapies.
18. Matsunaga J, Bergman A, Bhatia NN. Genital condylomata acuminata in pregnancy: effectiveness, safety and pregnancy outcome following cryotherapy. *Br J Obstet Gynaecol* 1987;94:168.

Affected women were treated as outpatients every 2 weeks until the warts were resolved. Labor and delivery were unaffected, even by cervical cryotherapy.
19. Schwartz DB, et al. Genital condylomas in pregnancy: use of trichloroacetic acid and laser therapy. *Am J Obstet Gynecol* 1988;158:1407.
   This combination therapy was effective in controlling condylomata in 97% of the patients. The complication and recurrence rates were low.
20. Krebs H, Helmkamp F. Chronic ulcerations following topical therapy with 5-fluorouracil for vaginal human papillomavirus-associated lesions. *Obstet Gynecol* 1991;78:205.
   A pyrimidine antimetabolite, 5-fluorouracil, causes sloughing of growing tissue. It is usually applied into the vagina or vestibule weekly for 12 weeks.
21. Hernandez E, et al. Interferon as an adjunct to laser therapy in the treatment of recalcitrant vulvar condylomata acuminata: a pilot study. *Am J Gynecol Health* 1992;6:35.
   The interferons, a family of glycoproteins with antiviral, antiprolific, and immunomodulatory properties, may be administered by either intralesional or intramuscular injection, alone or in combination with other therapies.
22. Beutner KR, et al. Imiquimod, a patient-applied immune-response modifier for treatment of external genital warts. *Antimicrob Agents Chemother* 1998;42:789.
   Iquimod stimulates production of interferon and other cytokines, and mild to moderate local inflammatory reactions are common.
23. Hines JF, Ghim SJ, Jenson AB. Prospects for human papillomavirus vaccine development: emerging HPV vaccines. *Curr Opin Obstet Gynecol* 1998;10:15.
   No evidence indicates that currently available treatments eradicate or affect the natural history of HPV infection.

---

60. ACQUIRED IMMUNODEFICIENCY SYNDROME

Michel E. Rivlin

When acquired immunodeficiency syndrome (AIDS) first came to the medical attention of the medical community in the United States in 1981, the affected groups seemed to comprise a sort of "4-H club" of homosexual and bisexual men, heroin and other illicit intravenous drug users, hemophiliacs, and Haitians. Since then, it has become clear that the sexual partners of patients with the infection are at risk for developing AIDS (horizontal transmission) and that pregnant women can transmit the disease to their children (vertical transmission). The occurrence of a disease that is at least moderately predictive of a defect in cell-mediated immunity in an individual with no other known source of diminished resistance to that disease constitutes the core concept of AIDS. However, AIDS is just one facet of the many manifestations of infection with the human immunodeficiency virus (HIV) and represents only the tip of the large iceberg of infection with HIV. Diseases that indicate immunocompromise include both opportunistic infections (e.g., *Pneumocystis carinii* pneumonia, cytomegalovirus infection, and toxoplasmosis) and neoplasias such as Kaposi's sarcoma and non-Hodgkin's lymphoma.

The HIV virion has a diameter of about 10 nm. It is classified as a retrovirus because its genetic material is ribonucleic acid (RNA), which directs production of deoxyribonucleic acid (DNA) (the reverse of the usual pattern), which then directs production of RNA, and this, in turn, directs production of viral proteins. The virus survives in the host in a latent state, during which viral genes are integrated into the DNA of host cells. Survival outside the host is limited, and the fragile organism is readily destroyed by simple disinfection. The virus most readily attacks cells with receptors for the T peptide, such as helper T_4 lymphocytes (CD4-positive cells) and neural cells. Helper cells play a key role in coordinating a variety of immune functions, including B-lymphocyte activity and the induction of natural killer cells. When helper cells are inactivated, the immune system is effectively disabled. The system is further damaged by HIV infection of the monocytes/macrophages. The striking lymphopenia typically found is specifically due to a quantitative and qualitative defect in the T4-inducer or -helper subset of T-lymphocytes, with a consequent reversal of the normal ratio to T8 suppressor-cytotoxic cells.

The effect of HIV on the nervous system is manifested by subacute encephalitis, vacuolar myelopathy, chronic meningitis, and peripheral neuropathy. Histologic studies reveal demyelination, focal necrosis, and the presence of multinucleated giant cells. The virus resides in the lymphocytes in semen and also has been isolated from cervical/vaginal secretions and breast milk. These fluids and blood have all been implicated in the transmission of the virus. Saliva, spinal fluid, urine, tears, and amniotic fluid also contain smaller amounts of virus but have not been implicated in transmission. Thus, any sexual act that can injure the mucosa, thereby providing a portal of entry for the virus, involves risk of transmission. Although oral intercourse and deep kissing pose theoretic risks, the exact probability of transmission is unknown. No evidence of casual transmission exists (e.g., by the sharing of utensils, or shaking hands). Accidental transmission to health-care workers has been infrequent and has always been related to direct inoculation or exposure of the skin to infected blood.

Between 1991 and 1995, the number of women in the United States with AIDS increased by 63%, more than any other group reported. At the end of this period there were an estimated 160,000 HIV-positive women, of whom about 45,000 had an AIDS-defining opportunistic illness (OI). Latin American and African-American women represent 14% of the population but constitute about 75% of the AIDS cases in women. In 1995, of women 25 to 44 years of age, one in 1,100 African-American women, one in 2,500 Hispanic women, and one in 15,000 white women were HIV-infected. Although it appears that most patients with AIDS are residents of large urban areas, the proportion of rural and suburban cases is increasing. Two major reasons for women's greater susceptibility to HIV infection during heterosexual intercourse are that (1) more men than women in the United States are infected and (2) HIV appears to be more easily transmitted from men to women than the reverse.

The majority of women with AIDS are intravenous drug users; the second most commonly affected group are those who have heterosexual contact with a person at risk for AIDS. Most childhood cases occur as perinatal infections, in most cases from mothers who abuse intravenous drugs or whose partners do. Since the screening of all blood and blood products for transfusions was implemented in 1985, the risk associated with transfusions has now become minimal. At this time, the three major risk groups are the sex partners of HIV-infected persons, infants born to infected mothers, and needle-sharing partners (or others with de facto parenteral contact) of those infected. Although the nature of transmission of HIV is similar to that of hepatitis B, HIV is less readily transmitted. In one report, the risk of transmission of hepatitis B from a needlestick-like exposure is 6% to 30%; the risk associated with HIV was 0.49%. Factors associated with an increased risk of transmission include an increased number of sex partners, the presence of genital ulcers (syphilis, herpes), and anal-receptive intercourse. An estimated 20% to 40% of the infants born to untreated infected mothers acquire HIV.

Antibodies to HIV are detected weeks to months after initial infection; viral culture and viral antigen studies show that virus is present and transmissible before antibody is detectable. It is therefore postulated that the clinical course of HIV infection commences with an initial asymptomatic incubation period, followed by a mild, self-limited, acute mononucleosis-like infection, probably occurring from 2 weeks to 3 months after exposure. This is followed by a period of asymptomatic seropositivity consisting in some patients of the development of generalized persistent lymphadenopathy and, in others, of severe systemic manifestations. Manifestations include anorexia, weight loss, fever, night sweats, rashes, fatigue, diarrhea, susceptibility to infection, or lymphadenopathy, or a combination of these. When lymphocytes are stimulated by a secondary infection, the latent virus replicates and breaks out of the lymphocytes, resulting in a depletion of T4 cells and leaving the patient vulnerable to OIs. Each infected lymphocyte can produce thousands of virus particles. OIs often stem from the reactivation of childhood infections that were latent until the immunosuppression occurs, such as in the case of *P. carinii*. Protozoal infections also include cryptosporidiosis and toxoplasmosis. Viral diseases consist of cytomegalovirus and herpes. Bacterial infections comprise tuberculosis, nocardiosis, and atypical mycobacteria. Fungal infections include *Candida,* histoplasmosis, and cryptococcosis. The immunologic and hematologic abnormalities encountered include hemolytic anemia, thrombocytopenia, and lymphadenopathy. In addition to the central nervous system manifestations of OI, many neurologic findings reflect a direct effect of HIV infection.

Tests for the immunoglobulin G (IgG) antibody to HIV begin with a serologic test of high, but not 100%, sensitivity (i.e., percentage of diseased patients with a positive test result). This is an enzyme-linked immunosorbent assay (ELISA) and is used as a screen. The results of these tests may be falsely positive, sometimes reflecting either autoimmune disease or the existence of cross-reacting antibodies resulting from transfusion or other viral infections. Tests are repeated if results are positive and, if results are again positive, usually a Western blot assay or a fluorescent method is used for confirmation. The Western blot is highly specific but is technically demanding to perform and requires subjective interpretation. The plasma HIV viral load is quantitated by measuring HIV DNA or RNA using polymerase chain reaction (PCR) technology. Virus culture is available only in specialized laboratories and is not generally available for diagnostic purposes. Although these positive test results for HIV indicate HIV infection, the diagnosis of AIDS requires the additional demonstration of an OI and the exclusion of other causes of immunodeficiency. If testing programs are developed, consent for testing must be obtained and seropositive patients must be provided with counseling given by properly trained persons. Knowledge of test results must be confined to those directly involved in the patient's care, or as required by law, with assurance of confidentiality. Infected patients must be provided with needed optimal care. HIV is a chronic infection with a variable course; it takes about 10 years from the time of infection for AIDS to develop in 50% of infected persons.

Several laboratory and clinical markers predict the risk of progression from asymptomatic HIV infection to AIDS, and the most useful of these are the absolute CD4 lymphocyte count and quantitative viral load. Antiretroviral therapies interfere with the replication of HIV. There are three major drug groups. The nucleoside reverse transcriptase inhibitors (nRTIs) prevent translation of RNA to DNA. Examples include zidovudine (AZT), didanosine (ddI), and zalcitabine (ddC). The major limiting toxicity of AZT is bone marrow suppression, and that of ddI is pancreatitis. AZT side effects also include headaches, nausea and vomiting, muscle weakness, and fatigue. Standard therapy of HIV infections includes multiple drugs in an attempt to limit drug resistance. Dual nRTI combinations usually form the basis of the regimens. The second group is composed of the nonnucleoside reverse transcriptase inhibitors. These include nevirapine and delaverdine and may be used with a dual nRTI regimen. The third group is composed of the protease inhibitors, including indinavir, ritonavir, nelfinavir, and sequinovir. These may be given as dual therapy, or with a dual nRTI regimen. Gastrointestinal adverse effects are common, and there may be long-term metabolic disturbances, including hyperlipidemia, lipodystrophy, and insulin resistance resulting in accelerated atherosclerosis. The combination regimens are very effective, but close adherence to dosage schedules is imperative and requires multiple pills at different times of the day, and the drugs are extremely expensive. Drug resistance and severe interdrug reactions are common, as is nonadherence to the schedules, especially as general health improves. Both primary prophylaxis (prevention of illness) and secondary prophylaxis (prevention of recurrence) for opportunistic infections are available and indicated for the suppression of several diseases, including pneumocystic pneumonia, candidiasis, herpes, tuberculosis, toxoplasmosis, cryptococcosis, cytomegalovirus, and the *Mycobacterium avium intracellulare* complex. Guidelines are given for initiating antiretroviral treatment and pneumocystic pneumonia prophylaxis based on a plasma HIV-1 RNA level above 5,000 to 10,000 copies/ml and on CD4 counts, generally less than 500/µl for antivirals and less than 200/µl for trimethoprim-sulfamethoxazole. The T-cell levels decline slowly, such that 3- to 6-monthly testing intervals are generally acceptable. Patients should be screened for the existence of syphilis, hepatitis, cervical dysplasia, tuberculosis, and fungal disorders. Vaccine schedules should be updated, nutritional needs met, and mental health and substance abuse interventions supplied.

The available strategy for preventing the spread of HIV is to eliminate the vectors that are responsible for spreading the disease: sex or needle-sharing with infected persons, births to infected persons, injections of HIV by means of transfusions or needlestick injuries, and unusual de facto parenteral transfer. The combined use of education, motivation, and skill building; serologic screening; and contact tracing and notification could substantially reduce the rate of transmission. The message that should be communicated is that any sexual intercourse (outside of mutually monogamous or HIV antibody-negative relationships) must be protected with a condom. Unsterile needles or syringes should not be shared, and all exposed women should be tested before pregnancy and, if positive, should avoid pregnancy. Because medical history and examination cannot reliably identify all infected patients, blood and body fluid precautions should be consistently adopted for all patients (universal precautions). Barriers should be used to prevent skin and mucous membrane exposure when contact with blood or body fluids of any patient is anticipated. Gloves may protect the hands, masks and protective eyewear may protect the head, and gowns or aprons may protect against splashes. The hands or other skin should be washed immediately after contamination. Needles should not be recapped or manipulated by hand. After use, sharp instruments should be discarded in readily available puncture-proof containers. In order to avoid contact with body fluids during resuscitation, specially designed ventilation devices should be readily available, and wall suction devices should be employed for clearing the airway. Blood spills should be cleaned off with 0.5% sodium hypochlorite solution (diluted bleach). Isolation is required only if the patient's hygiene is poor. If a needlestick injury occurs, the health-care worker should be assessed and receive routine care for hepatitis B exposure. Prophylaxis with antiretroviral medication is indicated in certain situations. Antibody testing should be conducted and repeated at 6 weeks, 3 months, and 6 months; if this proves HIV-seronegative, follow-up may be discontinued. The care of pregnant women infected with HIV and of their children is detailed in Chapter 9.

Any communicable disease that affects primarily young, previously healthy individuals and has a mortality rate in excess of 80% clearly requires an urgent remedy. Unfortunately, until effective treatment and control programs are developed, the incidence of AIDS will continue to increase and its impact on human health and health-care resources will be felt throughout the world.

Reviews
1. Klirsfeld D. HIV disease and women. *Med Clin North Am* 1998;82:335.
   For all adults with HIV infection, routine immunization against influenza, Pneumococcus, Haemophilus influenza B, hepatitis B, tetanus, and diphtheria is indicated and advised.
2. Centers for Disease Control. Revised classification system and expanded AIDS surveillance definition for adolescents and adults. *MMWR* 1992;41:RR-17.
   The revised system emphasizes CD4 lymphocyte testing and is based on three ranges of CD4 counts and three clinical categories, giving a matrix of nine exclusive categories.
3. Kotler DP. HIV in pregnancy. *Gastroenterol Clin North Am* 1998;27:269.
   Most babies born to HIV-infected mothers will test positive because of the passive transmission of maternal IgG antibodies. A definitive diagnosis requires evidence of HIV in blood or tissues by culture, nucleic acid, or antigen detection.
4. Report of the NIH panel to define principles of therapy of HIV infection. *Ann Intern Med* 1998;128(Pt 2):1057.
   This report includes guidelines for the use of antiretroviral agents in HIV-infected adults and adolescents.

Epidemiology
5. Wortley PM, Fleming PL. AIDS in women in the United States. Recent trends. *JAMA* 1997;278:911.
   In 1995 women accounted for 19% of AIDS cases in adults. AIDS is the fourth leading cause of death in women between the ages of 25 and 44 years.
6. Mocroft A, et al. The incidence of AIDS-defining illnesses in 4883 patients with human immunodeficiency virus infection. *Arch Intern Med* 1998;158:491.
   Knowing the incidence of AIDS-defining illnesses across a wide range of CD4 lymphocyte counts enables disease-specific prophylaxis for the most appropriate population.
7. Public Health Service guidelines for the management of health-care worker exposures to HIV and recommendations for post exposure prophylaxis. *MMWR* 1998;47:RR-7.
   The occupational risk of acquiring HIV in health-care settings is low and is most often associated with the percutaneous inoculation of blood from an infected patient.
8. AIDS among persons aged > or = 50 years—United States, 1991–1996. *MMWR* 1998;47:21.
   Individuals over the age of 50 account for 11% of AIDS cases, of whom 16% are female. These older individuals are more likely to have advanced disease, probably because of diagnostic delay related to age.

Diagnostic Testing
9. De Cock KM, Johnson AM. From exceptionalism to normalisation: a reappraisal of attitudes and practice around HIV testing. *BMJ* 1998;316:290.
   Testing should be made available to all those whose behavior puts them at risk— pretest and posttest counseling is integral to the testing procedure, and informed consent must be obtained before testing. Patients should be offered testing that is both anonymous and confidential.
10. Centers for Disease Control. Update: serologic testing for antibody to human immunodeficiency virus. *JAMA* 1988;259:653.
    The ELISA has a sensitivity and specificity of better than 98%. Repeated reactive tests must be confirmed by another test, generally the Western blot. Positive blot reactions should be to three bands: P24, gp 41, and gp 120/60.
11. Sebire K, et al. Stability of human immunodeficiency virus RNA in blood specimens as measured by a commercial PCR-based assay. *J Clin Microbiol* 1998; 36:493.
    Not only does PCR HIV testing provide diagnostic information, but quantitative viral load monitoring also guides therapy and provides prognostic information.

Therapy and Prevention
12. Carpenter CC, et al. Antiretroviral therapy for HIV infection in 1998: updated recommendations of the International AIDS Society-USA Panel. *JAMA* 1998; 280:78.
    Potential advantages and disadvantages of aggressive, early therapy versus conservative management in which therapy is withheld until agreed-on CD4 cell counts or viral load limits present in the individual patient.
13. Luzuriaga K, Sullivan JL. Prevention and treatment of pediatric HIV infection. *JAMA* 1998;280:17.
    Infants born to HIV-1–infected women should be tested at birth by HIV-1 DNA PCR and repeatedly during the first months of life to ensure identification of infection and prompt treatment with potent combination antiretroviral therapies.
14. Public Health Service Task Force recommendations for the use of antiretroviral drugs in pregnant women infected with HIV-1 for maternal health and for reducing perinatal HIV-1 transmission in the United States. Centers for Disease Control and Prevention. *MMWR* 1998;47(RR-2):1.
    Recommendations include oral AZT from 14 weeks' gestation, IV zidovudine in labor, and neonatal oral AZT. Multiple drug therapy is indicated in certain women after expert consultation.

15. Yerly S, et al. A critical assessment of the prognostic value of HIV-1 RNA levels and CD4$^\pm$ cell counts in HIV-infected patients. *Arch Intern Med* 1998;158:247.
    The ratio of viral load over CD4$^\pm$ cell count provided the most useful predictor of clinical outcome.

16. Rosenstein IJ, et al. Effect on normal flora of three intravaginal microbicidal agents potentially active against human immunodeficiency virus type 1. *J Infect Dis* 1998;177:1386.
    Chemical irritation of the vaginal mucosa may actually enhance transmission of HIV, and an optimal dose or agent would inactivate the virus without irritation of the mucosa.

17. Newell ML. A randomised trial of mode of delivery in women infected with the human immunodeficiency virus. *Br J Obstet Gynaecol* 1998;105:281.
    Medical therapy is very effective in prevention of vertical HIV transmission, and cesarean delivery also may be effective, but the surgical risk appears unwarranted for the possibly marginal benefit.

18. Evans B, Darbyshire J, Cartledge J. Should preventive antiretroviral treatment be offered following sexual exposure to HIV? Not yet! *Sex Transm Infect* 1998; 74:146.
    Needle exchange programs, safe sex counseling, routine prophylaxis after occupational exposure, and perhaps postcoital prophylaxis will be added to these standard prophylactic recommendations, particularly in the context of sexual assault.

General
19. Schaker TW, et al. Biological and virologic characteristics of primary HIV infection. *Ann Intern Med* 1998;128:613.
    Plasma HIV RNA levels decrease to a nadir within 120 days of acquisition, after which they gradually increase. Acute infection is associated with clinical syndromes ranging from heterophil-negative mononucleosis to aseptic meningitis.

20. Palella FJ, et al. Declining morbidity and mortality among patients with advanced human immunodeficiency virus infection. HIV Outpatient Study Investigators. *N Engl J Med* 1998;338:853.
    Potent antivirals provide long-term control of viral replication with possible recovery of the immune system and the potential for converting HIV infection to a chronic controllable disease rather than one that is invariably fatal.

21. Plummer FA. Heterosexual transmission of human immunodeficiency virus type 1 (HIV): interactions of conventional sexually transmitted diseases, hormonal contraception and HIV-1. *AIDS Res Hum Retrovir* 1998;14[Suppl 1]:5.
    Cervical ectopy, common with exogenous hormones, and / or an infected, inflamed genital tract, common with STDs, increase exposure of HIV-susceptible cells to any HIV-infected material in the vagina, thus increasing the risk of HIV infection.

22. Maiman M. Prevalence, risk factors, and accuracy of cytologic screening for cervical intraepithelial neoplasia in women with the human immunodeficiency virus. *Gynecol Oncol* 1998;68:233.
    Most caregivers of HIV-infected women perform 6 monthly Pap smears and readily refer for colposcopy.

23. Perry S, et al. Effectiveness of psychoeducational interventions in reducing emotional distress after human immunodeficiency virus antibody testing. *Arch Gen Psychiatry* 1991;48:143.
    This article considers the value of supportive and cognitive counseling, the treatment of severe anxiety and depression, stress management techniques, and the merits of support groups and assistance that meet practical stage-specific needs at different points in the course of HIV infection.

61. VAGINITIS

Abraham Rubin

Vaginal discharge is the most common gynecologic complaint, but it is important to distinguish between leukorrhea and an infected vaginal discharge. Leukorrhea may be mucinous, due to reactive hypersecretion, resulting from the presence of cervical polyps or "erosions"; hyperestrogenic or postovulatory, resulting from the use of birth control pills; or caused by hyperdesquamation stemming from an exaggerated response of the vaginal mucosa to normal or abnormal hormonal stimulation. Hyperdesquamation is classically associated with a nonadherent, abundant, whitish discharge. There may be an associated itch in 30% of such patients. Therapy may be confined to reassuring the patient and confirming the noninfective nature of the condition. A subgroup of purulent vaginitis (desquamative inflammatory vaginitis), characterized by excessive epithelial cell exfoliation and a diffuse vaginitis, has been identified. It is associated with malodor, often only experienced during intercourse, and occasional dyspareunia. A microbiological, possibly gram-positive cocci, etiology is suspected. There is 95% clinical improvement with 2% topical clindamycin ointment.

A nonspecific vaginal discharge in adult women may be related to the presence of foreign materials, such as forgotten diaphragms, cotton balls, sponges, tampons, or even condoms. There is also an increased discharge associated with the use of an intrauterine device (IUD). Tight underwear or nylon may cause chafing, thus producing itching, vulvitis, and vaginitis with an excessive discharge. Allergies to various types of clothing fabrics, feminine deodorant sprays, detergents, soaps, and douches may produce a profuse leukorrhea. These conditions frequently become secondarily infected, stemming from damage to the epithelium caused by chemicals or after scratching in response to the intense pruritus. Atrophic vaginitis results from the loss of natural estrogens. It is seen in women after radiation therapy or oophorectomy and in menopausal women. The mucosa is easily fractured in these settings, and initially there is a nonspecific, often blood-stained discharge. Invasion by pathogenic organisms may follow.

The three most common vaginal infections in women of reproductive age are *Trichomonas vaginalis, Candida albicans,* and bacterial vaginosis, previously called *Gardnerella* vaginitis. *T. vaginalis* is transmitted sexually, usually in the immediate postmenstrual phase. The discharge involved is characteristically malodorous, frothy, and yellow and has a pH of 5.0 to 5.5. The infection may produce vulvovaginal erythema and edema. In its most severe form, petechiae with swollen vaginal papillae (strawberry vagina) may be seen. It must be stressed, however, that many infections cause reddened vaginas in conjunction with malodorous discharges, and *T. vaginalis* infection should therefore not be assumed based solely on these findings. Specimens for examination should be obtained from fairly high up on the posterior vaginal wall. The swab is placed in a saline tube and rotated several times, then applied to a slide and a coverslip placed over the area of the application. Motile trichomonads can be seen without the use of a specific stain. Trichomonads also can be seen on routine Papanicolaou (Pap) smears. Either metronidazole or analogs, 500 mg taken twice daily for 7 days or 2 g as a single dose, can cure 90% of the cases. It is important that the male partner also be treated. Oral metronidazole should not be used in the first trimester of pregnancy, although there is no definite evidence of teratogenesis. Metronidazole vaginal gel (0.75%) is preferred (even though there is some absorption). It is inserted twice daily for 5 days. If alcohol is consumed, metronidazole can produce side effects such as nausea and dizziness. In pregnant women, 15% of *T. vaginalis* infections are combined with candidiasis.

Candida albicans is the most common of the specific agents causing vaginitis in pregnant or diabetic women; however, it can be present in the vagina as a commensal organism, inciting neither reactions nor symptoms. In the past two decades, there has been a worldwide increase in the incidence of fungal diseases. This is ascribed to the increased use of antibiotics, corticosteroids, cytotoxic agents, and oral contraceptives. Candidiasis occurs in 6% to 28% of women, but its incidence doubles in pregnant women. Typical complaints include leukorrhea, pruritus, and dyspareunia. Examination usually reveals the classic features of a red, edematous vulva and vagina with a thick, creamy discharge that adheres in patches to the vaginal wall. Removal of these patches may leave petechiae. The malodor is usually due to associated bacterial vaginosis or trichomoniasis. Diagnosis is based on the microscopic examination of the discharge, which is mixed with 10% potassium hydrochloride. Distinct translucent spores and hyphae (filaments) are seen after the potassium hydrochloride destroys the cellular elements. Confirmatory cultures can be made by plating the discharge on Nickerson's medium. Nightly insertions of miconazole cream or equivalent agents placed high up into the vagina for a week are usually quite efficacious, although a repeat course is sometimes necessary. Single-dose oral therapy with fluconazole (150 mg) has been highly effective. It is not used in pregnant patients. Symptoms are not improved more rapidly with the oral medication.

Recurrent *C. albicans* infections are associated with cell-mediated immunization responses, and there is a 50% decrease in the luteal phase. Maintenance low-dose oral ketoconazole for 6 months can effectively prevent recurrences, although relapses may occur when therapy is stopped. Long-term treatment with ketoconazole may be hepatotoxic. The microwave sterilization of underwear at a high setting kills all the organisms in 5 minutes, thereby reducing the risks of reinfection. Depo-provera (medroxyprogesterone) injections substantially reduce the number of recurrences. Topical flucytosine can be used for strains that are resistant to common preparations. Refractory infections may be treated by painting the whole vagina with 1% gentian violet.

Bacterial vaginosis is probably a sexually transmitted disease, but there have been many reports of nonsexually transmitted infections. It occurs when the pH in the vagina is high between 5.0 and 5.5. Concomitant treatment of the male partner has not been shown to be beneficial. There is a significant association between bacterial vaginosis in pregnancy and both low-mean-birth-weight infants and premature rupture of membranes. If the leukorrhea is heavy, this usually indicates a mixed infection. Many patients are asymptomatic, whereas others have mild pruritus and burning. The discharge is malodorous, grayish, and homogenous. The symptoms and the odor are probably related to the effects of anaerobes, and *G. vaginalis* may be only a "marker" organism. Because it is a surface infection, inflammation is rare. A wet mount shows clumps of dark, stippled epithelium ("clue cells"), but at least 20% must be present to establish the diagnosis. There are few pus cells and often no lactobacilli. The addition of 10% potassium hydrochloride to the discharge accentuates the malodor ("whiff test").

Papanicolaou smears have a sensitivity of 90% and a specificity of 97% in the detection of bacterial vaginosis. Oligonucleotide probes (30-minute test) are now commercially available for the detection of the organism with a 94% sensitivity and 81% specificity for diagnosis.

Two species of motile, curved gram-negative anaerobic rods (*Mobiluncus mulieris* and *curtisi*) have been isolated from patients with bacterial vaginosis. Vaginitis emphysematosa (bullous vaginitis) is associated with *Trichomonas* and *G. vaginalis* infection in immunocompromised patients. Metronidazole is very effective at a dose of 500 mg twice daily for a week. Vaginal metronidazole gel is only 2% absorbed, thus reducing the side effects and making it suitable for use in pregnancy. Twice-daily application for 5 days is very effective. An alternative regimen is clindamycin (300 mg twice daily for 7 days or intravaginally as a cream).

Atrophic vaginitis is characterized by a pale, thin, diffuse redness. The mucosa is smooth with ecchymoses and petechiae and loss of the normal rugae. The discharge is variable, ranging from blood-stained, thick, or watery to purulent. The pH is only slightly acidic. Cultures reveal mixed, nonspecific bacterial flora. Vaginal cytologic examination reveals the presence of abundant parabasal or basal epithelial cells. Rapid relief of the burning, itching, and dyspareunia is obtained with the local application of estrogen cream. In severe cases in which there are other symptoms of menopause, orally administered estrogens also may be used. Postmenopausal patients with atrophic vaginitis and cervicitis may have abnormal cytology on Pap smears, which disappears after treatment with estrogens. Secondary infection, like any nonspecific infection, can be treated with local sulfonamide preparations. Allergic and chemical vulvovaginitis may be treated with local corticosteroid preparations. The prolonged use of antibiotics may allow fungal overgrowth to take place, and therapy should be combined with an antifungal cream in such cases. Intercourse should be avoided during any treatment for vaginitis.

Reviews
1. Sparks JM. Vaginitis. *J Reprod Med* 1991;36:745.
   This is an excellent review article on vaginitis.
2. Martius J, et al. The role of bacterial vaginosis as a cause of amniotic fluid infection, chorioamnionitis and prematurity. A review article. *Arch Gynecol Obstet* 1990;247:1.
   A higher incidence of infections has been observed if bacterial vaginosis is present.
3. Ross CA. Postmenopausal vaginitis. *J Med Microbiol* 1975;11:209.
   In this survey, infected and noninfected postmenopausal vaginitis is discussed.
4. Moi H, et al. Mobiluncus species in bacterial vaginosis: aspects of pathogenesis. *APMJS* 1991;99:1049.
   The role of these organisms in the causation of vaginitis is unclear.
5. Fong IW, McCleary P, Read S. Cellular immunity of patients with recurrent or refractory vulvo-vaginal moniliasis. *Am J Obstet Gynecol* 1992;166:887.
   There is normal cellular immunity in most women with recurrent moniliasis.
6. Josey WE, Campbell WG Jr. Vaginitis emphysematosa. A report of 4 cases. *J Reprod Med* 1990;35:974.
   The association between vaginitis emphysematosa and infectious vaginitis is well demonstrated. It may be a feature of these infections in the immunosuppressed patient.
7. Sobel JD. Desquamative inflammatory vaginitis: a new subgroup of purulent vaginitis responsive to topical 2% clindamycin therapy. *Am J Obstet Gynecol* 1994;171:1215.
   Estrogen deficiency may also be a factor.
8. Riethdorf L, et al. Vaginitis emphysematosa during immunosuppression therapy. *Arch Gynecol Obstet* 1995;256:39.
   Further evidence is provided of the association between immunosuppression and vaginitis emphysematosa.

Epidemiology
9. Holst E. Reservoir of four organisms associated with bacterial vaginosis suggests lack of sexual transmission. *J Clin Microbiol* 1990;28:2035.
   The infection is frequently unrelated to sexual activity.
10. Spinillo A, et al. Epidemiologic characteristics of women with idiopathic recurrent vulvovaginal candidiasis. *Obstet Gynecol* 1993;81:721.
    Appropriate counseling about contraception, sexual activity, and personal hygiene habits could be an important preventive measure in these women.
11. De Oliveira JM, et al. Prevalence of *Candida albicans* in vaginal fluid of asymptomatic Portuguese women. *J Reprod Med* 1993;38:41.
    The overall prevalence of infection was 10.4%, and rates were lower in women taking birth control pills (6.8%).
12. Kent HL. Epidemiology of vaginitis. *Am J Obstet Gynecol* 1991;165:1168.
    This article reviews the epidemiology of three major causes of vaginitis in the United States and Scandinavia. There has been an increase in non-albicans monilia and a decrease in trichomonas.

Diagnosis
13. Wolner-Hanssen P, et al. Clinical manifestations of vaginal trichomoniasis. *JAMA* 1989;261:571.
    The sensitivity of symptoms and signs is relatively low.
14. Schoomaker JN, et al. A new proline aminopeptide assay for diagnosis of bacterial vaginosis. *Am J Obstet Gynecol* 1991;165:737.
    This is a useful objective test.

15. Hiller SL. Diagnostic microbiology of bacterial vaginosis. *Am J Obstet Gynecol* 1993;169(Pt 2):455.
    Detailed descriptions of diagnostic methods and sensitivity and specificity results are offered for the detection of bacterial vaginosis.
16. Platz-Christensen J, et al. Detection of bacterial vaginosis in Papanicolaou smears. *Acta Obstet Gynecol Scand* 1994;74:67.
    Pap tests are an excellent method for detecting bacterial vaginosis.

Risk Factors
17. Soper DE, Bump RC, Hurt WG. Bacterial vaginosis and *Trichomoniasis* vaginitis are risk factors for cuff cellulitis after abdominal hysterectomy. *Am J Obstet Gynecol* 1990;163:1016.
    Patients with bacterial vaginosis were found to have a dramatic increase in anaerobic bacterial counts. The authors advise pH and wet mount evaluation prior to hysterectomy.
18. Barbone F, et al. A follow-up study of method of contraception, sexual activity and rates of trichomoniasis, candidiasis and bacterial vaginosis. *Am J Obstet Gynecol* 1990;163:510.
    There was 40% lower incidence of T. vaginalis infection in association with oral contraceptive use than with the use of IUD or tubal ligation. There was a reduced incidence (15%–20%) of trichomoniasis and bacterial vaginosis associated with spermicidal use.

Treatment
19. Sobel JD, Schmitt C, Meriwether C. Clotrimazole treatment of recurrent and chronic *Candida* vulvovaginitis. *Obstet Gynecol* 1989;73:330.
    There was initial clinical remission in 90% of the cases; however, only a modest long-term protective effect was observed for intermittent prophylaxis.
20. Sobel JD. Recurrent vulvovaginal candidiasis. A prospective study of the efficacy of maintenance ketaconazole therapy. *N Engl J Med* 1986;312:1455.
    This discusses the topic of elective treatment in preventing recurrences. Relapses commence when treatment is stopped. Long-term therapy may be hepatotoxic.
21. Livengoode CH, Thomason JL, Hill GB. Bacterial vaginosis: treatment with topical intravaginal clindamycin phosphate. *Obstet Gynecol* 1990;76:118.
    Topical clindamycin cured 93.5% of the infections with 5-day treatment. There was little absorption and few side effects.
22. Ison CA, et al. Local treatment for bacterial vaginosis. *Br Med J* 1987;295:886.
    Vaginal chlorhexidine is as effective as oral metronidazole in the cure of bacterial vaginosis.
23. Dennerstein GJ. Depo-provera in the treatment of recurrent vulvovaginal candidiasis. *J Reprod Med* 1986;31:801.
    Long-acting injectable progestogen (evaluated in a pilot study) appeared to substantially reduce women's susceptibility and recurrence.
24. Josef MR, et al. Bacterial vaginosis: review of treatment options and potential clinical indications for therapy. *Clin Infect Dis* 1995;1:572.
    This is a good review of the available management and outcomes of therapy.

62. TOXIC SHOCK SYNDROME

Michel E. Rivlin

Toxic shock syndrome (TSS) gained great notoriety in 1980 when the connection between menses, tampon use, and disease was recognized, resulting in the withdrawal of certain high-absorbency tampons from the market. It soon became clear that the syndrome was also associated with a wide variety of surgical conditions unrelated to menses, and in recent years almost one case in three has been nonmenstrual, caused by *Staphylococcus aureus* infections at other sites. For epidemiologic and clinical identification of TSS, a case definition was formulated by the Centers for Disease Control and Prevention (CDC). According to this definition, a patient must have the following four major signs: fever (>38.9°C), rash (diffuse macular erythroderma), hypotension (<90 mm Hg), and desquamation (1–2 weeks from onset, particularly affecting the palms and soles). In addition, at least three organ systems must be involved with characteristic abnormalities: gastrointestinal (nausea, vomiting, or diarrhea at onset of illness), mucous membranes (vaginal, oropharyngeal, or conjunctival hyperemia), muscular (severe myalgia, creatine kinase at least twice normal), renal (creatinine at least twice normal or pyuria without infection), hepatic (bilirubin, serum glutamic-oxaloacetic transaminase, serum glutamic-pyruvic transaminase levels at least twice normal), hematologic (thrombocytopenia or leukocytosis with left shift), or nervous system (disorientation or altered consciousness). In addition, specific diagnostic tests for other possible causes must yield negative results. These include blood, throat, or cerebrospinal fluid cultures (blood culture may be positive for *S. aureus*). Such tests also include a search for increasing antibody titers for Rocky Mountain spotted fever, leptospirosis, or rubeola, or the presence of any bacteria other than *S. aureus*, such as group A streptococcal infections. Use of this strict case definition probably eliminates a large number of milder cases of the disease, but it is important to diagnose these mild cases in order to prevent recurrence.

The syndrome is caused by infection with strains of *S. aureus* having a unique phenotype, high levels of proteolytic activity, and the production of an exoprotein called toxic shock syndrome toxin-1 (TSST-1), either alone or in combination with one or more enterotoxins. Whereas colonization with, and antibody formation to, these organisms is common, TSS is relatively uncommon. Women who suffer from TSS have absent or low levels of serum antibody to TSST-1. The formation of antibodies after a bout with TSS is variable, and those persons who do not form them are prone to relapse. The syndrome is associated with a potential focus of infection (e.g., abscess or menses with a tampon in use), and focal growth conditions may play a major role. For instance, some tampon fibers that have high absorbency for water also absorb ions, particularly magnesium. Low concentrations of magnesium promote greater production of TSST-1 by *S. aureus*, perhaps explaining the increased risk of TSS associated with high-absorbency tampons. It therefore appears that TSS reflects a multifactorial pathogenic process that includes exposure to a toxin-producing organism, absence of preexisting immunity, and growth under optimal conditions for toxin production. The toxins cause direct cell membrane damage and activate vasodilators, resulting in increased permeability and decreased vasomotor tone with subsequent tissue hypoxia, metabolic acidosis, and ischemia. The gastrointestinal, epidermal, and mucous membrane manifestations are caused by direct toxin damage. The toxins also exert a direct effect on the myocardium, resulting in impaired contractility. The ischemia can lead to renal shutdown and central nervous system dysfunction.

The incidence of TSS declined from 890 cases in 1980 to 61 cases in 1990. The percentage of menstrual cases is stable at about two thirds of all cases in women. At highest risk are women in the 15- to 34-year-old group. The mortality rate, previously in the range of 5.6% to 8.3%, is currently 2.7% to 3.3% and is twice as high (8%) in men for reasons that are not clear. Nonmenstrual TSS can be associated with a wide variety of infections caused by *S. aureus*, including skin, bone, and soft tissue infections. Postpartum and postoperative obstetric cases have occurred, and rare instances of TSS complicating contraceptive diaphragm and sponge use have been described. Oral contraceptives may be protective for reasons that are not known, but this is possibly related to changes they effect in the vaginal environment because staphylococci are part of the normal vaginal flora in 10% of women.

Typically the onset of TSS is during menses, and a vaginal tampon may be found in place in such women. It may also appear 1 or 2 days after menses. The clinical presentation of menstrual and nonmenstrual TSS is essentially the same, but patient characteristics and onset of disease differ. The most common presentation consists of fever, myalgias, headache, dizziness, diarrhea, and vomiting. Physical examination reveals fever, hypotension, or orthostasis, and the existence of a diffuse sunburnlike erythroderma that blanches with pressure. Scleral or conjunctival infection is also common, and diffuse abdominal tenderness without rebound may be present. Thereafter, changes in the patient's sensorium and profound shock may develop. The characteristic desquamation begins at about day 7 and progresses to become a cast-like desquamation, with cleavage at the basal layer, particularly of the fingers, palms, toes, and soles between days 10 and 14.

The multisystem organ involvement caused both directly by the toxin and indirectly by the hypotension may lead to many laboratory abnormalities that are reflected in the blood count, liver and renal functions, and serum electrolyte levels. In arriving at the diagnosis, the critical finding is diffuse erythroderma, which is not found in other comparable diseases. If the erythroderma, which may be evanescent, is not seen, any bacteremic disease is possible and must be considered. Finding a site of *S. aureus* infection in nonmenstrual cases is strong evidence for a presumptive diagnosis of TSS in cases that may be otherwise somewhat atypical. Unfortunately, there are as yet no simple laboratory tests to confirm the diagnosis. Several complications have been reported that are related to disease severity and a delay in therapy. These include adult respiratory distress syndrome (ARDS), reversible acute oliguric and nonoliguric renal failure, myoglobinuria, myocardial dysfunction, disseminated intravascular coagulopathy (DIC), tetany with hypocalcemia, arthritis, and vasculitis. Survivors generally begin to recover within 7 to 10 days. The three major causes of death are ARDS, intractable hypotension, and DIC.

Patients must undergo aggressive fluid resuscitation in an intensive care area. A Swan-Ganz catheter should be inserted, and fluid challenges should be given until the wedge pressure is elevated to 15 to 20 mm Hg. Urine output should be kept above 20 ml/h. Positive-pressure ventilation may be needed to prevent respiratory failure and ARDS. If adequate blood pressure cannot be maintained, vasopressor drugs may be required. The administration of corticosteroids may decrease the severity of illness, if given early, but their efficacy has not been proved. Once the patient's condition is stabilized and the source of infection has been identified, the source of the toxin must be eliminated through drainage of infected wounds, debridement, or removal of an infected nidus such as surgical packings. Vaginal examination with removal of tampons, diaphragms, and other contraceptive devices is essential. Cultures of blood, mucous membranes, discharges, and foreign devices must be performed. There are few data to suggest that antibiotics affect the course of TSS. However, their use does lead to a decrease in the recurrence rate and can benefit those rare patients with *S. aureus* bacteremia. A penicillinase-resistant semisynthetic penicillin (nafcillin, oxacillin) given in a dose of 1 or 2 g administered intravenously every 4 hours for 10 to 14 days, is recommended. A first-generation cephalosporin or, in penicillin-allergic patients, vancomycin, may be used. Patients with sequestered infections, such as osteomyelitis, may require more prolonged therapy.

Toxic shock syndrome may recur within the first 2 to 3 months after the initial episode in 25% to 30% of patients. The cornerstone of prevention is education of the patient, in conjunction with effective antimicrobial therapy of the initial infection and avoidance of tampon use. Women who choose to use tampons should be advised to use them intermittently throughout menses, and for the shortest period consistent with personal comfort, perhaps alternating with pads. Tampons with the lowest absorbency compatible with hygienic protection should be used. Women who use tampons should be made aware of the syndrome and should be reassured that it is an uncommon disease. They should be familiar with early symptoms and signs and know to remove the tampon and seek medical care if an illness associated with fever, dizziness, rash, or diarrhea develops. Women with a history of TSS should be urged not to resume tampon use at all. If they insist on using them, *S. aureus* should first be eliminated from the lower genital tract and, if necessary, from the sexual partner. Nonmenstrual TSS may be largely prevented by the prompt institution of medical and surgical treatment of localized suppurative staphylococcal infection.

In recent years, there have been numerous descriptions of a similar constellation of findings associated with group A streptococci. This syndrome, termed the toxic streptococcal syndrome or toxic shock–like syndrome, may stem from a general reemergence of invasive streptococcal infections. Factors associated with the syndrome include the serotype, especially M types 1 and 3, pyrogenic exotoxins, and proteinases. Immunologic factors, such as preexisting M type–specific antibody and other host characteristics also may be important. The diagnosis and management are similar to those applied in the setting of staphylococcal TSS. However, tissue necrosis, rare with staphylococcal infections, is common, as is bacteremia (60%). Pain is a prominent feature, and the mortality rate ranges from 30% to 70%.

Reviews

1. Stevens DL. The toxic shock syndromes. *Infect Dis Clin North Am* 1996;10:727.
   The many similarities between TSS and gram-negative septic shock suggest that endotoxin may play a role in the disease.
2. Parsonnet J. Nonmenstrual toxic shock syndrome: new insights into diagnosis, pathogenesis, and treatment. *Curr Clin Top Infect Dis* 1996;16:1.
   Toxic shock syndrome occurs most commonly in the healthy patient with an intact immune system. Both S. pyogenes and S. aureus cause a variety of distinctive infections that may or may not be associated with a TSS.

Etiology

3. Todd J, et al. Toxic-shock syndrome associated with phage-group 1 staphylococci. *Lancet* 1978;2:1116.
   This is the original report describing TSS. Phage-group 1, types 29 and 52, was originally implicated, but since then, many phage groups have been involved and may represent a regional distribution rather than a genetic association of the disease with a specific phage.
4. Hirose Y, et al. Toxic shock–like syndrome caused by non-group A beta-hemolytic streptococci. *Arch Intern Med* 1997;157:1891.
   The authors describe two fatal cases associated with streptococcal groups G and C.
5. Inagaki Y, et al. Serotyping of *Streptococcus pyogenes* isolated from common and severe invasive infections in Japan, 1990–5: implication of the T3 serotype strain-expansion in TSLS. The working group for group A streptococci in Japan. *Epidemiol Infect* 1997;119:41.
   Toxic shock syndrome patients may have an immunodeficiency that inhibits the production, maintenance, or both, of antibodies to the staphylococcal enterotoxins and TSST-1.
6. Hockett SP, Stevens DL. Superantigens associated with staphylococcal and streptococcal toxic shock syndromes are potent inducers of tumor necrosis factor beta synthesis. *J Infect Dis* 1993;168:232.
   Streptococcal pyrogenic exotoxins A through C are similar to TSST-1 and staphylococcal enterotoxins A through E in their ability to stimulate cytokine release.

Menstrual TSS

7. Sagraves R. Menstrual toxic shock syndrome. *Am Pharm* 1996;NS35:12.
   In arriving at the diagnosis, there should be reasonable evidence for the absence of other bacterial, viral, or rickettsial infections, drug reactions, or autoimmune disorders.
8. Garland SM, Peel MM. Tampons and toxic shock syndrome. *Med J Aust* 1995;163:8.
   Toxic shock syndrome may not be an important public health problem at this time, probably due to the removal of polyacrylate rayon tampons from the market and accompanying reductions in tampon absorbency.
9. Hanrahan SN. Historical review of menstrual toxic shock syndrome. *Women Health* 1994;21:141.
   The peak of reported cases of staph TSS in 1980 has been followed by a marked and persistent decline.

Nonmenstrual TSS

10. Graham DR, et al. Postoperative toxic shock syndrome. *Clin Infect Dis* 1995;
    20:895.
    *Nonmenstrual TSS begins a median of 2 days after operation in patients with sur-
    gical wound infections; from 1 day to 8 weeks in patients with nonsurgical, skin,
    subcutaneous, or soft tissue infections; and in postpartum and postabortion cases.*
11. Gutierrez RF, et al. Staphylococcal toxic shock syndrome associated with human
    immunodeficiency virus infection: report of a case with bacteremia. *Clin Infect
    Dis* 1996;22:875.
    The authors add immunoincompetence to the equation.
12. Toxic shock syndrome and related conditions in the United Kingdom: 1992 and
    1993. *Commun Dis Rep CDR Wkly* 1994;4:65.
    *Reliable estimates of the incidence of nonmenstrual TSS are largely unavailable,
    and systematic studies of risk factors have not been done.*
13. Walker LE, Breiner MJ, Goodman CM. Toxic shock syndrome after explantation
    of breast implants: a case report and review of the literature. *Plast Reconstr Surg*
    1997;99:875.
    *The greater the delay, the greater the need for extensive surgery. The rapid onset
    of shock and organ failure may even preclude surgical intervention.*

Streptococcal TSS

14. Stanford DG, et al. Toxic streptococcal syndrome. *Aust J Dermatol* 1997;38:158.
    Necrotizing fasciitis is commonly associated with strep TSS.
15. Sellers BJ, et al. Necrotizing group A streptococcal infections associated with
    streptococcal toxic shock syndrome. *Am J Surg* 1996;172:523.
    Massive debridement to healthy tissue is necessary for necrotizing infections.
16. Perez CM, et al. Adjunctive treatment of streptococcal toxic shock syndrome using
    intravenous immunoglobulin: a case report and review. *Am J Med* 1997;102:111.
    *The use of immunoglobulin for TSS is logical because patients with TSS have low
    to absent antibody titers, whereas the general population usually has high titers
    against the toxins.*

63. PELVIC INFLAMMATORY DISEASE

Michel E. Rivlin

Pelvic inflammatory disease (PID) is defined as the acute clinical syndrome attributed to the ascending spread of microorganisms from the vagina and endocervix to
the endometrium, fallopian tubes, one or both ovaries, and the pelvic and perhaps abdominal peritoneum. The suprahepatic space also may be involved. In most cases, it
is a community-acquired bacterial infection presumed to be initiated by sexual activity. Infections related to pregnancy or surgical procedures are usually not included in
the definition and are regarded as separate entities. There are an estimated 1 million
cases per year in the United States. Late sequelae develop in one fourth of the women
with acute PID, including involuntary infertility, which occurs in 15% to 20%. Other
sequelae include chronic pelvic pain, dyspareunia, and inflammatory masses, which
require surgical intervention in 15% to 20% of cases. In addition, the incidence of ectopic pregnancy is increased severalfold to about 8% in women who have had PID.

Several risk factors for PID can be identified. Previous PID damages endothelial
resistance and predisposes to recurrence. Women with multiple sex partners have a
relative risk factor of 4.6. The microbiologic causes of PID vary greatly. In general,
Neisseria gonorrhoeae has been estimated to account for 10% to 66% of cases, whereas,

at least in the United States, *Chlamydia trachomatis* is causally linked to approximately 20% of cases. Infection with *N. gonorrhoeae* or *Chlamydia* is associated with an approximate 10% to 20% risk of developing clinically recognizable PID. Oral contraceptive users have an increased risk of chlamydial cervicitis but a lesser risk of overt PID. Pill use does not affect the risk of tubal infertility. The use of an intrauterine device (IUD) increases the risk of PID by seven- to ninefold, chiefly in young nulliparous women, whereas the risk is much lower in older women who are multiparous and have only one partner. On the other hand, barrier contraceptives combined with spermicides reduce the risk of PID.

Pelvic inflammatory disease frequently has a polymicrobial etiology, no matter what organisms are cultured from the cervix. The traditional role of *N. gonorrhoeae* as the initiator of infection that paves the way for a subsequent invasion by gram-positive and -negative aerobic and anaerobic vaginal or enteric organisms has become less tenable because it now seems probable that all the organisms enter the upper tracts at the same time. Many studies have demonstrated a poor correlation between the bacteria obtained by cervical culture and those grown from cul-de-sac or laparoscopic samples, taken at the same time. In addition, genital mycoplasmas (e.g., *Mycoplasma hominis* and *Ureaplasma urealyticum*) may play a role in some cases of PID. Although the traditional division of PID into gonococcal and nongonococcal forms is therefore no longer widely alluded to, there is a difference between *N. gonorrhoeae* and chlamydial infections in that *Chlamydia* infection appears to be associated with a more indolent, less acute, and less severe clinical picture, with more potential for permanent tubal damage and its sequea, tubal infertility. Both *N. gonorrhoeae* and *Chlamydia* spread along the endocervix to the endometrium and then to the tubal mucosa. Characteristically (in 66%–77% of cases), gonococcal PID presents in the first postmenstrual week. There is also some evidence that bacteria may attach to sperm and reach the upper tract by means of bacteriospermia. The mechanism of spread appears to differ from that seen for IUD use. Here, the string may act as a wick (especially the multifilament string of the Dalkon shield), and the chronic local endometritis generated by the device may breach host defenses, leading to a lymphatic spread into the parametrium similar to that seen for postabortal or postpartum infections.

For the purposes of clinical management, PID may be subdivided into two major types: uncomplicated, which is not associated with an adnexal mass or inflammatory complex; and complicated, which is associated with an adnexal complex or more advanced condition. The presence of abdominal, adnexal, and cervical motion tenderness in a patient with a history of abdominal pain constitutes the clinical criteria recommended for establishing the diagnosis of PID. Objective indications of infection or inflammation, such as fever (>38.3°C; 100.4°F), leukocytosis (>10,500/mm²), or an elevated erythrocyte sedimentation rate (>20 mm/hour), add to the accuracy of diagnosis. Further objective evidence supporting the diagnosis includes the presence of gram-negative intracellular diplococci on endocervical smear, purulent material obtained from the peritoneal cavity by culdocentesis or laparoscopy, and an adnexal mass found during bimanual or sonographic examination. Endocervical tests for *Chlamydia* and gonorrhea and the estimation of C-reactive protein levels provide further important diagnostic information. Endometrial biopsy samples are obtained by some clinicians, with findings of plasma cell endometritis reported for almost all patients with proven PID. The clinical diagnosis of PID is incorrect in up to 35% of women, and the differential diagnosis is broad and includes ectopic pregnancy, appendicitis, ovarian cyst accidents, endometriosis, and, not infrequently, a normal pelvis. As a consequence, laparoscopy is increasingly used in doubtful cases because it exhibits a near 100% sensitivity and affords access to the tubes for culture. However, economic factors and logistic difficulties have, until now, prevented the routine use of laparoscopy diagnosis in all suspected PID cases in the United States. If laparoscopy is used, PID is deemed mild if the tubes are edematous, erythematous, and freely mobile, and as moderate if spontaneous gross purulence is seen with tubes that may not be mobile and stomata that may not be patent. In severe disease, there is an inflammatory complex or abscess (pyosalpinx, tuboovarian abscess) that may be leaking.

The goals of therapy are to cure the present illness and to prevent infertility and other chronic sequelae. Women with mild disease receive ambulatory therapy. The criteria for hospital admission include a suspected pelvic abscess, uncertain diagnosis, severe illness, and failure to respond to outpatient care within 48 hours; those patients who are unable to follow or tolerate the regimen or to be seen for follow-up within 48 to 72 hours should be hospitalized. In many areas, the hospitalization criteria are more liberal, especially with regard to nulliparous women with first infections. Because no single antibiotic is active against all possible pathogens, the Centers for Disease Control and Prevention (CDC) recommend several possible combination regimens that are directed against *N. gonorrhoeae*, including penicillinase-producing strains and *Chlamydia*. Cefoxitin, or an equally effective cephalosporin, plus doxycycline or tetracycline, is an example of a regimen that provides this activity. Therapy is maintained for 7 to 10 days. An alternative outpatient regimen also recommended by the CDC includes ofloxacin and either clindamycin or metronidazole for 14 days. Bed rest, sexual abstinence, analgesics, referral of sexual partners for examination and possible treatment, removal of an IUD if present, and contraceptive counseling are further important measures. If specific pathogens are cultured, the cultures should be repeated after therapy is completed. The CDC recommends two regimens for inpatient therapy: (1) cefoxitin or cefotetan plus doxycycline or (2) clindamycin plus gentamicin, followed by doxycycline. It is recommended that intravenous therapy be maintained for at least 48 hours after clinical improvement takes place.

Unfortunately, the clinical efficacy and even the efficacy of ambulatory versus inpatient therapy are not well established. In practice, those patients requiring hospitalization but who do not have an adnexal mass are often treated with single-agent regimens, with results equal to those observed for the CDC recommendations, but with lower costs and side effects. The drugs include the newer broad-spectrum cephalosporins and the expanded-spectrum penicillins. Adnexal inflammatory masses are usually treated with combinations of agents, including an aminoglycoside or aztreonam and an agent with specific anti-anaerobic activity (clindamycin, chloramphenicol, or metronidazole). Existing data do not establish the need for lengthy parenteral therapy, and many clinicians discontinue intravenous therapy when patients have become afebrile and asymptomatic. In general, fever is a poor prognosticator of response, unless it is elevated or rising. Instead, reduced abdominal pain and degree of peritonism and decreased cervical motion tenderness are better guides. About 15% of patients fail to respond to the initial medication, requiring a change of agents. Surgical treatment is not indicated for acute PID, other than to rule out possible surgical emergencies or in the event of pelvic abscess formation in certain circumstances. The surgical management of PID is reviewed in Chapter 64.

The relationship of infertility to the number of episodes is linear, with 11% of the patients infertile after one attack, 23% after two attacks, and 54% after three or more attacks. It is also related to the severity of disease, with 6% infertile after mild changes, 13% after moderately severe inflammation, and 30% after severe disease. PID recurs in 25% of the patients. In women who suffer one episode of salpingitis, the risk of ectopic pregnancy increases to 5% of live births (normally 1%–2%); in those with multiple previous episodes, the risk may be as high as 20%. Good results of therapy depend on early diagnosis and rational antibiotic selection and administration, together with the prevention of reinfection by means of patient education and the treatment of sexual partners. At issue is the reproductive capacity of an unfortunately ever-increasing group of young women.

Review
1. Pelvic inflammatory disease: guidelines for prevention and management. *MMWR* 1991;40:1.
   Differentiating lower from upper genital tract infections is often difficult.
2. Ivey JB. The adolescent with pelvic inflammatory disease: assessment and management. *Nurse Pract* 1997;22:78.
   The existence of chronic tubal infection is often only diagnosed in conjunction with ectopic pregnancy or infertility investigation.

Etiology
3. Hillis SD, et al. Recurrent chlamydial infections increase the risks of hospitalization for ectopic pregnancy and pelvic inflammatory disease. *Am J Obstet Gynecol* 1997;176(Pt 1):103.
   The greater the number of chlamydial infections, the higher the risk of PID or ectopic pregnancy.
4. Brunham RC, et al. Prevalence and correlates of antibody to chlamydial heat shock protein in women attending sexually transmitted disease clinics and women with confirmed pelvic inflammatory disease. *J Infect Dis* 1997;175:1453.
   Antibody to chlamydial heat shock protein is correlated with confirmed PID and upper tract pathology but not with acute chlamydial infection.
5. Khomassuridze AG, Tsertsvadze GL, Tsereteli TG. Intrauterine device and pelvic inflammatory disease. *Adv Contracept* 1997;13:71.
   The IUD is associated with PID in those women at high risk for STD, but not in women with mutually monogamous relationships.
6. Zhang J, Thomas AG, Leybovich E. Vaginal douching and adverse health effects: a meta-analysis. *Am J Public Health* 1997;87:1207.
   Frequent douching was highly associated with PID and modestly associated with ectopic pregnancy and cervical neoplasia.
7. Clarke LM, et al. Recovery of cytomegalovirus and herpes simplex virus from upper and lower genital tract specimens obtained from women with pelvic inflammatory disease. *J Infect Dis* 1997;176:286.
   CMV virus was recovered from 20% of upper and lower tracts of women with PID and therefore may be a factor in the pathogenesis of PID. HSV was not isolated from the upper tract.
8. Abele-Horn M, et al. Association of *Ureaplasma urealyticum* biovars with clinical outcome for neonates, obstetric patients, and gynecological patients with pelvic inflammatory disease. *J Clin Microbiol* 1997;35:1199.
   The T960 biovar seemed to be associated with chronic infections that cause or support PID. These strains also correlated with tetracycline resistance.
9. Peipert JF, et al. Bacterial vaginosis as a risk factor for upper genital tract infection. *Am J Obstet Gynecol* 1997;177:1184.
   The presence of bacterial vaginosis was associated with a threefold increased risk of upper genital tract infections.
10. Ness RB, et al. Oral contraception and the recognition of endometritis. *Am J Obstet Gynecol* 1997;176:580.
    Birth control pill use doubles the risk of chlamydial cervicitis but significantly reduces the risk of symptomatic PID. The risk to fertility is unknown.

Clinical Features
11. Hager WD, et al. Criteria for diagnosis and grading of salpingitis. *Obstet Gynecol* 1983;61:113.
    The article tabulates the clinical criteria required for diagnosis and the grading of severity based on the findings from clinical and laparoscopic examination as recommended by the Infectious Disease Society for Obstetrics and Gynecology.
12. Eschenbach DA, et al. Acute pelvic inflammatory disease: associations of clinical and laboratory findings with laparoscopic findings. *Obstet Gynecol* 1997;89:184.
    Clinical and laboratory findings have low predictive value for clinical severity as established with laparoscopy.
13. Munday PE. Clinical aspects of pelvic inflammatory disease. *Hum Reprod* 1997;12[Suppl]:121.
    The diagnosis and management of other common causes of lower abdominal pain are unlikely to be impaired by initiating empiric therapy for PID.
14. Velebil P, et al. Rate of hospitalization for gynecologic disorders among reproductive-age women in the United States. *Obstet Gynecol* 1995;86:764.
    Pelvic inflammatory disease was one of the five most frequent diagnostic groups. The highest rates were for non-white women, ages 25–39.
15. Barbosa C, et al. Pelvic inflammatory disease and human immunodeficiency virus infection. *Obstet Gynecol* 1997;89:65.

Successful treatment with standard regimens despite more severe initial presentation and a prolonged hospital course.

16. Abbuhl SB, Muskin EB, Shofer FS. Pelvic inflammatory disease in patients with bilateral tubal ligation. *Am J Emerg Med* 1997;15:271.
   Salpingitis can occur after tubal ligation.
17. Blanchard AC, Pastorek JG II, Weeks T. Pelvic inflammatory disease during pregnancy. *South Med J* 1987;880:1363.
   Pelvic inflammatory disease is a rare complication, generally amenable to antibiotic therapy, although the diagnosis may only be made at exploratory laparotomy.
18. Omens S, et al. Laparoscopic treatment of painful perihepatic adhesions in Fitz-Hugh-Curtis syndrome. *Obstet Gynecol* 1991;78:542.
   This paper describes a form of PID associated with perihepatitis and, on occasion, perisplenitis and perinephritis. Chlamydia and N. gonorrhoeae have been implicated as etiologic agents.
19. Safrin S, et al. Long-term sequelae of acute pelvic inflammatory disease: a retrospective cohort study. *Am J Obstet Gynecol* 1992;166:1300.
   Subsequent PID occurred in 43% of the patients, 24% experienced pelvic pain for 6 months or more, and 40% were involuntarily infertile after hospitalization for acute PID.

Treatment
20. Centers for Disease Control. 1998 Guidelines for treatment of sexually transmitted diseases. *MMWR* 1998;47(RR-1).
   Alternative parenteral regimens include ofloxacin plus metronidazole, ampicillin / sulbactam plus doxycycline, and ciprofloxacin plus doxycycline plus metronidazole.
21. Hemsell DL, et al. A multicenter study comparing intravenous meropenem with clindamycin plus gentamicin for the treatment of acute gynecologic and obstetric pelvic infections in hospitalized women. *Clin Infect Dis* 1997;24[Suppl 2]:222.
   Hospitalization times have been shortened with the availability of home parenteral therapy even in patients with tuboovarian abscesses.
22. Arredondo JL, et al. Oral clindamycin and ciprofloxacin versus intramuscular ceftriaxone and oral doxycycline in the treatment of mild-to-moderate pelvic inflammatory disease in outpatients. *Clin Infect Dis* 1997;24:170.
   No difference in efficacy or side effects between the two regimens was detected.
23. Howell MR, Kassler WH, Haddix A. Partner notification to prevent pelvic inflammatory disease in women. Cost-effectiveness of two strategies. *Sex Transm Dis* 1997;24:287.
   The best strategies for preventing PID are (1) prevention of Chlamydia infection and gonorrhea in both sexes, and (2) when this fails, early detection and treatment of lower-tract infection.
24. Carey M, Brown S. Infertility surgery for pelvic inflammatory disease: success rates after salpingolysis and salpingostomy. *Am J Obstet Gynecol* 1987;156:296.
   Adhesiolysis led to an intrauterine gestation in 41% and an ectopic pregnancy in 23%. Adhesiolysis in combination with terminal salpingostomy resulted in an intrauterine gestation in 18% and an ectopic pregnancy in 9%.

---

64. PELVIC ABSCESS

Michel E. Rivlin

Most pelvic abscesses are a sequela of infection in the upper genital tract originating as pelvic inflammatory disease (PID). Abscesses usually form as a result of inadequate treatment or patient delay in seeking care and are more commonly seen in women who have had multiple episodes of PID. Less frequently, pelvic abscesses are a complication of appendicitis, diverticulitis, or gynecologic or obstetric surgical procedures. The abscess may be largely confined to the uterine tube (pyosalpinx) but more commonly involves a tuboovarian complex. In some instances, purulent material will extend into the posterior pelvis and becomes walled off by multiple structures, including the tubes, ovaries, broad ligaments, small bowel, and omentum. Whereas PID is almost always a bilateral process, an abscess may be unilateral in up to 71% of the cases, especially if an intrauterine device (IUD) is present. Adnexal masses in the presence of pelvic infections are not necessarily abscesses, but frequently represent conglutination of the tubes and ovaries to the adjacent pelvic and abdominal structures as a reaction to the purulent exudate from the inflamed tube. This condition is better described as a tuboovarian complex rather than an abscess, for it lacks the classic abscess wall. The appropriate use of broad-spectrum antibiotics has led to a marked decreased in the incidence of tuboovarian abscess (TOA). An intraovarian abscess, contained within the parenchyma of the ovary, may arise through inoculation of an open wound, such as that produced by ovulation or by surgical procedures. This variety of pelvic abscess is relatively uncommon. Rupture into the general peritoneal cavity, with subsequent diffuse peritonitis, is the major complication of a pelvic abscess. The rupture may either be spontaneous or precipitated by trauma, such as that produced by a pelvic examination or barium enema, a fall, or abdominal blow. If not diagnosed and correctly treated within 24 to 48 hours, septicemia and septic shock follow with a resultant high mortality. Pelvic thrombophlebitis and ovarian vein thrombosis are other late complications of major pelvic infections that may be associated with significant morbidity and mortality.

The bacteria responsible are those normally found in the lower genital tract, including aerobes such as *Streptococcus* and *Escherichia coli*; anaerobes such as *Peptococcus, Peptostreptococcus,* and *Bacteroides*; and, rarely, *Clostridia* or *Actinomyces*. The infection is virtually always polymicrobial, with three or more organisms commonly recovered. The sexually transmitted organisms such as *Neisseria gonorrhoeae* and *Chlamydia* are usually not present in the abscess but may be recovered from the cervix in approximately one third of cases. The onset of symptoms is usually insidious, with the most common complaints pelvic pain and tenderness. Patients frequently experience fever and tachycardia, and some patients may complain of abnormal vaginal bleeding, vaginal discharge, nausea, anorexia, or diarrhea. On examination, lower abdominal and pelvic tenderness with or without evidence of peritonism may be present. An abnormal mass may not be found by clinical means, depending on its location, the woman's weight, and the degree of tenderness. Some patients may be afebrile, and the white blood count may be normal. Ultrasonography can usually show a complex adnexal mass, although a purely cystic lesion may be seen. Sonography will usually demonstrate the mass, and computed tomography (CT), or magnetic resonance imaging (MRI), which are probably the most accurate techniques for localizing intraabdominal abscesses, can be reserved for cases in which other diagnostic procedures have failed to confirm the diagnosis. The clinician must determine whether the abscess is confined to the pelvis and lower abdomen, or whether there is evidence of leakage or rupture. For the former to be the case, evidence of peritoneal irritation should be limited to the pelvis or lower abdomen; peritoneal signs above the umbilicus suggest leakage or rupture, which constitutes a surgical emergency. The differential diagnosis includes appendicitis, diverticulitis, ectopic pregnancy, twisted ovarian cyst, and septic abortion. In this respect, serum pregnancy tests are most helpful in identifying problems associated with pregnancy. The physical findings of endometriosis may be very similar to those of chronic adnexal sepsis, but in the acute phase, the systemic evidence of infection provides the diagnostic clue.

The initial approach to treatment in the patient with an unruptured abscess should usually be medical, consisting of antibiotics effective against anaerobes and aerobes, including *E. coli*. A commonly used regimen comprises an aminoglycoside in combination with clindamycin or metronidazole. The monocyclic beta-lactam aztreonam may be used in place of the aminoglycoside, which thus avoids potential nephrotoxicity. Fluid and electrolyte balance are maintained with intravenous fluids and nasogastric suction. Such conservative management may be successful in 33% to 74% of the cases. Surgical management is urgently indicated for patients with a ruptured abscess and in those whose condition deteriorates rapidly while they are being treated, with evidence of increasing peritonitis. Abscesses that are situated in the cul-de-sac and dissect down the rectovaginal septum should be drained via a colpotomy. Surgical intervention is also indicated for patients who do not respond to medical therapy, as evidenced by persistent fever and leukocytosis, pain, enlarging masses (based on the findings by examination, ultrasonography, or CT), and persistent ileus. Many clinicians set a time limit and proceed to surgical intervention if there has not been a good response within 48 to 72 hours. Surgical treatment is also indicated for those patients who, after discharge, continue to have pain and a persistent tender mass. Removal of the uterus and both adnexa may confer the least risk of postoperative morbidity and the least risk of the need for reoperation for an unresolved infection, but this results in castration, often at a young age. An operation that preserves the uterus and some ovarian tissue offers at least a possibility of childbearing, but a greater likelihood of recurrent or persistent infection. Consultation with the woman and her family with an explanation of the risks and benefits involved is an important factor in choosing the best operation for the particular patient. Novel approaches in the management of pelvic abscesses that may be more widely used in the future include laparoscopic drainage as well as sonographically or CT-directed percutaneous aspiration or catheter drainage.

The clinical picture exhibited by a woman with a ruptured abscess is highly variable. In some, the rupture is heralded by a severe and sudden exacerbation of pain, tachycardia that is out of proportion to the temperature, and signs of peritonitis and shock. Operative intervention is imperative as soon as the patient's condition has been stabilized through the administration of intravenous fluids. The placement of a central line or Swan-Ganz catheter may be helpful for this purpose. Conservative surgical treatment may be indicated under selected circumstances when preservation of reproductive function is a high priority and the patient is willing to accept the possibility of reoperation. In most instances, the patient is best served by a complete hysterectomy with bilateral adnexectomy. If the abscess is unilateral, an adnexectomy of the involved side may be sufficient. Careful exploration of the whole abdomen and examination of the entire bowel is necessary for achieving complete drainage, followed by copious irrigation and the liberal use of suction drains or drainage via the vaginal cuff. Mass closure of the abdominal incision with nonabsorbable sutures and delayed closure of the subcutaneous tissue and skin are advisable. Postoperative ileus is to be expected, requiring continued nasogastric drainage and possible total parenteral nutrition.

Pregnancy rates in patients treated for pelvic abscesses after all methods of treatment appear to range from about 10% to 20%. It is becoming apparent that the most appropriate approach to management is individual therapy that takes into account the age, clinical status, and desires of the properly informed patient.

Reviews
  1. Osborne NG. Tubo-ovarian abscess: pathogenesis and management. *J Natl Med Assoc* 1986;78:937.
     Pelvic thrombophlebitis is of late onset in the course of the disease. It presents like a resistant infection with tachycardia, fever, and dull, low abdominal pain. The clinical response to a therapeutic trial of heparin provides the presumptive diagnosis.
  2. Murthy JH, Hiremagalur SR. Differentiation of tubo-ovarian abscess from pelvic inflammatory disease, and recent trends in the management of tubo-ovarian abscess. *J Tenn Med Assoc* 1995;88:136.
     Clinical response to antibiotics was achieved in about 70% of patients. Surgery was required in 60% if the mass was larger than 10 cm, in 35% if 7 to 9 cm, and in under 20% if 4 to 6 cm. Conservative surgery was used in about 50%.
  3. Huang A, Jay MS, Uhler M. Tuboovarian abscess in the adolescent. *J Pediatr Adolesc Gynecol* 1997;10:73.
     Tuboovarian abscess (TOA) was found in one third of hospitalized PID patients. One fourth of TOAs require surgery, 100,000 patients are admitted per year with TOA, and 22% to 50% of TOAs are associated with PID.

Etiology / Diagnosis
4. Ha HK, et al. MR imaging of tubo-ovarian abscess. *Acta Radiol* 1995;36:510.
   The potential for demonstrating disease extent, characterizing the lesions, and making a specific diagnosis are discussed.
5. Kubota T, Ishi K, Takeuchi H. A study of tubo-ovarian abscesses, with a focus on cases with endometrioma. *J Obstet Gynecol Res* 1997;23:421.
   Sonographic diagnosis of TOA is 93% sensitive and 98% specific. The characteristic appearance is that of a complex cystic adnexal or cul-de-sac mass with thick irregular walls, septations and internal debris.
6. Fiorino AS, et al. Intrauterine contraceptive device–associated actinomycotic abscess and *Actinomyces* detection on cervical smear. *Obstet Gynecol* 1996;87:142.
   The literature reports 92 cases of actinomycotic pelvic abscesses associated with IUDs. If diagnosis is made before surgery, high-dose penicillin therapy may be curative.
7. Lau M, et al. Ovarian abscess 15 months after vaginal hysterectomy. *J Reprod Med* 1997;42:669.
   Adnexal abscesses after hysterectomy probably follow bacterial seeding during the surgery. Alternatively, prior PID, extension from adjacent infected organs, or hematogenous spread may be the causative mechanisms.
8. Maldjian PD, Zurlow J. Ovarian vein thrombosis associated with a tubo-ovarian abscess. *Arch Gynecol Obstet* 1997;261:55.
   Ovarian vein thrombosis is generally associated with pregnancy but can complicate PID. It may be diagnosed at surgery or by CT imaging. Therapy usually consists of IV heparin and antibiotics, but surgery may be required.
9. Sirotnak AP, Eppes SC, Klein JD. Tuboovarian abscess and peritonitis caused by *Streptococcus pneumoniae* serotype 1 in young girls. *Clin Infect Dis* 1996;22:993.
   Serotype 1 may have a unique predilection for the female genital tract and produce TOA in young girls. Sexual abuse must be ruled out.
10. Hoogewoud HM, et al. The role of computerized tomography in fever, septicemia and multiple system organ failure after laparotomy. *Surg Gynecol Obstet* 1986; 162:539.
    As soon as sepsis is suspected, an abdominal and pelvic CT study should be performed so that therapeutic procedures may be carried out at a stage when no organ is yet failing, that is, in a period when the risk of mortality is lowest.

Series
11. Landers BV, Sweet RL. Current trends in the diagnosis and treatment of tuboovarian abscess. *Am J Obstet Gynecol* 1985;151:1098.
    The failure to respond to adequate medical therapy may be the most reliable way of distinguishing those patients with true adnexal abscess from those with an adnexal inflammatory complex or salpingitis alone.
12. Kaplan AL, Jacobs WM, Ehresman JB. Aggressive management of pelvic abscess. *Am J Obstet Gynecol* 1967;98:482.
    The authors advocate routine hysterectomy with adnexectomy (often referred to as "pelvic clean-out," "pelvic sweep," "pelvic clearance"), to prevent long-term complications.

Therapy
13. Reed SD, Landers DV, Sweet RL. Antibiotic treatment of tuboovarian abscess: comparison of broad-spectrum beta-lactam agents versus clindamycin-containing regimens. *Am J Obstet Gynecol* 1991;164:1556.
    Extended-spectrum antibiotic coverage exhibited an efficacy equivalent to that of clindamycin-containing regimens.
14. Rivlin ME. Conservative surgery for adnexal abscess. *J Reprod Med* 1985;30:726.
    This article reviews the reoperation and pregnancy rates after conservative surgical treatment.
15. Rivlin ME. Clinical outcome following vaginal drainage of pelvic abscess. *Obstet Gynecol* 1983;61:169.
    The likelihood of pregnancy after colpotomy drainage when the uterus is left in place is thought to be about 10%.

16. Raiga J, et al. Laparoscopic management of adnexal abscesses: consequences for fertility. *Fertil Steril* 1996;66:712.
    Early laparoscopy with a second-look procedure 3 to 6 months later is associated with a 60% spontaneous pregnancy rate.
17. Aboulghar MA, Mansour RT, Serour GI. Ultrasonographically guided transvaginal aspiration of tuboovarian abscesses and pyosalpinges: an optional treatment for acute pelvic inflammatory disease. *Am J Obstet Gynecol* 1995;172:1501.
    The results of small studies that compare laparoscopic and percutaneous drainage are encouraging, but studies that compare antibiotic therapy alone versus therapy with antibiotics and drainage procedures, or that compare different drainage techniques, have not yet been attempted. There also have been no long-term fertility studies.
18. Wroblicka JT, Kuligowska E. One-step needle aspiration and lavage for the treatment of abdominal and pelvic abscesses. *Am J Roentgenol* 1998;170:1197.
    Computed tomography scanning, fluoroscopy, and transabdominal or transvaginal ultrasonography have all been successfully used for guidance in draining pelvic abscesses per vaginam, per rectum, or transabdominally.
19. Ramondetta LM, et al. Percutaneous abscess drainage in gynecologic cancer patients. *Gynecol Oncol* 1996;62:366.
    Complication rates of 2% to 10% include septicemia, hemorrhage, and bowel laceration. The success rates for TOAs were in the range of 77% to 93%. Surgery was avoided in 80%.
20. Sterghos SN Jr, Hoffman MS. Primary wound closure after laparotomy for tuboovarian abscess. *J Gynecol Surg* 1992;8:73.
    There was no increased risk of wound infection associated with immediate skin closure after laparotomy for a TOA.

Ruptured Tuboovarian Abscess
21. Vermeeren J, Te Linde RW. Intra-abdominal rupture of pelvic abscesses. *Am J Obstet Gynecol* 1954;68:402.
    This is the classic paper on the topic; the mortality rate was reduced from 90% to 12%.
22. Pedowitz P, Bloomfield RD. Ruptured adnexal abscess (tuboovarian) with generalized peritonitis. *Am J Obstet Gynecol* 1964;88:721.
    The authors report the best results ever published; a survival rate of 96.9% was obtained.
23. Rivlin ME, Hunt JA. Ruptured tuboovarian abscess. Is hysterectomy necessary? *Obstet Gynecol* 1977;50:518.
    Conservative procedures directed at the preservation of reproductive potential are possible, even in the most severe forms of PID.

65. GENITAL TUBERCULOSIS

Michel E. Rivlin

Infection of the genital tract with *Mycobacterium tuberculosis* is almost always secondary to a primary lesion elsewhere, usually in the lungs. Although rare in developed countries, the possibility of pelvic tuberculosis (TB) must be kept in mind, especially in foreign-born patients or in those living in conditions of poverty, overcrowding, and poor health care.

The incidence of pelvic TB varies widely, depending on the source of the estimation. For instance, in patients with problems of infertility living in India, the incidence is 5% to 10%; in a similar group in the United States, the incidence is under 0.5%. Ten percent to 50% of the patients with genital TB either have a history of pulmonary TB or x-ray evidence of the disease. The age range for patients with the disease is between 20 and 40 years in 80% to 90% of cases, although it may occur in the young and in women after menopause.

The decline in TB in the United States ceased in 1984; since then, the incidence has increased 18%, with 26,283 cases reported in 1991. This increase is largely due to the activation of latent disease in immunosuppressed persons and the rapid development of newly acquired infections in this group. The disease disproportionately affects young black and Hispanic people, many of them human immunodeficiency virus (HIV)-positive intravenous drug and alcohol abusers. TB is included in the list of acquired immunodeficiency syndrome (AIDS)-defining diseases; in some 30% of the new TB cases, the patients also have AIDS. The chance of an HIV-positive, TB-infected person suffering active disease is about 10% each year. Poor compliance with treatment also has resulted in multidrug-resistant TB, which is now found in up to 20% of the patients with active disease. Although pulmonary disease accounts for most of these infections, as many as 25% of the patients have extrapulmonary disease.

The fallopian tubes usually bear the brunt of the hematogenous spread from the primary lesion. Less commonly, there may be direct or lymphatic spread from adjacent viscera or peritoneal surfaces. The earliest tubal lesions are generally mucosal and bilateral and may spread to the uterus and ovaries by direct extension. The endometrium is thus repeatedly reinfected from the tubes. The reported rates of infection for the various pelvic organs are as follows: tubes, 90%–100%; uterus, 50%; ovaries, 30%; cervix, 5%–15%; and vagina/vulva, 1%.

The appearance of tubes affected by tuberculous salpingitis varies. In severe infections, they are distended with caseous material; in milder cases, they are not enlarged, but small tubercles may be seen on the serosal surface. The microscopic findings in the tubes and endometrium are similar, and they are characterized by tuberculous granulomas consisting of epithelioid cells surrounded by a zone of lymphocytes and plasma cells, together with the presence of giant cells and areas of caseating necrosis. The fimbrial end of the tube often remains patent, and the fimbria is everted, producing the so-called tobacco pouch appearance.

There is a family history of TB in about 20% of patients; 50% have had pleurisy, peritonitis, erythema nodosum, or renal, osseous, or pulmonary TB. Up to 85% of patients have never been pregnant, and half of the remaining 15% manifest symptoms within a year of their last delivery.

The most common complaint is infertility; the most common symptom is pelvic pain. The pain is seldom severe, unless there is secondary infection. The pain may be worsened by coitus, exercise, and menses. Menstrual disorders, which often occur, include menorrhagia and metrorrhagia; amenorrhea is most frequent in the setting of advanced endometrial disease. In 2% of cases, postmenopausal bleeding occurs. Frequently, there is a history of poor health that includes weight loss, fatigue, and malaise. A diagnosis of pelvic inflammatory disease (PID) nonresponsive to antibiotics is characteristic.

There may be no abnormalities encountered during physical examination. If abdominal involvement is present, there may be ascites with a doughy abdomen and irregular masses. The pelvic findings may be difficult to distinguish from those of nontuberculous PID. The bilateral masses, however, may be less tender and have a less-uniform consistency. The finding of bilateral inflammatory tuboovarian masses in a virgin constitutes strong presumptive evidence of genital TB.

The diagnosis depends on either the demonstration of the organism or the characteristic tubercles, usually on endometrial curetted specimens. The optimal time to perform biopsy or culture is during the late secretory phase. Direct microscopy and culture performed on selective media are especially valuable, not only to establish the diagnosis but also to ascertain the antibiotic sensitivities of the organism. Enzyme-linked immunosorbent assay (ELISA) and polymerase chain reaction (PCR) identification of the organism are available at some centers, providing rapid diagnosis of TB; however, they are costly, false-positive results occur, and they do not replace standard tests. It may take from 6 to 8 weeks for the bacteriologic results to become available, so therapy is usually begun based on the histologic findings. It also must be kept in mind that other conditions cause granulomas with giant cells. These include sarcoidosis, foreign body reactions, and actinomycosis. Furthermore, because there is no endometrial involvement in 50% of cases, curettage findings do not establish the diagnosis in at least half the cases. Other diagnostic methods include culturing menstrual blood, hysterosalpingography, and laparoscopy. Unfortunately, many cases are diagnosed only at the time of laparotomy performed to evaluate suspected PID or of tuboplasty to treat suspected blocked tubes. If the diagnosis is not then appreciated, the surgical procedure is associated with a high complication rate, including recrudescence of the infection and fistula formation.

The workup in the patient with suspected genital TB should include a chest x-ray film, but the original lesion may have healed by the time the genital lesion appears, so negative findings should not be interpreted to rule out TB. A tuberculin skin test should also be performed, and it is rare for a patient to have TB without a positive skin reaction. Active extragenital disease should be sought in proved cases, and this includes bacteriologic examination of sputum and urine. Persons with TB should be tested for HIV.

The therapy for genital TB, with or without extragenital lesions, primarily consists of continuous, long-term, combined drug therapy lasting 1 to 2 years. The drugs available for treatment include isoniazid, ethambutol, rifampin, pyrazinamide, and streptomycin. Because of the problem of drug resistance, it is currently recommended that therapy start with isoniazid, rifampin, pyrazinamide, and either ethambutol or streptomycin, and the four drugs should be continued until the complete results of drug-susceptibility tests are available. Two new agents, ciprofloxacin and capreomycin, are available for drug-resistant infections. All patients at risk for noncompliance or in locales with low treatment completion rates should receive directly observed therapy if possible. General therapeutic measures, including adequate diet and rest, should not be neglected. It is essential to include an experienced chest physician on the therapeutic team. Most patients may be treated on an outpatient basis. Response to therapy is monitored by endometrial biopsy or curettage findings, obtained at 6 and 12 months, as well as by clinical observation, including pelvic examination. Long-term follow-up is essential because late recurrence is not uncommon.

Surgical intervention is indicated if endometrial TB persists or recurs after a year of therapy or if pelvic symptoms do not abate with long-term treatment. Further indications for surgical treatment include persistent adnexal masses or masses that enlarge during therapy. Less commonly, surgical measures may be indicated for patients who do not comply with medical therapy or for those with persistent fistulas. If genital TB is encountered unexpectedly at operation, only biopsy should be performed, because procedures performed after 3 to 4 months of antimicrobial therapy are technically much easier and hence less prone to complications. For the same reason, operation should be delayed until chemotherapy has been carried out for 3 to 4 months, whenever possible.

If surgical intervention is necessary, patients over 40 years of age should undergo a total hysterectomy with bilateral salpingo-oophorectomy. In younger patients, if menstrual function is desired, the uterus and one or both of the ovaries may be conserved, provided they are free of TB. Drug therapy must be resumed after operation. The prognosis for further pregnancy is extremely poor. As of 1976, only 31 cases of well-documented, successful pregnancy out of 7,000 cases of genital TB had been reported in the literature. Thus, although the prognosis for cure is good, the prospects for pregnancy are negligible, although some centers have reported successful pregnancies with in vitro fertilization, which would appear to be the only treatment with any possibility of success.

Reviews
1. Sutherland AM. Gynaecological tuberculosis: analysis of a personal series of 710 cases. *Aust N Z J Obstet Gynaecol* 1985;25:203.
   A high level of suspicion is necessary to achieving a high detection rate of genital TB.
2. Saracoglu O, Mungan T, Tanzer F. Pelvic tuberculosis. *Int J Gynecol Obstet* 1992; 37:115.
   Of 72 cases, salpingogram in 34 showed blocked tubes in 32, and chest x-ray was negative in 81%.
3. Wehner JH, et al. Pulmonary tuberculosis, amenorrhea, and a pelvic mass. *West J Med* 1994;161:515.

This case report includes a review of the clinical manifestations, diagnosis, and treatment of pelvic tuberculosis.
4. Figueroa-Damian R, et al. Tuberculosis of the female reproductive tract: effect on function. *Int J Fertil Stud* 1996;41:430.
   The authors recommend three negative endometrial biopsies before ending therapy.

Diagnosis
5. Sahmay S, et al. Endometrial biopsy findings in infertility: analysis of 12,949 cases. *Int J Fertil Menopausal Stud* 1995;40:316.
   Prevalence of TB endometritis in this series from Turkey was 5.4%.
6. Seigler AM, Kontopoulos V. Female genital tuberculosis and the role of hysterosalpingography. *Semin Roentgenol* 1979;14:295.
   A hysterosalpingogram is useful, although not diagnostic. Pelvic calcification or irregular filling defects along the tube should arouse suspicion. Endometrial adhesions and deformity may be found.
7. Crowley JJ, Ramji FG, Amundson GM. Genital tract tuberculosis with peritoneal involvement: MR appearance. *Abdom Imaging* 1997;22:445.
   Ultrasound, CT, and MR provide invaluable imaging information but are rarely diagnostic.
8. Miranda P, Jacobs AJ, Roseff L. Pelvic tuberculosis presenting as an asymptomatic pelvic mass with rising serum CA-125 levels. A case report. *J Reprod Med* 1996;41:273.
   CA-125 levels may be elevated in women with pelvic tuberculosis.
9. Srivastava N, Manaktala U, Baveja CP. Role of ELISA (enzyme-linked immunosorbent assay) in genital tuberculosis. *Int J Gynaecol Obstet* 1997;57:205.
   This article reviews the role of ELISA for antimycobacterial IgM and IgG antibodies against A-60 antigen of TB.
10. Pietrzak J, et al. Comparison of polymerase chain reaction with standard methods in the diagnosis of Mycobacterium tuberculosis infection. *Eur J Clin Microbiol Infect Dis* 1994;13:1079.
    Polymerase chain reaction testing has a sensitivity of 93% and yields a result in 3 days, but it is difficult to perform and expensive.
11. Marana R, et al. Incidence of genital tuberculosis in infertile patients submitted to diagnostic laparoscopy: recent experience in an Italian University Hospital. *Int J Fertil* 1991;36:104.
    Laparoscopy appears to be an excellent diagnostic modality for abdominal and genital TB.

Therapy
12. American Thoracic Society. Treatment of tuberculosis and tuberculosis infection in adults and children. *Am J Respir Crit Care Med* 1994;149:1359.
    Problems of compliance contribute to treatment failure and drug resistance. Directly observed therapy, in which a designated person actually observes the patient ingest the prescribed drugs, is recommended.
13. Centers for Disease Control and Prevention. Initial therapy for tuberculosis in the era of multidrug resistance. *MMWR* 1993;42(RR-7):1.
    Rifampicin inhibits the effectiveness of oral contraceptives and several other drugs by accelerating their hepatic degradation.
14. Sutherland AM. Surgical treatment of tuberculosis of the female genital tract. *Br J Obstet Gynaecol* 1980;87:610.
    There is probably no place in tuberculosis for tubal reconstructive procedures.
15. Marcus SF, et al. Tuberculous infertility and in vitro fertilization. *Am J Obstet Gynecol* 1994;171:1593.
    Of 10 women with 22 in vitro fertilization cycles, three had live births. No pregnancies occurred if the endometrium was atrophic.
16. Schenker JG. Etiology of and therapeutic approach to synechia uteri. *Eur J Obstet Gynecol Reprod Biol* 1996;65:109.

Tuberculous endometritis is an important cause of intrauterine synechia and may present as dysmenorrheic amenorrhea.

17. Lifson AR, et al. Classification of HIV infection and disease in women from Rwanda. Evaluation of the World Health Organization HIV staging system and recommended modifications. *Ann Intern Med* 1995;122:262.

    In addition to death directly caused by TB, progression of HIV may be accelerated if TB adversely affects the immune system or enhances HIV expression.

Less Common Forms

18. Chakraborty P, et al. Tuberculous cervicitis: a clinicopathological and bacteriological study. *J Indian Med Assoc* 1995;93:167.

    Granulomatous diseases of the cervix include syphilis, granuloma inguinale, and tuberculosis.

19. Chaudray SK, Kapoor N, Jagtawat J. Tuberculosis of the vulva. *J Indian Med Assoc* 1996;94:357.

    In a woman with an ascending infection, the possibility that the husband has an active genital lesion should not be overlooked.

20. Sutherland AM. Gynaecological tuberculosis after the age of 40. *J Obstet Gynaecol* 1991;11:445.

    Eighty-one of the 711 cases occurred in women older than 40 years, 55 were premenopausal and 26 were postmenopausal. Fifty-seven percent of the patients had irregular bleeding, and 20% had pelvic pain.

Pregnancy

21. Nogales-Ortiz F, Tarancon I, Nogales FF. The pathology of female genital tuberculosis. A 31-year study of 1436 cases. *Obstet Gynecol* 1979;53:422.

    Four cases of active female genital TB were found that coexisted with intrauterine or ectopic pregnancies.

22. Gurgan T, Urman B, Yarali H. Results of in vitro fertilization and embryo transfer in women with infertility due to genital tuberculosis. *Fertil Steril* 1996;65:367.

    There was one live birth after 44 cycles in 24 women.

23. Bate TWP, Sinclair RE, Robinson MJ. Neonatal tuberculosis. *Arch Dis Child* 1986;61:512.

    The diagnosis of congenital or neonatal TB is difficult; the purified protein skin test derivative result is usually negative initially and only becomes positive some 6 weeks to 4 months later.

XII. CONTRACEPTION

66. HORMONAL CONTRACEPTION

Michel E. Rivlin

Combination oral contraceptives are the most widely used form of reversible contraception in the United States. The major mechanism of action of oral contraceptives consists of an alteration in the gonadotropin sequence, resulting in the suppression of ovulation. Other mechanisms include an atrophic effect on the endometrium and endocervical mucus that renders them hostile to sperm. The pregnancy failure rate is about 0.5%–2%, and this usually stems from compliance problems rather than from method failure, or results from interactions with other medications that lessen the contraceptive effect. These medications include anticonvulsants, nonsteroidal antiinflammatory agents, and antibiotics, particularly rifampicin. By comparison, pregnancy failure rates associated with condom contraception range from 2% to 10% and, with no method, up to 90%.

The modern combination pill contains estrogen in the form of ethinyl estradiol or mestranol, both of which appear to have virtually identical pharmacologic activity; the dose in each pill is 30–50 μg. The progestin component is provided by one of five synthetic progestins, all derivatives of 19-nortestosterone. They are norethindrone, ethynodial diacetate, norethindrone acetate, norethynodrel, and norgestrel. Three recently developed progestins that are claimed to have lesser androgenic properties, norgestimate, desogestrel, and gestodene, are now also available. Whether they represent a clinical improvement over the older formulations is as yet uncertain. Monophasic pills contain constant doses of the two components, and multiphasic or varying-dose pills combine a steady or slightly varied dose of estrogen with varying doses of progestins in an effort to lower the total steroid dose. Lower doses of estrogen and progestins are associated with more breakthrough bleeding and amenorrhea; higher doses, especially of estrogens, are associated with the more serious complications.

Common minor side effects include nausea and vomiting (in approximately 10% of users in the first cycle), breakthrough bleeding and spotting, amenorrhea, mastalgia, weight gain and edema, and depression. These cause more discomfort than real harm, but account for much of the discontinuation of the method (about 35% in the first year). Most symptoms usually subside after 3 months. More serious side effects include a worsening of migraine headaches; a worsening of asthma or epilepsy; growth of preexisting fibroids; or a worsening of kidney or heart disease. These side effects necessitate medical evaluation of the individual patient. Oral contraceptives decrease carbohydrate tolerance; therefore, diabetic and prediabetic patients must be carefully monitored. There is also an increase in the levels of triglycerides and total phospholipids of unknown clinical significance, but with important implications in terms of possible atherogenic effects. There may be an increased risk of gallbladder disease after only 6–12 months of use, possibly with cholelithiasis. Ocular lesions, including optic neuritis or retinal thrombosis, may be associated with use of the pill.

The complications that have received the most attention are cardiovascular disease and cancer, though the data are often conflicting. Most of the mortality statistics offer little evidence for a relationship between the pill and cardiovascular events. Multiple variables, such as age, smoking, and differences in the pills, have not been allowed for in these studies; nevertheless, the risk must be considered when counseling individual patients.

Hypertension develops in an estimated 1%–5% of pill users and usually resolves when use is discontinued. The risk of venous thromboembolism may be increased by from three to eleven times; however, heavy smoking may be the major factor here. Estrogen is thought to be the cause, and the effect disappears 4–6 weeks after discontinuation, as the levels of coagulation factors, increased by estrogens, return to normal. It is therefore recommended that pill use cease at least 2 weeks before a woman undergoes a major surgical procedure or during prolonged immobilization.

The risk of thrombotic stroke appears to be approximately doubled in users, and, as with the other circulatory diseases, the risk of myocardial infarction (MI) is largely confined to those women older than 35 years who smoke. In younger women, the mortality risk of MI is less than that of pregnancy; however, longer duration of use increases the risk of MI, and this risk persists after the discontinuance of pill use, particularly in older women who have taken the pill for more than 5 years and those who are heavy smokers. The atherosclerotic change responsible for MI and stroke appears to be related to the progestin component, as progestins decrease the level of HDL (high-density lipoprotein) cholesterol and increase the level of low-density lipoprotein (LDL) cholesterol, an effect that promotes the development of heart disease. Estrogens have the opposite effect. There is no clinical evidence as yet regarding the relationship between these lipid changes and vascular diseases; however, the strong relationship between vascular disease and lipoprotein concentrations cannot be ignored. Furthermore, the risk associated with low HDL cholesterol levels is exaggerated when combined with other risks such as hypertension and elevated LDL cholesterol levels.

The data on the role of the pill and cancer are fairly clear. There is little evidence that oral contraceptives adversely affect the risk of breast cancer. Although there is some evidence of a higher incidence of cervical neoplasia, the influence of sexual activity could not be eliminated and the relationship to pill use is unclear. Pill use for 12 months or longer is protective against all three major subtypes of endometrial cancer, an effect persisting for at least 15 years after the discontinuation of pill use. There is also a protective effect against ovarian cancer. There does appear to be an increased incidence of rare liver tumors associated with pill use, including benign hepatic adenomas and hepatocellular cancers, and an increasing duration of pill use increases the risk, though the incidence is still very low. Pill use does not appear to have any bearing on the incidence of pituitary adenoma or malignant melanoma. The inadvertent use of contraceptive steroids during early pregnancy does not appear to lead to fetal anomalies. Beneficial side effects of pill use include a significantly decreased incidence of benign breast disorders, functional ovarian cysts, gonococcal pelvic inflammatory disease, iron-deficiency anemia, dysmenorrhea, and ectopic pregnancy.

Absolute contraindications to pill use include the existence of thrombophlebitis or thromboembolism or a history of these disorders; cerebral, vascular, or coronary artery disease; known or suspected breast or endometrial cancer; undiagnosed abnormal genital bleeding; pregnancy; and the presence of a benign or malignant liver tumor. The pill is virtually contraindicated in women older than 35 years who smoke or who have other high-risk factors such as hypertension or abnormal carbohydrate or lipid laboratory values, or both. Current recommendations are to use a multiphasic or low-dose monophasic pill in the 85% of women who are acceptable candidates for pill use. Women taking the high-dose pills should be stepped down to low-dose preparations. Blood pressure together with glucose and lipid levels should be monitored in women with risk factors who nevertheless wish to use the pill. One suggestion is that pills should not be prescribed if the total cholesterol level is over 300 mg/dl, the LDL cholesterol concentration is over 190 mg/dl, the HDL cholesterol level is less than 35 mg/dl, or the triglyceride content exceeds 500 mg/dl. Among the few reasons for considering use of a 50-μg pill are persistent breakthrough bleeding or amenorrhea (alternatives include switching from a low-dose monophasic to a multiphasic pill, or vice versa, or the intermittent use of estrogen); use of anticonvulsants; and long-term antibiotics, as used in acne therapy. Counseling is the key to the successful use and selection of oral contraceptives. Considering that fewer than 23% of women are well educated about health matters and that the average reading level in the United States is sixth grade, ensuring comprehension is a serious issue. For most women who meet the medical criteria, the benefits of the pill outweigh the risks, particularly the risks associated with pregnancy.

The pill may be started on the first day of menses or the first Sunday after the period commences. Seven days of continuous use are sufficient for full protection. Active pills are taken for 21 days, with either no pill or placebo taken during days 22–28. Withdrawal bleeding, usually light and painless, generally occurs between courses.

If a patient has had an abortion, the pill should be started a week later; with a viable gestation, a 2-week interval is allowed after delivery. The pill is excreted in breast milk and also decreases milk volume, so it should not be used by breast-feeding mothers. If a patient misses a pill for 2 days in a row, she should add barrier contraception for 7 days. If three or more pills are missed, or two pills are missed in the third week of the cycle, the next pill pack should be started directly. If a patient misses two consecutive periods, pregnancy must be ruled out. A pill with greater estrogen content may then be required.

About 65% of women conceive within 3 months of stopping the pill; however, about 1% have amenorrhea that persists for 6–12 months afterward. About 15% of these have associated galactorrhea. These patients require evaluation to rule out pituitary microadenoma. With therapy (e.g., clomiphene or gonadotropins), about 42% conceive.

Many clinicians advise delaying fertilization after pill discontinuation, because, in those patients who become pregnant within 1 to 2 months of stopping the pill, the risk of congenital anomalies may be slightly increased, although this finding is controversial. There is also a possible association between congenital abnormalities and use of the pill in the first trimester. Therefore, progestin-estrogen withdrawal bleeding should not be used as a pregnancy test.

The minipill (progestin alone) is taken daily in low doses. It is generally used for patients in whom estrogen is a risk factor (e.g., those with fibroids, hypertension, diabetes, or epilepsy). Because it does not suppress lactation, it may be given to lactating mothers. Unfortunately, irregular bleeding occurs in 70% of the patients, and the pregnancy rate is three per 100 users per year, with an increased incidence of ectopic gestation.

Progestin-only contraception may also be given either by intermittent intramuscular injection using depot medroxyprogesterone acetate (150 mg every 3 months) or by the subdermal placement of levonorgestrel-releasing implants (Norplant), which provide protection for 5 years. Circulating levels of progestin are adequate to block ovulation, and the failure rate is below 1%. Side effects include menstrual irregularity, amenorrhea, weight gain, headache, breast tenderness, and psychologic complaints such as depression, nervousness, fatigue, and loss of libido. Progestin-only methods are generally reserved for patients who refuse combination oral contraception or in whom estrogen is contraindicated.

The postcoital or morning-after pill may be taken within 72 hours of unprotected intercourse to prevent normal implantation. Generally, diethylstilbestrol (25 mg), or an equivalent estrogen, is taken twice daily for 4 days. An alternative that does not cause the nausea associated with a high estrogen dosage is to administer ethinyl estradiol (0.2 mg) and norgestrel (2.0 mg) in two doses over 24 hours. The antiprogestational agent mifepristone (RU-486) is also highly effective, but is not available for use in the United States at this time. Although postcoital pills are very effective, the drawback is that, if pregnancy occurs, the fetus has been exposed to exogenous hormones and termination may have to be considered.

Reviews
1. Fauser BC, Van Heudsen AM. Manipulation of human ovarian function: physiological concepts and clinical consequences. *Endocrinol Rev* 1997;18:71.
   Low-dose oral contraception is characterized by extensive residual ovarian activity and, hence, reduced tolerance for omission of pill intake.
2. Bromham DR. Long-acting hormonal contraception. *Ann NY Acad Sci* 1997; 816:432.
   Parenteral long-term progesterone release provides highly effective contraception with less emphasis on patient compliance.

Metabolic Changes
3. Kluft C, Lansink M. Effect of oral contraceptives on haemostasis variables. *Thromb Haemost* 1997;78:315.
   Oral contraceptives should not be prescribed in women with known thrombophilic states such as deficiency of protein C and S, and antithrombin III and factor V Leiden mutation.

4. Godsland IF, et al. Insulin resistance, secretion, and metabolism in users of oral contraceptives. *J Clin Endocrinol Metab* 1992;74:64.
   The general metabolic effects of the pill are similar to those found in pregnancy, although to a lesser degree. Carbohydrate metabolism is affected, with a resultant decrease in glucose tolerance, increased insulin resistance, and increased pancreatic insulin secretion.
5. Knopp R, Arosa JL, Burkman RT. Contraception in dyslipidemia. *Am J Obstet Gynecol* 1993;168:1994.
   Increased levels of triglycerides and low-density lipoprotein cholesterol, and decreased levels of high-density lipoprotein cholesterol are all changes linked with atherogenesis and associated with pill use; however, the newer formulations appear to minimize these changes.

Adverse Reactions
6. Burkman RT. The estrogen component of OCs: cardiovascular benefits and risks. *Int J Fertil Womens Med* 1997;1:145.
   Vascular-related contraindications include systemic lupus erythematosus, uncontrolled hypertension, and diabetic vascular disease.
7. Kay CR. The Royal College of General Practitioners' Oral Contraception Study: some recent observations. *Clin Obstet Gynecol* 1984;11:759.
   The mortality rates for various groups of women aged 40–44 were as follows: 6.6/100,000, nonsmoking pill users; 58.4/100,000, smoking and pill users; and 71.4/100,000, associated with pregnancy and childbirth. (These figures are based on the use of older pill formulations.)
8. Douketis JD, et al. A reevaluation of the risk for venous thromboembolism with the use of oral contraceptives and hormone replacement therapy. *Arch Intern Med* 1997;157:1522.
   The risk ratio with oral contraceptives was 1.6–4.2. With a gonane progestin, it was 5; however, this may reflect prescribing bias, with low-androgen progestin pills being prescribed for high-risk women.
9. Carr BR, Ory H. Estrogen and progestin components of oral contraceptives: relationship to vascular disease. *Contraception* 1997;55:267.
   The newer progestins, possessing little or no androgenic activity, appear to have less effect on lipid and lipoprotein metabolism than the older, more androgenic progestins.
10. Klein BEK, Moss SE, Klein R. Oral contraceptives in women with diabetes. *Diabetes Care* 1990;13:895.
    Contraception in the diabetic represents a difficult choice, and the risks versus benefits must be weighed for the individual.
11. Becker WJ. Migraine and oral contraceptives. *Can J Neurol Sci* 1997;24:16.
    This article describes a relative contraindication, especially in smokers.
12. Rosenberg L, et al. A case-control study of the risk of breast cancer in relation to oral contraceptive use. *Am J Epidemiol* 1992;136:1437.
    Family history of breast cancer and previous biopsy for benign breast disease are not contraindications to hormonal contraception.
13. Gram IT, Macaluso M, Stalsberg H. Oral contraceptive use and the evidence of cervical intraepithelial neoplasia. *Am J Obstet Gynecol* 1992;167:40.
    There is probably no increased risk of invasive cancer, but a possible increased risk of precursor lesions in pill users. Women on oral contraceptives require annual Papanicolaou smears.
14. Scott LD, et al. Oral contraceptives, pregnancy, and focal nodular hyperplasia of the liver. *JAMA* 1984;251:1461.
    Rarely, hyperplasia or hepatoma may occur. The major danger is rupture with intraabdominal bleeding.
15. Lammer EJ, Cordero JF. Exogenous sex hormone exposure and the risk for major malformations. *JAMA* 1986;255:3128.
    Exposure to oral contraceptives during pregnancy does not appear to increase the risk for birth defects in the offspring.

16. Moore LL, et al. A comparative study of one-year weight gain among users of medroxyprogesterone acetate, levonorgestrel implants, and oral contraceptives. *Contraception* 1995;52:215.
    Significant weight gain was not found in any of the treatment groups.
17. Branham J. Oral contraceptives and depression. *BMJ* 1970;1:237.
    An underlying cause of this depression may be a disturbance in tryptophan metabolism precipitated by a pill-related pyridoxine deficiency. Therapy with vitamin B₆ may be useful to counteract these effects.

Benefits
18. DeCherney A. Bone-sparing properties of oral contraceptives. *Am J Obstet Gynecol* 1996;174:15.
    There is an increased bone mineral density in women using oral contraceptives, implying possible protection against osteoporosis.
19. Rosenberg L, et al. A case-control study of oral contraceptive use and invasive epithelial ovarian cancer. *Am J Epidemiol* 1994;139:654.
    An estimated 1,700 cases of ovarian cancer are averted in the United States annually by the use of oral contraceptives.
20. Williams JK. Oral contraceptives and reproductive system cancer. Benefits and risks. *J Reprod Med* 1991;36:247.
    An estimated 2,000 cases of endometrial cancer are averted in the United States every year by the use of oral contraceptives.

Other Hormonal Contraceptives
21. Graham S, Fraser IS. The progestogen-only minipill. *Contraception* 1982;26:373.
    Findings indicate that the method is reasonably efficacious and the side effects are minor. The authors suggest use in diabetics, cardiac patients, breast-feeding patients, and older patients, as well as in those who suffer the depression and loss of libido associated with combination drugs.
22. Chi IC. The safety and efficacy issues of progestin-only oral contraceptives—an epidemiologic perspective. *Contraception* 1993;47:1.
    This agent is particularly helpful for use as a contraceptive in lactating women.
23. Cromer BA, et al. A prospective comparison of bone density in adolescent girls receiving depot medroxyprogesterone acetate (Depo-Provera), levonorgestrel (Norplant), or oral contraceptives. *J Pediatr* 1996;129:671.
    The degree of estrogen deficiency induced by depot medroxyprogesterone acetate may adversely affect bone density. Women using the drug exhibit bone density values intermediate between normal premenopausal and postmenopausal controls.
24. del Carmen Cravioto M, et al. A multicenter comparative study on the efficacy, safety, and acceptability of the contraceptive subdermal implants Norplant and Norplant-II. *Contraception* 1997;55:359.
    Flexible Silastic capsules placed subcutaneously in the inner surface of the upper arm release 30 µg of levonorgestrel daily. Both implant systems are equally effective, safe, and acceptable.
25. Ledipo OA. Norplant use by women with sickle cell disease. *Int J Gynaecol Obstet* 1993;41:85.
    Appears to be safe for women with mild to moderate sickle cell disease.
26. Trussell J, Ellertson C, Rodriguez G. The Yuzpe regimen of emergency contraception: how long after the morning after? *Obstet Gynecol* 1996;88:150.
    Alternatives include the insertion of a copper intrauterine device, high-dose estrogen, or progesterone-only pills.

67. INTRAUTERINE DEVICES

Michel E. Rivlin

Product liability and medical malpractice issues in the United States have resulted in a marked decline in the use of the intrauterine device (IUD). At this time, the only IUDs available in the United States are the Progestasert and the Copper T 380A (ParaGard). The manufacturers of these devices have developed extremely detailed informed consent forms, which must be read and completed by the patient with guidance from her physician. These forms also have the effect of defining those patients at least risk for complications and those in whom the device is contraindicated. Partly as a result, there have been few if any medicolegal problems associated with the Progestasert or the ParaGard device.

Intrauterine contraception is very popular outside the United States and is used by up to 100 million women worldwide. The IUD is convenient, effective, and relatively safe, with failure rates only slightly higher than those for oral contraceptives. Approximately 80% of the women continue use through the first year, and about 60% use it through the second year.

The IUD is a foreign body that is placed in the uterus to prevent pregnancy. Devices may be either nonmedicated or medicated. Medicated devices contain progesterone (Progestasert) or copper (T 380A). A mild inflammatory reaction occurs around the IUD. However, the mechanism of action is uncertain. It appears to stem from the interference with fertilization rather than from implantation. Progestaserts are reinserted annually, and the copper devices are reinserted after 10 years when medication is exhausted. Inert devices can be left in for longer periods if there are no complications. Contraindications to IUD use include pregnancy; uterine abnormalities that distort the cavity; uterine malignancy; abnormal bleeding; acute cervicitis; and a history of pelvic inflammatory disease (PID), sexually transmitted disease (STD), postpartum endometritis, or infected abortion. Relative contraindications include hypermenorrhea, severe dysmenorrhea, nonmonogamous relationship, congenital or valvular heart disease, and nulliparity. Approximately 20% of the women require removal of the device during the first year because of side effects, such as bleeding, cramping, and pain.

Insertion is usually carried out during menses, so as not to disturb a pregnancy. Use of a careful aseptic technique performed by experienced personnel, prior sounding of the uterine cavity (it should be more than 6 cm and less than 9 cm in length), and atraumatic fundal placement in the correct plane are all measures that minimize complications. The IUD tail string is cut approximately 3 cm from the external os, and the patient is instructed in the technique of checking for the string. She should be informed of minor side effects, including cramping, intermenstrual bleeding, increased menstrual flow, and increased vaginal secretions. Women should be reexamined after their next menses and thereafter at least annually.

If at follow-up the IUD string cannot be felt or seen, it must be determined whether pregnancy, expulsion, or perforation has taken place. Once pregnancy is ruled out, the device may be palpated with a sound or localized by ultrasound or x-ray, with the cavity indicated by placement of an instrument or dye. Hysteroscopy or laparoscopy may be required for this in some instances. Uterine perforation occurs in one per 1,000 insertions. Because all devices are capable of eliciting peritonitis, adhesions, and organ penetration, the IUD must be removed by means of laparoscopy, hysteroscopy, or laparotomy when perforation is diagnosed. Expulsion occurs in 3–12 per 100 women per year, usually in the first few months after insertion.

There is an increased risk of PID associated with the use of IUDs, though the risk is much lower if the Dalkon Shield figures are removed from the overall statistics. The risk of infection is highest in the first 4 months after insertion. The women at greatest risk are those at risk for STDs—that is, those who have more than one sexual partner or whose partner has multiple consorts. IUD use is not recommended in such women. If symptoms of PID do occur, antibiotics should be administered and the IUD should be removed. Actinomyces, an anaerobic gram-positive bacterium, is occasionally detected in IUD users by the appearance of the characteristic Gupta bodies on Papanicolaou (Pap) smears. In the absence of PID, penicillin therapy should be instituted and the IUD left in place. If PID is present or the Actinomyces infection does not respond to penicillin, the IUD should be removed. Actual Actinomyces infection of the pelvic organs is rare; however, the risk of pelvic Actinomyces infection increases with the duration of IUD use.

The pregnancy rate for users of the IUD varies from 1.8 to 2.8 per 100 women per year. Women who become pregnant with an IUD in place must be advised of the increased risk of spontaneous abortion, together with an increased risk of septic abortion, septicemia, septic shock, and death. If the woman decides on pregnancy termination, the IUD can be removed at that time. If she decides to proceed with the pregnancy, the IUD should be removed if the strings are visible. She must be warned that abortion may follow removal. If any signs of infection or impending abortion appear, vigorous treatment with intravenous broad-spectrum antibiotics must be mounted. If the IUD is removed in the first trimester, the risk of a second- or third-trimester fetal loss is not increased. If the IUD remains in place, there is an increased risk of both first-trimester abortion and septic abortion, especially in the second trimester, and of premature birth in the third trimester. There does not appear to be an association between IUD use and an increased risk of congenital abnormalities in the offspring. Although most IUDs do not promote ectopic pregnancy, they do not offer protection against an ectopic gestation. In the case of the Progestasert, the likelihood of ectopic pregnancy appears to be increased, and users should be warned of this enhanced risk. In patients with IUDs who do become pregnant, there is a 1:20 ratio of ectopic to intrauterine gestation (1:200 in the general population) as a result of the contraceptive effect of the devices. These women must therefore be evaluated for this complication. The pregnancy rates in women after removal of IUDs appear to be similar to those in women who discontinue the use of other types of contraceptives. The outcome of pregnancies conceived after the removal of an IUD appears to be no different than that in women discontinuing use of other contraceptive methods.

Unrecognized PID may, however, partially or completely interfere with the restoration of fertility among former IUD users, as it does among non-IUD users.

Reviews
1. Mishell Jr DR. Intrauterine devices. *Curr Ther Endocrinol Metab* 1997;6:285.
   The Food and Drug Administration, the United States Agency for International Development, and the World Health Organization still consider the IUD to be safe and effective.
2. Kaunitz AM. Reappearance of the intrauterine device: a user-friendly contraceptive. *Int J Fertil Womens Med* 1997;42:120.
   For appropriately informed and selected candidates, IUDs represent a safe, effective, convenient, and low-cost contraceptive option.

Complications / Benefits
3. Spinnato II JA. Mechanism of action of intrauterine contraceptive devices and its relation to informed consent. *Am J Obstet Gynecol* 1997;176:503.
   The article suggests that the contraceptive effectiveness of intrauterine contraceptive devices is achieved by both a prefertilization spermicidal action and a postfertilization inhibition of uterine implantation.
4. Transabdominal and transvaginal ultrasound detection of levonorgestrel IUD in the uterus. *Acta Obstet Gynecol Scand* 1997;76:244.
   Ultrasonography is well suited for determining the location of an IUD within the uterus.
5. McKenna PJ, Mylotte MJ. Laparoscopic removal of translocated intrauterine contraceptive devices. *Br J Obstet Gynaecol* 1982;89:163.
   There is an increased risk of perforation after pregnancy. Laparoscopic removal was successful in 77% overall and in 44% for copper IUDs.

6. Skjeldestad FE. How effectively do copper intrauterine devices prevent ectopic pregnancy? *Acta Obstet Gynecol Scand* 1997;76:684.
   Relative to nonusers of contraception, current copper IUD users had a 91% protection against ectopic pregnancy.
7. Hill DA, et al. Endometrial cancer in relation to intrauterine device use. *Int J Cancer* 1997;70:278.
   With IUD use, there is a reduced risk of endometrial cancer for reasons that are unclear.
8. Coleman M, McCowan L, Farquhar C. The levonorgestrel-releasing intrauterine device: a wider role than contraception. *Aust NZ J Obstet Gynaecol* 1997;37:195.
   The IUD has a potential role in managing heavy and painful menstruation, and the symptoms of the climacteric.

Pregnancy
9. Herbertsson G, Magnusson SS, Benediktsdottir K. Ovarian pregnancy and IUCD use in a defined complete population. *Acta Obstet Gynecol Scand* 1987;66:607.
   Women who have an ectopic pregnancy while using an IUD appear to be at significantly higher risk of having an ovarian implantation.
10. Sivin I, et al. Rates and outcomes of planned pregnancy after use of Norplant capsules, Norplant II rods, or levonorgestrel-releasing or copper TCu 380Ag intrauterine contraceptive devices. *Am J Obstet Gynecol* 1992;166:1208.
    Normal fertility and pregnancy outcomes were unrelated to the method and duration of use.
11. Biggerstaff ED, et al. Maternal midtrimester sepsis in association with the intrauterine contraceptive device: early histopathologic findings. *Am J Obstet Gynecol* 1976;124:207.
    The insidious onset of a flulike syndrome, with a rapidly developing fulminant infection and an absence of pelvic findings, culminated in severe sepsis, septic shock, and maternal death within 72 hours.
12. Foreman H, Stadel BV, Schlesselman S. Intrauterine device usage and fetal loss. *Obstet Gynecol* 1981;58:669.
    Pregnancy with an IUD in place at the beginning of the second trimester carries a 10-fold increased risk of fetal loss. Third-trimester risk of fetal loss is also increased, but the magnitude is uncertain.
13. Sivin I, et al. Contraceptives for lactating women: a comparative trial of a progesterone-releasing vaginal ring and the copper T 380A IUD. *Contraception* 1997;55:225.
    The ring, with a 1-year pregnancy rate of 1.5 per 100, did not differ significantly from the IUD with respect to contraceptive effectiveness.

Pelvic Inflammatory Disease
14. Grimes DA. The intrauterine device, pelvic inflammatory disease, and infertility: the confusion between hypothesis and knowledge. *Fertil Steril* 1992;58:670.
    Epidemiologic studies of IUD use and pelvic inflammatory disease (PID) were biased by overdiagnosis of PID in IUD users.
15. Farley TNM, Rosenberg MJ, Rowe J, et al. Intrauterine devices and pelvic inflammatory disease: an international perspective. *Lancet* 1992;339:785.
    This study found no increased risk of pelvic inflammatory disease among IUD users who were at low risk of sexually transmitted disease.
16. Khomassuridze AG, Tsertsvadze GL, Tsereteli TG. Intrauterine device and pelvic inflammatory disease. *Adv Contracept* 1997;13:71.
    Careful selection of patients and bacteriological screening can effectively reduce the risk of bacterial contamination and subsequent development of pelvic inflammatory disease.
17. Yoonessi M, et al. Association of Actinomyces and intrauterine contraceptive devices. *J Reprod Med* 1985;30:48.
    A total of 4%–8% of IUD users may have Actinomyces-like organisms on a Pap smear, but this finding has not been equated with pelvic actinomycosis, nor has the risk of subsequent pelvic infection been quantified.

68. BARRIER AND CHEMICAL CONTRACEPTIVES

Marc Vatin

Barrier methods of contraception seek to prevent conception by interposing a mechanical, chemical, or combination barrier between the spermatic ejaculate and the cervical os. Barrier methods are nonsystemic, have distinct advantages such as safety in lactating mothers, and can be quite effective if used properly.

One must distinguish between the theoretic effectiveness of a birth-control method and its use effectiveness. Theoretic effectiveness is the antifertility action of a contraceptive if used under ideal conditions without human error or negligence. Its use effectiveness is that action achieved in real-life conditions. Effectiveness is measured in terms of failure rates by the pregnancy rate (PR) or pearl index. The index is calculated by the number of pregnancies multiplied by the months of exposure. In a population that does not use any contraceptive method the PR is 80 pregnancies per 100 woman-years. The theoretic effectiveness of barrier methods is very high, with a PR of 1–7 pregnancies per 100 woman-years, but the effectiveness varies widely with motivation and education. The PR can reach 30 per 100 woman-years.

Modern mechanical barriers include the condom, the diaphragm, the cervical cap, the contraceptive sponge, and the most recent development, the "female condom." Chemical barriers are the topical spermicides.

The condom is a disposable sheath used to cover the erect penis during intercourse and collect the ejaculate. Condoms are made of latex of various colors, textures, thicknesses, and perfumes. They are the most widely used and available contraceptive in the world. Their theoretic effectiveness is very high, at about one pregnancy per 100 woman-years; their use effectiveness is 6–18 pregnancies per 100 woman-years. Method failure occurs when the condom breaks; this is rare. Most failures are due to "user failure." Condoms should be stored in a cool, dry place and checked for tears before use. The condom must be applied before there is any contact between the penis and the vagina, with a space left at the tip as a reservoir for the ejaculate. The penis must be withdrawn before detumescence, while the rim of the condom is held manually to prevent spillage of semen. Petroleum or oil-based products should not be used for lubrication, since they weaken the latex. There are rare side effects of local irritation. In addition to its contraceptive role, the condom has recently received tremendous publicity for its protective role in sexually transmitted diseases (STDs), including the acquired immunodeficiency syndrome (AIDS), and cervical neoplasia. Laboratory studies have shown that latex condoms can block the passage of Chlamydia and Neisseria organisms, the human immunodeficiency virus (HIV), herpes simplex virus (HSV), cytomegalovirus (CMV), and hepatitis B virus (HBV). Proper use of latex condoms can reduce, although not eliminate, the risk of transmission of STDs. The use of spermicide-containing condoms may provide additional protection. Latex allergy has led to the development of nonlatex condoms made of polyurethane (Avanti condoms) or Tactylon, a nonlatex synthetic rubber material.

The diaphragm is a soft rubber cup with a metal-reinforced rim that is inserted into the vagina before intercourse to cover the cervix and thus prevent penetration of sperm into the uterus. It is also a receptacle for spermicidal cream or jelly. Diaphragms range in size from 50 to 105 mm in diameter. Most women can be fitted with a size 70–80-mm diaphragm. The most commonly used types of diaphragms are the coil spring and flat spring for the woman with good pelvic support, and the arcing spring for the woman with poor vaginal muscle tone or cystocele. It is essential that the diaphragm be fitted properly. After a pelvic examination, the diagonal length of the vaginal canal, from the posterior aspect of the symphysis pubis to the posterior vaginal fornix, is assessed by digital examination and the correct size diaphragm chosen. Alternately, several sizes of fitting rings can be inserted and tried for determination of the correct size. The largest diaphragm that can be tolerated comfortably should be chosen. It should fit snugly between the symphysis pubis and the cul-de-sac, covering the cervix and a great part of the anterior vaginal wall. A postpartum woman should not be fitted until 6 weeks after delivery. After the fitting, the user must be taught how to insert and remove the diaphragm and how to check placement by feeling the cervix.

The diaphragm can be inserted up to 8 hours before intercourse, but additional spermicide should be used if more than 2 hours elapse before coitus. Adding more spermicide prior to each coital act is also recommended. The diaphragm must be left in place for at least 8 hours after intercourse, but leaving it for more than 24 hours may result in infection. An 8-hour delay is necessary before douching, since douching soon after intercourse dilutes the spermicide.

The theoretic effectiveness of the diaphragm used with spermicidal agents is high, with a PR of three pregnancies per 100 woman-years. Use effectiveness varies, ranging from 6 to 25 pregnancies per 100 woman-years. Method failures occur when the diaphragm is displaced in certain coital positions or when it is defective.

The diaphragm is contraindicated in certain clinical conditions such as complete uterine prolapse, severe cystocele, or rectocele. Minor side effects are local irritation or allergic reactions. Diaphragm users may have more frequent urinary tract infections (UTIs) but do not appear to be at increased risk for toxic shock syndrome (TSS). A beneficial side effect may be a degree of protection against cervical cancer, pelvic infections, and STDs.

The cervical cap is a reusable, thimble-shaped rubber cup that blocks only the cervix and is held in place by suction. It is available in several sizes and should be initially fitted by a physician. Spermicidal cream or jelly should be placed inside the cap before each insertion. It can remain in place for 48 hours, during which reapplication of spermicide is not necessary. However, it could be displaced during coitus. The cap is comparable to the diaphragm in effectiveness. The cap can be used by women with poor muscle tone or prolapse, but not when there is cervical malformation, cervicitis, or abnormal Papanicolaou (Pap) smear. There is an increased rate of conversion to an abnormal Pap test during the first 3 months of cervical cap wear; therefore, a follow-up Pap test should be done after the first 3 months and if it is abnormal, the cap is discontinued. The Pap test must be repeated annually thereafter. The cap cannot be used during menstrual periods or during the postpartum and postabortal periods. There may be a slight increase in the risk of TSS. New caps awaiting FDA approval include Lea's Shield, Fem cap, and Oves, a disposable cap that could sell like male condoms. The main difficulty is that users need to locate their cervix. The best users will be women who have used the diaphragm in the past.

The disposable contraceptive sponge, made of polyurethane impregnated with spermicide, is shaped like a mushroom cap and fits in the upper vagina with a concave side covering the cervix. It is left in place to provide continuous protection for 24 hours, then discarded. It is about as effective as topical spermicides but less effective than diaphragm plus spermicide. Side effects are allergic-type reactions and vaginal irritation; there may also be an increased risk of TSS. Sponges have a tendency to tear and can be difficult to remove from the vagina. Discontinuation of the Today sponge and fear of lawsuits connected with use of silicone are forces discouraging research. A new sponge, Protectaid, is now available in Canada. It works in two ways. First it acts as a physical barrier blocking and absorbing semen and preventing sperm from entering the uterus. Second, it contains three spermicides and functions as a chemical barrier. In addition, since the spermicides exhibit antiviral properties in vitro it may work for the prevention of STDs.

The recently approved "female condom" combines features of male condoms and diaphragms. Also called a vaginal pouch, it is a lubricated polyurethane pouch that lines the vagina and is inserted like a tampon. There is a flexible ring at the closed end of the pouch which covers the cervix, like a diaphragm. Another ring at the open end remains outside the body and helps keep the pouch in place during intercourse. This device gives the woman more control since she can easily insert it in advance and is not dependent on the male's willingness to use a condom. Since the external genitalia are also covered, there should also be increased protection against STDs. During clinical trials, it was found to be very acceptable to both men and women, although there were some complaints that the device was cumbersome and unaesthetic. On the positive side, it does not seem to increase the risk of UTIs. And one size fits all. New models of female condoms are being tested. The Bikini condom looks like a G string. The perineal shield contains a rolled-up condom that the male partner pushes up the vagina at the time of intercourse. It is made of latex and prelubricated. Women's Choice requires an applicator for insertion.

Vaginal chemical contraceptives or spermicides are packaged in four basic forms: foams (including aerosol and tablets), creams and jellies, suppositories, and soluble films. The spermicide is inserted high into the vagina prior to intercourse, allowing time for the spermicidal agent to disperse and block the cervix. Another application is required prior to each coital act if more than 1 hour elapses before coitus. No douching is permitted for 6 hours after the last coital act. Occasionally, there are side effects of local irritation. Spermicides tend to have high failure rates (PR up to 30 pregnancies per 100 woman-years) but are readily available and easy to use. The most commonly used spermicidal agents are surfactants that destroy sperm cell membranes.

There has been some concern about the potential teratogenicity of spermicides. Most epidemiologic studies addressing this problem have found no evidence of an association between spermicides and congenital malformations or spontaneous abortion.

On the positive side, spermicides have been shown to provide some protection against STDs, including AIDS. Public health experts suggest the use of spermicides along with condoms to reduce the transmission of STDs.

Must Read
1. Trussell J, Sturgen K, Strichler J, et al. Comparative contraceptive efficacy of the female condom and other barrier methods. *Fam Plann Perspect* 1994;26:66.
   Comparing the contraceptive efficacies of different methods is problematic in the absence of randomized clinical trials. The female condom appears to have great potential for reducing a woman's risk of acquiring HIV.

Reviews
2. Connell E. Barrier contraceptives. *Clin Obstet Gynecol* 1989;32:377.
   Adverse publicity has damaged the image of oral contraceptives and IUDs, making barrier contraceptives more attractive. Moreover, the rapid spread of sexually transmitted diseases and HIV make them the first line of defense against major morbidity and infertility.
3. Glasier A, Gebbie A. Contraception for the older woman. *Ballieres Clin Obstet Gynecol* 1996;10:121.
   Barrier methods figure prominently among the choices of this category of women.

New Products
4. Dannemiller Memorial Foundation. Future barrier methods. *Contracept Rep* 1997;8:9.
   A rapid review of research in the pipeline, including the Protectaid sponge, Lea's shield, the Fem cap, and polyurethane condoms.
5. Mauck C, Glover L, Miller E, et al. Lea's Shield: a study of the safety and efficacy of a new vaginal barrier contraceptive used with and without spermicide. *Contraception* 1996;53:329.
   This article reviews a new one-size-fits-all silicone device. Fitting is not required. It is equipped with a valve that allows the passage of cervical secretions and air. It creates a better fit over the cervix. Failure rates are similar to the diaphragm or the cap. It is already available in Canada, Australia, and Germany.
6. Rosenberg MJ, Waugh MS, Solomon HM, et al. The male polyurethane condom: a review of current knowledge. *Contraception* 1996;53:141.
   The polyurethane condom was significantly more acceptable in appearance, lack of smell, comfort, sensitivity, and natural feel. Further evidence is needed on the device efficacy in pregnancy and sexually transmitted disease prevention.
7. Trussell J, Warner DC, Hatcher RA. Condom performance during vaginal intercourse. Comparisons of Trojan-Enz and Tactylon condoms. *Contraception* 1992; 45:11.

Tactylon, a nonlatex synthetic rubber, is being developed to enhance sensitivity during intercourse. The material may be more resistant than latex, and have a longer shelf or wallet life.

8. New barrier methods for women in development. Family Health International, Research Triangle Park, NC. *Network* 1994;14:12.

New types of vaginal spermicidal film, including benzalkonium chloride, instead of Nonoxynol, as the active agent are being tested for safety. Stability in tropical climates is a problem. Praneem cream and suppositories are made from extracts of three plants. Advantage 24 is a new Nonoxynol gel, which contains an agent that adheres to the vaginal surface, maintaining the spermicide activity for up to 24 hours.

9. Mauck CK, Baker JM, Bari SP. A phase I study of Fem cap used with and without spermicide postcoital testing. *Contraception* 1997;56:111.

The Fem cap is made of silicone rubber. It is shaped like a US sailor's hat; the bowl of the cap covers the cervix completely, while the rim fits into the vaginal fornices. The result is a complete seal over the cervix. The groove between the surface of the bowl and the rim provides a storage area for spermicide and traps sperm. It can be used by patients with latex allergy, can be sterilized, and can be worn for up to 48 hours. It can be used as a delivery system for a broad range of microbicides for sexually transmitted diseases, including HIV.

Beneficial Effects

10. Wiltkowski KM, Sussar E, Dretzk, et al. The protective effects of condoms and nonoxynol 9 against HIV infection. *Am Med J Public Health* 1998;88;590.

This article recommends the use of condoms and spermicides to reduce the transmission of HIV.

11. Alexander NJ. Barriers to sexually transmitted diseases. *Sci Am* 1996;3:32.

This article reviews the mechanism of barrier methods in the fight against sexually transmitted diseases.

69. FEMALE STERILIZATION

Marc Vatin

Sterilization is the voluntary destruction of the reproductive function. It can apply either to the male or female partner, but, in practice, female sterilization is performed more frequently than male sterilization.

The most frequent indication is multiparity. The woman has completed her family and wants a permanent method of contraception. Another obvious indication is the presence of any disease process in which pregnancies would endanger the patient, such as cardiac disease. Generally, an adult woman (regardless of parity or marital status) can request sterilization, but the laws governing sterilization vary from state to state, and the physician should be familiar with them. Alternatives to sterilization, failure rates, complications, and possible long-term effects of sterilization should all be discussed with the patient. Approximately half a million female sterilizations are performed annually in the United States. It is estimated that 1% of those women will seek reversal of the procedure within the subsequent 5 years; the usual reason given is a change in partner. Regret of sterilization is thus a public health problem. The most important risk factor for regret is age at time of sterilization (less than 30 whatever the parity). There is also a much higher incidence of regret in postpartum sterilization rather than interval sterilization.

A great variety of techniques have been used to prevent the union of the sperm and the ovum, generally by interrupting the fallopian tube. Unless there is concomitant pelvic pathology, hysterectomy is not usually considered an acceptable method of sterilization owing to its potential risks and morbidity. Tubal "ligation" is a misnomer. In fact, it is a partial salpingectomy, through a standard laparotomy incision; a small, 2.5–3.0-cm, suprapubic incision (minilaparotomy); or a 3–5-cm incision through the posterior cul-de-sac (colpotomy). Both colpotomy and minilaparotomy can be done under local anesthesia. The colpotomy technique has been found to have a significantly higher infectious morbidity than the abdominal approach.

The postpartum period is very convenient for sterilization, since the fundus is near the umbilicus and the fallopian tubes are easily accessible through a mini-infraumbilical incision; failure rates are higher than for interval procedures, however. In the interval procedure (sterilization done in the absence of pregnancy), the key to success is the elevation of the uterine fundus against the anterior abdominal wall. The most popular partial salpingectomy method is the Pomeroy, because of its simplicity and effectiveness (0.0–0.4% failure rate). A 2.5-cm midportion loop of tube is picked up and ligated at its base with absorbable suture, after which the loop is excised. The stumps are left tied together, but absorption of the ligature leads to their separation after a few weeks. Many other techniques have been described: Madlener, Irving, and Uchida, to name a few.

The most popular approach to interval sterilization in the United States uses laparoscopy. It is rapid, it allows visualization of the pelvic cavity, and it can be done under local anesthesia on an outpatient basis. First, the abdomen is insufflated with 2–4 liters of gas administered through a Veress needle inserted into the subumbilical area. A sharp trocar is then placed to allow introduction of the laparoscope. Alternately, the trocar can be inserted first and the pneumoperitoneum created through the trocar. Both methods are acceptable. Disposable shielded trocars can now be used to ensure sharpness and reduce the risk of injury. The fallopian tube is then identified, its midportion is grasped with the forceps, and it is destroyed by fulguration or occluded by mechanical devices.

Complications include injury to major vessels or bowels during the blind insertion of the needle or trocar, bleeding from mesosalpingeal tears during manipulation of the tubes, and bowel burns resulting from electrical methods. Burns often go undetected at the time of laparoscopy. Only compatible electrosurgical units should be used, and the manufacturer's recommendations followed. Failures and complications have been traced to unauthorized "mixing" of bipolar forceps and generators. The risk of burn is now greatly reduced through the use of bipolar forceps. With another method, endo- or thermocoagulation, no current enters the body. The coagulation instrument is merely heated to effect coagulation, though the failure rates associated with the use of this method are higher than those observed with bipolar current. Transection or resection of a segment of tube, in addition to electric coagulation, does not improve the effectiveness of the procedure and increases the risk of hemorrhage. Coagulation alone is very effective, if a minimum 3-cm length of tube is destroyed by creating multiple coagulation points.

For the nonelectrical or mechanical methods of laparoscopic sterilization, a special applicator is used to occlude the fallopian tube with a mechanical device. The Yoon band, or Falope ring, is a small Silastic ring that is slipped onto the base of a loop of the fallopian tube. If a tube is inadvertently transected, the ring can be applied to each stump or the stumps can be electrocoagulated. The clips (the spring-loaded clip of the Hulka and the titanium-silicone rubber clip of the Filshie) destroy the least amount of tissue (0.5 cm) and preserve the continuity of the utero-ovarian vascular anastomosis. Compared with the otherwise very efficient Falope ring and Hulka clip, the Filshie clip can accommodate thick tubes with less trauma. Because of the minimal tissue destruction, clips have better reversibility potential. This should be an important consideration, given the number of such requests.

The data on failure rates used to be derived from small series reported by individual institutions. They reported failure rates of 3–4 per 1,000 procedures within the first 2 years. Recently though, the CREST study (U.S. Collaborative review of sterilization) followed 10,685 US women for 8–14 years poststerilization. It is regrettable that the Filshie clip was approved too late in the United States to be included in the study. The 10-year cumulative failure rates vary from 1.8/1000 to 54.3/1000 depending upon the method used and the characteristics of the patient. The CREST study was carried out at teaching institutions where the providers may have had less experience. The Filshie clip has a failure rate of 2.6/1000 over 24 months in data submitted to the FDA. The most serious complication of laparoscopic sterilization failure is ectopic pregnancy. It appears that electrocoagulation techniques lead to a higher rate of ectopic pregnancies.

Overall, laparoscopic sterilization is a safe procedure with very low morbidity. In the United States, figures of 0.27% morbidity and two per 100,000 mortality rates have been cited.

Many experimental methods of sterilization are now being tested. In hysteroscopic coagulation, a small endoscope is inserted via the cervix into the endometrial cavity, which is then distended by gas or liquid for proper visualization of the internal ostia. An electrode or a thermoprobe is passed into the tubal orifices, which are fulgurated at the uterotubal junction. It is a procedure fraught with technical difficulties and potential life-threatening complications (e.g., uterine perforations and burns, and interstitial or cornual pregnancies following failures) as well as a high failure rate (11%–35%).

In another method, which uses a transcervical route via a hysteroscope, various chemicals may be instilled into the fallopian tubes. They act either by destroying the inner lining of the tubes, with subsequent fibrosis (sclerosing agents), or by forming solid occluding plugs. If improved, these methods could have a future as a quick, inexpensive outpatient procedure. For the present, however, they still have a high failure rate.

Another promising avenue for research is in immunization of the female against sperm. Animal studies have shown that local cervical secretion of antisperm antibodies can be induced. Each coital act would then serve as a booster to keep antibody titers high.

Long-term effects of sterilization are difficult to evaluate because the data published to date lack adequate controls. A poststerilization syndrome has been described that is characterized by menorrhagia, pelvic discomfort, and ovarian cyst formation. Some uncontrolled studies report very high (25%–50%) rates of menstrual disturbance associated with electrocautery. This problem may be related to the fact that the blood flow to the ovaries undergoes cyclic changes and is correlated with the systemic progesterone level. The mechanism of such changes in the blood flow are unknown. Surgical sterilization seems to interfere with the vascular supply of the ovaries, especially if coagulation involving the mesosalpinx is used.

Some patients develop psychologic or sexual dysfunctions, or both, following sterilization. These problems are often related to ambivalence regarding the procedure. Furthermore, fertility is so intimately associated with femininity for many women that they cannot easily relate to the loss of the reproductive function. Careful preoperative counseling is essential if these problems are to be avoided.

Reviews and Methods
1. Peterson HB, et al. Tubal sterilization. In: Thompson JD, Rock JA, eds. *Te Linde's Operative gynecology*. Philadelphia: Lippincott, 1996.
   This is the gold standard of technical reviews.
2. Sterilization. *ACOG Tech Bull* no. 222, April, 1996.
   Every practitioner should read this article before attempting a sterilization.
3. Graf AH, et al. An evaluation of the Filshie clip for postpartum sterilization in Austria. *Contraception* 1996;54:309.
   There are only a few reports regarding the use of Filshie clips during the postpartum period when tubes are edematous and friable. Complications rates were low, and there were no pregnancies during the follow-up period (24 months).
4. Schnepper FW. Sterilization by open laparoscopy under local anesthesia in a private office. *J Am Assoc Gynecol Laparosc* 1997;4:469.
   A review of 813 sterilizations done by the author. Minor complications consisted of three superficial wound infections and two failed laparoscopies.
5. Johnson PL, et al. Laparoscopy. Gasless vs. CO_2 pneumoperitoneum. *J Reprod Med* 1997;42:255.

There is a marked increase in technical difficulty and an absence of clear clinical benefits. For the healthy patient, CO_2 is preferable.

6. Kaali SG, et al. Modified open laparoscopy through placement of an optical surgical obturator. *Fertil Steril* 1997;67:969.
   This new surgical approach may assist surgeons in avoiding injuries.

Counseling

7. Haws JM, et al. A comprehensive and efficient process for counseling patients desiring sterilization. *Nurse Pract* 1997;22:52.
   This article presents a 10-step process to ensure a comprehensive counseling session.
8. Wilcox LS, et al. Risk factors for regret after tubal sterilization: 5 years of follow-up in a prospective study. *Fertil Steril* 1991;55:927.
   In a study of 7,500 women followed for 5 years, Wilcox found that women younger than 30 at the time of sterilization were three times more likely to report regret than those between the ages of 30 and 35.

New Methods

9. Pelage JP, et al. Selective salpingography and fallopian tubal occlusion with n-butyl-2-cyano-acrylate: report of 2 cases. *Radiology* 1998;207:809.
   This is an interesting preliminary report from France. No other method of sterilization was possible, and a new pregnancy was considered life-threatening. After 4 years of follow-up, there was no pregnancy.
10. Steele SJ. The potential for improved abdominal procedures and approaches for tubal occlusion. *Int J Gynaecol Obstet* 1995;51:517.
    Methods are reviewed. Clip sterilization comes nearest to fulfilling the criteria of a satisfactory method. The development of the Cambridge clip offers an improvement in reliability, and a small clip would facilitate the use of local anesthesia.

Benefits

11. Mac Mahill HL, et al. Tubal ligation and fatal ovarian cancer in a large prospective cohort study. *Am J Epidemiol* 1997;145:349.
    Tubal ligation seems to reduce the risk of ovarian cancer. Is it due to alteration of the hormonal environment or physical destruction of a carcinogen's route to the ovary?
12. Green A, et al. Tubal sterilization, hysterectomy, and decreased risk of ovarian cancer. *Int J Cancer* 1997;71:948.
    Tubal sterilization was associated with a 39% reduction in the risk of ovarian cancer. Risk remained low 25 years after surgery and was reduced irrespective of sterilization technique or types of epithelial ovarian cancer. The author's theory is that contaminants from the vagina such as talc or from the uterus such as endometrium gain access to the peritoneal cavity through patent fallopian tubes and enhance the malignant transformation of ovarian surface epithelium. Tubal occlusion prevents the access of such agents.

Reversal

13. Stadtmaner L, Saner MV. Reversal of tubal sterilization using laparoscopically placed titanium staples, preliminary experience. *Hum Reprod* 1997;12:647.
    This study included only 14 cases, but the method used seems a viable alternative to open abdominal microsurgical approaches.
14. Kim JD, Kim S, Doojk R. A report on 387 cases of micro surgical tubal reversal. *Fertil Steril* 1997;68:875.
    The pregnancy success rate was significantly higher for the Falope ring sterilization than the cautery. Patients with tubal length 7 cm or greater had a better chance.

Complications

15. Peterson HB, et al. The risk of pregnancy after tubal sterilization: findings from the U.S. collaborative review of sterilization. *Am J Obstet Gynecol* 1996;174:1161.
    A multicenter, prospective cohort study. Cumulative 10-year probabilities of pregnancies were highest after clip sterilization (36.5 / 1000 procedures) and lowest

after unipolar coagulation (7.5 / 1000), and postpartum salpingectomy. The cumulative risk of pregnancy was highest for women sterilized at a young age with bipolar application (52.1 / 1000). These rates are higher than generally reported.
16. Peterson HB, et al. The risk of ectopic pregnancy after tubal sterilization. U.S. Collaborative review of sterilization working group. *N Engl J Med* 1997;336:762. *The 10-year cumulative probability of ectopic pregnancy for all methods of tubal sterilization combined was 7.3 per 1,000 procedures. Women sterilized by bipolar tubal coagulation before the age of 30 had a probability of ectopic pregnancy 27 times as high as women of similar age who underwent postpartum partial salpingectomy (31.9 versus 1.2 ectopics per 1,000 procedures).*
17. Kaplan DB, et al. Desmoid tumor arising in a laparoscopic trocar site. *Am Surg* 1998;64:388. *Desmoid tumors are fibrotic neoplasms of low metastatic potential. They have been associated with laparotomy incisions. This would be the first report of a tumor arising from a laparoscopic port.*
18. Sunniala S, et al. Increased uterine and ovarian vascular resistance following Filshie clip application. Preliminary findings obtained with color Doppler ultrasonography. *J Clin Ultrasound* 1995;23:511. *Preliminary findings imply that sterilization may cause an increase in the local vascular resistance.*
19. Sunniala S, et al. Salivary progesterone concentration after tubal sterilization. *Obstet Gynecol* 1996;88:792. *Although the menstrual pattern was not affected, laparoscopic tubal sterilization caused measurable changes in luteal function.*
20. Robson S, et al. Intractable pelvic pain following Filshie clip application. *Aust NZ J Obstet Gynaecol* 1997;37:242. *The title speaks for itself.*
21. Gentile GP, et al. Is there any evidence for a post tubal sterilization syndrome? *Fertil Steril* 1998;69:179. *A review of 200 articles in the English literature. Many study results are affected by the failure to control for age, parity, obesity, previous contraceptive use, interval since sterilization, or type of sterilization. The authors conclude that there is no increased risk of menstrual dysfunction, dysmenorrhea, or increased menstrual distress in women who are sterilized after age 30.*
22. Hillis SD, et al. Higher hysterectomy risk for sterilized than non-sterilized women: findings from the U.S. Collaborative Review of Sterilization. *Obstet Gynecol* 1998;91:241. *A significant risk of hysterectomy was observed for each method employed. But this data should be interpreted with caution considering the lack of proof to support an effect on menstrual disorder. Would there be a follow-up bias and a self-selection bias?*

XIII. INFERTILITY

70. EVALUATION OF THE INFERTILE COUPLE

John D. Isaacs Jr.

Infertility is defined as the inability of a couple to conceive after 1 year of unprotected intercourse. Approximately 10%–15% of couples in the United States are affected (3–5 million). The major causes of infertility include ovulatory dysfunction (30%), fallopian tube compromise (30–35%), and defects of sperm function or delivery (30%). The initial infertility evaluation is designed to address these major etiologies as efficiently as possible and will reveal the conditions responsible in most couples (90%). In approximately 10% of couples, the initial infertility evaluation will yield normal findings; these couples are said to have unexplained infertility. With careful planning, the infertility evaluation can be completed in 2–3 months.

Important historical items to be elicited include pelvic infection, use of an intrauterine device, previous surgery, or recent changes in body weight. Physical examination of the female partner may reveal evidence of genetic defects, genital malformations, galactorrhea, androgen excess, or other factors contributing to female infertility. Information to be elicited from the male partner includes previous fathered pregnancies, urogenital surgery, impotence, diabetes, or mumps orchitis.

Confirmation of ovulation relies on detection of progesterone, which is secreted by the corpus luteum. Menstrual cycles occurring at regular intervals of 25–35 days preceded by moliminal symptoms (breast tenderness, etc.) predict ovulation reliably (95%). Progesterone is a thermogenic hormone; therefore, its secretion by the corpus luteum produces an elevation in the basal body temperature. Basal body temperature records that show an increase of 0.4° F for 12–15 days provide retrospective evidence of ovulation and duration of the luteal phase of the cycle. A serum progesterone greater than 10 ng/ml during the midluteal portion of the menstrual cycle provides confirmation of ovulation.

Patients with ovulatory dysfunction require investigation. Common causes of ovulatory dysfunction include hyperprolactinemia, androgen excess, polycystic ovarian disease, and thyroid dysfunction. Laboratory evaluation of prolactin, thyroid stimulating hormone (TSH), testosterone, dehydroepiandrosterone-sulfate (DHEAS), luteinizing hormone (LH), and follicle stimulating hormone (FSH) may be helpful in determining the etiology of ovulatory dysfunction in these patients.

A hysterosalpingogram performed during the follicular phase of the menstrual cycle permits evaluation of the uterine cavity and fallopian tubes. Contrast medium is injected transcervically into the uterus and tubes under fluoroscopic visualization, allowing assessment of tubal patency and intrauterine contour. Laparoscopy and hysteroscopy provide for direct visualization of the endometrial cavity, fallopian tubes, and pelvic peritoneum. Disorders such as endometriosis and peritubal adhesions, which may impair fecundity, cannot be seen on hysterosalpingography and require laparoscopy for diagnosis. Laparoscopy not only enables the physician to make these diagnoses but also provides an opportunity to treat these disorders.

A semen sample is obtained from the male partner for microscopic analysis of ejaculate volume (2–5 cc), sperm density (20 million/ml), motility (50%), and morphology (50%) as well as evidence of infection (white blood cells). Abnormal findings should be confirmed with a second test in 90 days. If an abnormal semen analysis is present, the gynecologist or urologist should evaluate the male for evidence of varicocele, testicular atrophy, or other urogenital malformations.

Identification of abnormalities provides for directed therapy. Ovulatory dysfunction may be treated with clomiphene citrate or human menopausal gonadotropins. Intrauterine insemination may improve fertility in cases of male factor infertility and may be done with semen from either the husband or a donor. In vitro fertilization combined with intracytoplasmic sperm injection provides good fertilization and pregnancy rates in couples with male factor abnormalities who do not conceive or are not candidates for therapy with other abnormalities. Pelvic adhesions, endometriosis, and other tuboperitoneal factors are usually treated surgically. Couples who do not conceive following these initial therapies may be treated with in vitro fertilization. Approximately 5%–10% of couples will remain without an explanation for their infertility after completion of this basic evaluation.

General
 1. Collins JA, et al. The prognosis for live birth among untreated infertile couples. *Fertil Steril* 1995;60:22.
    Approximately 2% of couples with unexplained infertility can be expected to conceive each month without therapy. Treatment efficacy must be evaluated in light of such factors.
 2. Hull MGR. Review. Infertility treatment: relative effectiveness of conventional and assisted conception methods. *Hum Reprod* 1992;7:785.
    An excellent overview of the relative efficacy of commonly used treatments for infertility.

Male Factor
 3. Barratt CLR. On the accuracy and clinical value of semen laboratory tests. *Hum Reprod* 1995;10:250.
    Where do we derive the definition for an abnormal semen analysis? This paper examines the relevance of the conventional semen analysis.
 4. Crosignani PG, et al. Clinical pregnancy and male subfertility: the ESHRE multicentre trial on the treatment of male subfertility. *Hum Reprod* 1994;9:1112.
    A large European report on experience with conventional treatments for male subfertility.

Tubal Factor
 5. Swart P, et al. The accuracy of hysterosalpingography in the diagnosis of tubal pathology: a meta-analysis. *Fertil Steril* 1995;64:486.
    Hysterosalpingography is the traditional method for evaluation of tubal patency and endometrial contour. This paper provides estimates of predictive values for this test.
 6. Adamson GD, Pasta DJ. Surgical treatment of endometriosis-associated infertility: meta-analysis compared with survival analysis. *Am J Obstet Gynecol* 1994; 171:1488.
    Does surgical therapy for endometriosis improve fecundity postoperatively? This meta-analysis suggests that women with mild and moderate endometriosis have an improved fecundity if their disease is treated surgically.
 7. Canis M, et al. Laparoscopic distal tuboplasty: report of 87 cases and a 4-year experience. *Fertil Steril* 1991;56:616.
    In vitro fertilization is widely used for the treatment of tubal infertility. Laparoscopic tuboplasty remains an acceptable alternative for many women.

Ovulation Factor
 8. Moghissi KS. Ovulation detection. *Endocrinol Metab Clin North Am* 1992;21:39.
    An excellent overview of the most widely used methods for detection of ovulation.
 9. Gysler M, et al. A decade's experience with an individualized clomiphene treatment regimen including its effect on the postcoital test. *Fertil Steril* 1982;37:161.
    A classic paper detailing expectations for ovulation and pregnancy in anovulatory women treated with clomiphene citrate.
10. Fluker MR, et al. Exogenous gonadotropin therapy in World Health Organization Groups I and II ovulatory disorders. *Obstet Gynecol* 1994;83:189.
    Details pregnancy rates in women treated with gonadotropins.
11. Blackwell RE. Hyperprolactinemia. Evaluation and management. *Endocrinol Metab Clin North Am* 1992;21:105.
    Hyperprolactinemia is present in 10%–15% of women with ovulation defects. This is an excellent review of the evaluation and treatment of these patients.

71. TREATMENT OF MALE-ASSOCIATED INFERTILITY

John D. Isaacs Jr.

Infertility affects 10%–15% of couples attempting to conceive in the United States. At least one third of infertility cases can be attributed to the male partner alone, and another 15%–25% are a combination of male and female factors. In general, when compared to female infertility, less is known about male infertility, and treatment outcomes have been poorer. A precise definition of male infertility is difficult because as long as motile sperm can be found in the ejaculate, pregnancies have occurred. Additionally, the criteria for a "normal" or acceptable semen analysis have become less strict with time. This makes comparisons between scientific efforts aimed at investigating male infertility treatments difficult to interpret.

The evaluation of male infertility requires a history, physical examination, and semen analysis at a minimum. The history is important (see Chapter 70) and may reveal toxic insults to spermatogenesis. The identification of such insults often merely gives the patient and physician a diagnosis since treatment is rarely available unless the offending agent can be removed prior to complete destruction of the seminiferous tubules. Antineoplastic agents, cimetidine, sulfasalazine, nitrofurantoin, alcohol, marijuana, androgenic steroids, radiation, insecticides, and a host of industrial chemicals are known spermatogenic toxins. The history of testicular trauma is only significant for infertility if resultant edema occurred or hospitalization was necessary. Sexual history should include lubricant use (many are spermicidal), coital frequency and timing in the menstrual cycle, and impotence. Men should be reassured that the use of boxer shorts as opposed to tight briefs and the frequency of hot baths have never been conclusively implicated in infertility. Galactorrhea, anosmia, or visual disturbances would point to more unusual disorders of the hypothalamic pituitary axis. The presence of severe chronic or metabolic diseases such as uremia, cirrhosis, sickle cell disease, etc. should be sought since they can also impair fertility.

The blood pressure, pulse, body habitus, hair and fat distribution, breast examination for gynecomastia, evaluation of smell, and visual fields are components of the physical examination useful in identifying endocrine causes of infertility such as hyperthyroidism, Kallmann's syndrome, and pituitary disorders. The presence of inguinal herniorrhaphy scars may herald previous damage to components of the spermatic cord. Careful genital examination should include evaluation for the presence of hypospadias, bilateral vas deferentia, varicocele, and the size and consistency of the testicles. Normal testicular volume is 15–25 cc (best determined by comparison to sized plastic models), while length should be greater than 4.5 cm with moderately firm consistency. Small soft testicles are associated with loss of normal seminiferous tubules, while small extremely firm testicles are found in Klinefelter's syndrome. Rectal examination to evaluate the prostate is important. If urethral secretion is noted after examination, it should be viewed microscopically and cultured when necessary.

The hallmark of laboratory evaluation for male infertility is the semen analysis. Generally accepted normal values are more than 1 ml of total volume, 15–20 million sperm per milliliter, 30% motility after 2 hours, 60% normal morphology, and liquefaction within 60 minutes. Morphology and velocity (linear and curvilinear) are most closely correlated with pregnancy outcome. Samples should be collected within 2 hours of collection, and prior abstinence is recommended for a minimum of 2–3 days. Since even a normal man will have significant variation in semen parameters over time, abnormal samples should be repeated twice, no closer than monthly. Normal spermatogenesis occurs over a 72-day period such that the initial semen analysis reflects events which may have occurred several months in the past.

Testosterone, follicle-stimulating hormone (FSH), and luteinizing hormone (LH) levels should be obtained on all patients with oligospermia (<20 million sperm per milliliter) or azoospermia (absence of sperm in semen). Antisperm antibodies are indicated for patients with gross sperm agglutination, abnormal postcoital tests, a previous vasectomy reversal, and history of cryptorchidism or significant trauma. A testicular biopsy is obtained to differentiate between gonadal failure and ductal obstruction or agenesis in patients with azoospermia (total absence of sperm) and a normal FSH. Karyotype analysis should be obtained to evaluate males with an elevated FSH.

Klinefelter's syndrome is the most common genetic abnormality associated with male infertility. It consists of decreased androgenicity, eunuchoid habitus, gynecomastia, azoospermia, and small firm testes less than 3.5 cm in length. FSH is elevated, and testosterone is typically low but can be normal. This syndrome is associated with an XXY karyotype and lacks specific therapy. Other genetic causes of male infertility such as mosaicism and translocations are extremely rare.

Varicoceles, discovered on scrotal examination as a "bag of worms," are simply varicosities of the spermatic venous system. Ninety percent of varicoceles are left sided, presumably due to increased hydrostatic pressure associated with the higher insertion of the left testicular vein into the left renal vein. Infertility, it has been proposed, results from either increased temperature of the testicles, decreased testosterone production, or reflux of adrenal byproducts to the testes through the testicular vein. Varicoceles are found in 41% of infertile males, yet they are also present in 15% of fertile men, which has raised questions concerning their true role in infertility. Some studies have shown improved semen parameters, a 50% increase in testosterone, and better pregnancy rates following repair. Others fail to show an improvement after surgical repair, but since the procedure is minimally invasive, many feel that surgery is warranted when other measures have failed.

The most common reversible anatomic defect results from male sterilization (vasectomy). Using current microsurgical techniques, pregnancy rates of 45%–60% can be expected. Prognostic factors for success include proximity to sterilization (<10 years is optimal), finding sperm in the proximal segment at surgery, and the absence of antisperm antibodies. Nearly all men develop some level of antisperm antibodies poststerilization, and the level increases over time. Congenital absence of the vas deferens and/or seminal vesicles is suspected when azoospermia and lack of seminal fructose are discovered. Congenital absence of the vas deferens is associated with an increased incidence of cystic fibrosis carrier status. All men with this diagnosis should be screened for cystic fibrosis mutations, and, if positive, the female partner should be screened prior to attempts at pregnancy.

Antisperm antibodies have been detected in the male and found to decrease motility and interfere with zona pellucida penetration. They are present most commonly after sterilization reversal. The recent widespread use of immunobead antibody identification techniques allows the detection of antibodies on the sperm surface itself, differentiating between immunoglobulin A and immunoglobulin G. This technique also allows for indirect localization of antibody to serum, prostatic, and seminal vesical fluid. Treatments include high-dose corticosteroid regimens (associated with significant side effects such as aseptic necrosis of the femoral head) and ejaculation directly into buffer solution to reduce the antibody binding from seminal vesicle or prostatic secretions. Neither of these regimens have consistently shown improved pregnancy rates when compared to no therapy.

Neurologic integrity of the male genital system is required for normal erection and external ejaculation to occur. To simplify, the parasympathetic system is responsible for erection while the sympathetic system regulates ejaculatory contractions. Any neurologic condition such as diabetes or spinal cord injury resulting in disruption of this system can cause retrograde ejaculation, impotence, or ejaculatory failure. Retrograde ejaculation has been effectively treated with the separation of sperm from postejaculatory urine followed by intrauterine insemination (IUI). In the absence of confounding infertility variables, this technique has enjoyed excellent results. Ejaculatory failure has been treated by electroejaculation where a transrectal probe is used to electrically stimulate the ejaculatory sequence. In this situation, if semen parameters are poor, combination with in vitro fertilization and intracytoplasmic sperm injection has improved pregnancy outcome.

Less than 5% of male infertility patients are found to have an endocrinopathy responsible for their inability to achieve a pregnancy. Men with oligospermia/azoospermia can be divided into hypergonadotropic (testicular failure) and hypogonadotropic (hypothalamic or pituitary failure) groups using measurements of testosterone, LH, and FSH. Patients with hypergonadotropic hypogonadism (low testosterone, elevated FSH and LH) generally have irreversible testicular damage due to genetic factors previously mentioned, congenital absence of germ cells, or exogenous toxic insults to the testes including chronic diseases, all of which carry an extremely poor prognosis. In contrast, hypogonadotropic hypogonadism (low testosterone with normal FSH and LH) is generally associated with an excellent treatment prognosis. Causes of this disorder include Kallmann's syndrome (hypogonadism, anosmia, and midline somatic defects), isolated gonadotropin deficiency, pituitary failure (tumors, infarctions, infiltrative disease), excessive hormones (body building anabolic steroids, Cushing's syndrome, congenital adrenal hyperplasia), thyroid disease, and hyperprolactinemia. Prior to any therapy, imaging the pituitary and hypothalamus with computed tomographic scan or magnetic resonance imaging is an absolute necessity to rule out the presence of a tumor. For specific disorders, treatment alone usually results in return of normal spermatogenesis. If spermatogenesis fails to resume or the cause is idiopathic then gonadotropic replacement is indicated. An accepted regimen begins with human chorionic gonadotropin (mimics LH), 2,500–5,000 IU three times weekly for 8–12 months to stimulate testosterone production. Generally, in men with postpubertal onset of hypogonadism, this is the only treatment required to normalize the semen analysis. If this fails or if hypogonadism had its onset in the prepubertal period, then human menopausal gonadotropins (hMG, containing FSH and LH in equal proportions) are added at a dose of 75 units three times weekly for 4 months followed by 150 units three times weekly for 4 months. Results of therapy are excellent, although expensive, and may take 6–12 months to be realized.

Unfortunately, after a thorough evaluation as described above, most patients are given the diagnosis of idiopathic infertility. Empiric therapies such as intrauterine insemination alone or in combination with ovarian stimulation with either clomiphene citrate or hMG, or assisted reproductive technologies including in vitro fertilization (IVF), gamete intrafallopian transfer (GIFT), and zygote intrafallopian transfer (ZIFT) have all been used as treatments in this situation. The literature is mixed on the efficacy of these treatments; some demonstrate improvement while others show no improvement in pregnancy rates. Many studies fail to include control groups. Without treatment, couples with isolated male factor have a 9%–18% chance of pregnancy over at least a 24-month follow-up period. Despite the disparity among investigators concerning overall pregnancy rates, most feel that these treatments shorten the time to pregnancy. To some couples, this may in fact be the most pressing goal in their pursuit of infertility treatment.

The IVF and ZIFT procedures both involve "in vitro" fertilization and allow physicians to visualize fertilization prior to replacing zygotes into the female partner. Thus, these procedures provide the most accurate method of testing the fertilizing capacity of sperm. Using these techniques, pregnancy rates as high as 10%–20% per cycle have been achieved. Often however, sperm from men with oligospermia fail to fertilize in vitro. For this reason, intracytoplasmic sperm injection (ICSI) was developed. With this procedure a single sperm cell is injected directly into an oocyte. Fertilization rates of 70% with this procedure compare favorably with those seen in couples undergoing IVF for non–male factor-related diagnoses. This procedure has revolutionized treatment of male factor infertility and now makes IVF feasible if even a small number of sperm are available either in the ejaculate or surgically aspirated directly from the testicle or vas deferens.

Lastly, and most importantly, the practitioner must know when to recommend cessation of therapy and counsel patients about adoption or donor insemination. Adoption laws are different in every state but invariably there are several different options available to couples choosing this avenue.

Artificial insemination by donor is indicated in cases of failed treatment as well as cases involving a genetic disorder in the male genome or when there is no desire to undergo vasectomy reversal. After a normal semen analysis, donors undergo history, physical examination, screening tests for human immunodeficiency virus (HIV), hepatitis B, and cytomegalovirus, as well as routine screening tests. Donated specimens are frozen and held until a second HIV test is negative 6 months later. Donors are then screened on a 6-month basis for HIV. In the absence of female infertility factors, monthly fecundity rates are 8%–10%. Timing of insemination is accomplished through the use of basal body temperature charting or urinary LH ovulation predictor kits administered at home.

Diagnosis

1. Rowe PJ, et al. *WHO manual for the standardized investigation of the infertile couple.* Cambridge: Cambridge University Press, 1993.
   Defines the limits of normal used in the laboratory diagnosis of male factor infertility.
2. Faslery TNM. The prevalence and aetiology of infertility. In: *Biological components of fertility. Vol. 1.* Liege: Belgium, 1988.
   Details the diagnoses present in 7,057 men among couples seeking treatment for infertility.

Treatment

3. Schlesinger MH, et al. Treatment outcome after varicocelectomy: a critical analysis. *Urol Clin North Am* 1994;21:517.
   A review of treatment outcomes following surgical therapy for varicocele-related infertility.
4. O'Donovan PA, et al. Treatment of male infertility: is it effective? Review and meta-analyses of published randomized controlled trials. *Hum Reprod* 1993; 8:1209.
   This comprehensive review concludes that few conventional treatments for male infertility confer any benefit as measured by improved fertility. Not considered in the analysis were donor insemination and in vitro fertilization.
5. Palermo G, et al. Intracytoplasmic sperm injection: a novel treatment for all forms of male factor infertility. *Fertil Steril* 1995;63:1231.
   Chronicles the development of this remarkable advance in the treatment of male factor infertility.
6. Le Lannov D, et al. Artificial procreation with frozen donor semen: experience of the French Federation CECOS. *Hum Reprod* 1989;4:757.
   Reviews the factors associated with success following the use of donor semen as a treatment for male infertility.

---

72. TREATMENT OF FEMALE-ASSOCIATED INFERTILITY

John D. Isaacs Jr.

Counseling patients about treatment options for infertility is difficult due to confusion in the literature regarding efficacy. Since term pregnancy rates are the only true indicators of success, many studies that have end points such as fertilization, ovulation, or chemical pregnancy do not necessarily support the efficacy of a particular therapy. Additionally, very few studies contain adequate numbers of patients. The background (treatment-independent) pregnancy rate is high for infertility patients, and therefore large numbers are required to demonstrate differences. For example, in patients who have no cause identified after routine evaluation, as many as 60%–80% will achieve a pregnancy after 3 years, even without treatment.

Tuboperitoneal factors are responsible for 30%–40% of female infertility and prior to the introduction of in vitro fertilization were very difficult to treat effectively. Etiologies include pelvic adhesive disease from endometriosis or previous infection, hydrosalpinx, proximal tubal obstruction, and obstruction due to previous sterilization. Laparoscopic surgical approaches for the correction of these defects have begun to replace traditional laparotomy microsurgical procedures, as success rates are similar for both methods. Results are best with simple adhesiolysis or ablation of mild or moderate endometriosis where pregnancy rates of 40%–60% have been obtained. Severe tubal disease or severe endometriosis has a much poorer outcome following surgical therapy. The poor prognosis seen with surgical therapy for severe tubal or peritoneal disease has made in vitro fertilization with embryo transfer the preferred mode of therapy.

Endometriosis is a common finding in infertility patients. For those who undergo laparoscopy as part of the evaluation, 50% will have endometriosis. Mechanisms proposed for endometriosis-associated infertility include adhesions with disrupted oocyte pickup, alterations in peritoneal fluid composition (increased in prostaglandin F and protein content), and an increase in peritoneal macrophages and their activation. Medical and surgical treatments, a combination of the two, and observation have all been used in endometriosis-associated infertility. Medical treatments for endometriosis include progestational agents (medroxyprogesterone), danazol, and gonadotropin-releasing hormone agonists (GnRHa). Medical therapy of endometriosis provides excellent control of pain symptoms but offers no improvement in pregnancy rates over observation alone. Surgical treatment, however, improves postoperative fecundity when compared to patients who undergo a purely diagnostic procedure. Surgical therapy is therefore the preferred method of treatment for patients with endometriosis-associated infertility.

Ovulatory dysfunction, present in some 20% of couples seeking infertility treatment, has the best prognosis with therapy. History, basal body temperature (BBT) charting, urinary luteinizing hormone (LH) monitoring, and serum progesterone are all methods utilized to confirm the diagnosis. First-line treatment consists of clomiphene citrate 50 mg daily for 5 days during the early follicular phase of the cycle beginning 3–5 days after spontaneous or progesterone-induced menses. BBT charting, urinary LH, or serum progesterone can be used to follow patients and if ovulation does not result the dose may be increased by 50 mg per cycle up to 150–200 mg before abandoning clomiphene citrate therapy.

Clomiphene citrate is a nonsteroidal antiestrogen which acts at the level of the hypothalamus by interrupting the negative feedback mechanism of estrogen. Clomiphene therapy induces ovulation in 85% of patients and results in pregnancy in 50%. Side effects such as vasomotor symptoms, abdominal discomfort, and abnormal ovarian enlargement are unusual. The multiple gestation rate is less than 10%, and the vast majority are twins.

Human menopausal gonadotropin (hMG) is the next therapeutic step in cases of clomiphene resistance, hypogonadotropic hypogonadism, and as empiric therapy for unexplained infertility. Due to the high cost and the potential for severe and even life-threatening side effects, this therapy should not be undertaken until a complete diagnostic evaluation is performed and other less complex methods have been attempted. hMG is a urinary extract of follicle stimulating hormone (FSH) and LH (1:1) from postmenopausal women. Several formulations (ratios) are available including a nearly pure FSH preparation, all of which appear to have similar efficacy. A multitude of protocols exists for administration of gonadotropins. In general, early in the follicular phase hMG is administered at a beginning dose of 150 units IM daily. Every 3 days estrogen determinations and ultrasounds are performed to monitor follicular development. The frequency of monitoring and dose is adjusted according to response. When the dominant follicle reaches 16 mm or greater and the estrogen level is acceptable (200–300 pg per follicle > 14 mm), human chorionic gonadotropin (hCG) 5,000 IU is given followed by natural or intrauterine insemination. Pregnancy rates for this therapy after six cycles range from 65% for anovulatory or hypogonadotropic patients to 25% in the case of unexplained infertility. Side effects include multiple gestation and ovarian hyperstimulation syndrome.

A controversial aspect of the infertility evaluation is the postcoital test for cervical mucous and sperm competence. Proponents of postcoital testing hold that abnormal results can identify couples with coital abnormalities, abnormal cervical mucous, and those with either male- or female-derived immunologic infertility. The test is performed in the periovulatory period and involves examination of the cervical mucous 2–12 hours after coitus. The amount, clarity, stretchability, cellularity, and sperm presence in the endocervical mucous are recorded. Additionally, observations regarding sperm numbers and motility in the cervical mucous are noted. Abnormal postcoital tests are usually repeated, as the most common cause of an abnormal test is poor timing with respect to ovulation. Persistent abnormal findings are usually treated with intrauterine insemination. Unfortunately analyses of outcome following an abnormal postcoital test reveal that pregnancy occurs as often without therapy in patients with an abnormal postcoital test as in patients with a normal postcoital test. This lack of discrimination has led to decreased utilization of this test.

Assisted reproductive technology (ART) is the final common pathway for infertility patients with a variety of diagnoses. Despite its expense, it offers the only hope for patients who without it would have little chance for pregnancy. Tubal occlusion, severe pelvic adhesions unlikely to respond to surgery, male factor abnormalities, failure of conventional treatment for any of the above conditions, and unexplained infertility are all indications for the use of ART.

In vitro fertilization with embryo transfer (IVF-ET), gamete intrafallopian transfer (GIFT), and zygote intrafallopian transfer (ZIFT) are the most commonly used ART methods. All use a stimulation protocol similar to that described above for hMG therapy with the addition of GnRHa in the luteal phase of the preceding cycle to prevent a premature LH surge. When follicular maturity is attained, hCG injection is given and oocyte recovery is performed 36 hours later. At this point the three above-mentioned procedures diverge. In IVF-ET, oocytes are recovered transvaginally in an outpatient setting under ultrasound-guided needle aspiration of the follicles. The gametes are cultured together in supportive media. Fertilization is easily documented by the presence of two pronuclei at 16–20 hours. Most programs transfer embryos after 48–72 hours; however, pregnancies have been obtained when embryos are transferred as late as the blastocyst stage. Transfer is accomplished by careful injection of embryos into the uterine cavity via a thin plastic catheter. ZIFT and GIFT are only useful in patients with normal tubal architecture. These procedures offer the advantage of allowing fertilization in GIFT and early embryo development in ZIFT to occur in the tube, which is felt to be advantageous due to an unknown secretory factor. ZIFT differs from IVF-ET only in the location of the transfer. In ZIFT, embryos are transferred into the tube either by laparoscopy or by a transcervical route using ultrasound guidance. In the case of GIFT the patient must undergo a procedure to harvest oocytes, which are combined with sperm, loaded into a flexible catheter, and replaced into the distal tube at the time of surgery.

Success of the ART procedures is variable depending on the cause for infertility and the procedure used. For IVF-ET, the best prognosis is seen in endometriosis and unexplained infertility patients while the worst prognosis is seen in the male factor group. Overall success rates of 15%–20% term pregnancy per transfer procedure have been noted. Pregnancy rate increases with the number of embryos transferred; with more than four embryos multiple pregnancy rates rise without an improvement in pregnancy rate. The multiple gestation rate has been 20%–25%, of which 25% are triplets or higher. Patients with more than two gestations can undergo selective reduction to triplets or twins. Five percent to 7% of pregnancies are ectopic. Reports of results with GIFT and ZIFT have been somewhat better than IVF-ET; however, these procedures are relatively new and are still undergoing evaluation.

A simple extension of ART is oocyte donation, which is occasionally used in women with ovarian failure. In this situation, the donor undergoes the stimulation with hMG and oocyte retrieval while the recipient is given exogenous estradiol and progesterone to mimic a normal cycle in synchrony with the donor's cycle. Term pregnancy rates with oocyte donation have approached 50%. This obvious improvement is thought to be due to lower levels of estrogen stimulation in the recipient's endometrium.

Since large numbers of embryos are often produced with ART procedures, methods of cryopreservation of oocytes and embryos have been developed. Social and ethical issues associated with cryopreserved embryos are currently being addressed. Today, the survival rate for thawed embryos is low but likely to improve in the future.

General
1. Masana R, et al. Distal tubal occlusion: microsurgery versus in vitro fertilization— a review. *Int J Fertil* 1988;33:107.
   This article presents a summary of 14 clinical trials examining pregnancy rates following surgical therapy for tubal disease.
2. Holst N, et al. Handling of tubal infertility after introduction of in vitro fertilization: changes and consequences. *Fertil Steril* 1991;55:140.
   This large series from Norway reveals that the liberal use of in vitro fertilization for the treatment of tubal infertility actually lowers the cost per pregnancy compared to tubal surgery.
3. Hughes EG. A quantitative overview of controlled trials in endometriosis-associated infertility. *Fertil Steril* 1993;59:963.
   This article discusses a meta-analysis of 25 trials of medical and surgical therapies for endometriosis. Ovulation suppression with gonadotropin-releasing hormone agonist or danazol was found ineffective for treatment of endometriosis-associated infertility.
4. Mascovx S. Laparoscopic surgery in infertile women with minimal or mild endometriosis. *N Engl J Med* 1997;337:217.
   This article reports on a randomized trial of surgical therapy versus diagnosis alone at the time of laparoscopy in 341 women with endometriosis. Surgical therapy increased pregnancy rates postoperatively to 30.7% compared to 17.7% in the group not treated during 9 months of postoperative follow-up.
5. Hammond MG, et al. Factors affecting the pregnancy rate in clomiphene citrate induction of ovulation. *Obstet Gynecol* 1983;62:196.
   This article presents a comprehensive review of cumulative success rates following therapy with clomiphene citrate as well as recommendations for monitoring therapy.
6. Dor J, et al. Cumulative conception rates following gonadotropin therapy. *Am J Obstet Gynecol* 1980;136:102.
   Diagnosis-specific pregnancy rates are detailed for a large cohort of patients treated with gonadotropin therapy.
7. Society for Assisted Reproductive Technology and The American Society for Reproductive Medicine. Assisted reproductive technology in the United States and Canada: 1994 results generated from the American Society for Reproductive Medicine/Society for Assisted Reproductive Technology registry. *Fertil Steril* 1996;66:697.
   Approximately 40,000 cycles of assisted reproductive technology are performed annually in the United States. Twenty percent to 30% of couples undergoing an egg retrieval will conceive and deliver a pregnancy.

---

73. ANOVULATORY INFERTILITY

Bryan D. Cowan

Repeated ovulation failure is manifested clinically as amenorrhea, menstrual irregularity, or infertility. An inability to conceive owing to failed ovulation accounts for 20%–40% of women complaining of infertility. The integrated function of the hypothalamic-pituitary-ovarian (HPO)–endometrial axis can be disrupted either by endogenous means (within the HPO axis) or by a perturbation of peripheral endocrine dysfunctions. In general, dysfunctions of the hypothalamic/pituitary system occur as a consequence of psychogenic causes, or develop as a result of structural defects or lesions within the central nervous system; on the other hand, peripheral endocrine disorders that cause ovulatory dysfunction do so by attenuating the normal cyclic sex steroids that signal the responding elements of the HPO axis.

Control of the self-regulated ovarian menstrual cycle is entrained in the "ovarian clock" conceptualized by Yen. In this model, nonlinear feedback of incremental estradiol (E_2) is generated over a well-defined time course. The two principal sources of circulating estrogen are gonadal (ovary) and extragonadal (adipose tissue). In the ovary, gonadotropin-dependent cyclic estrogen production occurs when granulosa cells respond to follicle-stimulating hormone (FSH), and stimulate androgen (androstenedione and testosterone [T]) conversion to estrogens (estrone and estradiol). The extraglandular gonadotropin-independent conversion of androgens to estrogens provides a second and steady-state mechanism for estrogen production. The predominant estrogen produced by peripheral conversion of androgens is estrone (E_1). The "E_1/E_2" ratio is often used to compare the relative contributions of extraglandular (E_1) and ovarian (E_2) estrogen to the circulation. High E_1/E_2 ratios (>1) are associated with excess extraglandular conversion of androgens and anovulation.

In addition to estrogens, androgens significantly affect the ability of the HPO axis to respond properly to feedback signals. In women, there are two sources of circulating androgens. The first, gonadotropin-stimulated ovarian stroma, primarily produces androstenedione and testosterone, whereas the second corticotropin, adrenocorticotropic hormone (ACTH)-stimulated adrenal zona reticularis, produces androstenedione, testosterone, dehydroepiandrosterone (DHEA), and DHEA-sulfate (DHEA-s). The most biologically important androgen produced by these two organs is testosterone. The ovary produces 25% of the circulating testosterone; 25% more is contributed by the adrenal glands; and a final 50% is derived by peripheral metabolism of testosterone precursors. The principal testosterone precursor is androstenedione, which is transformed to testosterone at several sites.

While estradiol and testosterone are important mediators of HPO responses, hormone-binding globulins unquestionably modulate the peripheral hormone effects of these steroids. In general, specific binding globulins exist for all biologically potent hormones, and the bulk of steroid hormones that circulate in the plasma are bound by such proteins. Sex hormone–binding globulin (SHBG), also named testosterone-estradiol-binding globulin (TeBG) has a high affinity for T, estradiol, and 5-alpha dihydrotestosterone. In addition to the specific steroid-binding hormone SHBG, albumin plays an additional major role in the binding of sex steroids. Approximately 60% of the circulating hormone is bound to albumin, 40% is bound to SHBG, while only 2% of estradiol is free in circulation. SHBG-bound steroids are generally not available for target tissue binding and action.

Polycystic ovarian syndrome (PCOS) is the most common cause of chronic anovulation. The term polycystic ovarian syndrome, or PCOS, emphasizes the heterogenicity of this entity, as ovulatory failure, infertility, hirsutism, obesity, and bilateral polycystic ovaries are not unique to PCOS. Although hyperandrogenism is a well-established feature of PCOS, the issue of its source (adrenal versus ovarian) has been the subject of several studies. The findings yielded by direct adrenal or ovarian vein catheterization studies suggest that the androgen excess in PCOS patients has a combined adrenal and ovarian origin. Furthermore, selective "medical ovariectomy" using the gonadotropin-releasing hormone (GnRH) agonist has been used as a probe to determine the respective contributions of ovarian and adrenal androgens to this syndrome. After the suppression of ovarian function with the GnRH agonist, the subsequent measurements of peripheral androgens reveal that ovarian hormones (androstenedione, testosterone, and 17-hydroxyprogesterone) are reduced to castrate levels, whereas the concentrations of the adrenal hormones (DHEA and DHEA-s) are unaffected. Thus, biglandular excess production of both ovarian and adrenal androgens contributes to the overall androgen excess present in patients with PCOS.

The secretion of excessive amounts of androgen, with subsequent conversion to estrogen, constitutes the basis for the chronic anovulation observed in PCOS. Relatively constant levels of estrogen are reflected mainly by chronically elevated levels of estrone (rather than estradiol), which is derived from extraglandular conversion of androstenedione. This chronically elevated estrogen environment perpetuates acyclic feedback and the inappropriate secretion of luteinizing hormone (LH) and FSH by the hypothalamic-pituitary system. Patients with PCOS typically demonstrate elevated blood LH concentrations together with relatively constant or low FSH levels, and the

LH-FSH ratio is usually greater than 3. The disparity between LH and FSH secretion in patients with PCOS can be explained by the following: (1) the negative feedback inhibition of both estradiol and estrone has greater impact on FSH than on LH; (2) FSH release is relatively insensitive to GnRH stimulation; and (3) a multicystic ovary in PCOS patients may secrete large amounts of follicular inhibin (an inhibitor of FSH release), which further inhibits the release of FSH.

In addition to abnormal androgen/estrogen metabolism, PCOS is associated with a peripheral resistance to insulin and glucose intolerance. Both obese and nonobese women with PCOS demonstrate a positive correlation between hyperinsulinemia and hyperandrogenism, implying that androgen excess may somehow mediate peripheral insulin resistance.

The genesis of PCOS is not related to an inherent defect in the HPO axis, but rather it is initiated and then sustained by elevated circulating androgen levels arising from any source. Increased androgen production then leads to increased acyclic peripheral estrogen formation. Peripheral estrogen preferentially inhibits pituitary FSH secretion and causes a high LH-FSH ratio to be established that sustains the acyclic nonincremental estrogen feedback on the HPO axis. LH stimulation of the ovarian stroma cells in conjunction with an associated excess secretion of ovarian androgens then ensues. The excess production of adrenal and ovarian androgens causes SHBG production to diminish, and this alteration further augments the biologic activity of the circulating androgens. In addition, the increased availability of circulating androgens for end-organ action makes them more available for peripheral conversion to estrogen. Thus, elevated androgen concentrations induce an acyclic steady-state of estrogen production (predominantly E_1), which perpetuates chronic anovulation. Ovarian changes, such as inadequate follicular maturation and increased follicular atresia, are secondary events that stem from both inadequate FSH and excess LH stimulation of the follicle.

The association between amenorrhea and galactorrhea has long been known, and its relationship with prolactin excess is well established. Prolactin is secreted by the lactotrophs of the anterior pituitary, mainly under the control of the prolactin-inhibiting factor, dopamine. The mechanism by which hyperprolactinemia is associated with hypogonadism is not yet well established. Dopamine agonists such as levo-dopa and the ergot alkaloids (e.g., bromocriptine and pergolide) decrease the serum prolactin level, whereas antagonists increase it. Many pharmacologic agents induce hyperprolactinemia, including estrogens, neuroleptics, antiemetics, antihypertensives, hallucinogens, and anesthetic agents. Removing or replacing these drugs is frequently sufficient therapy to restore ovulation. Pituitary prolactinomas are generally small (microadenomas) and are commonly treated with bromocriptine, with good fertility outcomes. Side effects from medical therapy are common and include postural hypotension and gastrointestinal symptoms. The cessation of therapy is usually followed by return of the prolactin excess. Larger tumors (macroadenomas) may require surgical removal. However, medical therapy alone or in combination with surgery has been used with success for some macroadenomas. The diagnosis and follow-up of patients with pituitary tumors are best conducted with computed tomographic (CT) scanning of the pituitary fossa, magnetic resonance imaging (MRI), and a visual field test to rule out pressure effects on the optic chiasma.

Central neuroendocrine failure (hypothalamic-pituitary) results in hypogonadotropic hypogonadism (World Health Organization [WHO] I) amenorrhea. Gonadotropins are depressed, and estrogen activity is absent. Ovarian failure is manifested by hypergonadotropic hypogonadism, with elevated gonadotropins and insufficient estrogen activity (WHO III) amenorrhea. Asynchronous gonadotropin and estrogen production results in anovulation and presents with varying clinical features (WHO II amenorrhea). The estrogen, LH, and FSH levels are usually normal in WHO II women, but the menstrual cycles are disrupted. Depending on the type of impairment, the clinical spectrum of anovulation therefore encompasses amenorrhea, dysfunctional uterine bleeding, and infertility.

The treatment of PCOS or chronic anovulation depends on the clinical diagnosis rendered and the wishes of the patient. If pregnancy is not desired, therapy is directed at protecting the endometrium from unopposed estrogen stimulation, which either could produce endometrial hyperplasia/adenocarcinoma or result in dramatic dysfunctional bleeding. Therapy usually consists of cyclic endometrial shedding, which can be initiated with medroxyprogesterone (10-mg tablet taken orally for 10–13 days every month) or with oral contraceptive pills (OCP). If androgen excess is also present, ovarian suppression through the use of oral contraceptive pills is usually the treatment of choice.

Women with chronic anovulation who wish to get pregnant require ovulation induction. Clomiphene citrate (CC) has been shown to be effective for this purpose in such women. CC is a novel synthetic preparation that acts as a strong antiestrogen as well as a weak estrogen. It predominantly affects hypothalamic-pituitary receptors for estrogen and promotes an increase in pituitary gonadotropin release, which stimulates follicular development and maturation. We initiate therapy with the administration of 50 mg CC on days 5–9 of the cycle, after a progestin withdrawal. Because approximately 75% of clomiphene-induced pregnancies occur during the first 3–4 months of treatment, a full infertility work-up need not be pursued until the woman fails to conceive after several ovulatory cycles. Efficacy (ovulation) can be monitored with basal body temperature charts, luteal-phase progesterone measurements, or endometrial histology. If ovulation does not occur at a 50-mg dose, the dose should be increased by 50 mg after each anovulatory cycle to a maximum of 150 mg. Side effects from clomiphene therapy include ovarian enlargement (13%), vasomotor flushes (10%), and abdominal discomfort (5%). The incidence of multiple gestation is 5%–10%. In patients with ovarian enlargement, therapy should be withheld until ovaries are a normal size. Occasionally, mild adrenal androgen suppression is also desirable in such patients. Our choice for this has been to administer 2.5–5.0 mg of prednisone at 10–11 p.m. and to monitor the clinical responses with DHEA-s measurements. Prednisone is a potent glucocorticoid with a short duration of action. As such, the risks of adrenal insufficiency resulting from lengthy chronic exposure to low doses of this preparation are small, but efficacy at low doses can be achieved only if the prednisone is given at night (a few hours before the endogenous nocturnal ACTH rise).

Patients who fail to respond to clomiphene are candidates for gonadotropin therapy. This medication is expensive, requires daily injections, and carries a substantial complication rate. For these reasons, patients must have an infertility work-up before gonadotropin therapy is begun. In particular, the uterotubal and male factors must be investigated and ovarian failure excluded. Patient counseling and instruction are essential.

Gonadotropin therapy requires only an ovary with responsive oocytes; about 90% of the patients ovulate with therapy. Women with hypogonadotropic hypogonadism have a 70%–90% chance of conception after 3 to 4 successful inductions. Unfortunately, PCOS patients will only have a 30%–40% rate during the same time interval. Multiple gestation is the major complication of the method, with an incidence of 20%–35%. Three or more fetuses per pregnancy will occur in 5% of women. Superovulation can be kept to a minimum by withholding human chorionic gonadotropin if the estrogen levels are excessive. The second major drawback of gonadotropin treatment is the ovarian hyperstimulation syndrome. The severe form is rare, consisting of large theca lutein cysts, ascites, hypovolemia, hypercoagulability, and even mortality. Ovarian rupture or hemorrhage may occur, necessitating laparotomy. A mild ovarian enlargement of 5–10 cm occurs in 30% of the ovulatory cycles.

GnRH, a hypothalamic decapeptide, is the neurohormone responsible for gonadotropin release. This decapeptide has been synthesized and its analogues used for ovulation induction. Physiologic GnRH secretion is pulsatile in nature, and thus its clinical use requires that the GnRH be administered by long-term pulsatile infusion. The early results of this method have proved promising in selected patients, generally women with hypothalamic amenorrhea.

Finally, surgical ablation of ovarian stromal follicles has been effective in restoring ovulation and establishing pregnancies in about 60% of cases of PCOS. Surgery is usually laparoscopically directed, and laser or endocoagulation is applied to several areas of the ovary.

General
1. Cowan BD. Anovulation. In: Collins RL, ed. *Clinical perspectives in obstetrics and gynecology: ovulation induction.* New York: Springer-Verlag, 1990:41–52.
   Current review of etiology and evaluation of anovulation.
2. Yen SSC. Chronic anovulation caused by peripheral endocrine disorders. In: Yen SSC, Jaffe RB, eds. *Reproductive endocrinology, physiology, pathophysiology, and clinical management.* Philadelphia: Saunders, 1986: 441–499.
   Exceptionally thorough treatise on anovulation.
3. Botwood N, et al. Sex hormone–binding globulin and female reproductive function. *J Steroid Mol Biol* 1995;56:529.
   Although sex steroids have long been known to influence serum concentrations of sex hormone–binding globulin (SHBG), it is now recognized that nutritional factors may be more important in the regulation of SHBG in women. Thus, SHBG concentrations are negatively correlated with body mass index (BMI) and, more particularly, with indices of central adiposity. Weight reduction in obese, hyperandrogenaemic women with polycystic ovarian syndrome is important in the management of both anovulation and hirsutism.

Polycystic Ovarian Syndrome
4. Kirschner MA, Jacobs JB. Combined ovarian and adrenal vein catheterization to determine the site(s) of androgen overproduction in hirsute women. *J Clin Endocrinol Metab* 1971;33:199.
   In general, the ovary is the major source of androgens in women with polycystic ovarian syndrome or idiopathic hirsutism.
5. Chang RJ, et al. Steroid secretion in polycystic ovarian disease after ovarian suppression by a long-acting gonadotropin-releasing hormone agonist. *J Clin Endocrinol Metab* 1983;56:897.
   Suppression of pituitary luteinizing hormone and follicle-stimulating hormone secretion reduces ovarian but not adrenal androgen secretion.
6. Chang R, et al. Insulin resistance in nonobese patients with polycystic ovarian disease. *J Clin Endocrinol Metab* 1983;57:356.
   Women with androgen excess demonstrate peripheral resistance to insulin.
7. Takai T, et al. Three types of polycystic ovarian syndrome in relation to androgenic function. *Fertil Steril* 1991;56:856.
   Possible subsets of polycystic ovarian syndrome based on extent of hirsutism and androgen excess.

Treatment
8. Blacker CM. Ovulation stimulation and induction. *Endocrinol Metab Clin North Am* 1992;21:57.
   Protocols for follicular stimulation.
9. Garcia-Flores RF, Vasquez-Mendez J. Progressive dosages of clomiphene citrate in hypothalamic anovulation. *Fertil Steril* 1984;42:543.
   Extended therapy with clomiphene citrate may induce ovulation when standard therapy fails.
10. Adashi EY. Clomiphene citrate: mechanism(s) and site(s) of action—a hypothesis revisited. *Fertil Steril* 1984;42:331.
    A well-written review describing the history of development and mechanisms of action of clomiphene citrate.
11. Nakamura Y, et al. Clinical experience in the induction of ovulation and pregnancy with pulsatile subcutaneous administration of human menopausal gonadotropin: a low incidence of multiple pregnancy. *Fertil Steril* 1989;51:423.
    Administration of gonadotropins in a pulsatile mode by means of a portable peristaltic pump via a subcutaneous catheter inserted in the lower abdominal wall.
12. Kousta E, White DM, Franks S. Modern use of clomiphene citrate in induction of ovulation. *Hum Reprod Update* 1997;3:359.
    Clomiphene citrate (CC) is the treatment of first choice in the management of infertility in normally estrogenized, anovulatory women (World Health Organization

*group II). The majority of women with pure anovulatory infertility respond to treat-
ment with CC. The rates of pregnancy and miscarriage are close to those expected
in a normal fertile population. Basal hormone concentrations do not predict outcome. When couples with other factors contributing to subfertility are excluded,
the cumulative conception rate continues to rise after 6 months of treatment with
CC, and reaches a plateau by treatment cycle 12.*

13. Pelosi MA. Laparoscopic electrosurgical furrowing technique for the treatment of
polycystic ovaries. *J Am Assoc Gynecol Laparosc* 1996;4:57.

*A retrospective analysis of reproductive outcomes was conducted in 30 anovula-
tory women treated with a new laparoscopic electrosurgical furrowing technique.
Regular ovulatory function resumed in 25 women (83.3%); the refractory patients
were administered clomiphene citrate (CC). Spontaneous conception occurred in
21 ovulatory patients (70.0%) and clomiphene-assisted conception occurred in
three of the five refractory women, for an overall pregnancy rate of 80% (24/30).
These results suggest that the laparoscopic electrosurgical furrowing technique for
the treatment of anovulatory infertility in women with polycystic ovary syndrome
refractory to CC and gonadotropin therapy is effective.*

14. Tadokoro N, et al. Cumulative pregnancy rates in couples with anovulatory infertility compared with unexplained infertility in an ovulation induction programme.
Hum Reprod 1997;12:1939.

*Using a retrospective analysis, the cumulative pregnancy rate (derived from life-
table analysis) after four ovulatory treatment cycles was 70% in the polycystic
ovarian syndrome group, 74% in the hypogonadism group, and 38% in the unexplained infertility group. Couples with unexplained infertility are less successfully
treated using human menopausal gonadotrophin (HMG).*

15. Isaacs JD Jr, Lincoln SR, Cowan BD. Extended clomiphene citrate (CC) and prednisone for the treatment of chronic anovulation resistant to CC alone. *Fertil Steril*
1997;67:641.

*Women who had failed to ovulate with 150 mg clomiphene for 5 days were treated
with 150 mg clomiphene for 7 days and 5 mg prednisone each night. Logistic (two-
parameter) pregnancy occurrence over time (cycles) revealed a maximum pregnancy probability of 0.66 and a cycle fecundity of 0.36. This therapy offers a potential reduction in cost and risk and should be considered in this group of
patients before gonadotropin stimulation or surgery.*

XIV. HUMAN SEXUALITY

74. ADOLESCENT SEXUALITY

Michel E. Rivlin

Children and adolescents are sexual beings, and this is normal. Fetal sexuality begins when an X or Y chromosome directs the development of either testicles or ovaries. Starting in the eighth week of gestation, the gonads elaborate hormones governing sex differentiation and function. In the male, ultrasound imaging has shown that erections occur in the same 90-minute cycle in the 17-week fetus as in adult men. Adolescent sexuality derives from earlier development; the infant period (to 18 months) leads to an awareness of body parts, including the genitals, oral exploration and gratification, and a sense of trust in the primary caretaker. The toddler or training period (to 3 years) is associated with elimination functions, body control, awareness of sex differences, and interest in sex roles. The preschool, Oedipal, or genital period (to 6 years) is characterized by romantic attachment to the opposite sex parent, sexual play, self-manipulation, exhibitionism, and awareness of sex differences. The school age or latent period (to 9 years) is a time of intense curiosity, sexual thoughts are self-contained, information is obtained from friends or the media, and same-sex play predominates. The hormonal and physical changes of puberty (see Chapter 82) result in the metamorphosis from childhood to adolescence.

Early adolescence (to 14 years) is often characterized by same-sex friendships and opposite sex contacts; same sex sexual contacts may occur. Concern with physical changes and normality is intense. In mid-adolescence (to 18 years), there may be opposite-sex contacts and risk-taking sexual behavior. Masturbation is also related to exploration and autonomy in adolescence; by age 15, 33% of females masturbate, and by age 20, over 75%. During late adolescence (after 18 years), young women may become concerned about life-planning issues and acquire an increasing ability to consider the consequences of their own behavior. Along with adult sexual identity and concerns about future parenthood, the ability to be intimate with another in an emotionally rewarding manner may be attained.

Adolescence is regarded as a time of turmoil, with a significant disruption in psychologic equilibrium leading to a fluctuation in mood, confused thought, rebellion against parents, and unpredictable behavior. In fact, however, the percentage of disturbances among adolescents is similar to that found among adults—namely, 20%. This means that 80 percent cope well with the teenage years. At age 16, a third of the adolescents have attained the highest level of cognitive development (formal operations)—the same percentage as is found in adults. The decision-making ability is the same in both, and is based less on rationality than on training and habit. Thus, when it comes to choices made regarding drugs, sex, smoking, and drinking, social acceptance by peers and parental example are more important than is logical information provided by education. When the information is intrinsically conflictive, adolescents, like adults, accept only the message they believe will make them acceptable in their social environment.

Much of adolescent behavior consists of experimenting with a variety of activities, many potentially perilous, including sex, substance abuse, and violence. The adolescent group is the only age group exhibiting an increasing mortality rate in America, with accidents, suicides, and homicides responsible for more than 75% of teenage mortality. Substance abuse contributes to this phenomenon. Sexual experimentation results in millions of cases of sexually transmitted diseases and unwanted pregnancies each year, as adolescents show little insight into the consequences of their actions. Adolescents younger than age 16 think in present terms and find it difficult to consider the future or to truly comprehend their behavior in terms of cause and effect. Many of these risk-taking behaviors are interconnected with their origins in childhood experiences, parenting, peer pressure, timing of puberty, self-esteem, ethical and religious training, and education. It is important for adults to understand that thought processes continue to develop and change during adolescence.

National survey data indicate that age 16 is now the average age of first intercourse (coitarche). Rates of sexual activity continue to climb among the youngest adolescents at a rate faster than that of older adolescents. Sexual activity among adolescents is as common in Canada, England, and France as it is in the United States, but the United States teen pregnancy rate is twice as high (see Chapter 16). The critical difference is a lack of contraceptive knowledge and use. Compliance with contraception is difficult to assess; however, only the birth control pill has been shown to achieve high contraceptive efficacy in teenagers. The number of 15–19-year-old women who use oral contraceptives (about 1.5 million) is more than twice the number who rely on condoms, the next most popular method.

Because adolescence represents a time of sexual experimentation, the 15–19-year age interval appears to be the highest risk interval for multiple sex partners, and the earlier sexual activity begins, the greater the likelihood for multiple sex partners. Four factors are especially linked to the early onset of coitus: the less the mother's education, the weaker the religious affiliation, the younger the age at menarche, and the less stable the family at age 14 years, the earlier the age at first intercourse.

Denial is a particular characteristic of adolescence, and risk taking is a natural behavioral sequela; this adds to the likelihood of acquiring and transmitting sexually transmitted diseases. Some 18%–30% of sexually active adolescents are infected with the human papillomavirus and some 5%–30% with chlamydial cervicitis. Forty percent of the cases of gonorrhea occur in adolescents, as do 47% of the reported cases of genital herpes. Adolescents account for 1% of the cases of the acquired immunodeficiency syndrome (AIDS), and the incidence is increasing. Age-specific rates of pelvic inflammatory disease are highest for adolescent females and the risk of it in the sexually active 15-year-old girl is estimated to be one in eight.

The data for substance abuse are equally discouraging. About 71% of Americans aged 12–17 years have used cigarettes (21% are daily smokers), 93% have consumed alcohol (5.5% are daily drinkers), 57% have smoked marijuana (5.5% are daily smokers), 35% have used stimulants, and 16% have used cocaine.

Fortunately, not all teenagers are the alcoholic, sex-crazed, reefer-pulling aliens that many adults think they are. The important sources of the data show inevitable flaws, such as those related to self-reporting. Furthermore, there is a steady increase in the use of contraception by teenagers. Nearly half of the sexually active girls have had only a single partner, and nearly 85% of the remaining half have had no more than three partners. Up to 25% have had intercourse only once or twice; 39% of sexually experienced teens think that premarital sex is wrong; and 83% cite a best age for intercourse older than the age at which they experienced it. The same conventional view is found with regard to substance abuse, in that teenage drug use may be a time-limited pattern of behavior that for many will be abandoned or lessened in young adulthood.

The physician has an important role in encouraging adolescents to be responsible for their own health care. Confidentiality is essential, so that the teen can speak freely and openly. Because most adolescents learn about sexual matters from their peers, peer group values are usually the dominant force in their lives. The physician and parents should attempt to keep their own values out of the picture. A nonjudgmental and supportive parental attitude can spare the teenager enormous emotional stress and pain, and the physician, provided that confidentiality is not breached, can provide valuable support to both the parents and the child.

More effective than sermons about the dangers of sex is a relationship in which the young person believes her physician is concerned, and that concern is manifested by the sharing of accurate information. Conversations may address concerns about obesity, acne, and other body image issues, as sexual intercourse is often sought as a means of gaining reassurance about appearance. Adolescents of all ages, regardless of sexual activity, often need to be reassured that they are normal. Discussions of ways to handle peer pressure may also be helpful at all stages of adolescence. Questions or concerns about sexual orientation require the provision of accurate information and the opportunity to deal with these feelings and fears. If the physician is uncomfortable dealing with these issues, timely referral to a knowledgeable professional is essential.

Generally, the clinician functions best in a climate of parental knowledge, but, if confidentiality is requested, treatment need not be withheld. The mature minor rule allows the physician to supply full medical care if the minor is considered capable of understanding the nature, extent, and consequences of the invasion of her body. Full documentation is essential.

Contraceptive-based sex education for adolescents in the United States has been shown to increase knowledge, but to have little impact on behavior, birth control use, and pregnancy. However, countries in which sex education has been accepted and combined with widespread free family-planning services and abortion on demand have the lowest pregnancy and abortion rates in the world.

Reviews
1. Sugar M. Female adolescent sexuality. *J Pediatr Adolesc Gynecol* 1996;9:175.
   Without specifying socioeconomic status, it is inaccurate to compare sexual activity of different groups.
2. Goldfarb AF. Adolescent sexuality. *Acad Sci* 1997;816:395.
   Education regarding sexual activity, sexually transmitted disease, and contraception place Western European adolescents at lower risk for the many problems commonly seen in the United States.
3. Haka-Ikse K. Female adolescent sexuality. The risks and management. *Acad Sci* 1997;816:466.
   Society reaps the adolescents it sows. Adults themselves have been licentious in the past several decades.

Biology
4. Tanner JM. *Growth of adolescence*, 2nd ed. Oxford: Blackwell, 1962.
   The staging of secondary sex characteristics allows the prediction of future events based on present developmental status.
5. Piaget J. Intellectual evolution from adolescence to adulthood. *Hum Dev* 1972;15:1.
   This discusses the development of the ability to plan and consider alternatives and their possible results before embarking on any action. This development is affected by genetics, environment, stimulation, education, and economics.
6. Malasonos TH. Sexual development of the fetus and pubertal child. *Clin Obstet Gynecol* 1997;40:153.
   Adolescent sexuality is based on the preceding phases with increasing hormone levels, body changes, and attendant anxieties, proceeding in a fairly regular developmental fashion.

Statistical Sources
7. Centers for Disease Control. Premarital sexual experience among adolescent women, United States, 1970–1988. *MMWR* 1990;39:929.
   By 1988, over one-fourth of both black and white 15-year-old females had experienced coitus; by age 19 years, over four-fifths of both races were sexually experienced.
8. Neal JJ, et al. Trends in heterosexually acquired AIDS in the United States, 1988 through 1995. *J Acquir Immune Defic Syndr Hum Retrovirol* 1997;14:465.
   Blacks and Hispanics accounted for 75% of persons with AIDS due to heterosexual contact and should be prioritized for education and prevention programs.

Contraception
9. Adler N, et al. Adolescent contraceptive behavior: an assessment of decision processes. *J Pediatr* 1990;116:463.
   One study of metropolitan area teenagers revealed that there was a mean delay between first intercourse and first use of a prescription method of contraception of 11 months for clinic patients and 13 months for private patients.
10. Moore SM, Rosenthal DA. Condoms and coitus: adolescents attitudes to AIDS and safe sex behavior. *J Adolesc* 1991;14:211.

If teenagers are concerned about becoming infected with the human immunodeficiency virus (HIV), if they believe condoms are protective, if they are not embarrassed to discuss the issue with the partner, if they have discussed the use of condoms with a physician, and if they carry them, they are more likely to use them consistently.

11. Lauchli S, et al. Safer sex behavior and alcohol consumption. Research Group of the Swiss HIV Prevention Study. *Ann Epidemiol* 1996;6:357.
   This study found no significant difference between sex with or without alcohol in terms of safer sexual behavior. This study was set in Switzerland; however, it may not be applicable to other populations.

Problems

12. Taylor SE, et al. A comparison of AIDS-related sexual risk behaviors among African-American college students. *J Natl Med Assoc* 1997;89:397.
   This article demonstrates the need to convey to African-American male students the reality that AIDS does not discriminate.

13. Moore NB, Davidson JK Sr. Guilt about first intercourse: an antecedent of sexual dissatisfaction among college women. *J Sex Marital Ther* 1997;23:29.
   Significant variables included uncommunicative parents, overstrict fathers, and uncomfortableness with sexuality.

14. Sugar M. Adolescent pregnancy in the U.S.A.: problems and prospects. *Adolesc Pediatr Gynecol* 1991;4:171.
   One million teenage pregnancies occur each year, 400,000 of which end with induced abortion; 85% of teens are already sexually active when they first request contraception.

15. Comerci GD, Macdonald DI. Prevention of substance abuse in children and adolescents. *Adolesc Med* 1990;1:127.
   Sexual practices as well as drug use are biologically based and complex behaviors. Sexual activity can be spontaneous and unplanned and can take place when judgment is impaired by the effects of alcohol and / or other drugs.

16. Rosenthal SL, Biro FM. A preliminary investigation of the psychological impact of sexually transmitted diseases in adolescent females. *Adolesc Pediatr Gynecol* 1991;4:198.
   Adolescent females were grouped according to whether they had cervical dysplasia or gonorrhea / Chlamydia infection. Rates of psychopathologic conditions and the impact of the diagnosis were compared. Overall, the patients were more likely to have avoidance rather than intrusive thoughts.

17. Moscicki AB, et al. The association between human papillomavirus deoxyribonucleic acid status and the results of cytologic rescreening tests in young, sexually active women. *Am J Obstet Gynecol* 1991;165:67.
   In early puberty, columnar epithelium extends into the vagina. Infection with human papillomavirus involving the transformation zone at an early age apparently results in cervical cytologic changes during the teenage years.

18. Remafedi G. Adolescent homosexuality: psychosocial and medical implications. *Pediatrics* 1987;79:331.
   The majority of adolescents in this study had experienced school problems related to sexuality, substance abuse, and emotional difficulties. Nearly half gave a history of having sexually transmitted diseases, running away from home, or conflicts with the law.

19. Rousso H. Affirming adolescent women's sexuality. *West J Med* 1991;154:629.
   Although many disabled teenage women have less satisfying social lives than do their nondisabled counterparts, this is not the inevitable consequence of disability.

20. Chamberlain A, et al. Issues in fertility control for mentally retarded female adolescents. I. Sexual activity, sexual abuse, and contraception. *Pediatrics* 1984; 73:445.
   The proportion of retarded female adolescents who had intercourse was comparable to that seen in the general adolescent population. The currently available contraception methods did not appear to be adequate.

Education

21. Ruusuvaara L. Adolescent sexuality: an educational and counseling challenge. *Ann NY Acad Sci* 1997;846:411.
   The focus is on avoiding high-risk behaviors with little concern shown for promoting more communicative, pleasurable, and egalitarian sexual relations.
22. Wilson MD, Manoff S, Joffe A. Residents self-assessed skills in providing sexuality-related care to teenagers. *Arch Pediatr Adolesc Med* 1997;151:418.
   Skills assessed included a pubertal and sexual history, sexual preference, examination, diagnosis, and counseling. Female residents were less comfortable with male teenagers.
23. Card JJ, et al. The program archive on sexuality, health and adolescence: promising prevention programs in a box. *Fam Plann Perspect* 1996;28:210.
   Effective programs are identified, archived, and distributed.
24. Ansuini CG, Fiddler-Woite J, Woite RS. The source, accuracy, and impact of initial sexuality information on lifetime wellness. *Adolescence* 1996;31;283.
   Ignorance was found to have produced guilt and illness in the majority of respondents.

---

75. ALTERATIONS IN SEXUALITY WITH AGING, DRUGS, AND DISEASE

Michel E. Rivlin

The aging process affects the entire body, with sexuality being among the last functions to decline. These involutional changes occur gradually and at different rates for different people. At menopause, reproduction ceases in women, whereas men may retain fertility throughout their lives. Men reach their sexual peak in late adolescence, and this is followed by a gradual decline. Female peaks are reached in the late thirties and the subsequent decline is less than that in the male. Postmenopausal changes in the vagina include epithelial atrophy, disappearance of the rugae, elevation in pH, decrease in lubrication, reduced elasticity, vascular fragility, and narrowing of the outlet. There is also an increased susceptibility to vaginitis and dyspareunia. All these changes may be prevented or reversed to a major extent by estrogen replacement. In the male, the ejaculatory demand decreases as, too, do the expulsive force, seminal volume, erectile rigidity, and maintenance. However, although erection is slower and physical stimulation may be necessary, erection may be maintained for extended periods. The decline in the frequency of intercourse associated with aging is related primarily to male sexual dysfunction.

These alterations in sexuality with aging involve all three phases of sexual response. Men show a much greater decline in the sex drive (desire) than do women. Thus, at age 17, the average is four to 10 ejaculations a week; this rate falls to about one a week at age 60. The sex drive in the male is very sensitive to stress and depression, and declining levels of testosterone may also be a factor. In contrast, many women have an increase in libido at menopause, perhaps associated with the unopposed action of adrenal testosterone when the ovarian supply of estrogen declines. Older men generally require both psychic and tactile stimuli to produce erection in the excitement phase. In the female, lubrication and swelling may diminish, but frequent intercourse, hormone replacement, and the use of lubricants readily restore adequate function. The phase of orgasm is shorter in older women, and, in older males, the refractory period usually increases substantially. The combination of declining physical capacity and a maintained psychologic need for sex in the male leads to his becoming more vulnerable sexually and more dependent on his partner.

A great number of aged people have an active sexual life. There is a large range of sexual behavior, including erotic fantasy, masturbation, coitus, and nongenital erotic pleasuring, that remains as satisfactory in later years as it does for the young. Social and economic factors have an important influence on the sexual life of the elderly, so that, for instance, married women and wealthy men (single or married) maintain a higher frequency of sexual activity. A relatively high level of sexual activity over the years sets the pattern in old age also.

Primary care physicians can promote sexual health in older women by always taking a sexual history. A wide variety of physical, emotional, and pharmaceutically induced disorders may influence sexuality. Physicians can reassure patients that sexual dysfunction is not inevitable with advancing age. If problems are identified, management is directed at reducing specific contributory organic, hormonal, psychologic, and social stresses. Because a lack of suitable male partners is common for older women, acceptable alternatives of sexual expression must be sought. If possible, older women should be encouraged to discard unnecessary strictures against masturbation. The staff of long-term care facilities should be nonjudgmental, understanding, and supportive. Privacy and the opportunity to express sexual desires should be provided. Most elderly people cease engaging in sexual activity because of psychological and societal misconceptions, not because of aging processes or disease. In women, as in men, androgens are more important for sustaining sexual desire than physiologic responsiveness. The longer it has been since sexuality has ceased, the more difficult it is to resume; therefore, therapy should be prompt and vigorous.

The physiologic mechanisms involved in the normal sexual response include psychogenic, vascular, neurogenic, and hormonal factors, which are coordinated by centers in the hypothalamus, limbic system, and cerebral cortex. Many commonly used drugs can interfere with sexual function in either sex, causing a loss of libido, interfering with erection or ejaculation in men, and delaying or preventing orgasm in women. The pharmacologic mechanisms proposed to explain these adverse effects include anticholinergic activity, alterations in adrenergic tone, and changes in central serotonin and catecholamine levels, in addition to endocrine and sedative effects. Drug-related changes may be difficult to distinguish from sexual dysfunction stemming from the disease state per se; for instance, untreated hypertensive and depressed patients exhibit a higher incidence of sexual difficulties than does the general population. Patients experiencing drug-related sexual dysfunction may be able to discontinue the therapy responsible, and it is vital to inform them about this possibility and to reassure them that the changes are reversible. If possible, symptoms may be alleviated by either switching agents or lowering the dosage without loss of the desired therapeutic effect. Most reports concern male patients, and it is not known whether women's sexual functioning is less vulnerable to drug changes or whether information on these alterations has not been volunteered.

Antihypertensive agents are probably the most frequent offenders. Thiazides, drugs with peripheral sympatholytic action, and centrally acting sympatholytics can all cause impotence and ejaculatory failure. Beta-adrenergic-blocking agents can produce loss of libido and impotence. Drugs less likely to cause sexual dysfunction include the angiotensin-converting enzyme inhibitors, calcium channel blockers, and the arteriolar dilator hydralazine. The antipsychotic drugs, most antidepressant drugs, and central nervous system depressants including sedatives may impair sexual function in both men and women. Many of these medications also cause hyperprolactinemia. They can diminish desire, cause anorgasmy, impair erection, and interfere with ejaculation. Antineoplastic drugs can cause gonadal damage and progressive loss of libido in both sexes.

If noncompliance or drug misuse to promote an aphrodisiac effect (alcohol, marijuana, benzodiazepines, or yohimbine) is suspected, sexual function should be assessed. Furthermore, a baseline sexual history should be obtained before high-risk agents are prescribed. If an organic basis for sexual dysfunction is identified, agents known to aggravate the problem should be avoided. A high index of suspicion is particularly important in the elderly, because inappropriate drug use in this group is not uncommon. In this way, many serious problems that result from active or passive underuse, misuse, or excessive use of either prescribed or over-the-counter drugs may be avoided.

The range of physical and mental illness and disability that may affect sexual function is enormous. In some instances, there is organic sexual dysfunction; in others, psychosocial factors induce the dysfunction; and, in yet a third group, sexual activity is modified as a result of physical illness. Here again, these changes have been studied mainly in men.

Adequate sexual function requires intact vascular, neurologic, and endocrine function. Neurologic disorders, including spinal cord injury and multiple sclerosis, severely impair function. Diabetes is a common cause of sexual dysfunction, probably as a result of peripheral autonomic neuropathy. Vascular disease, particularly affecting the pelvic arteries and veins, may compromise engorgement enough to cause impotence. Endocrine disorders can influence sexuality; commonly, pituitary, adrenal, and ovarian disorders affect sexuality adversely because of the hormonal imbalance involved.

Either illness or a surgical procedure that involves the genitalia also causes sexual problems. These include urologic and gynecologic disorders, pelvic cancer, and congenital and acquired anatomic defects, as well as sexually transmitted diseases. Procedures commonly implicated include hysterectomy, prostatectomy, mastectomy, sterilization, castration, and radiotherapy.

Many chronic illnesses require marked sexual adjustments. These include painful conditions such as arthritis and the aftermath of major trauma, as well as disabling chronic respiratory disease, chronic renal failure, and chronic alcoholism. Cardiac disease, especially after a myocardial infarction, frequently interferes with sexual activity.

Physical illness normally causes marked anxiety, anger, grief, and depression, all of which frequently impair sexual function. This is particularly true when illness, trauma, or surgical procedure involves a change in body image or a loss of body parts that have a sexual connotation. For instance, mastectomy and ostomy patients are often left with sexual maladjustment, even though they are physiologically intact.

In managing such patients, both organic and psychogenic factors must be assessed, and the impact on the family must be evaluated. Counseling should have a preventive intent wherever possible (e.g., before operation) and should be specific and fitted to the individual. The spouse must be included in the process, because his or her role is crucial to therapeutic success. Treatment is generally behavioral in focus, but can also be educational, informative, and psychotherapeutic where indicated. In some instances, surgical measures play an important role in the treatment of sexual dysfunction with an organic cause, as in the construction of a neovagina, the insertion of a penile prosthesis, or postmastectomy breast reconstruction.

Aging

1. Loehr J, Verma S, Seguin R. Issues of sexuality in older women. *J Womens Health* 1997;4:451.

   In the absence of disease and with the availability of a sexually active partner, a woman's overall sexual behavior does not necessarily change with age.

2. Mueller IW. Common questions about sex and sexuality in elders. *Am J Nurs* 1997;97:61.

   The effects of estrogen on female sexual activity are largely unknown. In both sexes, testosterone has a positive effect on sexual motivation but does not affect sexual function.

3. Barber HR. Sexuality and the art of arousal in the geriatric woman. *Clin Obstet Gynecol* 1996;39:970.

   Neither aging men nor aging women can afford long, continued periods of coital continence if they are to continue as physically effective sexual partners.

4. Schow DA, Redmon B, Pryor JL. Male menopause. How to define it, how to treat it. *Postgrad Med J* 1997;101:62–64,67–68,71–74.

   Concept of male menopause and the dos, don'ts, and unknowns of treating it with testosterone.

Drugs
5. Shen WW, Sata LS. Drugs that cause sexual dysfunction. *Med Lett Drugs Ther* 1987;29:65.
   Includes a list of 92 medications reported to adversely affect sexual function.
6. Schiavi RC, Segraves RT. The biology of sexual function. *Psychiatr Clin North Am* 1995;18:7.
   The chronic use of most recreational drugs leads to sexual impairment, including diminished libido, erectile dysfunction, and delayed orgasm.
7. Shen WW, Sata LS. Inhibited female orgasm resulting from psychotropic drugs: a five-year, updated, clinical review. *J Reprod Med* 1990;35:11.
   Iatrogenic sexual dysfunction is a major reason for noncompliance with antihypertensive and antipsychotic agents.
8. Lane RM. A critical review of selective serotonin reuptake inhibitor-related sexual dysfunction; incidence, possible aetiology and implications for management. *J Psychopharmacol* 1997;11:72.
   Selective serotonin reuptake blockers may impair libido or orgasmic capacity in both sexes.

Diseases
9. Goldmeier D, et al. Prevalence of sexual dysfunction in heterosexual patients attending a central London genitourinary medicine clinic. *Int J STD AIDS* 1997;8:303.
   Substantial prevalence of sexual dysfunction was found, the service implications of which need to be addressed.
10. Andersen BL, Woods XA, Copeland LJ. Sexual self-schema and sexual morbidity among gynecologic cancer survivors. *J Consult Clin Psychol* 1997;65:221.
    Cancer survivors can be helped by short-term counseling and by information on anatomic alterations and erroneous beliefs, along with recommendations on when and how to resume intercourse and ways to minimize the physical effects of cancer on sexual function.
11. Barni S, Mondin R. Sexual dysfunction in treated breast cancer patients. *Ann Oncol* 1997;2:149.
    Lumpectomy fosters a more intact body image, but no surgical procedure either produces or inhibits psychologic symptomatology.
12. Dupont S. Multiple sclerosis and sexual dysfunction, a review. *Clin Rehabil* 1995;9:183.
    Between 50% and 90% will develop sexual difficulties.
13. Mahlstedt PP. The psychologic component of infertility. *Fertil Steril* 1985;43:335.
    The focus on sex for procreation in the management of infertility may lead to sexual dysfunction.
14. Saxton M. Reclaiming sexual self-esteem—peer counseling for disabled women. *West J Med* 1991;154:629.
    The severely disabled are underserved by mental health providers because of inadequate training, attitudinal barriers, and inaccessible programs, particularly regarding sexual issues.
15. Banerjee A. Coital emergencies. *Postgrad Med J* 1996;72:653.
    Awareness of the presentation of coital emergencies is essential to allow appropriate medical management and sexual counseling.
16. Kreuter M, Sullivan M, Siosteen A. Sexual adjustment and quality of relationship in spinal paraplegia: a controlled study. *Arch Phys Med Rehabil* 1996;77:541.
    Psychosocial rather than physical factors were important for a satisfying sexual life and relationship.
17. Muller JE, et al. Triggering myocardial infarction by sexual activity. Low absolute risk and prevention by regular physical exertion. *JAMA* 1996;275:1405.
    If the patient can walk rapidly for 10 minutes and then climb two flights of steps in 10 seconds without symptoms, then sexual intercourse should not place undue stress on the heart.

76. INHIBITED FEMALE SEXUAL DESIRE, EXCITEMENT, AND ORGASM

Michel E. Rivlin

Sexual response is described in terms of three related phases: desire, excitement, and orgasm. Sexual dysfunction may effect one or another of these phases without affecting the others. Sexual desire appears to be a centrally situated appetite, part of the brain system responsible for emotion and reproduction. There appears to be an excitement center (dopamine sensitive) in balance with an inhibitory center (serotonin sensitive). Testosterone may be responsible for programming these centers in prenatal life. During the excitement phase, there is vascular engorgement and increased muscular tension. Vasocongestion results in vaginal lubrication by means of fluid transudation, as well as clitoral tumescence and expansion of the upper vagina. This phase is primarily under parasympathetic control, with afferent fibers originating from the clitoris and anterior labia and efferent fibers coming from the pelvic nerve. Marked extragenital reactions also take place, including tachycardia, tachypnea, increased blood pressure, and a sex flush, or a red rash that covers the chest, neck, and face. In the orgasmic phase, uterine contractions occur and the muscles around the vagina, anus, and uterus undergo a series of reflex clonic contractions while extragenital reactions reach their maximum. Orgasm is primarily under sympathetic control, with afferent fibers originating from the clitoris and labia and efferent fibers traveling via the pelvic plexuses and via the pudendal nerve to striated muscles. The sexual response cycle ends with the phase of resolution. Unlike men, women have no refractory period and may be multiorgasmic; however, their orgasm is reached less directly and more slowly. There does not appear to be a vaginal, as distinct from a clitoral, orgasm.

Sexual dysfunction may be primary (never satisfactory), secondary (previously satisfactory), or situational (satisfactory in some circumstances, but not in others). Problems generally affect the orgasmic phase, but, if neglected, may eventually involve the other phases. Primary problems are usually psychogenic in origin; secondary problems may be organic in nature or related to the use of pharmacologic agents. Situational problems are almost always psychogenic or relational in origin. The organic causes of sexual dysfunction include neurogenic and vascular diseases, local pelvic abnormalities, plus endocrine and general medical disorders. The psychologic causes may be intrapersonal, including depression, anxiety, and trauma such as rape or incest; or they may be interpersonal and characterized by poor communication, anger, and resentment. Common disorders include the secondary inhibition of sexual desire, which is usually related to interpersonal strife. Inhibited sexual excitement refers to the failure to obtain or maintain genital swelling and lubrication in spite of adequate sexual activity. A delay in, or absence of, orgasm during adequate sexual activity is referred to as inhibited orgasm. Reliable estimates of the prevalence of these disorders may never be attainable.

The primary care physician can deal with many of these problems based on the information obtained during a general and sexual history in conjunction with a full physical and pelvic examination. The finding of severe anxiety, depression, or psychosis necessitates psychiatric referral. A finding of major marital disharmony might prompt referral for sexual and marital therapy. Abnormal medical, surgical, or gynecologic findings would constitute reasons for other relevant referrals. When in doubt, therapy may be started and future management guided by the patient's response. Many concerns can be alleviated by reassuring the patient that certain sexual behaviors are in order (permission) and that such concerns are common. Every effort must be made to remain nonjudgmental and to avoid giving too hasty advice or reassurance regarding specific problems. Education is most important. Misconceptions need to be dispelled by factual information. Many sexual concerns may be prevented, for instance, by careful counseling prior to hysterectomy or mastectomy procedures commonly attended by sexual dysfunction. Some practitioners may not be comfortable dealing with sexual problems and may wish to refer all such patients. Sex therapy attempts to initiate or restore previously absent sexual function in an individual or a couple. Most problems have a multifactorial basis. The initial focus of therapy should be on immediate causes, using the behavioral techniques popularized by Masters and Johnson. These include an initial ban on intercourse, with emphasis on nongenital sensual pleasuring (sensate focus exercises), improving interpersonal communication skills, masturbation training, and general sex education. Treatment may be done on an individual or couple basis (the relationship is the patient), or it may be dealt with in group therapy. If progress is not made, remote causes may then be sought using a psychodynamically oriented program.

Primary anorgasmy with arousal may result in pelvic congestion and irritability, owing to the nonorgasmic sexual response. Secondary anorgasmy may occur in certain situations but not in others. Medical and gynecologic causes of painful or difficult intercourse may be the source of the problem, or a specific partner may play an important causal role. Therapy for primary anorgasmy includes body acceptance and exploration using self-touching and masturbation techniques, including the use of lubrication jellies and vibrators. Pubococcygeus pelvic muscle exercises enhance sexual function and should be taught and practiced regularly. Once orgasm by self-stimulation is achieved, couple counseling is needed with the intent to lead to orgasm with a partner.

In counseling the couple, discussion of the importance of foreplay and the desire of most women to be courted, plus advice regarding the time, place, and form of sexual contact, are outlined. If the problem is one of orgasm accomplished by clitoral stimulation rather than with intercourse, it may be possible to get the patient to accept the situation as normal. If not, continuation of manual or vibrator masturbation induced by the partner or patient during intercourse may be used as a bridging technique until, through the process of experimental learning, orgasm may occur during coitus. In general, better clitoral contact and stimulation are obtained in the female-superior position than in the more generally used missionary position.

The treatment of secondary anorgasmy is more complex. There should be an emphasis on the relationship, commitment, trust, and need for honesty about feelings. The female partner needs to communicate what she wants; the male partner must listen without being defensive. Define what is missing, create an emotionally safe environment for change, add whatever sexual information or technique is required.

No strong claims for the overall effectiveness of directive sex therapies are justified at the present time because of the great difficulties in defining, reporting, and sampling these patients. Undoubtedly, sexual and marital therapy can sometimes bring about an improvement in sexual responses by providing insight into the problems and allowing realistic communication to take place; appropriate home assignments can enhance the process. The intrinsic limitations of therapy must, however, be faced realistically.

Most clinicians have some patients who are homosexual. Homosexuality is best regarded as a status, like left-handedness. Lesbians or gay men must deal with homophobia, prejudice, ignorance, and apprehension. The therapist must clear his or her own incorrect beliefs and understand that intimacy and satisfaction are found in homosexual relationships just as in heterosexual.

Sexual problems that require expert referral include gender disorders, sexual variations, and sexual deviations. The gender identity disorders include transsexualism, an overpowering desire to be the other sex, and transvestism, which is cross-dressing. Fetishism is related to transvestism in that a specific set of objects is necessary for sexual arousal. The paraphilias refer to sexual preferences that are unwelcome to society. There is a disconnection between sex and affection, and the behavior per se becomes the erotic end. Included are exhibitionists and pedophiles, the latter of which prey on prepubertal children of either sex, and sadomasochists, who receive sexual gratification from inflicting or receiving pain. Paraphiliacs may be heterosexual, homosexual, or bisexual. They are almost always male.

Reviews
1. Watson JP, Davies T. ABC of mental health. Psychosexual problems. *BMJ* 1997; 315:239.
   The question is not whether this is physical or psychological, but how much of each factor operates in this case.
2. Lewin J, King M. Sexual medicine. *BMJ* 1997;314:1432.
   The sexual dysfunctions are classified by the American Psychiatric Association in the Diagnostics and Statistical Manual of Mental Disorders (DSM).
3. Ekland M, McBride K. Sexual health care: the role of the nurse. *Cancer Nurse* 1997;93:34.
   The authors suggest the "PLISS IT" therapeutic approach: P, permission; LI, limited information; SS, specific suggestions; and, in nonresponders, IT, referral for intensive therapy.

Physiology, Incidence, Etiology
4. Weisberg M. Physiology of female sexual function. *Clin Obstet Gynecol* 1984; 27:697.
   The classic works of Masters and Johnson, Human Sexual Response and Human Sexual Inadequacy, are somewhat difficult to read; fortunately, numerous excellent commentaries on them are readily available.
5. Darling CA, Davidson JK, Conwag-Welch C. Female ejaculation: perceived origins, the Grafenberg spot/area, and sexual responsiveness. *Arch Sex Behav* 1990;19:29.
   Heated controversy has surrounded the existence and nature of the Grafenberg (or G spot), a purported major erogenous zone distinct from the clitoris on the anterior vaginal wall, as well as the concept of female ejaculation.
6. Frank E, Anderson C, Rubinstein D. Frequency of sexual dysfunction in normal couples. *N Engl J Med* 1978;299:111.
   The authors suggest that there is an epidemic of sexual dysfunction and unhappiness.
7. Segraves KB, Segraves RT. Hypoactive sexual desire disorder: prevalence and comorbidity in 906 subjects. *J Sex Marital Ther* 1991;17:55.
   The prevalence of psychosexual dysfunctions in females is estimated to be as follows: inhibited orgasm, 5%–30%; inhibited sexual desire, 1%–35%; and inhibited sexual excitement, indeterminate.
8. Hyde JS, et al. Sexuality during pregnancy and the year postpartum. *J Sex Res* 1996;33:143.
   Average time to resumption of intercourse was 7 weeks postpartum; breastfeeding women were significantly less sexually satisfied than non-breastfeeding women.
9. Meana M., et al. Dyspareunia: more than bad sex. *Pain* 1997;71:211.
   This article suggests that dyspareunia should be integrated into mainstream pain research and thus benefit from the multidisciplinary perspective of recent approaches to the study of pain.
10. Lazarus JA. Ethical issues in doctor-patient sexual relationships. *Psychiatr Clin North Am* 1995;18:55.
    Surveys of all healthcare professionals indicate that 1%–10% have been sexually involved with patients.
11. Abel GG, Rouleau JL. Sexual abuses. *Psychiatr Clin North Am* 1995;18:139.
    In treating sexual dysfunction associated with prior sexual trauma, the guiding principles are to teach the person to be a survivor rather than a victim and to help the couple develop a functional and satisfying sexual style, because living well is the best revenge.
12. Wederman MW. Pretending orgasm during sexual intercourse: correlates in a sample of young adult women. *J Sex Marital Ther* 1997;23:131.
    Over half the women reported faking; only increased sexual esteem was uniquely related to this behavior.

Management
13. Kellett J. Functions of a sexual dysfunction clinic. *Int Rev Psychiatry* 1995;7:183.
    Specialist psychosexual services have arisen to assess and treat sexual dysfunctions that are considered to have psychological causes.

14. Rosen RC, Leiblum SR. Hypoactive sexual desire. *Psychiatr Clin North Am* 1995; 18:107.
   The pressure on individuals to be sexually interested, responsive, and enthusiastic within a committed relationship is at an all-time high.
15. Risen CB. A guide to taking a sexual history. *Psychiatr Clin North Am* 1995; 18:39.
   This guide counsels helping a patient tell her sexual story, including both historical narrative and a current expression in thoughts, feelings, and behaviors.
16. Kilmann PR, et al. The treatment of secondary orgasmic dysfunction II. *J Sex Marital Ther* 1987;13:93.
   The prognosis is less positive in patients with secondary orgasmic dysfunction than it is for those with primary anorgasmy, because nonsexual relationship problems are likely to be maintaining the orgasmic difficulty.
17. Christensen C. Prescribed masturbation in sex therapy: a critique. *J Sex Marital Ther* 1995;21:87.
   A contrarian view: masturbation may actually serve to further damage the openness and trust necessary for truly rewarding sexual expression.
18. Sarwer DB, Durlak JA. A field trial of the effectiveness of behavioral treatment for sexual dysfunctions. *J Sex Marital Ther* 1997;23:87.
   A 65% overall success rate is cited for behavioral treatment; however, most of the patients were well-educated dual-wage earners who held professional positions.
19. Kaplan HS. Sexual aversion, sexual phobias, and panic disorder. New York: Brunner/Mazel, 1987.
   These disorders involve avoidance of almost all genital contact with a sexual partner. Management was enhanced by the concomitant use of antidepressants and sexual therapy.

77. PROBLEMS OF ORGASMIC RESPONSE IN THE MALE

Michel E. Rivlin

The corpora cavernosa of the penis consist primarily of a trabecular network of lacunar spaces composed of smooth muscle and a fibroelastic frame. The walls of the arteries and arterioles that empty into the lacunar spaces are also primarily composed of smooth muscle. Engorgement and erection are due to relaxation of penile smooth muscle, with resulting dilatation of the penile arterial vessels leading to an increase of blood flow to the lacunar spaces. The increased flow expands the trabecular walls against the tunica albuginea, compressing the draining venous plexuses. As a consequence of the diminished venous drainage, there is an increase in pressure in the lacunar spaces, which leads to penile rigidity. Detumescence occurs as a result of penile smooth muscle contraction. Trabecular smooth muscle tone is controlled by three neurologic pathways. First, the adrenergic release of norepinephrine causes corporal smooth muscle contraction. Second, cholinergic stimuli have dilatory effects, as does the third pathway, which is neither cholinergic nor adrenergic and is mediated by nitric oxide (NO), which is also released from the vascular endothelium. The sympathetic pathways travel from T-11 through L-2 to the hypogastric and pelvic plexus, whereas the parasympathetic pathways (nervi erigentes) originate from S2 to S4 via the pelvic plexus; a third innervation comes from S2 to S4 via the pudendal nerve. Thereafter, prostatic secretions, sperm in the vasa and ampulla, and the fructose-rich seminal vesicle content are expressed by contraction of these organs into the posterior urethra (emission). The bladder neck and external sphincter are closed during this phase, resulting in increased urethral pressure; thereafter, rhythmic contractions of the pelvic floor and periurethral muscles, along with intermittent relaxation of the external sphincter and urogenital diaphragm, allow for expulsion of the ejaculate. The male orgasm is the cortical appreciation of the sympathetically and somatically coordinated events of ejaculation.

Erectile dysfunction (impotence), the inability to achieve and maintain an erection sufficient for vaginal penetration and intercourse, may be primary or secondary in origin. The latter always follows a period of normal erectile function. Situational impotence is experienced by all men at one time or another, and is commonly associated with fatigue, stress and alcohol consumption. The incidence of impotence is about 5% at age 40 and 15% at age 70.

Organic causes of erectile dysfunction include neurogenic and vascular diseases as well as many drugs, such as abused substances (alcohol and marijuana), antihypertensive agents (diuretics and methyldopa), and psychiatric medications (tricyclics and phenothiazines). Diabetes, probably stemming from both neurogenic and vascular involvement, as well as associated psychogenic factors, is associated with a 35% prevalence of impotence. Other endocrine disorders, including hyperprolactinemia, hypogonadism, and thyroid disease, have also been implicated as causal factors. Less common are the end-organ problems such as Peyronie's disease, phimosis, microphallus, and chordee, and almost all pelvic surgical procedures are associated with varying degrees of impotence postoperatively. The prevalence of psychogenic impotence ranges from 14% to 51%, so that most impotence would appear to be organic in origin.

Diagnosis depends on a careful history, with particular attention to possible physical factors such as diabetes, alcoholism, and drugs. A detailed psychosexual history is taken, and evidence of a depressive illness must be sought. A history of nocturnal and waking erections, as well as erections elicited by tactile stimulation, may indicate psychologic impotence, whereas a slowly progressive decline in erectile function suggests organic causes. Physical examination is directed specifically at searching for endocrine, neurologic, and vascular abnormalities. Palpation of the testes, penis, and prostate, with assessment of secondary sexual characteristics, is necessary. A minimal neurologic evaluation should include assessment of the cutaneous sensation of the saddle area (S1–S3), as well as testing of the bulbocavernosus and lower limb reflexes.

In most instances, a costly detailed evaluation is not necessary and, in general, the work-up should be directed toward the individual patient. For instance, a full and maintained erection after the intracavernous injection of vasoactive agents (i.e., papaverine, phentolamine, or prostaglandin E_1) largely rules out the existence of vascular abnormalities. Absence of this response might suggest the need for sophisticated measures of arterial inflow and venous drainage, such as dynamic infusion cavernosometry and cavernosography, duplex sonography, plethysmography, and interval pudendal angiography. Such studies may identify a group of patients amenable to corrective vascular procedures directed toward either improving arterial inflow or correcting abnormal increased venous leakage. If neurologic disease is suspected, neurologic review, biothesiometry (estimation of the penile vibratory threshold), and perhaps electromyography may be included in the diagnostic assessment.

Endocrine studies must include testing of the glucose tolerance. Thyroid studies, as well as measurement of serum testosterone, prolactin, luteinizing hormone (LH), and follicle-stimulating hormone (FSH) levels, may also be performed, although findings of thyroid disease, hypogonadism, or hyperprolactinemia are uncommon. Psychologic testing may be carried out, or a routine brief psychiatric consultation may be obtained to gauge the extent of the psychic component present. Nocturnal penile tumescence testing may be helpful in differentiating organic from psychic impotence.

Management should include medical, surgical, psychiatric, and sexual treatments, as well as marital counseling, all tailored to the needs of the individual patient. Defective sexual skills owing to either ignorance or misinformation and obsessive concerns over sexual performance are common and require correction through education and counseling. Behavioral alterations directed at removing performance anxiety include the use of self-stimulation and sensate focus exercises.

Initial therapy is generally with the newly introduced oral agents such as seldenafil. If this proves ineffective or is contraindicated, alternative approaches such as transurethral alprostadil or intracorporeal injections are available. Seldenafil is a selective inhibitor of cyclic guanosine monophosphate (cGMP)–specific phosphodiesterase type 5 (PDE 5). Nitrous oxide (NO) activates guanylate cyclase, which increases levels of cGMP, producing smooth muscle relaxation. By inhibiting PDE 5, which degrades cGMP, seldenafil enhances the action of NO. The drug is effective in a broad range of patients, including those with organic or nonphysical causes; however, as it potentiates the hypotensive effects of nitrates, it is absolutely contraindicated in patients receiving nitroglycerin or other organic nitrates. There is a degree of cardiac risk associated with sexual activity; therefore patient and physician must consider cardiovascular status before initiating any therapy.

Drug therapy may also be indicated for specific reasons. For instance, injections of testosterone can be administered in patients with clinical and biochemical evidence of hypogonadism, or bromocriptine can be given in some impotent men with hyperprolactinemia. The use of androgens in normal men remains highly controversial, and it must be realized that exogenous androgens inhibit spermatogenesis, may elevate cholesterol levels, and may cause polycythemia and cholestatic jaundice. The clinical experience with intracorporeal injections of vasodilators has been encouraging in the treatment of all forms of impotence. However, major complications (priapism, damage to the corpora, and systemic effects) may occur. Mechanical devices that can be used for the management of erectile dysfunction include externally positioned constriction bands, vacuum devices, and penile implants. The implantation of penile prostheses is indicated in those patients with a strong sexual desire in whom other modalities have failed and who understand that this measure will not restore libido, the ability to ejaculate, or penile sensation. There are two types of prostheses—semirigid rods and inflatable devices—each having advantages and disadvantages. Counseling before and after implantation of these devices is vital. Satisfaction rates of about 80% have been reported for both vacuum constriction devices and implants.

Premature ejaculation is the most common male sexual dysfunction, with a prevalence of up to 29%. It is defined as persistent or recurrent ejaculation with minimal stimulation before, upon, or shortly after penetration, resulting in distress and relationship difficulties. Lack of control of the ejaculatory response is the critical factor. Traditionally, psychological factors were thought to be preeminent and psychological therapy was felt to provide good results. However, it appears likely that men with the problem comprise a heterogeneous group, many with organic disorders linked to erectile dysfunction such that responses to behavioral therapy are often disappointing. Encouraging results have followed the use of pharmacologic agents such as the serotonergic antidepressant drugs (paroxetene, fluoxetine) in delaying ejaculation. If anxiety is a major etiologic factor, other medications such as benzodiazepines may be useful.

Psychologic therapy includes careful history-taking regarding both remote and recent factors that have fostered the condition, together with providing proper information and education, combined with behavioral techniques aimed at extending voluntary control over the ejaculatory reflex. These include vaginal containment without thrusting (to acclimate the penis) and the stop-and-go technique, in which intercourse is deliberately interrupted to allow arousal to diminish. Another valuable technique is firm squeezing of the glans penis to end excitement intermittently.

Inhibited sexual excitement or desire, or both, are common in both men and women. Hormonal factors are rare, and explanations are usually sought in terms of relationship dynamics and family-of-origin theories. Inhibited orgasm (retarded ejaculation and ejaculatory incompetence) is rare in males and is psychogenic in origin. Elements from the treatment of anorgasmic women, including the use of vibrators and behavior maneuvers that are orgasm triggers, have been used with some success in men in these situations.

Reviews
1. Lewis RW. Organic erectile dysfunction. *Curr Ther Endocrinol Metab* 1997;6:366. Erectile dysfunction *is a better term than* impotence, *but the two terms are used interchangeably.*
2. Burnett AL. Erectile dysfunction: a practical approach for primary care. *Geriatrics* 1998;53:34. *Good summary with useful tables.*

3. Easdly I. New oral therapies for the treatment of erectile dysfunction. *Br J Urol* 1998;81:122.
   These agents may act centrally (phentolamine, yohimbine, trazadone, bromocriptine) or within the penis (seldenafil, L-arginine).

Diagnosis
4. Rosen RC, et al. The international index of erectile function (IIEF): a multidimensional scale for assessment of erectile dysfunction. *Urology* 1997;49:822.
   Sex drive is related to general sexual interest; sexual desire is specifically oriented to a particular object; sexual satisfaction occurs when expectations are met.
5. Rajfer J. Impotence—the quick work-up. *J Urol* 1996;156:1951.
   Erection following intracavernosal injection with vasoactive drugs will not separate organic from psychogenic etiologies, but does provide treatment options.
6. Govier FE, McClure RD, Kramer-Levien D. Endocrine screening for sexual dysfunction using free testosterone determinations. *J Urol* 1996;156:405.
   The authors maintain that, if free testosterone is normal, there is no need to measure prolactin.
7. Moore CA, Fishman IJ, Hirshkowitz M. Evaluation of erectile dysfunction and sleep-related erections. *J Psychosom Res* 1997;42:531.
   A history of nocturnal and early morning erections is generally sufficient, and sleep laboratory testing is seldom indicated.
8. Kaufman JM, et al. Evaluation of erectile dysfunction by dynamic infusion cavernosometry and cavernosography: multi-institutional study. *Urology* 1993;41:445.
   Accurate preoperative evaluation is needed to identify candidates for revascularization procedures for the treatment of cavernosal artery insufficiency and corporeal venoocclusive dysfunction.

Treatment
9. Lue TF, et al. A study of seldenafil (Viagra™) a new oral agent for the treatment of male erectile dysfunction. *J Urol* 1997;157:701.
   Reversible side effects include headache, flushing, visual disturbances, and myalgia.
10. Dunsmuir WD, Holmes SA. The aetiology and management of erectile, ejaculatory, and fertility problems in men with diabetes mellitus. *Diabet Med* 1996;13:700.
    Up to 50% of older diabetics have these types of problems. Mechanisms probably include diabetic neuropathy and psychogenic factors.
11. Sunduram CP, et al. Long-term follow-up of patients receiving injection therapy for erectile dysfunction. *Urology* 1997;49:932.
    This therapy is effective, but there is a long-term dropout rate of 50%–80%.
12. Lewis RW, Witherington R. External vacuum therapy for erectile dysfunction: use and results. *World J Urol* 1997;15:78.
    This therapy is useful for any etiology but is cumbersome, and retrograde ejaculation is a disadvantage.
13. Garber BB. Inflatable penile prosthesis: results of 150 cases. *Br J Urol* 1996; 78:933.
    Surgical prostheses are successful when other methods fail, but are expensive and frequently require revisions. Satisfaction rates of up to 80% are reported.
14. Padma-Nathan H, et al. Treatment of erectile dysfunction by the medicated urethral system for erection (MUSE). *Urology* 1995;153:472.
    Intraurethral suppositories of prostaglandin E provide good results and avoid many of the problems associated with injections.
15. Stahl SM. How psychiatrists can build new therapies for impotence. *J Clin Psychiatry* 1998;59:47.
    Success rates of specific techniques have not been adequately quantified.
16. Levine FJ, Goldstein I. Vascular reconstructive surgery in the management of erectile dysfunction. *Int J Impotence Res* 1990;2:59.
    Surgical measures are directed at penile artery revascularization or at the prevention of venous leak, depending on the nature of the vascular problem.

17. Leiblum SR, Rosen RC. Couples therapy for erectile disorders: conceptual and clinical considerations. *J Sex Marital Ther* 1991;17:147.

The authors identify four key relationship variables (status and dominance, sexual attraction, intimacy and trust, and sexual scripts) of special importance in the management of erectile problems.

Abnormalities of Ejaculation

18. Ozturk B, et al. Erectile dysfunction in premature ejaculation. *Arch Ital Urol Androl* 1997;69:133.

This article states that there is a significant prevalence of organic dysfunction, especially with secondary premature ejaculation.

19. Xin ZC, et al. Somatosensory evoked potentials in patients with primary premature ejaculation. *J Urol* 1997;158:451.

Hypersensitivity and hyperexcitability of glans noted with objective testing provide organic implications for premature ejaculation.

20. Metz ME, et al. Premature ejaculation: a psychophysiological review. *J Sex Marital Ther* 1997;23:3.

Poor results of therapy may be due to heterogeneous patient groups receiving generalized treatment rather than therapy targeted to the specific type of problem.

21. Waldinger MD, Hengeveld MW, Zwinderman AH. Ejaculation-retarding properties of paroxetine in patients with primary premature ejaculation: a double-blind, randomized, dose-response study. *Br J Urol* 1997;79:592.

Antidepressants including clomipramine, fluoxetine, paroxetine, and sertraline appear to be effective in retarding ejaculation, whether or not depression is present.

---

78.   DYSPAREUNIA AND VAGINISMUS

Michel E. Rivlin

Dyspareunia may be defined as persistent and recurrent genital pain experienced during intercourse. The Diagnostic and Statistical Manual of Mental Disorders includes dyspareunia under the classification of psychosexual disorders. Dyspareunia and vaginismus are linked; either may be the cause of the other. The difference between the two is that, while intromission is usually painful in women with dyspareunia, it is virtually impossible in women with vaginismus because of the muscle spasm involved. If vaginismus is the cause of dyspareunia, the primary diagnosis is vaginismus. Dyspareunia and anorgasmy are often, but not always, linked. Primary dyspareunia exists throughout the patient's sexual lifetime, whereas secondary dyspareunia develops in a patient who had once enjoyed pain-free intercourse. The problem may be complete, that is, present under all circumstances, or selective, that is, occurring only in specific situations. In women with superficial dyspareunia, the pain is perceived at the introitus or in the vagina; in those with deep dyspareunia, the pain is experienced in the lower abdominal area.

The incidence of dyspareunia is not known, but it is thought to be one of the most common sexual dysfunctions and the most common in women of lower socioeconomic status. The literature presents two viewpoints regarding the etiology. In one, psychogenic or functional dyspareunia is considered uncommon; in the other, organic factors are regarded as usually temporary and easily correctable and rare as a cause of longstanding disorder. A recommended approach to adopt in such patients is to regard the causality on a continuum as primarily physical or psychogenic, with the potential for both to be equal contributors. Thus, an integrated diagnostic and therapeutic approach requires the careful evaluation of the emotional and psychologic aspects as well as the physical.

The physical causes of superficial pain on entry include vulvovaginitis, urethritis and urethral syndrome, cystitis or interstitial cystitis, vulvar vestibulitis, and bartholinitis. Postoperative tender or contracted scars, especially those resulting from episiotomy or vaginal surgical repair, are common causes. In older women, lack of estrogen or vulvar dystrophy frequently leads to discontinuation of intercourse because of pain. In younger patients, a rigid hymen or a developmental anomaly of the vagina may be another obvious etiologic factor. Traumatic factors include errors in sexual technique, such as an absence of foreplay, leading to poor lubrication. Allergic reactions to contraceptive chemicals, feminine sprays, and vaginal douches are also possible causes.

The physical causes of deeply situated coital pain include endometriosis and pelvic inflammatory disease stemming from inflammation, adhesions, and adnexal masses. The pain that may follow pelvic operations can be due to adhesions or scarring, or may result from an ovary that has become adherent to the vaginal cuff. Radiation therapy and radical pelvic operations or pelvic neoplasms may produce sufficient anatomic distortion as to cause dyspareunia and even apareunia (absent intercourse). Whereas a retrodisplaced uterus is a frequently encountered normal variation, occasionally, an ovary displaced to the cul-de-sac or a tender retroflexed uterine fundus may lead to deep thrust dyspareunia. Cervical lacerations and scars can also be significant etiologic factors. Rectal and orthopedic problems must be ruled out. The myofascial pain syndrome and pelvic varicocele are believed by some to be possible causes of dyspareunia.

During the assessment of dyspareunia, intrapersonal (intrapsychic) and interpersonal (relationship) problems must be sought and identified. In patients with intrapersonal problems, fear, trauma, ignorance, anxiety, and lack of sexual emancipation may be the primary reasons or may have an impact on a physical disorder. Interpersonal problems may be due to conflicts in the areas of contraception, relationship priorities, sexual frequency, sexual timing and technique, and sexual boredom. Struggle for control can be an issue, and these relationships are often characterized by poor communication in general, particularly with regard to feelings and sexual issues. Often these factors are interrelated; for instance, a physical problem can adversely affect the relationship or may coexist with an intrapersonal problem. Cases are classified according to the most obvious source of the problem. Faulty information and intrapsychic problems are more common in women with primary dyspareunia, and relationship issues may be more important in women with secondary dyspareunia.

The diagnosis depends on the woman's history, with particular reference to the site and duration of pain, and on the findings from physical examination, in which different maneuvers should be used to reproduce the same kind of pain that the patient feels during coitus. Special investigations may be helpful in certain circumstances, particularly laparoscopy, which may be essential in establishing the diagnosis of minimal endometriosis or in confirming the absence of genital pathology. Once the organic and psychologic components of the problem have been identified, therapy is directed toward ameliorating these factors. The patient and, if possible, her partner should be educated and reassured regarding the nature and of prognosis for the problem. Organic disease is dealt with using standard pharmacologic or surgical methods, for instance, estrogen therapy for atrophic vaginitis and hormonal manipulation or surgical ablation for endometriosis. When indicated, marital and sexual therapy should be offered, with particular emphasis on the couple's communication skills, sensate focus exercises, relaxation, and masturbatory techniques. Behavioral modifications include vaginal self-dilation with lubricated fingers and graduated dilators, Kegel's pelvic floor exercises, water-soluble lubricants, and changes in coital positioning. Specific surgical procedures indicated for eradicating introital dyspareunia include the excision of painful scars, with resuture in the transverse plane, or hymenotomy for an unruptured or inadequately ruptured hymen. Plastic surgical procedures may be required to correct congenital or surgically acquired disorders of the vulva or vagina (perineoplasty and vaginoplasty), or both, that are not amenable to progressive self-dilation. Specific surgical procedures for the treatment of deep dyspareunia unresponsive to standard therapy include ventral suspension of the retroverted uterus with ovaries prolapsed in the cul-de-sac, or even hysterectomy in a few carefully selected patients with disabling symptomatology who have no wish to conceive. In patients with postoperative adhesions or with ovaries trapped in the cul-de-sac, lysis of the adhesions and removal or resuspension of the ovaries may be indicated. All surgical procedures also require concomitant psychologic, marital, and sexual therapy, as indicated.

Vaginismus is a condition characterized by an involuntary conditioned reflex spasm of the musculature surrounding the vaginal outlet and outer third of the vagina—that is, the perineal and levator muscles and even the adductor muscles of the thighs. The spasm is stimulated by real or imaginary attempts at vaginal penetration of any sort. It has been compared with the blink reflex elicited when corneal contact is anticipated. it is termed *primary* when coitus has never been achieved and *secondary* if successful intercourse has preceded onset of the problem. It is the least common of the female sexual dysfunctions but the most disabling; in the absence of organic pathology, it represents a prime example of a psychosomatic condition consisting of phobic features and somatically expressed vaginospasm. There are varying degrees of severity, and it may be absolute or situational in occurrence.

Reported etiologic factors include a history of genital or psychic trauma (especially incest), religious beliefs, sexual misinformation, and anxiety. Vaginismus and dyspareunia are inevitably linked. Although vaginismus may cause dyspareunia, repeated episodes of dyspareunia may result in secondary vaginismus. An organic cause of vaginismus must always be ruled out before initiating therapy. The most frequent presenting complaints of the condition include unconsummated marriage (primary apareunia), secondary apareunia, an inability to use tampons or undergo pelvic examination, exposure to male sexual dysfunction, and infertility. Low libido may be a factor, but women with vaginismus are at least as frequently able to achieve orgasm as normal women, because the patient usually chooses partners for their passivity, and alternative, noncoital sexual release may be substituted.

Therapy consists of desensitization techniques involving Kegel's exercises and the use of passive vaginal dilatation using either a set of graduated plastic dilators (syringe barrels may be substituted) or the patient's fingers. She is encouraged to observe the pubococcygeal muscle contraction using a mirror and a finger to palpate the contracted muscle. By tightening and relaxing the muscle she is helped to understand the source of the problem. This combined deconditioning of the abnormal physical response and the behavior modification techniques then progress to include the partner and the eventual attempt at male passive coitus in the female-superior position. Because vaginismus is a hysterical condition and a type of conversion reaction, management of the phobic element is essential. Both partners must be involved and must be instructed in normal sexuality and the nature of their problem. Treatment takes about 6 to 8 weeks and usually yields good results. If progress is limited after three or four treatment sessions, psychiatric or psychologic referral to deal with patient resistance should be considered.

Reviews
1. Steege JF, Ling FW. Dyspareunia: a special type of chronic pelvic pain. *Obstet Gynecol Clin North Am* 1993;20:779.
   Associated psychologic disorders include fear, anxiety, phobic reactions, conscious reactions, partner hostility, and psychologic trauma.
2. Jones KD, Lehr ST, Hewell SW. Dyspareunia: three case reports. *J Obstet Gynecol Neonatal Nurs* 1997;26:19.
   This article describes how to elicit an accurate sexual history and 12 common causes of dyspareunia, which is a symptom, not a diagnosis.

Dyspareunia
3. Jamieson DJ, Steege JF. The prevalence of dysmenorrhea, dyspareunia, pelvic pain, and irritable bowel syndrome in primary care practices. *Obstet Gynecol* 1996;87:55.
   The self-reported prevalence was 90%, 46%, 39%, and 12%, respectively. Low income was a risk factor for dysmenorrhea and dyspareunia, and African-American race was a risk factor for pelvic pain.

4. Weber AM, et al. Vaginal anatomy and sexual function. *Obstet Gynecol* 1995; 86:946.
   Introital caliber, vaginal length, and vulvovaginal atrophy do not correlate well with sexual function, particularly as regards dyspareunia and dryness.
5. Loprinzi CL, et al. Phase III randomized double-blind study to evaluate the efficacy of a polycarbophil-based vaginal moisturizer in women with breast cancer. *J Clin Oncol* 1997;15:969.
   Both the study moisturizer and the placebo lubricator substantially relieved vaginal dryness and dyspareunia in breast cancer survivors.
6. van Lankeld JJ, et al. Difficulties in the differential diagnosis of vaginismus, dyspareunia and mixed sexual pain disorder. *J Psychosom Obstet Gynecol* 1995; 16:201.
   No univariate differences were found between members of the three groups or between their partners. It was not possible to make a multivariate prediction of group membership.
7. Yoong AF. Laparoscopic ventrosuspensions. A review of 72 cases. *Am J Obstet Gynecol* 1990;163:1151.
   The success of laparoscopic ventrosuspension for the treatment of deep dyspareunia or pelvic pain associated with a retroverted uterus varies from 18% to 42%. Prior use of a Hodge pessary did not predict success of the procedure.
8. Lamont JA. Dyspareunia and vaginismus. In: Sciarra JJ, ed. *Gynecology and obstetrics. Vol. 6*. Hagerstown, MD: Harper & Row, 1992:1–8.
   The term apareunia refers to the inability to experience vaginal containment of the penis.
9. Scholl GM. Prognostic variables in treating vaginismus. *Obstet Gynecol* 1988; 72:231.
   The worst prognostic sign was a fixed belief on the woman's part that her vagina was anatomically abnormal. Previous attempts to correct the vaginismus surgically were particularly detrimental to the success of sex therapy.

Vaginismus
10. Sexual function after pelvic surgery in women. *Ann Acad Med Singapore* 1995;24:755.
    Vaginismus was treated with a rapid desensitization program using vaginal moulds and resulted in all patients achieving satisfactory intercourse within 2–6 weeks.
11. Shaw J. Treatment of primary vaginismus: a new perspective. *J Sex Marital Ther* 1994;20:46.
    The article challenges the efficacy of cognitive-behavioral therapy. A case is made for sexual competence based on self-competence.

79. RAPE, INCEST, AND ABUSE

Michel E. Rivlin

Sexual assault may be defined as any sexual act committed by one person on another without that person's consent, using either force or the threat of force. The inability to give appropriate consent, because of age or mental condition, is deemed to be a lack of appropriate consent (statutory rape). The presence of semen is not necessary. Common situations include abduction rape, spousal rape, date rape, and rape of the most vulnerable, including children, the elderly, and those with physical or mental disabilities. Males may also be rape victims. Sexual molestation is a noncoital sexual contact performed without consent.

Rape is reported to be the fastest growing violent crime in the United States. In 1987, the annual incidence was 73 per 100,000 females. It is estimated that 10 times that number go unreported. Rape victims are generally young, unmarried women, many of them younger than 18 years of age. A substantial number are prepubertal. Adult women tend to be raped at home—60% by a stranger. A weapon is used in approximately one third of the alleged assaults, and about 1% of the victims require hospitalization. The assault generally occurs in the late night or early morning hours. Physical injury is present in eight to 45% of the victims. The average rapist commits about 12 offenses before being caught. Rapists are mostly male (98%) and come from all walks of life. The personality and character traits of rapists are separate and distinct from their sexual orientation and interests. The rapist does not want consensual sex; because of anger, his wish is to overpower, humiliate, and degrade the victim. Most follow certain patterns in their assaults; the conclusion of sexual activity, generally in the first 10 minutes, is usually followed by further physical and psychologic abuse lasting for another 45 minutes on average. In offender programs, it has been found that it takes rapists approximately 1 year to believe that they are indeed rapists or child molesters. Rape has far-reaching effects on the victim and her family; about half of married rape victims are divorced within 1–2 years of the assault.

Those involved in any kind of trauma—war, flood, fires, and the like—tend to experience similar reactions afterward. Symptoms can arise both immediately after the event and later, and often last for years. This kind of reaction is called *posttraumatic stress disorder*. Sexual assault can produce similar effects, which have been described as the rape trauma syndrome. Reactions can be divided into two phases. An acute phase, lasting for hours or days, is associated with disorganization of usual behavior patterns as well as emotional and somatic symptoms. In the expressed style, fear and anxiety are manifested through crying, restlessness, or tenseness. In the controlled style, a subdued affect masks the victim's true feelings. Somatic reactions include headaches, fatigue, sleep disturbance, and urinary or bowel upset. Emotional reactions include anger, self-blame, fear, and humiliation. The long-term second phase starts two to three weeks after the trauma. It consists of reorganization with return toward normal function. Dreams and nightmares, fears, phobias, and sexual anxieties are common. Major life-style changes may be instituted. Some victims never fully recover; they suffer chronic stress disorders and loss of security, with a significant long-term morbidity.

In evaluating the patient, medical concerns include documentation of the pertinent history, physical examination, prompt treatment of any physical injuries, and psychologic support and follow-up. Laboratory specimens must be collected and preserved so they may be used in court, and prophylaxis against venereal disease and pregnancy must be offered. Informed consent is necessary to permit the examination to be performed, and also to allow the alleged assault to be reported and the records and specimens released to law enforcement authorities. In practice, a careful protocol should be available at a center such as a large emergency room, where office-based physicians can refer rape victims to avoid the legal, social, and psychologic consequences of an inappropriate work-up.

The history includes the specifics of the alleged assault, and information on the last voluntary sexual experience, drug use, contraceptive practice, and the menstrual record. The physical examination includes determination of the patient's mental status, relevant photographs, and collection of significant stains and clothing. Combing of the pubic hairs can yield foreign material, and the pelvic examination should include rectal examination. Wet samples from the vagina, rectum, and mouth should be examined for the presence of motile sperm, as indicated by the patient's history. If no sperm are seen, the acid phosphatase level should be checked. A saliva sample for the determination of blood group antigens is obtained to see whether the victim is a secretor or not (85% secrete blood type in all body fluids). Drug screening, blood typing, serology, and serum pregnancy tests are carried out. The specimens obtained must conform to legal protocol, known as the chain of evidence, with documentation of acceptance and transference of materials.

The risk of acquiring gonorrhea ranges from 6% to 12%, and of syphilis up to 3%. Because 40%–90% of the patients are lost to follow-up, treatment should be given presumptively and be sufficient to cure persistent gonorrhea, incubating syphilis, and Chlamydia infection. Single doses of ceftriaxone and azythromycin provide the necessary coverage. Testing for sexually transmitted disease should be repeated at 6 weeks. Acquired immunodeficiency syndrome testing should be offered. Although pregnancy resulting from rape is rare (the probability of pregnancy resulting from any one unprotected coital act is 4%), pregnancy prophylaxis should be offered. Two 50 μg estrogen-containing combination oral contraceptive tablets given initially, and taken again in 12 hours, if carried out within 72 hours of intercourse, have a 1% failure rate and are used in preference to high-dose estrogens, which are associated with nausea and the risk of causing fetal injury in the event of failure. Some women may prefer to wait and, if pregnancy occurs, may then elect to terminate. In either event, a followup pregnancy test should be performed. Subsequent visits at 1 and 6 weeks should be scheduled so that the patient's emotional condition and the need for further counseling or psychiatric intervention can be assessed, in addition to the general medical follow-up.

Child sexual abuse includes rape, incest, and molestation. The latter two are grossly underreported. An estimated 2% of natural fathers and 17% of stepfathers are likely to have sexual contact with their daughters. In all cases of sexual abuse, the appropriate authorities (e.g., Child Protective Services) must be notified immediately.

A sexual offense is the performance of any sexual act prohibited by law. Sexual deviation (perversion) is a predominant and unconventional sexual interest in a particular activity, object, or individual. These activities are currently referred to as para philias. Deviations may not be offenses, as in the case of habitual cross-dressing (transvestism), or they may be, as in the case of pedophilia, in which adult males are attracted to and sexually abuse young boys. Some authorities maintain that sexual offenders can be treated just as successfully as alcoholics, and that effective treatment reduces the rate of recidivism. Treatment includes the administration of drugs such as medroxyprogesterone acetate or gonadotropin agonists, behavior modification, and psychologic counseling or therapy. It is often necessary to institutionalize or incarcerate offenders.

In 85% of child sexual assault cases, the molester is known to the child and has an important relationship with the child (e.g., a child care provider). The history is frequently difficult to obtain, and it may be advisable to work with the children's protection agency. Although occasional coaching by a parent or guardian may be evident, in general, false reporting is uncommon. The medical examination performs an important psychologic function and helps to allay unrealistic fears and fantasies in the child. After the examination, the parents need to be informed of the findings and plan, keeping the discussion open and nonjudgmental.

Incest and molestation differ from rape in that the abuse often takes place over a period of years and the victim has an ongoing relationship with the assailant. Frequently, other adults give covert permission to the activity. The clinical presentation is often typical, and consists of sexually transmitted disease, pregnancy, and various emotional and social disorders. A child who is physically abused may also be a victim of sexual abuse. Physical examination may reveal the existence of signs such as a spacious introitus in a premenstrual child or the presence of healed lacerations, leukorrhea, and cervicitis. Frequently, child assailants were themselves assaulted as children, and child victims of sexual abuse, when adult, often experience difficulty in establishing stable relationships. Nevertheless, with proper intervention and help, most children can recover from the adverse experience; even adults who were abused as children can benefit from treatment and overcome their long-standing problems. Generally, the more trusted the assailant, the more damaging the experience. The reaction of other adults is also important in determining the degree of guilt felt by the child.

Sexual abuse is a specific area of the larger problem of physical violence. Up to 25% of the injured women seen in emergency rooms are victims of domestic battering. Physicians treating these patients recognize the presence of physical abuse only 3%

of the time, and often their approach to treatment consists only of prescribing pain medications or psychiatric referral. There are an estimated 500,000 to 2.5 million cases of abuse of an elderly person annually. This exceeds other forms of violence against the unprotected, and this problem will escalate as the numbers of elderly increase. The most common abuser is an adult child with whom the parent lives. One must be aware of the possibility when interviewing elderly patients who exhibit strange behaviors and apparently irrational fears. If suspected, community resources should be involved to remove the victims and counsel the abuser.

Review
1. Hampton HL. Care of the woman who has been raped. *N Engl J Med* 1995; 332:234.
   In obtaining the chain of evidence, each separate piece of evidence should be marked with the patient's name, hospital number, date, physician's name, and type of specimen. Each person in the chain must document acceptance and transference of material.
2. Royce CF, Coonan PR. Emergency! Adolescent rape. *Am J Nurs* 1997;97:45.
   The physician's legal responsibilities include the accurate recording of events, documentation of injuries, collection of samples, and reporting to authorities, as required.

The Rapist
3. Polaschek DL, Ward T, Hudson SM. Rape and rapists: theory and treatment. *Clin Psychol Rev* 1997;17:117.
   Rapists are significantly different from child molesters. Classification of rapists is essential for designing and evaluating treatment and in the prediction of future risks.
4. Kalichman SC. Affective and personality characteristics of MMPI profile subgroups of incarcerated rapists. *Arch Sex* 1990;19:443.
   Rape, although a sexual offense, is mainly concerned with anger, rage, revenge, power, and punishment. Sex is used as a weapon, and the assailant seldom experiences sexual gratification. Most sexual offenders should be dealt with by purely penal methods.

The Victim
5. Hilton MR, Mezey GC. Victims and perpetrators of child sexual abuse. *Br J Psychiatry* 1996;169:408.
   A single child molester may commit hundreds of sexual acts on hundreds of children. They were often themselves also victims of childhood abuse.
6. Slaughter L, et al. Patterns of genital injury in female sexual assault victims. *Am J Obstet Gynecol* 1997;176:609.
   A localized pattern of genital trauma can frequently be seen, usually minor, but nevertheless useful for the clinical forensic examiner.
7. McCauley J, et al. Clinical characteristics of women with a history of childhood abuse. *JAMA* 1997;277:1362.
   Adult health problems include physical symptoms, psychological problems, and substance abuse. The association may be as strong as for women experiencing current abuse.
8. Bohn DK, Holz KA. Sequelae of abuse. Health effects of childhood sexual abuse, domestic battering, and rape. *J Nurse Midwifery* 1996;41:442.
   Violence against women is endemic in the United States, where wife beating results in more injuries requiring medical treatment than do rape, auto accidents, and muggings combined.

Psychology
9. Burgess AW, Holmstrom LL. Rape trauma syndrome. *Am J Psychiatry* 1974;131:9.
   Two states were described: (1) an immediate, acute phase in which there were either expressed or controlled emotional responses to a life-threatening situation,

and (2) a long-term phase of reorganization, accompanied by changes in life-style, phobic reactions, dreams, and nightmares.
10. Darves-Bornoz JM. Rape-related psychotraumatic syndromes. *Eur J Obstet Gynecol Reprod Biol* 1997;71:59.
    In a study that followed 92 victims for 6 months, there was a high incidence of posttraumatic stress disorders associated with phobic, disassociative, and borderline disorders.
11. Duddle M. Emotional sequelae of sexual assault. *J R Soc Med* 1991;84:26.
    Immediate support seems to be a factor in alleviating later symptoms. There appears to be significantly more related distress in those women who did not receive help until later.
12. Moscarello R. Psychological management of victims of sexual assault. *Can J Psychiatry* 1990;35:25.
    During the first 6 weeks or so of disorganization, victims need someone to listen to their problems over and over again without getting impatient, as close friends and relatives often do.

Statutory Rape
13. Fleming JM. Prevalence of childhood sexual abuse in a community sample of Australian women. *Med J Aust* 1997;166:65.
    There are high rates of sexual abuse (20%); 10% of these involved intercourse. The perpetrator is usually male (98%) and known to the child.
14. Romans SE, Martin JL, Morris EM. Risk factors for adolescent pregnancy: how important is child sexual abuse? Otago Women's Health Study. *N Z Med J* 1997;110:30.
    The problem is not random but related to families with known psychosocial problems. If the abuse included intercourse, it was then predictive of pregnancy.
15. Donovan P. Can statutory rape laws be effective in preventing adolescent pregnancy? *Fam Plann Perspect* 1997;29:30.
    According to the authors, to reduce adolescent pregnancy, the need is to invest time and money in women, not in incarcerating men.
16. Sinal SH, et al. Clinician agreement on physical findings in child sexual abuse cases. *Arch Pediatr Adolesc Med* 1997;151:497.
    Experienced clinicians did not always agree on genital findings; thus, overemphasis on physical findings should be avoided.

Laboratory Evidence
17. Hooft PJ, van de Voorde HP. Bayesian evaluation of the modified zinc test and the acid phosphatase spot test for forensic semen investigation. *Am J Forensic Med Pathol* 1997;18:45.
    Zinc and acid phosphatase are present in seminal plasma and can be identified as presumptive evidence of the presence of semen.
18. Young WW, et al. Sexual assault: review of a national model protocol for forensic and medical evaluation. *Obstet Gynecol* 1992;80:878.
    The object of such a protocol is to minimize the physical and psychologic trauma while maximizing the probability of collecting and preserving physical evidence for potential use in the legal system.

Medical Management
19. Schwarca SK, Whittington WL. Sexual assault and sexually transmitted diseases: detection and management in adults and children. *Rev Infect Dis* 1990; 6:S682.
    The risk of acquiring a viral sexually transmitted disease may be less than the risk of a bacterial infection because of the episodic nature of viral shedding.
20. Yuzpe AA, Smith RP, Rademaker AW. A multicenter clinical investigation employing ethinyl estradiol combined with dl-norgesterol as postcoital contraceptive agent. *Fertil Steril* 1982;37:508.
    The 1% failure rate and teratogenicity of postcoital medications should be explained to the patient. All interventions are ineffective after 72 hours.

21. Lumley VA, Miltenberger RG. Sexual abuse prevention for persons with mental retardation. *Am J Ment Retard* 1997;101:459.
    This article reviews sexual abuse prevention training for persons at risk and for their care givers.
22. Hobbs C, Wynne J. Use of the colposcope in examination for sexual abuse. *Arch Dis Child* 1996;75:539.
    Normal anatomy and normal variations must be understood in order to determine whether a given finding is abnormal. However, clear guidelines as to the significance of anogenital findings with respect to sexual abuse have yet to be developed.

XV. GYNECOLOGIC ENDOCRINOLOGY

80. AMENORRHEA

Randall S. Hines

Amenorrhea is defined as the complete absence of vaginal bleeding in a woman of reproductive age; this term describes a symptom—not a diagnosis. Lack of menstruation is considered to be normal and physiologic prior to puberty, during pregnancy and lactation, and after menopause. Primary amenorrhea, or delayed puberty, refers to females who fail to undergo menarche or development of secondary sexual characteristics by age 14, or who have no menstrual period by age 16 regardless of the presence of secondary sexual characteristics. Secondary amenorrhea is defined as the absence of menstrual periods for 6 months, or a length of time equivalent to three normal menstrual cycles.

The approach to the patient with either secondary or primary amenorrhea is essentially the same. The reason for this is that there will be overlap in the etiologies of both conditions. Patients are categorized initially according to their endogenous estrogen status. This can be determined on the basis of physical exam in patients with delayed puberty (lack of secondary sexual characteristics) or by the presence or absence of a progestin-induced withdrawal bleed in patients with secondary sexual characteristics. Another technique involves the interpretation of a vaginal smear (estrogen will cause a predominance of superficial or large cells on a vaginal smear). Patients who are determined to be euestrogenic (having normal-circulating estrogen) will most commonly be found to have chronic anovulation (polycystic ovarian disease [PCOD]). If the patient fails to bleed in response to progestin she is hypoestrogenic, and gonadotropin levels should be measured. Direct measurement of estrogen levels is not recommended. Those patients with elevated gonadotropins are categorized as having hypergonadotropic hypogonadism. Those patients with low or normal gonadotropins are included in the category of hypogonadotropic hypogonadism.

In addition to PCOD, other disorders that cause chronic anovulation include hyperprolactinemia, thyroid disease, Cushing's syndrome, congenital adrenal hyperplasia, and androgen-secreting ovarian or adrenal tumors. In addition to chronic anovulation, patients with an apparent normal estrogen status also include those patients who have outflow tract abnormalities. These patients will present having never experienced menses and they will have normal breast development. Examination in some will reveal the absence of a vaginal opening. The differential diagnosis for such a patient includes: (1) complete absence of the vagina and uterus (müllerian agenesis, Mayer–Rokitansky–Kuster–Hauser syndrome); (2) transverse vaginal septum, in which incomplete canalization of the vagina has occurred; (3) imperforate hymen and (4) androgen insensitivity (formerly testicular feminization). Androgen insensitivity may be diagnosed in a patient with scant pubic hair, normal breast development, and absence of a vaginal opening. This disorder results from a mutation in the gene for the androgen receptor located on the X chromosome, and more in-depth discussion follows in chapter 88. Rarely, outflow tract obstruction can be acquired as in the case of cervical stenosis, typically from surgery or from intrauterine adhesions (Asherman's syndrome), which again most often follows either surgery or infection.

Patients with hypogonadotropic hypogonadism will require imaging of the central nervous system to exclude tumors. This may include prolactin-secreting adenomas, null cell tumors of the pituitary, and craniopharyngiomas. The latter may disrupt the normal communication between the hypothalamus and the pituitary. Patients with normal imaging studies may be found to have causes related to stress, weight loss, or exercise. Anorexia nervosa is a life-threatening condition which can result in amenorrhea. In addition, prolonged and extreme exercise may also cause cessation of menses. With a negative history and normal central nervous system imaging, a diagnosis of Kallmann's syndrome or idiopathic hypogonadotropic hypogonadism should be entertained. Kallmann's syndrome is associated with anosmia and has been best understood in the male patient with delayed puberty. Molecular etiologies for this type of disorder include mutations in the Kall gene. This gene encodes a protein that functions as a neural adhesion molecule and is important in the embryologic development of a normal hypothalamus. In addition, mutations in the gonadotropin-releasing hormone receptor have been documented.

Pituitary insufficiency may also result from Sheehan syndrome or postpartum pituitary necrosis following obstetrical hemorrhage. These patients will have hypogonadotropic hypogonadism, and the loss of pituitary function typically follows this pattern: prolactin, gonadotropins, growth hormones, thyroid hormones, and finally adrenocorticotropic hormones. Other various categories of hypothalamic pituitary amenorrhea include the empty sella syndrome, which may be congenital or surgically induced. Pressure from the cerebrospinal fluid flattens the pituitary gland against the sellar floor, producing absence of the gland on imaging.

The most common of the amenorrhea syndromes are found in the category of hypergonadotropic hypogonadism. These patients present with either delayed puberty or secondary amenorrhea. Elevated gonadotropins are obtained in the workup, and the next diagnostic step is a karyotype. This group of patients can then be divided into those with normal chromosomes for a female (46,XX) or abnormal chromosomes. The abnormal karyotype group is typically described as having gonadal dysgenesis because the absence of two normal X chromosomes results in failure of proper gonadal development. A large spectrum of karyotype abnormalities can be found. The most common is 45,X (Turner's syndrome). Patients will be found to have varying degrees of the typical features of Turner's, including webbed neck, coarctation of the aorta, high-arched palate, cubitus valgus, broad shield chest, and short fourth metacarpals, with cardiac and renal anomalies being the most significant finding. The most common phenotypic feature of patients with gonadal dysgenesis is short stature. In addition to the 45,X karyotype, mosaic karyotypes include 45,X/46,XX; 45,X/46,XY; and varying degrees of deletion of one of the X chromosomes. In addition, patients may be found to have a 46,XY karyotype (Swyer's syndrome). These patients present with delayed puberty and are of normal or tall stature. Despite the presence of a Y chromosome, they have a failure of normal function of the gene responsible for testicular development known as SRY. Without the normal function of this gene, they fail to form a normal testicle and will have streak gonads. Gonadectomy is necessary in any patient with evidence of Y material on karyotype. A 30% risk for tumor formation may occur.

In patients with a normal 46,XX karyotype the most common diagnosis is premature ovarian failure occurring in a patient who has previously normal menses. A variety of etiologies may be responsible, the most serious of which are autoimmune disorders affecting not only the ovary but potentially the adrenal and the pituitary. Other causes of 46,XX ovarian failure include 17, hydroxylase deficiency, radiation, infection, resistance to gonadotropins, and other autoimmune diseases such as myasthenia gravis.

The evaluation of the patient with amenorrhea includes first an exclusion of pregnancy. Next, prolactin and thyroid-stimulating hormone should be obtained. At the first visit, assessment of estrogen status should be determined through either physical characteristics (presence or absence of breast development), vaginal smear, or a progestin-induced withdrawal bleed to be ascertained over the next 2 weeks. In those patients with low estrogen status, gonadotropins should be obtained. In patients with elevated gonadotropins, a karyotype is necessary. In patients with low or normal gonadotropins, careful evaluation of the central nervous system is required.

General
1. Doody KM, Carr BR. Amenorrhea. *Obstet Gynecol Clin North Am* 1990;17:361.
   A general review of the topic of amenorrhea.
2. Mashchak CA, et al. Clinical and laboratory evaluation of patients with primary amenorrhea. *Obstet Gynecol* 1981;57:715.
   A review of the laboratory evaluation for patients with amenorrhea.
3. Rojers J. Menstruation and systemic diseases. *N Engl J Med* 1958;259:721.
   A review of the influence of systemic diseases on the menstrual cycle.

4. Reindollar RH, Byrd JR, McDonough PG. Delayed sexual development: a study of 252 patients. *Am J Obstet Gynecol* 1981;140:371.
   A review of delayed puberty.
5. Griffin JE, Wilson JD. The syndromes of androgen resistance. *N Engl J Med* 1980;302:198.
   A review of the subject of androgen insensitivity syndromes.

Hypothalamic Disorders
6. Lambalk CB, et al. The frequency of pulsatile luteinizing hormone-releasing hormone treatment and luteinizing hormone and follicle-stimulating hormone secretion in women with amenorrhea of suprapituitary origin. *Fertil Steril* 1989; 51:416.
   The pituitary needs to be stimulated in a pulsatile fashion by luteinizing hormone–releasing hormone to maintain luteinizing hormone and follicle-stimulating hormone secretion.
7. Frisch RE, Revell R. Height and weight at menarche and a hypothesis of menarche. *Arch Dis Child* 1971;46:695.
   This article discusses the impact of weight on the establishment of menarche.
8. Vigersky RA, et al. Hypothalamic dysfunction in secondary amenorrhea associated with simple weight loss. *N Engl J Med* 1977;297:1141.
   This article presents a detailed investigation of the hypothalamic alterations associated with weight loss.
9. Jonnavithula S, et al. Bone density is compromised in amenorrheic women despite return of menses: a 2-year study. *Obstet Gynecol* 1993;81:669.
   Bone mineral density was measured by single- and dual-photon absorptiometry in spine, wrist, and foot.
10. Warren MP, Vande Wiele RL. Clinical and metabolic features of anorexia nervosa. *Am J Obstet Gynecol* 1973;117:435.
    A comprehensive review of anorexia nervosa.
11. Tagatz G, et al. Hypogonadotropic hypogonadism associated with anosmia in the female. *N Engl J Med* 1970;282:1326.
    A review of Kallman's syndrome as a cause of primary amenorrhea.
12. Berga SL, et al. Neuroendocrine aberrations in women with functional hypothalamic amenorrhea. *J Clin Endocrinol Metab* 1989;68:301.
    Reproductive quiescence is associated with the presence of unfavorable environments.

Pituitary Disorders
13. Sheehan HL. Simmonds' disease due to postpartum necrosis of the anterior pituitary gland. *Q J Med* 1939;8:277.
    This article presents the original description of postpartum pituitary necrosis.

Ovarian Disorders
14. Kazer RR, Kessel B, Yen SSC. Circulating luteinizing hormone pulse frequency in women with polycystic ovary syndrome. *J Clin Endocrinol Metab* 1987;65:233.
    This article presents a discussion of the role of luteinizing hormone in polycystic ovarian disease.
15. Rosenfeld R, Grumbach MM, eds. *Turner syndrome.* New York: Marcel Dekker, 1990.
    This is an in-depth review of Turner's syndrome.
16. Mignot MH, et al. Premature ovarian failure: the association with autoimmunity. *Eur J Gynecol Reprod Biol* 1989;30:59.
    This article reviews autoimmune disorders resulting in premature ovarian failure.
17. Corenblum B, Rowe T, Taylor PJ. High-dose, short-term glucocorticoids for the treatment of infertility resulting from premature ovarian failure. *Fertil Steril* 1993;59:988.
    Results were best with ovarian failure of less than 2 years' duration and with concomitant autoimmune thyroid disease.

Outflow Tract Disorders

18. Frank RI. The formation of an artificial vagina without operation. *Am J Obstet Gynecol* 1938;35:1053.
    This article discusses treatment of the blind vaginal pouch with progressive dilatation.
19. Jones HW, Rock JA. *Reparative and constructive surgery of the female genital tract.* Baltimore: Williams & Wilkins, 1983.
    This article reviews surgical techniques for providing a functional vaginal passage.
20. Asherman JG. Traumatic intrauterine adhesions and their effects on fertility. *Int J Fertil* 1957;2:49.
    This article discusses amenorrhea related to intrauterine instrumentation.

81. HYPERPROLACTINEMIA

Cecil A. Long

Prolactin is a polypeptide hormone with 198 amino acids. Several biologic forms of prolactin are secreted that possess different molecular sizes; however, the small form (22,000 daltons) is the active hormone and represents approximately 80% of the molecules secreted. Prolactin is secreted by lactotropic cells located in the lateral wings of the anterior pituitary gland. The half-life of prolactin is approximately 20 minutes.

Prolactin is secreted in a sleep-related circadian rhythm. The level is highest between 3 and 5 a.m. and is also increased in the early afternoon. The secretion of prolactin from the anterior pituitary gland is controlled mainly by the inhibitory action of dopamine. Depending on individual laboratory methodology, the upper limits of prolactin levels range between 20 and 25 ng/ml.

Prolactin promotes lactogenesis. The concentration may increase 10- to 20-fold during pregnancy; however, it returns to baseline levels within approximately 6 weeks in nonnursing mothers and within 6–8 months in lactating mothers. Prolactin levels are also affected by various environmental factors including nipple stimulation, ingestion of food, and stress. The use of certain medications, such as antihypertensive agents, antidepressants, psychotropic drugs, sex steroids, and antiemetics, may lead to elevated prolactin levels. Inhibitors of prolactin secretion include dopamine. Prolactin secretion is sensitive to alterations of the hypothalamic-pituitary axis. Pathologic factors affecting the secretion of prolactin include endocrine disorders, prolactin-secreting adenomas, and nonpituitary tumors that interfere with the transport of hypothalamic hormones, and neural transmitters, resulting in pituitary dysfunction. Primary hypothyroidism results in elevated prolactin levels accompanied by galactorrhea in approximately 3% of all patients. These patients have a low serum thyroxine concentration that causes an increased secretion of thyroid-releasing hormone (TRH) from the hypothalamus. The TRH then overstimulates the thyrotropes and the lactotropes in the anterior pituitary gland, causing an increase in both thyroid-stimulating hormone (TSH) and prolactin levels.

Another common cause of hyperprolactinemia is a prolactin-secreting pituitary adenoma (prolactinoma). Most patients with pituitary prolactinomas have galactorrhea and prolactin levels approaching 100 ng/ml. As these tumors grow, they compress the pituitary stalk, leading to interruption of inhibitory dopamine action. When the tumor is 1 cm or greater, this is a macroadenoma; if less than 1 cm, it is a microadenoma.

Nonpituitary tumors can also affect prolactin secretion. Craniopharyngiomas arise from epithelial remnants of Rathke's pouch. These types of tumors, along with other space-occupying lesions, including germinomas and gliomas as well as infiltrative processes (tuberculosis, sarcoidosis, histiocytosis), lead to a loss of the inhibitory control exerted by dopamine by compressing the pituitary stalk. A variety of other disorders may also be responsible for hyperprolactinemia. These include chronic disease processes such as renal failure, adrenal insufficiency, and acromegaly.

Sheehan's syndrome is the only known entity that involves lower-than-normal prolactin levels. The insult to the pituitary gland that precipitates Sheehan's syndrome usually arises from hemorrhage in the immediate postpartum period. This results in ischemia of the lateral pituitary gland, which damages the lactotropes. These women may also have blunted luteinizing hormone (LH), follicle-stimulating hormone (FSH), and TSH responses.

Hyperprolactinemia should be suspected in the patient who presents with galactorrhea (more than 50%) and oligo-amenorrhea (20%). Hyperprolactinemia may also be responsible for a subtle ovulation dysfunction, manifested by an inadequate luteal phase. These patients typically have shortened luteal phases and lowered mid-luteal phase progesterone levels. Disruption of gonadotropin secretion from the anterior pituitary resulting from elevated prolactin levels is thought to be the source of anovulation and luteal phase defects in these women.

Prolactin levels should be measured in all patients seen because of menstrual cycle irregularities or galactorrhea. Because of the intricate relationship between prolactin and TSH secretion, thyroid evaluation (TSH and thyroid hormone levels) should also be carried out. The best time to collect serum for prolactin measurements is between 8 and 12 a.m. Elevated prolactin levels indicate the need for evaluation of the sella turcica. Magnetic resonance imaging (MRI) or computed tomography (CT) scan are the most reliable methods for this purpose.

There are four indications for treatment of the patient with hyperprolactinemia: (1) progressive pituitary enlargement (macroadenoma, greater than or equal to 1 cm in diameter); (2) persistent galactorrhea; (3) hypoestrogenemia; and (4) ovulation dysfunction in the patient who desires pregnancy. For these patients, dopamine agonists (bromocriptine, cabergoline) are the treatment of choice. The oral administration of these agents may produce gastrointestinal disturbances, especially nausea and vomiting. These side effects usually subside; however, in some women, the treatment has to be discontinued. When this situation arises, the vaginal administration of dopamine agonists may be considered to reduce the gastrointestinal side effects. Patients with pituitary macroadenomas usually respond well to dopamine therapy. Therapy must be continued indefinitely because discontinuation usually results in the return of hyperprolactinemia as well as growth of the adenoma. In patients who do not respond to dopamine agonists, surgical management may be required. Overall, there is an approximately 50% recurrence of pituitary adenomas after surgical ablation.

An understanding of the natural history of prolactinomas is evolving. In general, prolactin-secreting microadenomas progress in less than 10% of the cases; the balance of the tumors either remain the same or, in some cases, spontaneously reduce. There is only a minimal risk of complications from prolactinomas during pregnancy. Once pregnancy is confirmed, dopamine agonists should be discontinued. Evaluation during pregnancy should be reserved for the patient who starts to experience headaches or exhibit focal neurologic defects, indicating progression of the tumor. Imaging of the sella turcica is required when these symptoms develop. In the event of tumor progression in the setting of pregnancy, dopamine agonist treatment may be restarted. Medical management with bromocriptine can be extremely effective, and most women have a successful pregnancy outcome.

Prolactin Physiology
1. Hwang P, et al. Purification of human prolactin. *J Biol Chem* 1972;247:1955.
   This describes the biochemistry of prolactin.
2. Zacur HA, et al. Multifactorial regulation of prolactin secretion. *Lancet* 1976;
   1:410.
   This is a review of the numerous factors that stimulate or suppress prolactin secretion.

3. Sassin JF, et al. Human prolactin: 24 hr pattern with increased release during sleep. *Science* 1972;177:1205.
   Reviews the circadian secretion.

4. Robyn C, et al. *Physiological and pharmacological factors influencing prolactin secretion and their relation to human reproduction.* London: Academic Press, 1977.
   The role of prolactin in reproduction.

5. Kletzky OA, et al. Prolactin synthesis and release during pregnancy and puerperium. *Am J Obstet Gynecol* 1980;136:545.
   This discusses the topic of prolactin production in pregnancy.

6. Noel GL, et al. Prolactin release during nursing and breast stimulation in postpartum and non-postpartum subjects. *J Clin Endocrinol Metab* 1974;38:413.
   This article discusses postpartum prolactin secretion.

7. Okatani Y, et al. Role of melatonin in nocturnal prolactin secretion in women with normoprolactinemia and mild hyperprolactinemia. *Am J Obstet Gynecol* 1993; 168:854.
   Melatonin, a pineal gland secretion, can stimulate prolactin release and may be involved in the nocturnal increase in prolactin secretion noted in normal and mildly hyperprolactinemic women.

Management

8. Brant-Zawadski M, et al. Magnetic resonance imaging of the brain: the optimal screening technique. *Radiology* 1984;152:71.
   This discusses the applications of magnetic resonance imaging to pituitary evaluation.

9. Thorner MO, et al. Rapid regression of pituitary prolactinomas during bromocriptine treatment. *J Clin Endocrinol Metab* 1980;51:438.
   This article discusses bromocriptine therapy for pituitary prolactinomas.

10. Kletzky OA, et al. Effectiveness of vaginal bromocriptine in treating women with hyperprolactinemia. *Fertil Steril* 1989;51:269.
    This article considers the efficacy of vaginally administered bromocriptine in the treatment of hyperprolactinemia.

11. Lengyel AMJ, et al. Long-acting injectable bromocriptine (Parlodel LAR) in the chronic treatment of prolactin-secreting macroadenomas. *Fertil Steril* 1993;59:980.
    Monthly injections were well tolerated and highly effective in the study.

12. Schlechte J, et al. The natural history of untreated hyperprolactinemia: a prospective analysis. *J Clin Endocrinol Metab* 1989;68:412.
    Thirty women were followed an average of 5.2 years. Disease progression is unlikely, and improvement may occur.

13. Serri O, et al. Recurrence of hyperprolactinemia after selective transsphenoidal adenomectomy in women with prolactinoma. *N Engl J Med* 1983;309:280.
    This discusses the recurrence of prolactin-secreting tumors after surgical ablation.

14. Bergh T, et al. Clinical course and outcome of pregnancies in amenorrheic women with hyperprolactinemia and pituitary tumors. *BMJ* 1978;1:875.
    The clinical course of prolactinomas during pregnancy is considered.

15. Scanlon MF, for the Cabergoline Comparative Study Group. A comparison of cabergoline and bromocriptine in the treatment of hyperprolactinemic amenorrhea. *N Engl J Med* 1994;331:904.
    Cabergoline was more effective and better tolerated than bromocriptine; it has a very long intrapituitary half-life.

16. Biller BMK, et al. Treatment of prolactin-secreting macroadenomas with the once-weekly dopamine agonist cabergoline. *J Clin Endocrinol Metab* 1996;81:2338.
    There is limited experience with this treatment in pregnancy.

82. PRECOCIOUS PUBERTY

Harriette Hampton

The development of the capacity for reproduction commences in utero and continues through puberty. During the fetal stage, gonadotropin secretion increases progressively with patterns and levels comparable with the onset and first half of puberty. Gonadal steroidogenesis increases, and episodic release of gonadotropins indicates that negative feedback mechanisms and differentiation of the hypothalamic-pituitary-gonadal (HPG) axis are functional. During the neonatal phase, hormonal secretion is greater than during childhood. For a few weeks, secretion persists at pubertal levels but without overt physical changes. In the childhood phase, downregulation results in hormone levels equivalent to those in hypogonadotropic hypogonadal adults. The low levels of secretion are a function of decreased hypothalamic stimulation, which is under control by the central nervous system (CNS). The final phase of development is puberty, which is marked by a resurgence of gonadotropin and sex steroid secretion. This begins with pulsatile, sleep-coincident, pituitary gonadotropin release. With further maturation, the pattern becomes regularly episodic over the entire 24-hour period.

In girls, normal puberty is accompanied by an acceleration of growth and by breast development (thelarche). Pubic and axillary hair then develop (adrenarche), followed by menses (menarche). True or central precocious puberty indicates gonadotropin-dependent changes following production of gonadotropins with sex hormone elaboration. The normal clinical sequence of pubertal changes is preserved. In peripheral or gonadotropin-independent precocious puberty (precocious pseudopuberty), primary disease of the gonads or adrenals is implicated. Alterations in the normal sequence of pubertal changes may occur. Change consistent with the sex of the individual is called isosexual precocity, while heterosexual precocity indicates the presence of virilization in the female. Those disorders in which development is mild or not progressive, including the entities of precocious thelarche and adrenarche, are sometimes termed incomplete sexual precocity.

Precocious puberty in females has been traditionally defined as the appearance of secondary sexual characteristics before 8 years of age. This definition has been challenged by a large-scale cross-sectional study of pediatric practices in the United States. This study indicated that 27.2% of African-American females and 6.7% of Caucasian females exhibited breast or pubic hair development by 7 years of age. By 8 years of age, 48.3% of African-American girls and 14.7% of Caucasian girls had secondary sexual characteristics. The onset of puberty is frequently later in children suffering from chronic illness or malnutrition. However, contrasexual development requires evaluation regardless of the age of presentation.

In approximately 75% of cases of precocious puberty in females, the cause is idiopathic. A thorough evaluation must be performed, however, to eliminate gonadal, adrenal, or CNS dysfunction. The early development of secondary sexual characteristics may promote psychosocial problems for the child that should be carefully addressed. Typically, these girls are taller than their peers as children due to estrogen stimulation of long bone growth, but become short adults secondary to premature fusion of the long bone epiphyses. Radiologic determination of bone age is an important adjunct in the classification of precocious sexual development.

Various classification systems are proposed for female precocious puberty. For the purposes of our discussion, we will discuss premature thelarche, premature adrenarche, luteinizing hormone–releasing hormone (LHRH)–dependent precocious puberty, and LHRH-independent precocious puberty.

Isolated breast development and premature thelarche usually presents in a female child age 3 years or younger and arrests at Tanner stage III. The purpose of a careful history and physical examination is to identify other features of puberty that would suggest that the diagnosis is not simply premature thelarche. These findings include the presence of pubic or axillary hair, vaginal bleeding, a growth spurt, or acne and body odor. With confirmation of isolated thelarche and normal bone age, careful follow-up at 3–6-month intervals is appropriate until the child's lack of progression confirms the presumptive diagnosis of premature thelarche. Any progression of pubertal events should prompt a more complete evaluation.

Precocious isolated pubic hair development, premature adrenarche, usually results from early maturation of adrenal androgen pathways. Adrenal maturation normally begins at age 4–7 and ends at age 15–20. Isolated pubic hair development can also be associated with late onset 21-hydroxylase deficiency, or rarely 11-hydroxylase deficiency. The diagnosis of premature pubarche due to 21-hydroxylase deficiency will be confirmed by an elevated early morning serum 17-OH progesterone (17-OHP). Dehydroepiandrosterone sulfate (DHEAS) in the early to mid-adrenarchal range (60–200 μg/dl) confirms that adrenarche is in fact in progress. With this finding, it is appropriate to make a presumptive diagnosis of premature adrenarche and to re-evaluate the child carefully every 3–6 months until a typical pattern of premature adrenarche confirms the diagnosis. If plasma DHEAS is either preadrenarchal or above the adult range, further diagnostic studies must be undertaken to exclude adrenal hyperplasia or tumor.

Female isosexual development can be LHRH dependent or LHRH independent. To determine whether or not there has been pubertal activation of LHRH secretion an LHRH stimulation test must be performed. A prepubertal response (no LH release after LHRH) indicates that hypothalamus-pituitary maturation (puberty) has not occurred. A pubertal response, LH elevation, should be followed by evaluation of the pituitary and hypothalamus by computed tomography or magnetic resonance imaging scan. Midline CNS tumors may cause sexual precocity by impinging on the hypothalamus, resulting in gonadotropin-releasing hormone activation. Craniopharyngiomas and hamartomas are the most common CNS tumors to prematurely activate puberty. A negative scan implies idiopathic precocious puberty.

The evaluation of LHRH-independent precocity includes imaging of the adrenals and gonads to rule out neoplasia. Serum levels of 17-OHP and human chorionic gonadotropin (hCG) are required to exclude 21-hydroxylase deficiency (or 11-hydroxylase deficiency) or an hCG-secreting neoplasm. Thyroid function tests are an appropriate adjunct for considerations of primary hypothyroidism.

All forms of LHRH-dependent precocious puberty can be treated effectively with LHRH agonists. Treatment options include deslorelin (4 μg/kg body weight/day, s.c.), or histrelin (10 μg/kg/day, s.c.) or depot leuprolide (0.3 mg/kg q 2 weeks, IM for the first month, then 0.3 mg/kg q 3–4 weeks thereafter).

Precocious puberty resulting from an LHRH-independent mechanism requires treatment tailored to the particular case. Adrenal and gonadal tumors are treated surgically. Congenital adrenal hyperplasia due to 21-hydroxylase deficiency is treated conventionally with glucocorticoid and mineralocorticoid replacement.

The infrequent finding of sexual precocity warrants a thorough history, physical examination, and laboratory studies to distinguish benign from serious, even fatal causes. Appropriate therapy assures suppression of the pituitary-gonadal axis and allows long bone growth to progress at the normal rate.

General
1. Cutler GB Jr. Precocious puberty. In: Hurst JW, et al., eds. *Medicine for the practicing physician,* 3rd ed. Woburn, MA: Butterworth, 1992: 577–581.
   This is a well-written, clinically oriented chapter on the evaluation and treatment of precocious puberty.
2. Styne DM, Grumbach MM. Puberty in the male and female: its physiology and disorders. In: Yen SSC, Jaffe RB, eds. *Reproductive endocrinology: physiology, pathophysiology and clinical management,* 3rd ed. Philadelphia: Saunders, 1991: 511–554.
   This is a comprehensive chapter by leading authorities.

Normal Puberty
3. Tanner JM, ed. *Growth at adolescence,* 2nd ed. Oxford: Blackwell, 1962.
   This article describes the Tanner stage I–V classification of the changes of puberty,

including breasts and pubic hair, such that stage I is the infantile and stage V the adult appearance, with the other stages describing the intermediate morphology.

4. Marshall WA, Tanner JM. Variations in pattern of pubertal changes in girls. *Arch Dis Child* 1969;44:291.

Pubertal sexual development progresses in a predictable way; any deviation from this sequence may indicate abnormal development.

5. Tanner JM, Davies PSW. Clinical longitudinal standards for height and height velocity for North American children. *J Pediatr* 1985;107:317.

The peak height velocity is attained in the majority between ages 11 and 14. The average girl grows 2–3 inches over the 2 years following menarche.

6. Goji K. Pulsatile characteristics of spontaneous growth hormone (GH) concentration profiles in boys evaluated by an ultrasensitive immunoradiometric assay: evidence for ultradian periodicity of GH secretion. *J Clin Endocrinol Metab* 1993;76:667.

Human growth hormone secretion could have an ultradian rhythm with periodicities of 100–120 minutes under physiological conditions.

7. Lee PA. Pubertal neuroendocrine maturation: early differentiation and stages of development. *Adolesc Pediatr Gynecol* 1988;1:3.

The nature of the neuroendocrine mechanism that initiates puberty at the appropriate time is not known.

8. Oerter KE, et al. Gonadotropin secretory dynamics during puberty in normal girls and boys. *J Clin Endocrinol Metab* 1990;71:1390.

This article presents normative data for spontaneous and luteinizing hormone–releasing hormone–stimulated gonadotropin levels during puberty.

Abnormal Pubertal Development

9. Van Winter JT, et al. Natural history of premature thelarche in Olmsted County, Minnesota 1940 to 1984. *J Pediatr* 1990;116:278.

Idiopathic premature thelarche, in the absence of a source of exogenous estrogen, is usually a benign self-limiting disorder, and, in general, no therapy is indicated.

10. Ibanez L, et al. Natural history of premature pubarche: an auxological study. *J Clin Endocrinol Metab* 1992;74:254.

Controversies surround the etiology and diagnostic approach to the child with isolated pubic hair development. Premature adrenarche may be a normal variant of puberty.

11. White PC, New MI, Dupont B. Congenital adrenal hyperplasia. *N Engl J Med* 1987;316:1519.

This is a comprehensive review of this disorder.

12. Foster CM, et al. Absence of pubertal gonadotropin secretion in girls with McCune–Albright syndrome. *J Clin Endocrinol Metab* 1984;58:1161.

Polycystic fibrous dysplasia (McCune–Albright syndrome) may be associated with precocious puberty. The disorder is characterized by long bone cysts and cafe au lait spots.

13. Navarius C, et al. Paraneoplastic precocious puberty. Report of a new case with hepatoblastoma and review of the literature. *Cancer* 1985;56:1725.

Tumors that secrete human chorionic gonadotropin can cause precocious puberty. The hCG stimulates the gonads directly.

14. Cook CD, McArthur JW, Berenberg W. Pseudoprecocious puberty in girls as a result of estrogen ingestion. *N Engl J Med* 1953;248:671.

Estrogen-containing medications, including skin care products and therapeutic estrogen cream for vulvar agglutination can cause premature thelarche.

15. Hochman HI, Judge DM, Reichlin S. Precocious puberty and hypothalamic hamartoma. *Pediatrics* 1981;67:236.

Other central nervous system disorders associated with precocious puberty include Von Recklinghausen's disease (neurofibromatosis), which is characterized by cafe au lait spots and subcutaneous neurofibromas.

16. Sonis WA, et al. Behavior problems and social competence in girls with true precocious puberty. *J Pediatr* 1985;106:156.

This article presents the psychosocial consequences of early physical maturation.

Diagnosis and Treatment

17. Wilkins L, ed. *The diagnosis and treatment of endocrine disorders of childhood and adolescence,* 3rd ed. Springfield, IL: Charles C. Thomas, 1965.
    This article discusses a classic textbook with clinical insight.
18. Pescovitz OH, et al. The NIH experience in precocious puberty: diagnostic sub-groups and the response to short-term LHRH analogue therapy. *J Pediatr* 1986; 108:47.
    This article discusses a large series of patients referred to the National Institutes of Health following the introduction of luteinizing hormone–releasing hormone agonist.
19. Pescovitz OH, et al. Premature thelarche and central precocious puberty: the re-lationship between clinical presentation and the gonadotropin response to LHRH. *J Clin Endocrinol Metab* 1988;67:474.
    This article discusses premature thelarche: diagnosis and mechanisms.
20. Counts ER, Cutler GB Jr. Precocious puberty: pathogenesis and treatment. *Curr Opin Pediatr* 1992;4:674.
    A brief review of the recent literature.
21. Laue L, et al. Treatment of familial male precocious puberty with spironolactone, testolactone, and deslorelin. *J Clin Endocrinol Metab* 1993;76:151.
    Spironolactone is an antiandrogen, testolactone is an aromatase inhibitor that blocks the conversion of androgen to estrogen, and deslorelin is a luteinizing hormone–releasing hormone agonist.

---

83. HIRSUTISM AND VIRILIZATION

Bryan D. Cowan

The masculine distribution of hair in a girl or woman is a cosmetic catastrophe that generates anguish for the patient and her family. Excess growth of pigmented hair on the body surface of a woman where hair growth is ordinarily absent is known as hir-sutism. When clitoral hypertrophy, varying degrees of suppression of cephalic hair, deepening of the voice, increased muscle mass, and amenorrhea are present with hir-sutism, the symptom complex is called *virilism.* Virilism is almost always the accom-paniment of pathologic processes in which androgens are produced to extreme excess in women.

The human hair follicle lies more or less dormant until puberty and becomes fully activated only under the hormonal stimulation of androgenic hormones. In women, androgen production is biglandular, and these hormones are produced in roughly equal amounts by the adrenal glands and ovaries. The most important androgens are testosterone, dihydrotestosterone, androstenedione, dehydroepiandrosterone, and de-hydroepiandrosterone-sulfate (DHEA-s).

Approximately 25% of circulating testosterone in normal women is produced di-rectly by the ovary, an additional 25% of circulating testosterone is produced directly by the adrenal gland, and the remaining 50% is produced by the peripheral conver-sion of testosterone precursors. At target sites for androgen utilization (genital skin and hair follicles), the enzyme 5-alpha-reductase converts testosterone to the potent hormone 5-alpha-dihydrotestosterone (DHT). Both testosterone and DHT interact with androgen receptors to promote androgen-mediated cellular response. However, DHT has much greater affinity for the receptor and, hence, is the most potent of the two predominant androgens.

The clinician will often view every female with excess hair as an endocrine prob-lem. Such a conclusion is essentially correct if the hair follicle is viewed as an end-organ influenced and stimulated by androgens. However, most hirsute females do not manifest any obvious disorder of endocrine homeostasis. Secondary sexual characteristics such as body contour, breast development, muscle mass, and fat deposits are completely normal. Menstrual cycles may be regular and ovulatory, and the ability to bear children may not be impaired at all. Factors that can stimulate excess hair growth in the female who has no pathologic endocrine conditions include increased sensitivity of the pilosebaceous apparatus to androgens, abnormal distribution of circulating androgens (steroid bindings), and certain drugs.

Except for direct effects at the site of production, androgens are transported by plasma to target tissues before they can express a biologic effect. In plasma, almost all of the androgens are bound to one of two proteins: albumin or sex hormone-binding globulin (SHBG). Albumin has a low affinity for testosterone, whereas SHBG has a high affinity for testosterone. Only about 1%–2% of the measurable testosterone in circulation is free, and the remainder is bound to protein. SHBG is synthesized by the liver, and its plasma levels are determined by the balance between estrogens and androgens, thyroid hormone, and liver function. Abnormalities in SHBG function or production can affect the free testosterone concentration in plasma and produce clinical androgen excess without demonstrable biochemical abnormalities in total testosterone concentrations.

Women with abnormal hair growth can be classified into three groups. The first group is composed of women with pathologic androgen excess associated with ovarian and adrenal tumors, congenital adrenal hyperplasia (CAH), or Cushing's syndrome. The second group is represented by nonpathologic androgen excess seen in many variant forms of the polycystic ovarian syndrome (PCOS). Idiopathic or unexplained hirsutism, the last group, is composed of those patients who have no detectable hormonal abnormalities but do express excess hair growth.

The most important task of the physician caring for a patient with hirsutism or virilization, or both, is to disprove the presence of a pathologic condition producing androgen excess. Tumors of the adrenal gland are rare and, if malignant, occur only with an incidence approaching two per 1 million population per year. These neoplasms occur at any age of life, and the average age of diagnosis in one large series was 34 years. Unfortunately, only 10%–25% of adrenal carcinomas exhibit evidence of endocrine function. Of those, approximately two fifths demonstrate virilization; the remainder have signs of Cushing's syndrome. Virilizing ovarian tumors, like adrenal tumors, are uncommon. Although the true incidence and prevalence of virilizing ovarian tumors are unknown, such lesions compromise much less than 1% of all ovarian tumors.

Cushing's syndrome represents a systemic illness associated with a myriad of clinical and metabolic abnormalities and pathologic androgen excess. This syndrome develops from excess adrenal production of glucocorticoids and androgens. Endogenous hypercortisolism results from one of three disorders: (1) adrenocorticotropic hormone (ACTH) excess from hypothalamic or pituitary disease (referred to as Cushing's disease), (2) autonomous hypercortisolism from an adrenal neoplasm (Cushing's syndrome), or (3) ectopic ACTH from tumor (ectopic ACTH syndrome). Specific features of Cushing's syndrome include central obesity, pigmented stria, muscle weakness, hypokalemia, and ecchymosis. Diagnostic tools to determine whether pituitary, adrenal, or ectopic ACTH Cushing's syndrome is present include the overnight 1-mg dexamethasone suppression test (screening), measurements of urinary free cortisol, low- and high-dose dexamethasone suppression tests, and the measurement of plasma ACTH. Approximately 80% of patients with androgen-secreting ovarian tumors have palpable adnexal pathology on bimanual examination. Thus, the pelvic examination is of fundamental importance in the diagnosis of androgen-secreting ovarian tumors. An elevated serum testosterone greater than 2 ng/ml or palpable adnexal mass, or both, will be present in most women with a functional androgen-secreting ovarian tumor. Furthermore, there is a small residual group of patients in whom pelvic sonography will identify ovarian enlargement not detectable by pelvic examination. There are several varieties of histologically definable tumors of the ovaries that secrete androgens. These tumors are usually of stromal cell origin. The most common gonadal stromal tumors are represented by the thecoma and fibrothecoma. These lesions are almost always unilateral and benign. The androblastoma (arrhenoblastoma, gynandroblastoma) is also a gonadal stromal tumor. These tumors are principally benign but can be associated with the Peutz-Jeghers syndrome or mucinous cystadenoma. Sertoli cell tumors in the female do not produce virilization, but the Sertoli-Leydig cell tumor is associated with androgen excess.

In addition to ovarian or adrenal tumor, CAH is a source of pathologic androgen excess. Three inheritable enzymatic defects are recognized, all of which lead to a decrease of cortisol biosynthesis (and hence an increase in pituitary ACTH release). The most common is the 21-hydroxylase deficiency, which is referred to as the "salt-losing form." The next most common defect is the 11β-hydroxylase deficiency and is referred to as the "hypertensive form." The rarest form of all is the 3β-ol dehydrogenase deficiency. The source of androgen excess in each form of CAH is production of excess adrenal androgens driven by excess pituitary ACTH. The diagnosis is confirmed by detecting pathologic elevations of the precursor steroid hormone, which is normally converted by the enzyme in question.

In the course of evaluating affected women, menstrual irregularity should be noted. Of significance is the detection that menstrual irregularities are new in onset. Women with idiopathic hirsutism or PCOS, or both, have the onset of hirsutism and menstrual irregularities associated with menarche. Women who develop pathologic ovarian or adrenal tumors report that the onset of hair growth and menstrual irregularities are new. On physical examination, the location and extent of terminal hair on the face, neck, chest, upper back, upper abdomen, lower abdomen, and perineum should be determined. Clitoral inspection should be performed, and a clitoral index can serve as a good marker for the presence of androgen excess. A pelvic examination should be performed, and blood pressure should be recorded.

Women with clinically significant hirsutism or minimal hirsutism associated with changes in menstrual patterns, infertility, or pelvic masses, and women with infertility and anovulatory cycles should have serum androgen determinations. To properly evaluate patients with clinical signs and symptoms of androgen excess, measurements and interpretation of androgen hormones are essential. The most useful measurements for determining the status of androgen production in women are serum testosterone and DHEA-s. The purpose of the testosterone measurement is to determine the potential of an androgen-producing ovarian tumor. If the testosterone is greater than 2 ng/ml, the likelihood of an ovarian tumor is increased. DHEA-s is a steroid that reflects adrenal androgen production. Greater than 90% of circulating DHEA-s is produced by the adrenal gland, and measurements of this steroid display little diurnal variation. A value of greater than 8,000 ng/ml is highly suggestive of an adrenal neoplasm as the source of androgen excess.

Treatment of a pathologic androgen excess should be directed at correcting the pathologic condition responsible for aberrant hormone production. The treatment of androgen excess owing to PCOS or idiopathic causes is modulated somewhat by the short- and long-term goals of each patient. In general, combined pharmacologic and cosmetic treatments offer the most effective treatments. Pharmacologic options include oral contraception to reduce ovarian androgen production, glucocorticoids to reduce adrenal androgen secretion, and androgen receptor antagonists (spironolactone). In addition, gonadotropin-releasing hormone (GnRH) agonists have demonstrated remarkable efficacy in reducing ovarian androgens. Cosmetic adjuncts include shaving, waxing, depilatories, and electrolysis. Most patients respond well to these treatments but often do not achieve optimal results. New hair growth can be halted, but involution of established hair follicles is a slow process.

Androgen Production and Metabolism
1. Udoff LC, Adashi EY. Polycystic ovarian disease: current insights into an old problem. *J Pediatr Adolesc Gynecol* 1996;9:3.
   New data continue to implicate etiologic alterations in the hypothalamic-pituitary axis, beginning in the perimenarcheal period, as well as derangements in insulin and insulin-like growth factor metabolism. Current observations also support a role for an increase in adrenal androgen production and an increase in adrenal sensitivity to trophic hormone stimulation in the development of polycystic ovarian syndrome.

2. Barth JH. Investigations in the assessment and management of patients with hirsutism. *Curr Opin Obstet Gynecol* 1997;9:187.
Most hirsute women have polycystic ovaries. The few women who have a more sinister cause for their hirsutism can probably be identified by clinical symptoms and signs. Therefore, the purpose of investigation is to identify those women, and this can probably be best achieved by a first-line measurement of serum testosterone. It is probably unnecessary to measure any endocrine parameters once therapy has been initiated, since there is no relationship between these variables and hair growth.

3. Gilchrist VJ, Hecht BR. A practical approach to hirsutism. *Am Fam Physician* 1995;52:1837.
Women often express concern about what they consider to be excess body or facial hair. This surplus of hair may be normal or it may signal hirsutism. Hirsutism may be idiopathic, secondary to increased responsiveness of hair follicles to normal circulating levels of androgens, or it may result from an excess of androgens. The evaluation of hirsutism must include the identification, or exclusion, of androgen-producing tumors.

4. Rittmaster RS. Clinical relevance of testosterone and dihydrotestosterone metabolism in women. *Am J Med* 1995;98:17S.
In many hyperandrogenic women, there is no well-defined hormonal abnormality. Androgen sensitivity is determined, in part, by 5-alpha-reductase activity in the skin. This is a localized phenomenon, and there is no generalized increase in 5-alpha-reductase activity in these women. Dihydrotestosterone can be converted to glucuronide and sulfate conjugates, including androstanediol glucuronide. These androgen conjugates have been proposed to be serum markers of cutaneous androgen metabolism, but recent evidence indicates that they arise from adrenal precursors and are more likely to be markers of adrenal steroid production and metabolism.

Congenital Adrenal Hyperplasia

5. Pang S. Congenital adrenal hyperplasia. *Baillieres Clin Obstet Gynaecol* 1997;11:281.
A clinical spectrum, varying from prenatal onset to postnatal onset of symptoms, exists in all hyperandrogenic forms of congenital adrenal hyperplasia (CAH). Postnatal onset hyperandrogenic symptoms such as premature pubarche, clitoromegaly, hirsutism, menstrual disorders, and infertility are well-known manifestations of CAH due to 21-hydroxylase deficiency, 3 beta-hydroxysteroid dehydrogenase deficiency, or 11 beta-hydroxylase deficiency. These hyperandrogenic symptoms of CAH are clinically indistinguishable from other causes of hyperandrogenism. Specific hormonal criteria define the molecular proof of the disorder. Prevalence of the hyperandrogenic forms of CAH, as well as pubertal maturation and reproductive function in women with hyperandrogenic forms of CAH, are discussed.

6. Gonzalez F. Adrenal involvement in polycystic ovary syndrome. *Semin Reprod Endocrinol* 1997;15:137.
The etiology of hyperandrogenic chronic anovulation is heterogeneous and relatively unknown in the majority of cases. Affected individuals in this latter segment are considered to have polycystic ovarian syndrome (PCOS) of which 50%–60% exhibit androgen excess of adrenal origin. Since pituitary adrenocorticotropic hormone (ACTH) secretion promotes developmental growth and overall steroidogenic efficiency within the adrenal cortex, it is probable that these actions of ACTH along with the adrenal's unique centripetal circulation play a major role in the induction of adrenarche. This latter phenomenon is characterized by alterations in adrenocortical morphology and steroidogenic enzyme activities culminating in increases in adrenal androgens to normal circulating adult levels. Increases in 17,20-lyase activity and adrenal androgen hyperresponsiveness to ACTH in response to physiological ACTH may be promoted by the functional elevation of estrogen of ovarian origin in PCOS. The latest in vitro data suggest that the estro-

gen may elicit its effect on the adrenal cortex through a receptor-mediated mechanism. Therefore, the currently available data indicate that adrenal androgen excess in PCOS is also heterogeneous in etiology.

7. Baskin HG. Screening for late-onset congenital adrenal hyperplasia in hirsutism or amenorrhea. *Arch Intern Med* 1987;147:847.

This article describes the method and utility of the short adrenocorticotropic hormone stimulation test for the assessment of late-onset congenital adrenal hyperplasia.

Polycystic Ovarian Disease

8. Rosenfield RL. Current concepts of polycystic ovary syndrome. *Baillieres Clin Obstet Gynaecol* 1997;11:307.

Polycystic ovarian syndrome (PCOS) may be loosely defined as unexplained hyperandrogenism, with variable degrees of cutaneous symptoms, anovulatory symptoms, and obesity. The vast majority of patients with the full-blown Stein–Leventhal syndrome have functional ovarian hyperandrogenism (FOH). Dysregulation of androgen secretion may affect the ovary alone (isolated FOH), the adrenal alone, or both together. Modest insulin resistance is common in PCOS, and the resultant hyperinsulinemia is a major candidate as the cause of the dysregulation. PCOS should be viewed as an early manifestation of a hyperinsulinemic condition that will predispose to cardiovascular and metabolic complications later in life. A subset of PCOS patients appears to have not only insulin resistance but also beta-cell secretory dysfunction, which may indicate a relationship of the disorder to non–insulin-dependent diabetes mellitus. The fundamental genetic defects remain to be elucidated.

9. Goudas VT, Dumesic DA. Polycystic ovary syndrome. *Endocrinol Metab Clin North Am* 1997;26:893.

The cardinal clinical features of polycystic ovarian syndrome are hirsutism and menstrual irregularity from anovulation. Obesity occurs in approximately 50% of hyperandrogenic anovulatory women, some of whom also have non-insulin-dependent diabetes mellitus (NIDDM). Under-lying these clinical findings are several biochemical abnormalities, including LH hypersecretion, hyperandrogenism, acyclic estrogen production, decreased SHBG capacity, and hyperinsulinemia, all of which contribute to increased ovarian production of androgens, particularly testosterone. A careful history and physical examination guide the extent of diagnostic testing. The ultimate goals of therapy for hyperandrogenic anovulatory women are to normalize the endometrium, antagonize androgen action at target tissues, reduce insulin resistance, and correct anovulation, if necessary.

10. Grasinger CC, Wild RA, Parker IJ. Vulvar acanthosis nigricans: a marker for insulin resistance in hirsute women. *Fertil Steril* 1993;59:583.

Association between hyperandrogenism, insulin resistance, and acanthosis nigricans (thickened pigmented skin lesion) was first described as the "HAIR-AN" syndrome.

Treatment

11. Barnes RB. Diagnosis and therapy of hyperandrogenism. *Baillieres Clin Obstet Gynaecol* 1997;11:369.

Endometrial hyperplasia can be prevented in hyperandrogenic, anovulatory women by the oral contraceptive pill or progestins. Hirsutism is best treated by a combination of the oral contraceptive pill and an anti-androgen. The first line of therapy for ovulation induction is clomiphene citrate, with human menopausal gonadotropins or laparoscopic ovulation induction reserved for clomiphene failures. hMG together with gonadotropin-releasing hormone agonist may decrease the risk of spontaneous abortion following ovulation induction in polycystic ovarian syndrome (PCOS). Weight loss should be vigorously encouraged to ameliorate the metabolic consequences of PCOS.

12. Pucci E, Petraglia F. Treatment of androgen excess in females: yesterday, today and tomorrow. *Gynecol Endocrinol* 1997;11:411.

Hirsutism, acne, and androgenic alopecia represent, in females, some of the manifestations of the clinical spectrum of hyperandrogenism. Several pharmacologic *agents have recently shown the ability to block the androgen receptors at target organ sites, thus allowing a specific antiandrogenic treatment. In some cases, cosmetic measures could be of great value. Obesity accompanied by hyperinsulinemia can represent the main cause of ovary androgen hypersecretion; therefore a reduced body weight and muscle activity represent the basis of any treatment. Some other drugs, such as long-acting analogs of somatostatin, could be considered among possible drugs for the future.*

13. Richards RN, Meharg GE. Electrolysis: observations from 13 years and 140,000 hours of experience. *J Am Acad Dermatol* 1995;33:662.
    Electrolysis has been performed since 1875. Electrolysis satisfactorily removes hair from women with static hair growth, but women with hirsutism often require concomitant management of their hormonal problems. Scarring does not occur with properly performed electrolysis. Hair is not an electrical conductor, and electronic tweezers do not result in permanent hair removal. Shaving 1–5 days before electrolysis greatly increases efficacy because it ensures that only growing anagen hairs are epilated.

Androgen Excess Disorders in Childhood

14. Rittmaster RS, Thompson DL. Effect of leuprolide and dexamethasone on hair growth and hormone levels in hirsute women: the relative importance of the ovary and the adrenal in the pathogenesis of hirsutism. *J Clin Endocrinol Metab* 1990;70:1096.
    The ovary is the major source of androgens in polycystic ovarian syndrome.

15. Emans SJ, et al. Treatment with dexamethasone of androgen excess in adolescent patients. *J Pediatr* 1988;112:821.
    Free testosterone levels reflect efficacy of therapy.

---

84. DYSFUNCTIONAL UTERINE BLEEDING

Bryan D. Cowan

Cyclic menstruation is the culmination of programmed hormonal stimulation on the endometrium. This orchestrated event is referred to as the ovarian-menstrual cycle. In the course of a normal ovulatory cycle, follicle-stimulating hormone (FSH) stimulates an ovarian follicle to maturation. The responding ovarian follicle secretes increasing quantities of estradiol-17B (E_2) during the proliferative phase of the menstrual cycle. When the plasma concentration of E_2 reaches the threshold level necessary to induce a luteinizing hormone (LH) surge, ovulation follows and the follicle is transformed to a corpus luteum.

In response to increasing ovarian E_2 secretion, the endometrial epithelium proliferates, the stroma thickens and becomes compact, and the endometrial glands increase in number and length. If estrogen secretion were to continue unopposed by the action of progesterone, the endometrium would proliferate until eventually it would outgrow its blood supply and slough away from the myometrium. In the normal ovulatory cycle, however, ovulation is followed by the formation of a corpus luteum at the site of the ovarian follicle, and the corpus luteum begins secreting progesterone. Progesterone acts on the endometrium to suppress the mitogenic action of E_2 and converts the proliferative endometrium into secretory endometrium. The straight, narrow endometrial glands become tortuous and dilated, and the endometrial stroma is transformed to decidua. If fertilization of the ovum and implantation of the embryo do not occur, the corpus luteum fails approximately 12 days after it is formed. With corpus luteum regression, E_2 and progesterone production fall, hormonal stimulation of the endometrium is withdrawn, and menstruation begins. After hormone withdrawal from the endometrium at the end of corpus luteum function, the concentration of prostaglandins (PGE_2 and PGF_2) increase. The prostaglandins induce spiral arteriolar vasomotor responses, which induce epithelial ischemia with subsequent necrosis and shedding. The ovarian-menstrual cycle is repeated 10 to 13 times a year in nonpregnant, sexually mature women. The repetitive nature of the cycle depends on changes in the two main pituitary gonadotropins, FSH and LH, and the two ovarian steroid hormones, E_2 and progesterone. If any one of these four hormones becomes tonically elevated or suppressed, anovulation results. Uterine bleeding that is acyclic and associated with anovulation is termed dysfunctional uterine bleeding (DUB). Such endometrial sloughing can be focal, resulting in frequent episodes of vaginal spotting, or the endometrial sloughing can be extensive, resulting in frank menorrhagia. DUB should respond to appropriate steroid hormone therapy, which either corrects the hormonal aberration of the menstrual cycle or directly affects the endometrium.

Times or conditions in which anovulation can lead to DUB are (1) puberty, (2) climacteric, (3) polycystic ovarian disease (PCOD), and (4) obesity. At the time of puberty, the cyclic hormonal interactions are not fully established. Estradiol secretion is continuous, and irregular uterine bleeding occurs. In the climacteric, FSH and LH become tonically elevated, E_2 secretion becomes tonically low, ovulation fails, and irregular uterine bleeding occurs. In PCOD, LH and estrone are tonically elevated, the endometrium is chronically stimulated by estrogens, ovulation fails, and the endometrium sloughs at irregular intervals. In association with obesity, estrone and LH are tonically elevated, the endometrium is chronically stimulated by estrogens as in PCOD, and irregular uterine bleeding results.

In each of these conditions, the endometrium is stimulated by estrogens without the suppressive action of progesterone and without the withdrawal of progesterone that initiates cyclic bleeding. Thus, the usual treatment of DUB should be directed at the endometrium to suppress the action of unopposed estrogens.

Before therapy for DUB can be undertaken, organic disease of the uterus, cervix, or endometrium must be ruled out. In the adolescent girl, it would be unusual to find an organic disease of the reproductive tract, but hematologic diatheses are not unusual in this age group. In the sexually mature woman, chronic estrogen stimulation of the endometrium is often associated with endometrial polyps and endometrial hyperplasia. Endometrial sampling (biopsy, curettage) or visualization (hysteroscopy) should be considered as part of the diagnostic evaluation for these women. Pelvic examination or sonography may disclose uterine tumors (fibroids), another cause of pathologic uterine bleeding.

After an evaluation has excluded organic causes for irregular uterine bleeding, a regimen of medical therapy directed at suppressing chronic estrogen stimulation and restoring cyclic interactions between the pituitary gland and ovaries is begun. Medroxyprogesterone acctate (MPA), 10 mg daily for 5 to 10 days, is usually administered. MPA is an orally active synthetic progestin and, like progesterone, will transform proliferative endometrium into secretory endometrium. When the MPA is discontinued, withdrawal uterine bleeding will follow 2–14 days later. Women treated with MPA should be forewarned of the withdrawal bleeding; otherwise, they may think that the treatment has been a failure. After the dysfunctional uterine bleeding has been controlled by MPA therapy, the physician should develop a long-term therapeutic plan.

Adolescent girls can usually be reassured that the problem is self-limiting and will remit spontaneously when ovulatory cycles are established. Likewise, perimenopausal women can be reassured that irregular bleeding will subside with menopause (although other hormonal management may be required). Obese women of all ages should be encouraged to reduce their body weight to near ideal size. Spontaneous resumption of ovulatory cycles often follows weight reduction. PCOD, especially in nonobese women, tends to be chronic and requires long-term medical management in accordance with the patients' treatment goals. If control of irregular bleeding is the desired therapeutic goal, chronic ovarian suppression with an oral contraceptive agent will control most cases of bleeding. If fertility is the desired goal, ovulation induction with clomiphene citrate is indicated. Finally, endometrial ablation or hysterectomy may be performed to stop the bleeding in women who have completed child bearing.

Occasionally, young and mature women develop severe bleeding and anemia from dysfunctional anovulatory bleeding. This medical emergency usually requires hospitalization for treatment of the bleeding and anemia. High-dose estrogen treatment is usually efficacious as the first treatment before progestins. We recommend 25-mg conjugated equine estrogens (Premarin) intravenously every 4 hours for three doses or until the bleeding stops. Once the bleeding is stopped, progestin therapy must be initiated to mature and then slough the endometrium.

Management of chronic unopposed estrogen stimulation of the endometrium, such as that seen in PCOD or obesity, may require intermittent progestin therapy for years. We utilize 5–10 mg of MPA in cycle days 16–25 during each or every other month, or oral contraceptives. In addition, the use of a menstrual calendar greatly facilitates patient compliance with therapy and interpretation of clinical responses.

Normal Menstrual Cycle
1. Speroff L. Regulation of the menstrual cycle. In: Speroff L, Glass RH, Kase NG, eds. *Clinical gynecologic endocrinology and infertility*, 4th ed. Baltimore: Williams & Wilkins, 1989: 91–119.
   This is a comprehensive, clear presentation of the endocrine events of the normal menstrual cycle.
2. Sherman BW, Korenman SG. Hormonal characteristics of the human menstrual cycles throughout reproductive life. *J Clin Invest* 1975;55:699.
   This is a longitudinal study of the dynamics of gonadotropin and sex-steroid hormones during the reproductive years.
3. Noyes RW, Hertig AT, Rock J. Dating the endometrial biopsy. *Fertil Steril* 1950;1:3.
   This is the classic description of the dynamic events in endometrial maturation.

Adolescent Bleeding
4. Gidwani GP. Vaginal bleeding in adolescents. *J Reprod Med* 1984;29:417.
   Careful elimination of organic causes is necessary before the diagnosis of dysfunctional uterine bleeding in adolescents can be made.
5. Deligeoroglou E. Dysfunctional uterine bleeding. *Ann NY Acad Sci* 1997;816:158.
   Dysfunctional uterine bleeding (DUB) is a frequent gynecological problem during adolescence and the most frequent cause of urgent admission to the hospital over this period of life. The initial step in the evaluation of DUB includes a detailed clinical history, followed by a complete physical examination. Laboratory tests should include a coagulation profile, a complete blood count with platelet evaluation, and sometimes a serum pregnancy test. Surgical treatment, such as dilatation and curettage, is rarely indicated in the adolescent patient.

Management of Dysfunctional Uterine Bleeding
6. Kramer MG, Reiter RC. Hysterectomy: indications, alternatives and predictors. *Am Fam Physician* 1997;55:827.
   Hysterectomy, the most common major nonobstetric operation, is performed in more than 570,000 women in the United States each year. The main indications for hysterectomy include the following conditions: uterine leiomyomas, dysfunctional uterine bleeding, endometriosis / adenomyosis, chronic pelvic pain, and genital prolapse. Current literature, however, routinely recommends conservative management of most nonmalignant gynecologic conditions, with hysterectomy reserved for refractory cases.
7. Chuong CJ, Brenner PF. Management of abnormal uterine bleeding. *Am J Obstet Gynecol* 1996;175:787.
   Patients treated for dysfunctional uterine bleeding are separated into two groups: those with acute bleeding episodes and those with chronic repetitive bleeding problems. An acute bleeding episode is best controlled with the use of high-dose estrogen. The management of chronic anovulatory dysfunctional uterine bleeding is determined by the needs of the patient. The long-term therapy is directed at the

reduction in menstrual blood loss. For these patients prolonged progestin use, oral contraceptives, nonsteroidal antiinflammatory drugs, antifibrinolytic agents, danazol, and gonadotropin-releasing hormone agonists are part of the therapeutic armamentarium. For patients who no longer desire future fertility, hysterectomy may be considered. Patients with von Willebrand's disease and excessive menstrual blood loss may be misdiagnosed as having dysfunctional uterine bleeding. There are improved diagnostic tests to identify this disorder and, most important, there is a high-concentration desmopressin acetate nasal spray available as treatment.

8. Cowan BD, Morrison JC. Management of abnormal genital bleeding in girls and women. *N Engl J Med* 1991;324:1710.
   This is a review of the etiology and management of dysfunctional uterine bleeding (DUB) in both adolescents and women. Specific algorithms for the evaluation and treatment of DUB are presented in detail.
9. Zimmermann R. Dysfunctional uterine bleeding. *Obstet Gynecol Clin North Am* 1988;15:107.
   The judicious use of hysteroscopy to evaluate dysfunctional uterine bleeding adds a new dimension in handling this often perplexing problem.
10. DeVore GR, Owens O, Kase N. Use of intravenous Premarin in the treatment of dysfunctional uterine bleeding—a double-blind randomized control study. *Obstet Gynecol* 1982;59:285.
    Bleeding stopped in 72 percent of women who received intravenous Premarin compared to 38 percent who received a placebo.

---

85. PREMENSTRUAL SYNDROME

Michel E. Rivlin

Categorizing the physical and psychological complaints linked to the menstrual cycle is controversial. Molimina, the non-distressing but perceived changes occurring before menses, is identical to premenstrual syndrome (PMS) in terms of the kind of symptoms and timing but differs in intensity. It is estimated that up to 75% of all women experience some PMS-like symptoms but only 3%–8% of cycling women can be diagnosed with PMS. Only 40%–50% with the self-diagnosis meet the usual medical criteria.

PMS is included as a provisional diagnosis in the Diagnostic and Statistical Manual of Mental Disorders (DSM-IV), in which it is termed premenstrual dysphoric disorder (PMDD), replacing the older term, late luteal phase dysphoric disorder. For the diagnosis of PMDD, five of 11 listed symptoms must be severe premenstrually with postmenstrual remission. The five symptoms must include at least one dysphoric symptom (irritability, mood swings, anxiety, or depression), and multiple physical symptoms are counted as one symptom. The physical symptoms include mastalgia, headaches, bloating, weight gain, and joint or muscle pains. The disturbances must markedly interfere with work or usual social activities and relationships and must not be an exacerbation of the symptoms of another disorder (e.g., panic disorder, depression, personality disorder).

PMS symptoms are highly variable, and more than 150 have been reported. The most common are the typical psychologic symptoms of irritability, aggression, depression, tension, anxiety, poor coordination, and clumsiness. There are also the typical somatic or physical symptoms, including bloating, distention, feeling of weight gain, edema, breast swelling, headache, and others.

The cause, or causes, of PMS are unknown. Hypoglycemia has been thought to be a possible cause of the headaches, fainting, and food cravings typical of the syndrome.

Although this has not been proved, dietary changes that are recommended include a low intake of refined sugar and salt, meals eaten in six small portions throughout the day, and the avoidance of methylxanthine-containing substances such as coffee, tea, or chocolate. Substance abuse is not uncommon and, if present, requires therapy. Alcohol consumption frequently increases in the premenstruum, and this tendency should be discouraged. Fluid retention is a favorite hypothesis for explaining many of the symptoms, such as weight gain and bloating. The luteal-phase increase in the aldosterone level provides a rationale for diuretic therapy with spironolactone (an aldosterone antagonist diuretic). However, studies have not demonstrated the existence of either premenstrual water retention or weight gain.

For many years, PMS was postulated to be the result of an impaired corpus luteal function, and therapy with synthetic or natural progesterone has been widely used, but has not yielded results better than those observed for placebo therapy. In fact, when patients and controls have been compared, no differences in the levels or patterns of secretion of progesterone, estradiol, gonadotropins, androgens, prolactin, or cortisol have been observed for the various phases of the menstrual cycle, suggesting that PMS represents an abnormal response to normal endocrine levels. Another etiologic hypothesis proposes a role for endorphins, the endogenous opioids. Because endorphin levels peak during the luteal phase and decline with menses, it has been suggested that PMS is a consequence of endogenous narcotic withdrawal.

Cyclic PMS symptoms may resemble a bipolar affective disorder. Excessive norepinephrine activity, such as is thought to occur in manic states, is diminished by the use of clonidine. Opiate withdrawal results in norepinephrine release, which then produces withdrawal symptoms. Clonidine has therefore been used with success in treating manic states, opiate withdrawal, and PMS. By contrast, lithium has not proved useful in the management of PMS. Some PMS symptoms are associated with prostaglandin-induced dysmenorrhea. Treatment with an inhibitor of prostaglandin synthesis may therefore ameliorate the associated symptoms as well as the cramps. Prolactin levels are higher in the luteal phase than the follicular phase; however, although bromocriptine can relieve the mastalgia, other symptoms are not alleviated. Because PMS is characteristically associated with mood, cognitive, and behavioral disturbances, a special relationship with psychiatric disorders has been postulated. About 80% of the patients who complain of PMS, but who do not have PMS, suffer depression; about 40% of the patients investigated for PMS have had some affective disorder. Menstrual cycle-related events may modulate or exacerbate a preexisting psychopathologic condition, and the often complex interweaving of a neurotic disorder and PMS makes it difficult to determine which came first in individual cases.

Dysfunction of serotoninergic transmission may be involved in the pathogenesis of several neuropsychiatric disorders, including anxiety and depression. Central serotonin systems also regulate many functions, such as appetite. It is therefore possible that derangements in serotonin activity may be important in the pathophysiology of PMS, as there is a relationship between ovarian steroids and serotoninergic function. Pharmacologic agents that influence serotonin activity have therefore been used for the treatment of PMS and have yielded good results. These agents include clomipramine, buspirone, d-fenfluramine, and fluoxetine. Although the improvement obtained is maximal with regard to behavioral symptoms, somatic problems are also frequently relieved.

The premenstrual syndromes are associated with cyclic ovarian activity and do not occur before puberty, during pregnancy, or after menopause. Menstruation itself is incidental, as the cyclic symptoms continue after hysterectomy if ovarian function has been preserved. The corollary of considering cyclic ovarian activity as fundamental in the etiology of PMS is that the suppression of ovulation should therefore abolish the PMS symptoms. Anovulation may be achieved pharmaceutically through the use of estrogen-progestin combinations, gonadotropin agonists, or danazol, or by surgical means (oophorectomy). In practice, however, the outcome of therapy is by no means predictable, and, in the instance of oral contraceptive agents, although some women may experience improvement, the condition in many may deteriorate or PMS symptoms may even be precipitated by the medication. In the rare patient undergoing oophorectomy, hysterectomy should also be performed, as estrogen replacement is usually well tolerated, but symptoms may recur if a progestin is added.

The first step in diagnosis is to recognize that the woman has a genuine disorder related to biologic events. She is not imagining her symptoms. The next step is to rule out other physical causes. This requires a full physical and gynecologic examination, including a Papanicolaou smear, complete blood count, chemistry screen, fasting blood glucose determination, and thyroid studies. The importance of a thorough evaluation is obvious when considering the common physical complaints: fatigue, headaches, bowel problems, and abdominal bloating. Numerous previously undetected diseases may be diagnosed in this way. A psychiatric diagnostic interview is also required if an emotional illness is suspected that may be exacerbated premenstrually. It is important to document that the symptoms are related to the menstrual cycle, rather than to other factors such as family or work stress. This is done by having the patient keep a daily diary of her symptoms for at least three cycles. Several PMS charts and calendars are available for this purpose. If records show that a marked increase in symptoms takes place premenstrually for two consecutive cycles, then a diagnosis of PMDD is made at the end of 3 months' charting. For formal psychologic testing, the Minnesota Multiphasic Personality Inventory (MMPI) is ideal because of its ability to detect attempts by a patient to make herself appear emotionally healthier or more disturbed than she actually is. The MMPI is administered to the patient in both the follicular and luteal phases, and the results are compared as an aid to diagnosis and therapy.

The serotonin reuptake inhibitors are becoming the first line of therapy for PMS because they are effective, well tolerated, and free of major side effects. Other antidepressants, anxiolytics, and gonadotropin-releasing hormone agonists have also proven useful for PMS. General measures, including exercise, increasing control of one's life, a healthy diet, avoidance of caffeine, and vitamin supplementation, have not proven effective for PMS, but they should be promoted for their obvious general health benefits. A trial of medication for two or three cycles should be followed by other therapies if relief is not sufficient.

Both the physician and the patient should be aware of the placebo effect. PMS shows a strong response to placebo, often quoted as 50%–60%, but rates as high as 94% have been reported. The duration of the placebo response varies, but the patient is generally back to a pretreatment intensity of symptoms by 6 months. The psychosocial and subjective components of medical care make the placebo process a legitimate part of every patient-physician interaction. It is likely that successful therapy of PMS, regardless of the agent or method used, depends to a significant degree on the placebo process.

Reviews
1. Parry BL. Psychobiology of premenstrual dysphoric disorder. *Semin Reprod Endocrinol* 1997;15:55.
   There are three key elements of the diagnosis: (1) a symptom complex consistent with the diagnosis, (2) a luteal-phase pattern, and (3) severity sufficient to disrupt the woman's life.
2. Freeman EW. Premenstrual syndrome: current perspectives on treatment and etiology. *Curr Opin Obstet Gynecol* 1997;9:147.
   Premenstrual syndrome symptoms include mood (irritability, depression, mood swings, and hostility), somatic complaints (mastalgia, bloating, headache, fatigue, insomnia, appetite changes, and hot flashes), cognitive problems (confusion and poor concentration), and behavioral symptoms (hyperphagia, social withdrawal, and arguing).
3. Steiner M. Premenstrual syndromes. *Annu Rev Med* 1997;48:447.
   The true etiology probably involves complex interactions of ovarian hormones with neurotransmitter, neuroendocrine, and circadian systems that influence mood and behavior.

Pathophysiology
4. Hurt SW, et al. Late luteal phase dysphoric disorder in 670 women evaluated for premenstrual complaints. *Am J Psychiatry* 1992;149:525.

Premenstrual dysphoric disorder is not the extreme manifestation of a physiologic gradient of severity in the population but is a discrete disorder affecting a small subgroup, with an actual prevalence of about 3%–5%.

5. Rabin DS, et al. Hypothalamic-pituitary-adrenal function in patients with premenstrual syndrome. *J Clin Endocrinol Metab* 1990;71:1158.

The authors attempt to explain the regular cycles seen in premenstrual syndrome patients with the irregular cycles associated with depression, anorexia nervosa, and chronic strenuous exercise.

6. Backstrom T. Neuroendocrinology of premenstrual syndrome. *Clin Obstet Gynecol* 1992;35:612.

Several areas within the brain are affected by ovarian steroids. Some of the effects might be mediated via the gamma butyric acid receptor and others via the genome; other mechanisms are also possible.

7. Su TP, et al. Effect of menstrual cycle phase on neuroendocrine and behavioral responses to the serotonin agonist m-chlorophenylpiperazine in women with premenstrual syndrome and controls. *J Clin Endocrinol Metab* 1997;82:1220.

Many studies have identified a deficiency in the whole-blood serotonin, cerebrospinal fluid serotonin metabolite, and brain serotonin contents, as well as in the platelet uptake of serotonin, in various abnormal behavioral states in which the salient characteristics are depression, anxiety, and aggression.

8. Parry BL, et al. Plasma melatonin circadian rhythms during the menstrual cycle and after light therapy in premenstrual dysphoric disorder and normal control subjects. *J Biol Rhythms* 1997;12:47.

Serotonin and melatonin metabolism are depressed in premenstrual dysphoric disorder compared with healthy control subjects.

9. Hammarback S, Ekholm UB, Backstrom T. Spontaneous anovulation causing disappearance of cyclical symptoms in women with the premenstrual syndrome. *Acta Endocrinol (Copenh)* 1991;125:132.

This article describes significant worsening of symptoms during ovulatory cycles and disappearance of symptoms in anovulatory cycles. The authors suggest that premenstrual syndrome is related to corpus luteum factors.

10. Osborn MF, Gath DH. Psychological and physical determinants of premenstrual symptoms before and after hysterectomy. *Psychol Med* 1990;20:565.

Premenstrual syndrome symptoms were reduced after hysterectomy even though ovarian function continued normally, suggesting a major role for psychologic factors in many patients.

11. Yonkers KA. Anxiety symptoms and anxiety disorders: how are they related to premenstrual disorders? *J Clin Psychiatry* 1997;58:62.

This article describes challenge studies that evoke panic in patients with panic disorder and elicit the same response in women with premenstrual dysphoric disorder (PMDD). Therapy for anxiety is also useful in PMDD.

12. Ader DN, Browne MW. Prevalence and impact of cyclic mastalgia in a United States clinic-based sample. *Am J Obstet Gynecol* 1997;177:126.

Breast pain or tenderness is better established than is mood disorder as a premenstrual symptom. Reported prevalences in the general population range from 41% to 69%.

13. Sugawara M, et al. Premenstrual mood changes and maternal mental health in pregnancy and the postpartum period. *J Clin Psychol* 1997;53:225.

A history of premenstrual symptomatology correlated with unstable mental health throughout the perinatal period.

Management

14. Allen SS, McBride CM, Pirie PL. The shortened premenstrual assessment form. *J Reprod Med* 1991;36:769.

The MOOS Menstrual Distress Questionnaire and the premenstrual assessment form are widely used for assessing premenstrual distress. They are long and require extensive time to complete.

15. Yonkers KA. Treatment of premenstrual dysphoric disorder. *Curr Rev Mood Anxiety Disord* 1997;1:215.

Well-designed placebo-controlled trials using either progesterone or oral contraceptives suggest that these interventions are no more effective than placebo.

16. Prior JC, et al. Conditioning exercise decreases premenstrual symptoms: a prospective, controlled 6-month trial. *Fertil Steril* 1987;47:402.
Moliminal symptoms were found to decrease in association with increasing exercise, without the development of anovulatory cycles, loss of body weight, or measured decreases in gonadal steroid levels.

17. Kurzer MS. Women, food, and mood. *Nutr Rev* 1997;55:268.
Caffeine consumption has been associated with an increased prevalence and severity of premenstrual symptoms.

18. Burnet RB, et al. Premenstrual syndrome and spironolactone. *Aust NZ J Obstet Gynaecol* 1991;31;366.
In those patients who did respond to spironolactone treatment, there was a significant difference in the androgen levels from the follicular to the luteal phase of the cycle versus those before treatment was initiated.

19. Chuong CJ, et al. Clinical trial of naltrexone in premenstrual syndrome. *Obstet Gynecol* 1988;72:332.
An oral opioid agonist (naltrexone), given before the periovulatory beta-endorphin peak and before withdrawal to maintain a constant level of beta-endorphin, proved helpful in the patients in this study.

20. Freeman EW, Sondheimer SJ, Rickels K. Gonadotropin-releasing hormone agonist in the treatment of premenstrual symptoms with and without ongoing dysphoria: a controlled study. *Psychopharmacol Bull* 1997;33:303.
This therapy improved luteal phase symptomatology but did not improve the premenstrual exacerbation group, suggesting that premenstrual syndrome depression may have mechanisms different from those of other dysphoric mood disorders.

21. Berger CP, Presser B. Alprazolam in the treatment of two subsamples of patients with late luteal phase dysphoric disorder: a double-blind, placebo-controlled crossover study. *Obstet Gynecol* 1994;84:379.
Most, but not all, trials using the benzodiazepine alprazolam have been successful. Unfortunately, concerns about the dependence potential and the sedating adverse effects of alprazolam limit its applications.

22. Yonkers KA, et al. Symptomatic improvement of premenstrual dysphoric disorder with sertraline treatment: a randomized controlled trial. *JAMA* 1997; 278:983.
Antidepressant drugs that block serotonin reuptake can be effective. Such treatment can improve psychosocial functioning as well as symptoms.

23. Kornstein SG, Parker AJ. Menstrual migraines: etiology, treatment, and relationship to premenstrual syndrome. *Curr Opin Obstet Gynecol* 1997;9:154.
Hormonal changes, including those associated with the menstrual cycle or oral contraceptives, may exacerbate migraine headaches.

---

86. MENOPAUSE

Cecil A. Long

Menopause is defined as the cessation of menstruation due to failure of ovarian follicular development in a woman who had previously had regular menstrual cycles. The average age at menopause in the United States is approximately 51 years, with a range between ages 45 and 55 years. If a woman ceases menstruating before the age of 40, the condition is labeled premature ovarian failure. If this occurs before the age of 30, such patients should undergo karyotyping. The presence of mosaicism with a Y chromosome indicates a need for gonadectomy to prevent the malignant change of testicular components within the gonads. The chance of malignant tumor transformation approximates 25%. Because of the association of premature ovarian failure with autoimmune disorders, evaluation for thyroid and adrenal function as well as selective laboratory tests for autoimmune disease are indicated.

During embryologic and fetal development, germ cells migrate from the yolk sac to the genital ridge. By 20 weeks' gestation, 6 to 7 million oogonia are present. From this point on, there is a rapid depletion of oogonia by atresia, leaving approximately 1 to 2 million follicles at the time of birth. By puberty, the number of follicles has reduced to approximately 400,000. By the age of 50 years, the store of oogonia approaches exhaustion.

Symptomatic features of menopause include hot flushes, night sweats, insomnia, and hypoestrogenic changes of the urogenital tract. Hot flushes occur in 50% to 75% of the women who reach the age of menopause. The hot flush is characterized by a sensation of intense warmth, especially of the upper body, usually following a prodrome. Episodes can last from 30 seconds to 5 minutes, and rarely even longer. The vasomotor flush is due to an abrupt withdrawal from estrogen. The hot flush coincides with the luteinizing hormone (LH) surge. The most valuable laboratory value to determine whether menopause is taking place is an elevated follicule-stimulating hormone level (>40 mIU/ml).

The long-term effects of estrogen deprivation in a postmenopausal woman include osteoporosis and an increased risk of cardiovascular disease. To counteract these events, estrogen replacement therapy is usually recommended in postmenopausal women in whom there is no absolute contraindication.

In the United States, approximately 1.5 million fractures (primarily spinal and hip fractures) occur annually as a result of osteoporosis. This translates into approximately 8 to 10 billion dollars spent annually for the health-care costs related to osteoporosis. Menopausal women experience bone loss at a rate of up to 2.5% per year after menopause. Black women have greater bone density; thus, osteoporosis does not develop as rapidly in them as it does in white women. Measurement of the bone mineral density (BMD) at various body sites (spine, hip, and forearm) help to predict the risk of fractures. Dual-energy x-ray absorptiometry (DEXA) has a high degree of accuracy and has gained widespread acceptance as a screening tool.

The minimum daily dosage of estrogen needed to prevent osteoporosis is 0.625 mg of conjugated estrogen or 1 mg of micronized estradiol. Calcium replacement (1,000–1,500 mg of calcium per day) and vitamin D supplement (up to 400 IU/day) are also indicated. The combination of estrogen and calcium reduces bone resorption and stimulates osteoblastic activity in the bone. Synthetic calcitonin can be administered as a nasal spray and also has been used for the treatment of osteoporosis. Its mechanism of action is primarily a reduction of bone resorption. However, tolerance to calcitonin develops in 25% to 50% of patients. This, combined with the cost of calcitonin, limits its widespread use for the treatment of osteoporosis. Bisphosphonates (Alendronate) are also antiresorptives. As an alternative to estrogen replacement therapy, bisphosphonates have similar effectiveness in reducing bone fractures.

Estrogen also has been found to protect against cardiovascular disease. The results of studies have indicated that doses as low as 0.625 mg of conjugated estrogen daily significantly lower low-density lipoprotein levels and increase high-density lipoprotein levels. Epidemiologic studies have demonstrated that estrogen use decreases the relative risk of ischemic heart disease by approximately 50%.

Estrogen for replacement therapy is available in several forms, and several regimens have been developed for administration. The dose and form of estrogen depend on the reason for estrogen replacement, as well as the age at which estrogen replacement is required. Younger women who need estrogen replacement because of surgical castration or premature ovarian failure need much higher doses than women who reach menopause. These groups of younger patients need up to 2.5 mg of conjugated estrogen or 2 to 3 mg of micronized estrogen per day in order to achieve symptomatic relief of the hypoestrogenic effects. In the menopausal patient, a daily estrogen dose of 0.625 mg of conjugated estrogen or 1 to 2 mg of micronized estrogen (estradiol) confers both bone and cardiovascular protection. The doses must be titrated in order to completely resolve other symptoms of menopause, including hot flushes and insomnia, and to counteract atrophy of the urogenital tract. In women who have a uterus, it is important to add progestin to the estrogen replacement regimen to counteract the effects of unopposed estrogen on the endometrium, because endometrial hyperplasia and, ultimately, adenocarcinoma may ensue in the patient who receives estrogen only. Medroxyprogesterone acetate (10 mg), taken for 7 days, reduces these changes to approximately 3%. Treatment with progestin for 10 to 13 days reduces the incidence to essentially zero. The regimen most widely recommended for menopausal women consists of 25 days of estrogen therapy combined with 10 days of progestin therapy. Some dosages used consist of daily estrogen therapy, with 10 days of progestin starting on the first of each month. Other researchers advocate continuous progestin therapy (2.5–5.0 mg/day) throughout the entire cycle. Parenteral forms of replacement include transdermal estrogen therapy as well as transvaginal delivery, and both provide protection against osteoporosis and vascular disease.

Adverse effects of estrogen replacement therapy include gallbladder disease, thromboembolic disease, and a potential increased risk of breast cancer. Estrogen replacement has been found to double the incidence of gallbladder disease. Estrogen therapy is also associated with thromboembolic changes that exhibit a dose-response relationship. However, several studies have shown that there is no increase in incidence of thrombosis with minimal daily estrogen doses (0.625 mg of conjugated estrogen or 1 mg of micronized estradiol). Use of the vaginal and transdermal routes of delivery avoids the hepatic "first pass" effect. There is much controversy surrounding a potential increased incidence of breast cancer associated with estrogen replacement. More data are needed to clarify this issue. Smoking appears to potentiate all the adverse effects of estrogen replacement therapy. Contraindications to estrogen replacement include unexplained vaginal bleeding, breast cancer, endometrial carcinoma, estrogen-related thromboembolic processes, and liver failure. Estrogen replacement may be considered if these disorders resolve or if the patient with endometrial or breast cancer survives more than 2 years with no evidence of disease recurrence. Recently, selective estrogen receptor modulators (i.e., tamoxifen, raloxifene) have been entertained as an alternative to traditional estrogen replacement. Experience is limited and long-term clinical data are needed to determine the effectiveness of these designer drugs. For all patients, the known risks and potential benefits of hormonal replacement must be individually weighed before initiation of treatment.

Many women undergo a perimenopausal period lasting from 2 to 5 years prior to menopause. In this period, a woman begins to experience a change in the length of her cycles as well as the effects of estrogen deprivation. For these women, provided they are nonsmokers, the newer low-dose oral contraceptive pills have proved to be effective in this transitional period. Not only do they provide adequate estrogen replacement, but they also offer a method of contraception. Once the patient reaches the menopausal age, she may switch to conventional estrogen-progestin replacement.

General

1. Erlik Y, Meldrum DR, Judd HL. Estrogen levels in postmenopausal women with hot flashes. *Obstet Gynecol* 1982;59:403.
   Hot flashes may respond to other agents if estrogens are contraindicated. These include progestins and clonidine.
2. Brenner PF. The menopausal syndrome. *Obstet Gynecol* 1988;77[Suppl]:6.
   Because of increased life expectancy, modern women in industrialized countries can expect to spend a third of their lives in the menopausal period.
3. Gambrell RD Jr. The menopause: benefits and risks of estrogen-progestogen replacement therapy. *Fertil Steril* 1982;37:457.
   Hormonal replacement therapy in the form of continuous estrogen-progestin treatment is discussed.
4. Willett W, et al. Cigarette smoking, relative weight, and menopause. *Am J Epidemiol* 1983;117:651.
   Cigarette smokers have lower estrogen levels than do nonsmokers.
5. Session DR, Kelly AC, Jewelewicz R. Current concepts in estrogen replacement therapy in the menopause. *Fertil Steril* 1993;59:277.

The daily administration of an estrogen and progestin eliminates withdrawal bleeding and increases patient compliance.

6. Watts NB, et al. Comparison of oral estrogens and estrogens plus androgen on bone mineral density, menopausal symptoms, and lipid-lipoprotein profiles in surgical menopausal women. *Obstet Gynecol* 1995;85:529.
   Androgen levels also decrease in the menopause and there may be a place for androgen supplementation in selected postmenopausal patients.

Osteoporosis

7. Delmas PD, Bjarnason NH, Mitlak BH. Effects of raloxifene on bone mineral chemistry, serum cholesterol concentrations and uterine endometrium in postmenopausal women. *N Engl J Med* 1997;337:1641.
   Raloxifene does not appear to stimulate the endometrium.
8. Lindsay R. The menopause: sex steroids and osteoporosis. *Clin Obstet Gynecol* 1987;30:847.
   This describes the changes in serum sex steroid levels that lead to osteoporosis in the postmenopausal female.
9. Raisz LG. Local and systemic factors in the pathogenesis of osteoporosis. *N Engl J Med* 1988;318:818.
   The author presents a comprehensive review of osteoporosis.
10. Field CS, et al. Preventive effects of transdermal 17β-estradiol on osteoporotic changes after surgical menopause: a two-year placebo-controlled trial. *Am J Obstet Gynecol* 1993;168:114.
    Transdermal estrogen is a safe and effective regimen for preventing bone loss in recently postmenopausal women.
11. Kiel DP, et al. Hip fracture and the use of estrogens in postmenopausal women. The Framingham study. *N Engl J Med* 1987;317:1169.
    This article discusses a follow-up of the Framingham study on the role of estrogens in the prevention of hip fracture.
12. Civitelli R, et al. Bone turnover in postmenopausal osteoporosis. Effect of calcitonin treatment. *J Clin Invest* 1988;82:1268.
    The effects of calcitonin therapy for treatment of postmenopausal osteoporosis are discussed.
13. Johnston GC, Slemenda CW, Melton LS. Clinical use of bone densitometry. *N Engl J Med* 1991;324:1105.
    Diminished bone density is a better predictor of fracture than blood pressure elevation is of stroke or cholesterol elevation is of heart attack.
14. Bauer DC, et al. Broadband ultrasound attenuation predicts fractures strongly and independently of densitometry in older women. *Arch Intern Med* 1997; 157:629.
    Ultrasonographic studies of the appendicular skeleton provide reliable predictions of fracture risk.
15. Liberman UA, et al. Effect with oral alendronate on bone mineral density and the incidence of fractures in postmenopausal osteoporosis. *N Engl J Med* 1995; 22:1435.
    Bisphosphonates may irritate the upper gastrointestinal tract and are therefore contraindicated in women with esophagitis, hiatal reflux, and peptic ulcer disease.

Arteriosclerosis

16. Witteman JCM, et al. Increased risk of atherosclerosis in women after the menopause. *Br Med J* 1989;298:642.
    Women with a natural menopause were found to have a 3.4 times greater risk of atherosclerosis than did premenopausal women; women who had a bilateral oophorectomy had a 5.5 times greater risk.
17. Sullivan JM, et al. Postmenopausal estrogen use and coronary atherosclerosis. *Ann Intern Med* 1987;108:358.
    Postmenopausal women who receive estrogens have a reduced risk of coronary artery disease.

18. Paganini-Hill A, Ross RK, Henderson BE. Postmenopausal oestrogen treatment and stroke: a prospective study. *Br Med J* 1988;2:519.

The risk of stroke in women receiving estrogen is reduced compared with that in women not taking estrogens.

19. Writing Group for the PEPI Trial. Effects of estrogen or estrogen/progestin regimens on heart disease risk factors in postmenopausal women. *JAMA* 1995; 273:199.

In the Postmenopausal Estrogen-Progestin Interventions Trial, medroxyprogesterone acetate blunted the estrogen-associated increase in HDL cholesterol substantially more than did micronized progesterone.

20. Hulley S, et al. Randomized trial of estrogen plus progestin for secondary prevention of coronary heart disease in postmenopausal women. *JAMA* 1998; 280:605.

In contrast to previous observational studies indicating a beneficial effect, this trial did not show a benefit of estrogen / progestin therapy in women with established coronary heart disease.

87. GONADAL DYSGENESIS

Randall S. Hines

Gonadal dysgenesis is described as the involution of germ cells soon after migration into the undifferentiated gonad early in embryonic life, resulting in fibrous streaks where the ovaries are usually found. Loss or mutations of the genetic material essential for gonadal development is the cause of the dysgenesis, and a wide range of karyotypes can be found. The most common group, 45,X, includes phenotypic females who display short stature, webbed neck, primary amenorrhea, and sexual infantilism originally described by Turner. Other forms of gonadal dysgenesis may be characterized as mosaic chromosome abnormalities (45,X/46,XY) and partial deletions of a single X (45,X del Xp). A proposed classification system would include (1) X chromosome aneuploidy-45,X; mosaic 45,X/46,XY; 45,X/47,XYY and other X deletions; and (2) Y chromosome aneuploidy-45,X/46,XY and others containing a Y chromosome. Pure gonadal dysgenesis refers to individuals with bilateral streak gonads, regardless of karyotype.

Reportedly, one X chromosome is completely absent in half of the patients with gonadal dysgenesis, resulting in the 45,X karyotype referred to as Turner syndrome. The most common feature encountered is short stature, with virtually all patients less than 155 cm tall. A variety of other anomalies may be present, including a short webbed neck, shield chest with wide-set nipples, a low hairline, a high-arched palate, epicanthal folds, cubitus valgus (a wide carrying angle of the arms), hypoplastic nail beds, shortening of the fourth or fifth metacarpals, and renal anomalies in 30%. Cardiac anomalies also may occur, including coarctation of the aorta, atrial septal defects, and valvular defects. Lymphedema of the extremities can occur (30%) at birth, which may be referred to as Bonnevie-Ullrich syndrome. It is important to remember that many patients have few physical stigmata other than short stature.

Treatment of these individuals is focused on obtaining maximum height followed by the development of secondary sexual characteristics. If large doses of cyclic steroid hormones are given before the total height has been reached, premature closure of the epiphysis may occur. For this reason, only small doses of estrogen (0.3 mg/day) are given and may be given unopposed until bleeding occurs. After a year or more of low-dose estrogen therapy, total replacement doses of estrogen are given to maximize breast development and genital tract maturation. Progestins should be added in cyclic fashion after genital bleeding occurs.

Synthetic growth hormone has been used successfully to augment growth in gonadal dysgenesis. Dosages vary between 0.5 and 1.0 IU/kg/wk, given subcutaneously in three divided doses beginning around age 12. The long-term effects of growth hormone given at an earlier age are currently under investigation. In addition to hormonal therapy, patients with gonadal dysgenesis should undergo a thorough cardiac and renal evaluation because of the increased risks of anomalies in these organs. Other disorders may occur later in life, including diabetes, hypertension, and inflammatory bowel disease.

Patients with the stigmata of gonadal dysgenesis may have some form of mosaicism or structural abnormality of the X chromosome (X aneuploidy). Deletion of the short (XXp-) or long (XXq-) arm and an isochrome for the long arm of the X chromosome (XXqi) are the most common structural anomalies and may exist with or without mosaicism. Interestingly, patients with long arm deletion tend to be taller. The findings suggest that stature may be determined by genes on the short arm, whereas ovarian development may result from genes on both the long and short arm of the X chromosome.

Mosaicism, due to a mitotic error, results in the development of two or more cell lines in one individual. The most common form of mosaicism is 45,X/46,XX. Patients display a wide variety of phenotypes, and patients with 45,X as well as those with other forms of mosaicism may have breast development, menstruate, and rarely become pregnant.

Patients with Y aneuploidy include those with either mosaicism and a normal Y chromosome (such as 45,X/46,XY, 45,X/47,XYY, or 45,X/46,XY/47,XYY), or those with a structurally abnormal Y chromosome. As a consequence of its effect of gonadal differentiation, a Y-bearing cell line modifies the typical female phenotype of the syndrome by causing a variable degree of masculine differentiation of the genital tract in some patients. Clinically, most patients have at least one fallopian tube and a uterus, and many patients have sexual ambiguity of the genitalia. When a Y chromosome is found in patients with gonadal dysgenesis, there is an approximately 30% chance of gonadal malignancy. Gonadoblastoma is the most common neoplasm found, and dysgerminoma is the second most common metastatic lesion. Prophylactic gonadectomy by laparoscopy or laparotomy is indicated in patients with streak or dysgenetic gonads who have a Y chromosome. This should be performed at the time of diagnosis with no delay for attainment of a certain age.

Those individuals with a 46,XY karyotype, who have rudimentary streak gonads and remain sexually infertile, but are of normal stature and lack the somatic stigmata of Turner syndrome, have Swyer syndrome. These patients often come to medical attention at the time of expected puberty because of primary amenorrhea and are found to have elevated gonadotropin levels, as would individuals with prepubertal castration. The body habitus is eunuchoid. This condition may result from a mutation in the gene for testicular differentiation, termed *sex region on Y* (SRY). This condition in rare cases may be transmitted from a mosaic father. Other cases presumably arise from mutation in genes that would be acted upon by SRY. Incomplete forms of gonadal dysgenesis result in varying degrees of virilization and sexual ambiguity.

Patients who have a 46,XX karyotype, amenorrhea, and elevated gonadotropins will either have premature ovarian failure or streak gonads and gonadal dysgenesis. These patients are difficult to distinguish because definitive diagnosis might require surgery and direct observation of the gonad. If the karyotype is 46,XX, there is no clinical benefit to surgery and thus surgery is not recommended. In these unique cases, an evaluation for the various causes of premature ovarian failure should be performed.

Gonadal Dysgenesis

1. Grumbach MM, Conte FA. Disorders of sexual differentiation. In: Wilson JD, Foster DW, eds. *Williams textbook of endocrinology*. Philadelphia: WB Saunders, 1992.
   The sections of the chapter entitled "The Syndrome of Gonadal Dysgenesis: Turner Syndrome and Its Variants" is a comprehensive review of gonadal dysgenesis.
2. Jaffe RB. Disorders of sexual development. In: Yen SSC, Jaffe RB, eds. *Reproductive endocrinology*, 3rd ed. Philadelphia: WB Saunders, 1991.
   The section on "Gonadal Dysgenesis" is comprehensively reviewed.

3. Tsutsumi O, et al. Y chromosome analysis and laparoscopic surgery in XY pure gonadal dysgenesis: a case report and a review of the literature. *Asia-Oceania. J Obstet Gynaecol* 1993;19:95.
   The sex-determining region Y is a gene located in the sex-determining region of the Y chromosome, which has many of the properties expected of the testis-determining factor.
4. Plouffe L Jr, McDonough PG. Ovarian agenesis and dysgenesis. In: Adashi EY, Rock JA, Rosenwalks Z, eds. *Reproductive endocrinology, surgery, and technology.* Vol. 6. Philadelphia: Lippincott-Raven, 1996.
   This is an updated review of gonadal dysgenesis.
5. Hines RS, et al. Paternal somatic and germ-line mosaicism for an SRY missense mutation leading to recurrent 46,XY sex reversal. *Fertil Steril* 1997;67:675.
   Description of the mechanism for inherited Swyer syndrome.

88. ANDROGEN INSENSITIVITY AND DISORDERS OF ANDROGEN ACTION

Randall S. Hines

Androgen insensitivity results from a mutation in the gene for the androgen receptor. Because this gene is located on the X chromosome, 46,XY individuals are affected. When androgens cannot effectively induce virilization in a genetic male (46,XY), these individuals in the past have been termed *male pseudohermaphrodites* and are phenotypically female. With our current understanding of the molecular basis for these disorders, this term has become outdated. When androgen actions are incompletely impaired, a spectrum of phenotypes may arise, ranging from severely undervirilized males to normally virilized males with only infertility or even fertile men who are minimally undervirilized.

By understanding the embryology of genital development, the clinician is able to interpret the range of presentations of patients with androgen insensitivity. Until 7 weeks' gestation, the fetal gonad is indifferent and both wolffian (male) and müllerian (female) structures are present in all individuals. If the testis does not produce testosterone and müllerian inhibiting factor (MIF), the wolffian structures regress and the müllerian structures form the internal genitalia, including the fallopian tubes, uterus, cervix, and upper vagina. When a normal Y chromosome is present, production of a protein encoded by the gene SRY (sex region on Y) from the short arm of the Y chromosome signals the differentiation of the gonad to a testis. The Sertoli cells of the testes secrete MIF, thereby inducing regression of the müllerian structures. This hormone is also known as antimüllerian hormone and müllerian inhibiting substance. The Leydig cells of the testes produce testosterone, which directs differentiation of the wolffian structures into the vas deferens, epididymis, and seminal vesicles. Testosterone is also converted intracellularly to dihydrotestosterone (DHT) by the enzyme 5-alpha-reductase. DHT induces virilization of the external genitalia to produce male genitalia and the prostate. In the absence of DHT, the genitalia will develop along a female pathway.

All patients with androgen insensitivity are genetically 46XY, but the disorder may be grouped into complete and incomplete forms. Individuals with the complete form of androgen insensitivity are phenotypic females who present with primary amenorrhea and normal breast development. These patients have female external genitalia, a blind vaginal pouch, absent or vestigial müllerian structures (uterus and tubes), and testes that are located in the labia, inguinal canal, or intraabdominally. Wolffian duct derivatives are usually absent, but vestiges may exist in a rudimentary or hypoplastic form. Patients with complete androgen insensitivity have little or no pubic, axillary, or facial hair. In the past this phenotype was referred to as testicular feminization. Although often missed at birth and early childhood, the diagnosis should be suspected in the phenotypic female infant with an inguinal hernia and a mass in the labia or inguinal region.

The incomplete form of androgen resistance includes a heterogeneous group of 46,XY individuals who exhibit variable degrees of masculinization. All affected males lack müllerian structures, and wolffian duct derivatives are sometimes present but usually hypoplastic. The external genitalia may be ambiguous and range in form from a blind vaginal pouch to a hypoplastic male appearance to normal. The most common presentation found in infancy consists of an apparent male but with hypospadias, a small penis, and often cryptorchidism. These patients experience puberty but do not masculinize completely and frequently have gynecomastia. This combination of ambiguous genitalia and only small degrees of androgenation is often referred to as Lubs syndrome, whereas the disorder in phenotypic males with undervirilization is referred to as Reifenstein syndrome.

The androgen insensitivity syndrome is an X-linked recessive disorder. Hormonal profiles in such patients reveal elevated luteinizing hormone (LH) and testosterone, normal follicle-stimulating hormone (FSH), and increased estradiol (for male) levels. The increased secretion of estradiol as well as the peripheral conversion of elevated androgens to estrogens result in the formation of secondary female sexual characteristics.

The cause of the androgen insensitivity can occur at any step of the mechanism of action of androgens on their target cells. The androgen resistance may be due to insufficient numbers of androgen receptors in target tissues, defective receptor function, or a postreceptor defect. The gene responsible for encoding the androgen receptor has been identified on the long arm of the X chromosome. Absence or decreased numbers of androgen receptors may be caused by a deletion, insertion, or mutation in the gene. There also may be normal numbers of the androgen receptors, but the qualitative function of these receptors may be decreased or absent. This range of defects explains the variety of phenotypes seen, from the complete form of androgen insensitivity with female features to the incomplete form consisting of minimal undervirilization of the male phenotype.

A form of incomplete male pseudohermaphrodism often included in discussions on androgen insensitivity are entity referred to as 5-alpha-reductase deficiency. These individuals with 46,XY chromosomes and ambiguous genitalia are usually found at birth to have a small hypospadiac phallus and blind vaginal pouch. The testes are normally differentiated but located in the labioscrotal folds or inguinal canal. The internal male ducts are fully developed and end either in the vaginal pouch or the perineum. Because of the deficiency in the enzyme that converts testosterone to DHT, embryologic structures responsive to testosterone (wolffian system) develop normally but the structures responsive to DHT (external genitalia and peripheral target tissues) virilize incompletely. At puberty, these individuals undergo marked, although selective, masculinization, including deepening of the voice, an increase in muscle mass, and enlargement of the phallus. This disorder is very similar to the incomplete forms of androgen insensitivity, but gynecomastia does not occur at puberty. The 5-alpha-reductase deficiency syndrome is inherited as autosomal recessive, and the gene for the type 2 enzyme is located on the short arm of chromosome 2. As with androgen insensitivity, a wide number of mutations have been described.

The diagnosis of complete androgen insensitivity can be established after puberty based on clinical criteria alone. An adolescent with breast development, a short, blind-ending vagina without a cervix, amenorrhea, and scant pubic hair and axillary hair has complete androgen insensitivity that can be confirmed by the finding of a serum testosterone level in the male range. The diagnosis of complete androgen insensitivity in infants more than 6 months of age or in children can be made when a 46,XY female is found to have an inguinal hernia or labial mass together with elevated LH or testosterone levels, or both, without virilization. Incomplete androgen insensitivity may be more difficult to diagnose. If the methods are available, fibroblast cultures and molecular analysis are helpful for demonstrating androgen receptor defects.

Measuring the levels of LH and testosterone (and their precursors) after administration of human chorionic gonadotropin also may discern androgen insensitivity from other defects in androgen action such as 5-alpha-reductase deficiency (discussed already) or defects in testosterone biosynthesis (not discussed). Patients with 5-alpha-reductase deficiency will have elevated levels of precursors (dehydroepiandrosterone sulfate and androstenedione).

The therapy for patients with complete androgen insensitivity centers around reinforcing the female gender identity. The testes should be removed due to the risk of malignancy, but the risk is low before the age of 25. Therefore, surgical correction should generally be delayed until after puberty to allow the formation of secondary sexual characteristics. If the vagina is too short for intercourse, manual dilatation with a prosthesis or surgical repair in the form of a McIndoe vaginoplasty is indicated at the onset of sexual activity.

The therapy for incomplete forms of androgen insensitivity depends on the degree of masculinization of the external genitalia. Sex rearing depends on the patient's age at diagnosis and the degree of ambiguity. Patients diagnosed at birth with minimal degrees of undervirilization are best raised as males, but ambiguous genitalia patients may best be reared as females because of the varying response to high-dose androgens and the gynecomastia that occurs at puberty. Gonadectomy is often indicated, and plastic repair of genitalia also may be necessary. If gonadectomy is performed before puberty, estrogen replacement beginning at age 12 to 13 should be instituted to ensure development of female secondary sexual characteristics.

Androgen Sensitivity Syndromes
 1. Grumbach MM, Conte FA. Disorders of sex differentiation. In: Wilson JD, Foster DW, eds. *Williams textbook of endocrinology,* 8th ed. Philadelphia: WB Saunders, 1992.
 2. Santen RJ. Male hypogonadism. In: Yen SSC, Jaffe RB, eds. *Reproductive endocrinology—physiology, pathophysiology and clinical management,* 3rd ed. Philadelphia: WB Saunders, 1991.
 3. Jaffe RB. Disorders of sexual development. In: Yen SSC, Jaffe RB, eds. *Reproductive endocrinology—physiology, pathophysiology and clinical management,* 3rd ed. Philadelphia: WB Saunders, 1991.
    The above three works are comprehensive reviews of androgen insensitivity, including the complete and incomplete forms, as well as 5-alpha-reductase deficiency.
 4. Griffin JE, et al. The syndromes of androgen resistance. *N Engl J Med* 1980; 302:198.
    This is a review of the spectrum of androgen resistance.
 5. Lee PA, Brown TR, La Torre HA. Diagnosis of the partial androgen insensitivity syndrome during infancy. *JAMA* 1986;25:2207.
 6. Nagel BA, Lippe BM, Griffen JE. Androgen resistance in the neonate: use of hormones of hypothalamic-pituitary-gonadal axis for diagnosis. *J Pediatr* 1986; 109:486.
    These two articles review the diagnosis of androgen insensitivity in infants and children.
 7. Castro-Magana M, Angulo M, Uy J. Male hypogonadism with gynecomastia caused by late-onset deficiency of testicular 17-ketosteroid reductase. *N Engl J Med* 1993;328:1297.
    A late-onset form of testicular 17-ketosteroid reductase deficiency can cause gynecomastia and hypogonadism in men.

Molecular Genetics of the Androgen Receptor
 8. Brown CJ, et al. Androgen receptor locus in the human X chromosome: regional localization to Xq11-12 and description of a DNA polymorphism. *Am J Hum Genet* 1989;44:264.
 9. French FS, et al. The molecular basis of androgen insensitivity. *Rec Prog Horm Res* 1990;46:1.

*These two articles review recent research into the DNA sequencing of the andro-
gen receptor to the X chromosome.*
10. McPaul MJ, et al. The spectrum of mutations in the androgen receptor gene that
    causes androgen resistance. *J Clin Endocrinol Metab* 1993;76:17.
    *This is a molecular biologic analysis of androgen receptor gene mutations. The
    phenotypic abnormalities are the result of receptor function impairment or de-
    creases in receptor abundance, or both.*
11. Thigpen AE, Davis DL, Milatovich A, et al. Molecular genetics of steroid 5α-
    reductase 2 deficiency. *J Clin Invest* 1992;90:799.

Mechanisms of Sexual Differentiation
12. Jost A, et al. Studies on sex differentiation in mammals. *Rec Prog Horm Res*
    1973;29:1.
    This is a classic review of the role of the gonad in sexual differentiation.
13. Wilson JD. Testosterone uptake by the urogenital tract of the rabbit embryo.
    Endocrinology 1973;92:1192.
14. Wilson JD, et al. The role of gonadal steroids in sexual differentiation. *Rec Prog
    Horm Res* 1981;37:1.
    *The authors of these two articles discuss molecular and biochemical aspects of sex
    differentiation.*
15. Koopman P, et al. Male development of chromosomally female mice transgenic
    for SRY. *Nature* 1991;351:117.
    *Recent evidence of the testis determining factor location on the Y chromosome is
    the SRY region.*
16. Puscheck EE, Behzadian MA, McDonough PG. Molecular biology of sexual dif-
    ferentiation. *Infertil Reprod Med Clin North Am* 1994;5:69.
    This is a review of the genetics underlying sex determination.

XVI. GYNECOLOGIC ONCOLOGY

89. NON-NEOPLASTIC AND INTRAEPITHELIAL NEOPLASTIC VULVAL CONDITIONS

Michel E. Rivlin

Symptoms related to vulvar disorders include pruritus, vulval pain (vulvodynia), superficial dyspareunia, or the presence of a lesion that may be white, red, or pigmented, raised or ulcerated. These symptoms may be due to infections such as candida, herpes, or papilloma virus, or to dermatologic disorders such as contact dermatitis, lichen simplex, or lichen planus. Local reactions may be caused by hygiene measures such as bath salts, oils, vaginal sprays, and detergents used for laundering underwear. Non-neoplastic epithelial disorders including lichen sclerosis and squamous hyperplasia, as well as neoplastic conditions such as *vulval intraepithelial neoplasia* (VIN), may be the causative factors.

If the diagnosis is not readily apparent, colposcopic examination of the vulva may define areas of abnormality that may warrant biopsy using a Keyes punch or biopsy forceps under local anesthesia. The nuclear stain 1% toluidine blue also may be helpful in delineating sites for potential biopsy. Therapy of vulvar disorders frequently includes local topical treatment such as Burrow's solution or warm sitz baths. Topical medical treatment such as a hormone cream (e.g., estrogen, progesterone, testosterone), or local anesthetic (e.g., lidocaine gel 2%) or topical corticosteroid cream. Steroid creams are grouped according to antiinflammatory activity as low potency (e.g., 1% hydrocortisone), medium potency (e.g., 0.1% triamcinolone), or high potency (e.g., 0.05% clobetasol). Whatever topical steroid is used, it should be applied in a thin coat, and ointments are indicated for the management of thick chronic dermatitis but inflamed skin requires lotions or creams. In rare situations, surgery, including vestibuloplasty, may be necessary.

Lichen sclerosis involves the pudendum and often continues across the perineum and perianal area. The skin is white, thin, and crinkly, but may be thickened when there is concurrent squamous hyperplasia. The introitus may shrink with fusion of the labia minora. Microscopically there is epidermal atrophy, hyalinized superficial dermis, and an underlying lymphocytic infiltrate. The etiology is unknown, but there is evidence suggesting a familial incidence and an underlying autoimmune disorder. It is most common in postmenopausal women, although it does occur in prepubescent girls. Lichen sclerosis may be associated with squamous carcinoma; some studies found that 3% to 5% will subsequently develop carcinoma. A persistent ulcer or nodule in a field of lichen sclerosis should be examined via biopsy. Therapy of lichen sclerosis includes very high-potency topical corticosteroids applied twice daily for 2 to 3 weeks, then daily with usual improvement in a month or less. Long-term maintenance is appropriate with applications limited to one to three times per week. Topical testosterone and progesterone also have been used with varying results. Testosterone is systemically absorbed and may cause androgenic side effects and should not be used in children.

The diagnosis of squamous cell hyperplasia is one of exclusion. The involved areas are usually asymmetrical, and in color they may range from white to gray and appear coarse and thickened. Microscopically, epithelial thickening (hyperplasia), thickening of the keratin layer (hyperkeratosis), elongation and widening of the epithelial rete ridges (acanthosis), and retention of nuclear material in the keratin layer (parakeratosis) are noted. Included in the differential diagnosis are lichen simplex chronicus, condyloma acuminatum, psoriasis, lichen planus, and seborrhea. Treatment consists of topical medium-strength corticosteroids applied twice daily and decreased to once daily when symptoms resolve. Response within 2 to 3 weeks is usual, and treatment is usually curative.

Vulval intraepithelial neoplasia is classified as types I through III (severe atypia and carcinoma in situ [CIS]), in a manner similar to the system used for classifying cervical intraepithelial neoplasia (CIN). The incidence of VIN has increased sharply, and the mean age of affected women has decreased from over 50 years to under 38 years. There is an association between VIN and sexually transmitted infections and other forms of genital tract neoplasia. Of patients with VIN III, 30% have synchronous or metachronous neoplasia at another genital site. At least 20% of women with VIN III have associated CIN III. The tendency for multicentric disease to develop obviously influences management. The etiology of VIN is unknown, but the increased incidence parallels the increase in the incidence of genital infections with human papilloma virus (HPV). Molecular hybridization studies have shown HPV deoxyribonucleic acid (DNA) in 70% of the patients with VIN III and in 50% of those with vulvar carcinomas.

A continuum from preinvasive to invasive vulval neoplasia has not been clearly established, and the malignant potential is uncertain. The disease is as likely to regress as to progress, although the risk of progression is probably less than 5%. In older women, VIN tends to be unifocal and the malignant potential appears to be greater. Immunosuppressed women also seem to be at higher risk of rapid progression. Most VIN III lesions show an aneuploid DNA content, suggesting a malignant potential. About half of the patients are asymptomatic. Pruritus, burning, and pain are the most common complaints in the remainder. The appearance is variable: 60% are white plaques, and about 15% are hyperpigmented. The cytologic changes that take place in mild atypia include enlarged hyperchromatic nuclei; in moderate atypia, there is coarse chromatin clumping. In the moderate form, the increased cellularity and cellular disarray are confined to the inner two thirds of the epithelium. In severe atypia, more than two thirds are involved, cells of the parabasal type are found near the surface, and chromatin clumping is moderately coarse and irregular. CIS is characterized by full-thickness cellular disorientation (with the exception of the most superficial keratinized layers), in conjunction with giant cells, multinucleated cells, individual cell keratinization, corps ronds formation (a pale halo of cytoplasm around a pyknotic nucleus), abnormal mitoses, and squamous pearls at the tips of the rete pegs. Parakeratosis and hyperkeratosis may be present, and there is usually an inflammatory response in the dermis.

The three preferred treatments for VIN are wide local excision, carbon dioxide laser vaporization, and, in unusual circumstances, a skinning vulvectomy with a split-thickness skin graft. Laser ablation is well adapted to hairless areas, as is surgical excision to hairy sites; the two procedures may thus be combined to advantage. Recurrence of VIN is common regardless of the therapy but can be managed again using conservative therapy.

The symptom complex of chronic burning vulvar discomfort is termed vulvodynia. In some cases, point tenderness that is localized within the vestibule, together with severe pain in response to vestibular touch and physical findings confined to vestibular erythema, is termed the *vulvar vestibulitis syndrome,* a form of vulvodynia. When other causes of vulvodynia have been ruled out, a diagnosis of idiopathic or dysesthetic or essential vulvodynia is appropriate. Treatment is with a low-dose tricyclic antidepressant to reduce neural feedback. Long-term support and management are essential because medical treatment alone is frequently not curative.

Squamous Cell Hyperplasia / Lichen Sclerosis
1. MacLean AB, Reid WMN. Benign and premalignant disease of the vulva. *Br J Obstet Gynaecol* 1995;102:359.
   Symptoms may be due to hygiene measures including bath salts, oils, foams, deodorants, sprays, and antiseptics, or sensitivity to detergents used for washing underwear.
2. Report of the Committee on Terminology. New nomenclature for vulvar disease. *Am J Obstet Gynecol* 1989;160:769.
   Terms no longer acceptable included dystrophy, kraurosis, and leukoplakia. The et atrophicus was dropped from lichen sclerosis.
3. Paolo C, et al. Fibrogenic cytokines in vulvar lichen sclerosis. *J Reprod Med* 1997;42:161.

Dermal infiltrating cells may participate via cytokine production in the pathogenesis of fibrosis in lichen sclerosis.

4. Joura EA. Short-term effects of topical testosterone in vulvar lichen sclerosis. *Obstet Gynecol* 1997;89:297.

Androgen status should be evaluated, and dosage should be individualized to avoid virilization.

5. Leibowitch M, et al. The epithelial changes associated with squamous cell carcinoma of the vulva: a review of the clinical, histological and viral findings in 78 women. *Br J Obstet Gynaecol* 1990;97:1135.

Lichen sclerosis was found in 61% of the patients and half of these also had VIN III. Epithelial hyperplasia was noted in 25% of lichen sclerosis cases.

Vulvar Intraepithelial Neoplasia

6. Reid R. The management of genital condylomas, intraepithelial neoplasia, and vulvodynia. *Obstet Gynecol Clin North Am* 1996;23:917.

The management of HPV-induced disease is the strategy of repeated local destruction.

7. Jones RW, Baranyai J, Stables S. Trends in squamous cell carcinoma of the vulva: the influence of vulvar intraepithelial neoplasia. *Obstet Gynecol* 1997;90:448.

The increasing incidence of VIN in young women is being reflected in an increase in VIN-associated squamous cell carcinoma of the vulva in women under age 50.

8. Chiasson MA, et al. Increased prevalence of vulvovaginal condyloma and vulvar intraepithelial neoplasia in women infected with the human immunodeficiency virus. *Obstet Gynecol* 1997;89:690.

In this study, the prevalence was increased and more likely to be multicentric and to involve the vulva, vagina, and cervix.

9. Kuppers V, et al. Risk factors for recurrent VIN. *J Reprod Med* 1997;42:140.

The grade as well as the multifocality are important, and recurrence developed in 36% of the women in this study.

Vulvodynia and the Vulvar Vestibulitis Syndrome

10. Van Lankveld JJDM, Weijenborg PTM, Ter Kule MM. Psychologic profiles of and sexual function in women with vulvar vestibulitis and their partners. *Obstet Gynecol* 1996;88:65.

Women with vulvar vestibulitis and their partners seem to be psychologically healthy in general, but the condition may be associated with a situationally defined sexual dysfunction for the women.

11. Bornstein J, et al. Predicting the outcome of surgical treatment of vulvar vestibulitis. *Obstet Gynecol* 1997;89:695.

Treatment approaches other than surgery should be considered in women with primary dyspareunia and in those with associated persistent vulvar pain.

12. Edwards L, et al. Childhood sexual and physical abuse: incidence in patients with vulvodynia. *J Reprod Med* 1997;42:135.

Women with vulvodynia did not experience a higher incidence of sexual or physical abuse during childhood as compared with a control group.

13. Reid R, et al. Flashlamp-excited dye laser therapy of idiopathic vulvodynia is safe and efficacious. *Am J Obstet Gynecol* 1995;172:1684.

This article discusses an instrument designed specifically for the photocoagulation of small blood vessels within the superficial dermis, but that is ineffective in the presence of deep pain.

90. CARCINOMA OF THE VULVA

Michel E. Rivlin

Ninety percent of the invasive vulvar carcinomas are of the squamous cell type and account for about 5% of gynecologic malignancies. There is often a background of vulvar intraepithelial neoplasia (VIN) in these patients. However, progression from VIN to carcinoma in a manner analogous to that noted in the cervix has not been shown. Vulvar carcinoma is a disease of older women, with a peak incidence in the seventh decade of life. Seventy percent of the tumors develop anteriorly on the labia majora, although tumors on the labia minora, clitoris, and perineum also occur. The usual symptoms consist of pruritus, an ulcer or nodule, and bleeding with pain. Although often well localized, these lesions may be extensive because they are frequently neglected for prolonged periods. Grossly, the lesion assumes the appearance of an indurated ulcer with raised, rolled edges. Histologically, they are well differentiated as a rule, although anaplastic varieties occur in 5% to 10% of the cases. Cords of squamous cells extend into the dermis and subcutaneous tissue, forming keratinizing epithelial pearls. Rare adenosquamous variants occur. The cancer then spreads directly to adjacent vulvar, perineal, and perianal areas. Metastasis to the lymph nodes is common and often takes place early. Lymphatic spread is predictable, first to the inguinal nodes (superficial, then deep) and then to the femoral and deep pelvic nodes. Midline tumors may drain to contralateral nodes. Large or poorly differentiated tumors are more likely to metastasize to lymph nodes. However, the size of the tumor is not always an accurate guide to the presence of groin metastasis (10% of the lesions measuring <2 cm have nodal involvement). The 5-year survival rate in affected patients after treatment is quoted to be 70%, which increases to 90% if lymph nodes are not involved, decreases to 65% if inguinal nodes are involved, and decreases further to 10% to 15% if metastases are present in deep pelvic nodes.

The revised International Federation of Gynecology and Obstetrics (FIGO, 1989) staging system for vulvar cancer has changed from a clinical to a surgical system because the clinical assessment of groin nodes is often in error (13%–39% of cases). The staging includes designations regarding the primary tumor (T), regional lymph nodes (N), and distant metastases (M). Stage 0 (Tis) indicates an intraepithelial carcinoma. A stage 1 (T1 N0 M0) tumor is confined to the vulva or perineum, or both, is 2 cm or less in its greatest dimension, and nodes are not palpable. A stage II (T2 N0 M0) tumor is confined to the vulva or perineum, or both, is more than 2 cm in its greatest dimension, and nodes are not palpable. A stage III (T3 N0 M0) tumor is a lesion of any size showing (1) adjacent spread to the lower urethra and/or vagina, or the anus (T3 N1 M0) and/or (2) unilateral regional lymph node metastasis (T1 N1 M0; T2 N1 M0). A tumor is classified as stage IVA if it has invaded any of the following: the upper urethra, bladder, rectum, or pelvic bone, and/or shows bilateral nodal metastases (T1–4 N2 M0). A stage IVB tumor constitutes any distant metastases, including the pelvic nodes (any T, any N, M1).

There appears to be an interrelationship between the human papillomaviruses and the development of lower genital tract intraepithelial and invasive neoplasia. A high proportion of the cases of intraepithelial neoplasia in the lower genital tract are multicentric. Carcinoma of the vulva is therefore frequently found in association with intraepithelial carcinoma of the vagina and cervix. Papillomavirus infections of the male partner also may be found. Cigarette smoking may be an important factor. Diagnosis is based on biopsy findings, often with the aid of colposcopic findings or toluidine blue staining. The differential diagnosis includes lichen sclerosis, squamous hyperplasia, and sexually transmitted ulcerative or condylomatous lesions, as discussed in Chapter 57. The preoperative workup may include lymphangiography or computed tomography or magnetic resonance imaging, with or without needle biopsy, to demonstrate whether groin or deep pelvic lymph nodes are involved. Associated cervical or vaginal disease should be sought and assessed if present.

Obesity, hypertension, diabetes, and arteriosclerosis are common in these patients, which, together with their advanced age, complicate therapy. Nevertheless, the majority of patients are sufficiently healthy to permit definitive therapy, which is generally surgical because radiotherapy and chemotherapy are relatively unsuccessful in the treatment of vulvar cancer.

For many years, radical vulvectomy with bilateral inguinal lymphadenectomy was the standard surgical approach for the treatment of vulvar carcinoma. The procedure removes the tumor along with the lymphatics and nodes en bloc. The presence of tumor in Cloquet's node (the deepest femoral node in the femoral canal) was an indication to proceed to deep pelvic lymphadenectomy. This radical procedure brought about dramatically improved survival rates, but was associated with significant rates of mortality and morbidity and severe damage to sexual function, and hence the patient's self-image. As a result, there has been a trend toward using more conservative approaches in the management of early forms of this disease. The main source of postoperative morbidity is breakdown of the groin wound, although the use of myocutaneous flaps in some cases has decreased the incidence of this complication. Wound sloughs over the femoral vessels were sometimes complicated by heavy bleeding, but this problem can be minimized by transplantation of the sartorius muscles over these vessels. A common difficulty after vulvectomy, stress urinary incontinence and vaginal wall prolapse, also may be prevented by the use of appropriate repair procedures at the time of vulvectomy. Persistent lymphedema of the legs, another significant problem, is managed by elevation of the legs and prompt treatment of cellulitis, and preservation of the saphenous veins during groin dissection also helps to minimize the problem.

Modern treatment is individualized; there is no longer a standard operation. Vulvar conservation is indicated for patients with unifocal lesions and an otherwise normal vulva. Groin dissection is avoided for stage 1 tumors and less than 1 mm of stromal invasion. Contralateral groin dissection is eliminated in lateral T1 lesions with negative ipsilateral nodes. Separate incisions are used for groin dissections. In patients with advanced disease, preoperative radiation may reduce the need for exenteration or in patients with two or more positive groin nodes, postoperative radiation may decrease the incidence of groin recurrence.

Malignant melanoma accounts for less than 10% of all vulvar malignancies, occurring as a rule in the sixth or seventh decade of life. It is the second most common vulvar cancer, however, so it is advised that any suspicious pigmented nevus on the vulva should be excised. Neither the FIGO vulvar cancer staging system nor the Clark classification of malignant melanomas is appropriate for classifying vulvar melanoma. Prognosis is related to depth of penetration and nodal status. The overall outcome in these patients is poor (32% survival), and because radical resection does not appear to confer any greater benefit in terms of local control, a disease-free interval, or patient survival versus a less extensive resection, it seems likely that, as in the treatment of anorectal melanoma, the less radical resection should be the usual therapy. Verrucous carcinoma is an unusual variant of squamous cell carcinoma. It presents postmenopausally as a large fungating, locally invasive tumor with well-differentiated squamous epithelium and little cellular atypia. Wide local excision is sufficient because nodal metastasis is rare. Radiotherapy is contraindicated. Basal cell carcinoma is a localized tumor seen in postmenopausal women; typically it has the appearance of a slightly raised, ulcerated nodule with rolled margins. Downgrowths of cells from the basal layer of the epidermis are apparent. The tumor is only locally invasive, and wide local excision to negative margins is therapeutic, although 20% recur after removal. Bartholin's gland tumors account for about 5% of vulvar cancers, occur in persons 40 to 70 years of age, and may be either adenocarcinoma (46%) or squamous cell carcinoma (40%); metastasis to regional and distant nodes occurs. Paget's disease of the vulva is frequently associated with other malignancies, including underlying intraepithelial adenocarcinoma (20% of cases) and other vulvar cancers. Furthermore, there is a strong potential for a second urogenital primary tumor to develop (30% of cases), so thorough urogenital evaluation and follow-up are indicated.

Reviews
1. Rosen C, Malmstrom H. Invasive cancer of the vulva. *Gynecol Oncol* 1997;65:213.
   In this review of 328 patients, the most important prognostic features were tumor stage, patient age, and tumor differentiation.
2. Cavanagh D. Vulvar cancer—continuing evolution in management. *Gynecol Oncol* 1997;66:362.
   There is a trend toward conservative surgery with rational utilization of preoperative or postoperative radiation in selected patients.

Etiology
3. Iwasawa A, et al. Human papillomavirus in squamous cell carcinoma of the vulva by polymerase chain reaction. *Obstet Gynecol* 1997;89:81.
   In younger women, sexual factors, cigarette smoking, and human papillomavirus infections are significant associations; in older women, lichen sclerosis and squamous hyperplasia are associated. These findings confirm the diverse nature of vulvar cancer.
4. Iversen T, et al. Squamous cell carcinoma of the penis and of the cervix, vulva and vagina in spouses: is there any relationship? An epidemiological study from Norway, 1960–62. *Br J Cancer* 1997;76:658.
   The authors detected a strong relationship to cervical cancer and a weak relationship to vulvar cancer.
5. Crum CP, et al. Pathobiology of vulvar squamous neoplasia. *Curr Opin Obstet Gynecol* 1997;9:63.
   Progression to invasion is most common in the elderly and the immunosuppressed; however, a substantial proportion of vulvar cancers may not be related to a venereally transmitted agent.

Pathology
6. Creasman WT, Phillips JL, Menck HR. The National Cancer Data Base report on early stage invasive vulvar carcinoma. *Cancer* 1997;80:505.
   Lymph node metastasis is related to depth of invasion in T1 cases: for instance, less than 2 mm, 8% metastasis; more than 5 mm, 37% metastases.
7. Smyczek-Gargya B, et al. A multivariate analysis of clinical and morphological prognostic factors in squamous cell carcinoma of the vulva. *Gynecol Obstet Invest* 1997;43:261.
   Pelvic node metastases occur in about 5% of cases, and they usually occur when there are three or more positive groin nodes.
8. Johnson GA, et al. Epidermal growth factor receptor in vulvar malignancies and its relationship to metastasis and patient survival. *Gynecol Oncol* 1997;65:425.
   Increased expression of epidermal growth factor in vulvar cancer is associated with metastasis and decreased survival.

Treatment
9. Stehman FB, et al. Early stage I carcinoma of the vulva treated with ipsilateral superficial inguinal lymphadenectomy and modified radical hemivulvectomy: a prospective study of the Gynecologic Oncology Group. *Obstet Gynecol* 1992; 79:490.
   Inherent in any conservative approach is the fact that the benefits gained from the conservative procedure, versus the radical approach, in terms of the lessened risks of morbidity and mortality outweigh the risks of recurrence of the cancer treated conservatively.
10. Calame RJ. Pelvic relaxation as a complication of the radical vulvectomy. *Obstet Gynecol* 1980;55:716.
    Pelvic relaxation complicated 17% of 58 cases; the author recommends performing preventive or reconstructive procedures during the primary operation.
11. Anderson BL, Hacker NF. Psychosexual adjustment after vulvar surgery. *Obstet Gynecol* 1983;62:457.
    Following vulvectomy, compared with healthy women, sexual arousal was lowered (reduced to the 8th percentile) and there was poor body image (reduced to the 4th percentile).

12. Faul CM, et al. Adjuvant radiation for vulvar carcinoma: improved local control. *Int J Radiat Oncol Biol Phys* 1997;38:381.
    Clinicians may use external-beam therapy with or without intracavitary or interstitial irradiation.
13. Cunningham MJ, et al. Primary radiation, cisplatin, and 5-fluorouracil for advanced squamous carcinoma of the vulva. *Gynecol Oncol* 1997;66:258.
    Chemotherapy in combination with radiotherapy is also effective.

Other Vulvar Malignancies
14. Goldblum JR, Hart WR. Vulvar Paget's disease: a clinicopathologic and immunohistochemical study of 19 cases. *Am J Surg Pathol* 1997;21:1178.
    Treatment requires wide local excision, and evaluation of surgical margins to ensure adequate excision is necessary. Associated invasion or adenocarcinoma requires radical therapy.
15. Gonzalez-Bosquet J, et al. Malignant vulvo-vaginal melanoma: a report of 7 cases. *Eur J Gynaecol Oncol* 1997;18:63.
    The primary lesion should be removed via en bloc resection, with removal of regional nodes if the area of invasion is more than 0.75 mm.
16. Copeland LJ, et al. Bartholin gland carcinoma. *Obstet Gynecol* 1986;67:794.
    Wide excision or radical hemivulvectomy together with ipsilateral inguinal lymphadenectomy and adjunctive irradiation to the vulva and regional nodes provided an 84% survival rate despite there being a nearly 50% frequency of nodal metastasis.
17. Benedet JL, et al. Basal cell carcinoma of the vulva: clinical features and treatment results in 28 patients. *Obstet Gynecol* 1997;90:765.
    Nodal metastasis is extremely uncommon.
18. Japaze H, Van Dinh T, Woodruff JD. Verrucous carcinoma of the vulva: study of 24 cases. *Obstet Gynecol* 1982;60:462.
    Verrucous carcinoma is histologically similar to condyloma acuminatum. It occurs in the oral cavity as well as on the genitalia.

91. CERVICAL INTRAEPITHELIAL NEOPLASIA

Michel E. Rivlin

The junction between the squamous epithelium lining the ectocervix and the columnar epithelium lining the endocervix is called the *squamocolumnar junction* or *transitional zone* (TZ). In young adults, it is usually located on the ectocervix and may enlarge and become more distally located during pregnancy (ectopy). After menopause, the junction usually recedes and is frequently located in the endocervical canal. Throughout reproductive life, the more fragile red columnar glandular epithelium is gradually replaced by the more resistant pink squamous epithelium, a process termed *squamous metaplasia*. The significance of these observations is that all grades of cervical neoplasia originate in the TZ. Normal epithelial maturation proceeds outward from the basal cells on the basement membrane, and minor lesions involve this zone only.

All grades of abnormal epithelial maturation may evidence abnormalities in either the deoxyribonucleic acid (DNA) content or chromosome number. Various degrees of cytologic and histologic dedifferentiation are seen, and cytologic cervical smears (Papanicolaou's [Pap] smears) as well as cervical biopsy specimens are graded according to the degree and extent of the cellular abnormalities. The size, configuration, denseness of the chromatin, number of mitoses, pleomorphism, and percentage of abnormal cells form the basis for the cytologic and histologic grade of the lesions. If the undifferentiated neoplastic cells extend through the full thickness of the epithelium but do not penetrate the basement membrane, the lesion is called carcinoma in situ (CIS).

Mild, moderate, and severe cervical dysplasia, together with CIS, represent stages along a continuum of preinvasive lesions of the epithelium of the uterine cervix. These lesions differ in the degree of cellular abnormalities seen and in the thickness of the epithelium involved. In an alternative terminology, the term *cervical intraepithelial neoplasia* (CIN) is used, such that CIN I represents mild; CIN II, moderate; and CIN III, severe dysplasia and CIS. Unlike invasive cancer, these lesions are reversible or may arrest, and this is especially true of the earlier changes seen in the setting of CIN I and II.

Human papillomavirus (HPV) infection is the causative factor in preinvasive and invasive cancers of the cervix. Immature metaplastic cells of the transformation zone are affected and exhibit the characteristic features of koilocytotic atypia (perinuclear cavitation). The HPV types most associated with neoplasia are 16, 18, and 31. Diploidy is usual in condylomata, polyploidy in CIN I, and aneuploidy in CIN III. Epidemiologic studies indicating that HPV infection is far more common than neoplasia suggest the necessity of cofactors. Potential cofactors include cigarettes, oral contraceptives and pregnancy, immunosuppression, and chronic inflammation. Because HPV is a sexually transmitted virus, preinvasive and invasive cervical cancer exhibits many of the features of other sexually transmitted diseases (STDs), including the importance of a high-risk male partner, low socioeconomic status, early intercourse (before age 18), and the presence of other STDs.

Cervical cytologic study is basic to the diagnosis of dysplasia. A properly procured Pap smear must sample both the endocervix and ectocervix. False-negative rates vary from 20% to 40%, but the repetition of smears over time markedly improves the rates of pick-up. Historically, Pap test results were reported as being class I to V: class I being negative; class II, inflammation; and classes III, IV, and V, increasing grades of dysplasia. Since 1988, however, the Bethesda System has been adopted for the reporting of cervical and vaginal cytologic findings. This system introduced the term *low-grade squamous intraepithelial lesion* (SIL), to include cellular changes consistent with HPV infection with or without mild dysplasia (CIN I). Moderate dysplasia (CIN II), severe dysplasia, and CIS (CIN III) are now reported as a high-grade SIL. The system also requires a comment regarding the adequacy of the smear and includes the categories of abnormal squamous cells of uncertain significance (ASCUS) and abnormal glandular cells of uncertain significance (AGCUS) to include those smears in which the nature of the cells is unclear to the cytologist. Similar changes in histopathologic reporting may follow these changes in cytologic nomenclature. The prevalence of dysplasia found by cytologic examination varies from 5 to 65 per 1,000, depending on the population group being screened. The American College of Obstetricians and Gynecologists recommends annual Pap smears starting at age 18, or at the age when sexual activity starts if this is before 18 years of age.

Cervical cytologic study is a screening process only; definitive diagnosis requires tissue sampling. Colposcopy can delineate the extent of the cervical lesion and direct biopsy to the worst areas. Cone biopsy is required if colposcopic examination is deemed unsatisfactory for any of the following reasons: the entire TZ cannot be seen, the colposcopic biopsy sample reveals a lesser grade of disease than the smear, or the endocervical curettage finding is positive. Cone biopsy is used for therapy as well as for diagnosis. Women with a high-grade SIL should have a colposcopic assessment and biopsy. Women with ASCUS should have a repeat smear in 4 to 6 months and undergo colposcopy if the abnormality persists. Low-grade SIL may be managed by colposcopy or as for ASCUS, and other factors may influence that decision with patients who smoke, have high-risk HPV types, or may be unreliable as regards follow-up, being good candidates for immediate colposcopy.

The treatment of CIN must be individualized according to the extent and grade of the lesion, the age and parity of the patient, the presence or absence of pregnancy, and her desire for future childbearing. The patient's suitability for surgery, her reliability with regard to regular follow-up, and the cost of therapy also must be taken into account.

In general, less extensive and less severe lesions are treated on an outpatient basis using local methods, such as eradication of infections known to cause inflammatory cellular atypia (*Trichomonas*), cryosurgery, electrocautery, and laser therapy. The loop electrosurgical excision procedures, also referred to as loop excision of the transformation zone (LETZ), have largely replaced the laser because they are faster and less expensive. Both laser ablation and LETZ may be used for local destruction or cone biopsy, although the heat-induced artifact may make subsequent histologic interpretation difficult. More severe and more extensive lesions are usually treated by cone biopsy and, occasionally, especially if other indications exist in patients who have completed their families, by hysterectomy. A concomitant pregnancy poses a problem, and, if possible, treatment is postponed until after pregnancy in these women. Cone biopsy may be performed during pregnancy, if necessary. Generally, the initial follow-up examination is performed 4 months after therapy and repeated every 6 months for 2 years before reverting to an annual basis. CIN can recur many years after therapy, and, although the risk is small (3%), recurrence is more common in patients who have had high-grade lesions, emphasizing the importance of more intensive and prolonged follow-up for these patients.

Reviews
1. Morris M, et al. Cervical intraepithelial neoplasia and cervical cancer. *Obstet Gynecol Clin North Am* 1996;23:347.
   The causes of false-negative cytologic findings include sample error (cells not on slide), screening error (cells missed by the cytotechnologist), and interpretative error (the pathologist misjudged the cells).
2. 1988 Bethesda System for reporting cervical/vaginal cytological diagnoses. National Cancer Institute Workshop. *JAMA* 1989;262:931.
   The Bethesda System of terminology and classification for cervical and vaginal cytology is currently the standard method, but has provoked considerable controversy and will probably require modification.

Epidemiology
3. Singer A. Cervical cancer screening: state of the art. *Baillieres Clin Obstet Gynecol* 1995;9:39.
   Screening techniques include cytology, human papillomavirus testing, colposcopy, and cervicography.
4. Noller KL. Incident and demographic trends in cervical neoplasia. *Am J Obstet Gynecol* 1996;175:1088.
   Epidemiologic data concerning cervical cancer are obtained through cancer registries such as the surveillance epidemiology results reporting (SEER) program. The incidence of preinvasive lesions may be increasing in the United States.

Etiology / Pathogenesis
5. Turek LP, Smith EM. The genetic program of genital human papillomaviruses in infection and cancer. *Obstet Gynecol Clin North Am* 1996;23:735.
   Interplay of cellular and viral factors determines whether outcome is active infection, viral latency, or, ultimately, genital cancer.
6. Syrjänen K, et al. Natural history of cervical human papillomavirus lesions does not substantiate the biologic relevance of the Bethesda System. *Obstet Gynecol* 1992;79:675.
   All six HPV types (6, 11, 16, 18, 31, and 33) as well as double infections were encountered in both the low-grade and high-grade cases of squamous intraepithelial lesions; however, human papillomavirus (HPV) 16 infections have a fivefold risk for progression, versus the risk observed for HPV 6 or 11 lesions.
7. Gram IT, Macaluso M, Stalsberg H. Oral contraceptive use and the incidence of cervical intraepithelial neoplasia. *Am J Obstet Gynecol* 1992;167:40.
   A weak positive association was found; however, confounding sexual behavior and detection bias have yielded conflicting results, so that a definite causal association has not yet been established.
8. Robinson WR, et al. Histology/cytology discrepancies in HIV-infected obstetric patients with normal Pap smears. *Gynecol Oncol* 1997;65:430.

A significant false-negative rate in the presence of cervical intraepithelial neoplasia is associated with immunosuppression as measured by low CD4 counts.
9. Zweizig S, et al. Neoplasia associated with atypical glandular cells of undetermined significance on cervical cytology. *Gynecol Oncol* 1997;65:314.
Abnormal glandular cells of uncertain significance are a marker for neoplasia, and colposcopic biopsy (and in older women endometrial biopsy) is indicated.
10. Casper GR, Ostor AF, Quinn MA. A clinicopathologic study of glandular dysplasia of the cervix. *Gynecol Oncol* 1997;64:166.
Glandular dysplasia on biopsy should be further investigated with hysteroscopy and cone biopsy.

Diagnosis
11. Skehan M, et al. Reliability of colposcopy and directed punch biopsy. *Br J Obstet Gynaecol* 1990;97:811.
Laser and electrosurgical excisional therapy techniques provide a histopathologic quality control of colposcopic biopsy findings. The data indicate that biopsy is relatively unreliable and management should include consideration of the cytology and colposcopic findings.
12. Orr JW Jr, et al. The efficacy and safety of the cytobrush during pregnancy. *Gynecol Oncol* 1992;44:260.
Innovative techniques for endocervical cytologic sampling increase the endocervical cell yields, thus decreasing the prevalence of inadequate smears, and may improve the detection of abnormal smears.
13. Noller KL. Endocervical curettage: a technique in search of an indication?: debate. *Clin Obstet Gynecol* 1995;38:649.
Comparison of endocervical curettage with cytobrush showed that the predictive value of a positive test result is high, but a negative test result is not reassuring.
14. Lee KR, et al. Comparison of conventional Papanicolaou smears and a fluid-based, thin-layer system for cervical cancer screening. *Obstet Gynecol* 1997; 90:278.
The sample is collected into a vial containing a preservative solution. This study showed a significant improvement in specimen adequacy and cytologic diagnosis.
15. O'Leary TJ, et al. PAPNET-assisted rescreening of cervical smears: cost and accuracy compared with a 100% manual rescreening strategy. *JAMA* 1998;279:235.
Computerized image analysis automated techniques used for rescreening negative Pap smears to reduce false-negative rates were not found to be cost-effective in this study.
16. Kaufman RH, et al. Relevance of human papillomavirus screening in management of cervical intraepithelial neoplasia. *Am J Obstet Gynecol* 1997;176:87.
Identifying high- or low-risk viral types was not of value in identifying women who could be safely followed with cytology only.

Treatment
17. Eduardo AM, et al. Outpatient loop electrosurgical excision procedure for cervical intraepithelial neoplasia. Can it replace cold knife conization? *J Reprod Med* 1996;41:729.
The outpatient loop electrosurgical excision procedure for cervical intraepithelial neoplasia can replace cold knife conization, according to many clinicians.
18. Hatch KD. Cryotherapy. *Baillieres Clin Obstet Gynaecol* 1995;9:133.
Cryotherapy is suitable for the treatment of CIN 1 and 2, but often the transformation zone is not visible following cryosurgery, thus complicating follow-up.
19. Jones HW III. Cone biopsy and hysterectomy in the management of cervical intraepithelial neoplasia. *Baillieres Clin Obstet Gynaecol* 1995;9:221.
Problems sometimes encountered with cone biopsy include postoperative hemorrhage, unclear surgical margins, and adverse effects on future fertility. Advantages include definitive histologic diagnosis and retention of fertility in most cases.
20. Cullimore JE, et al. A prospective study of conization of the cervix in the management of cervical intraepithelial glandular neoplasia (CIGN)—a preliminary report. *Br J Obstet Gynaecol* 1992;99:314.

Cervical intraepithelial glandular neoplasia comprises cervical glandular atypia and adenocarcinoma in situ. The findings from this study suggest that further surgical treatment is unnecessary if the cone specimen margins are free of disease, but the authors recommend close follow-up with cytologic studies and colposcopy.

21. Robinson WR, et al. Management of cervical intraepithelial neoplasia during pregnancy with loop excision. *Gynecol Oncol* 1997;64:153.

Limited indications, significant morbidity, and residual disease are similar to those associated with cone biopsy.

22. Skjeldestad FE, et al. Residual and recurrent disease after laser conization for cervical intraepithelial neoplasia. *Obstet Gynecol* 1997;90:428.

Irrespective of conization technique, mild to moderate disease and free margins are associated with a low rate of residual disease.

23. Shafi MI, et al. Randomised trial of immediate versus deferred treatment strategies for the management of minor cervical cytological abnormalities. *Br J Obstet Gynaecol* 1997;104:590.

The authors recommend immediate therapy owing to high default rate and incorrect cytology reports.

24. Campion MJ, et al. Psychosexual trauma of an abnormal cervical smear. *Br J Obstet Gynaecol* 1988;95:175.

This study reports a significantly decreased frequency of intercourse, decreased vaginal lubrication, decreased sexual arousal, and decreased frequency of orgasm after the diagnosis and treatment of CIN.

25. Montz FJ. Impact of therapy for cervical intraepithelial neoplasia on fertility. *Am J Obstet Gynecol* 1996;175:1129.

After cone biopsy, the authors noted increased rates of second trimester abortions and preterm delivery. Few data are available for other commonly used therapies.

92. CARCINOMA OF THE CERVIX

Michel E. Rivlin

Widespread cytologic screening has had a major impact on the earlier detection and associated decrease in the incidence and mortality associated with cervical cancer. However, delay by some women in seeking health care will contribute significantly to the estimated 15,700 new cases and 4,900 deaths from the disease expected in the United States each year. Cervical cancer is the third most common female pelvic cancer, endometrial cancer being the most common. The average age at diagnosis is 45 years. Epidemiologic data indicate that the major risk factors for acquiring the disease include early age at first intercourse and multiple sexual partners. These patterns suggest a venereal form of transmission. There is a strong association between infection with human papillomavirus type 16 or 18 and the development of cervical dysplasia and carcinoma. If left untreated, carcinoma in situ (CIS) can develop into frankly invasive cancer over a period of from 3 to 20 years in 70% of patients. Squamous cell carcinoma accounts for about 87% of the cases, and adenocarcinoma for about 13%. Of the epidermoid cancers, 65% are large-cell nonkeratinizing, 23% are large-cell keratinizing, and 17% are small cell. Based on the degree of differentiation, the cancers are further graded I, II, or III, depending on whether they are well, moderately, or poorly differentiated.

It is important to estimate the extent of the disease as an aid to determining the prognosis, planning therapy, and comparing therapeutic approaches. The pretreatment clinical evaluation and staging of the cancer are based on the findings at pelvic examination. The remainder of the evaluation includes a chest x-ray study, intravenous pyelogram, and barium enema. Cystoscopy or sigmoidoscopy or both are indicated in patients with advanced-stage disease or with symptoms referable to those organs. Computed tomography and magnetic resonance imaging scans, as well as lymphangiography, may provide further information, especially in regard to lymph node involvement. Staging is usually reported using International Federation of Gynecology and Obstetrics (FIGO) definitions. In stage I, disease is confined to the cervix. Stage IA lesions are diagnosed only on the basis of microscopy findings, usually using a cone biopsy specimen: stage IA1 indicates invasion of stroma no greater than 3 mm deep and less than 7 mm wide, and stage IA2 signifies a depth of invasion of less than 5 mm from the base of the epithelium with a horizontal spread of less than 7 mm. These latter two patterns are often referred to as microinvasion. Vascular space involvement should not alter the staging. Stage IB includes lesions larger than those in stage IA2: IB1, less than 4 cm in size, IB2, greater than 4 cm in size. In stage II carcinoma, the disease extends beyond the cervix and may involve the upper two thirds of the vagina. In stage IIA, there is a lack of parametrial involvement, but, in stage IIB, there is obvious parametrial spread. In stage III, there is no cancer-free space between the tumor and pelvic wall, or the tumor involves the lower third of the vagina. In stage IIIA, the extension has not reached the pelvic wall but involves the lower vaginal third. In stage IIIB, there is extension to the wall, as evidenced by ureteric obstruction together with hydronephrosis or a nonfunctioning kidney. Stage IV carcinoma extends beyond the true pelvis and involves the bladder or rectal mucosa, with spread to adjacent organs classified as stage IVA, and to distant organs, stage IVB. Lymphatic spread is to the regional pelvic nodes (parametrial, hypogastric, obturator, and external iliac). Stage I cancers involve regional nodes in 15% to 20% of cases; stage II, 30% to 40% (10% of these patients have paraaortic node involvement as well). The paraaortic nodes are involved in 45% of stage III cancers. Blood-borne metastases are rare but may affect the lungs, brain, and bone. Unfortunately, it has been found that clinical understaging occurs in 30% to 40% of the cases; however, thorough surgical staging has had no clear impact on survival, such that staging laparotomy is not a routine procedure in patients with locally advanced disease, although many clinical trials have included this procedure. By convention, however, all cases retain their original clinical staging for the purpose of comparative data, even though the treatment may be altered by the surgical findings.

Intermenstrual, postcoital, and postmenopausal bleeding are the most common symptoms of invasive cancer, and a vaginal discharge is usually present. Pelvic pain, often unilateral and radiating to the hip or thigh, indicates late disease. Physical examination may reveal an exophytic or ulcerative growth with a firm consistency that is usually friable and hemorrhagic. A rectovaginal examination may reveal infiltration with nodular thickening of the uterosacral and cardinal ligaments. Urinary or fecal fistulas, or both, may be present with stage IV disease. Diagnosis in patients with a gross lesion is based on the findings yielded by a cervical punch biopsy specimen. Colposcopic and cone biopsies are indicated for patients with abnormal cytology and no gross lesion.

The treatment of microinvasive disease depends on the depth of stromal penetration. If it is no more than 3 mm, the probability of lymphatic involvement is under 2%, so that simple hysterectomy and, in rare instances where fertility is a factor, even cone biopsy is regarded as acceptable management. Cancer cure should approach 100% in this stage. If the depth of penetration exceeds 3 mm, the risk of nodal involvement increases to 5% to 10%, so radical hysterectomy and pelvic lymphadenectomy or radiotherapy is indicated. Stages IB and IIA disease can be treated either with radical hysterectomy and pelvic lymphadenectomy or radiotherapy, which comprises a combination of external-beam irradiation and brachytherapy (the temporary insertion of intrauterine and vaginal colpostats that are loaded with a radioisotope, usually cesium 137). Surgical treatment is usually selected for younger women to preserve ovarian function and avoid vaginal irradiation. Radiotherapy is used for older patients or those with medical contraindications to surgery. Results for both approaches are equivalent, with a 60% to 90% survival rate. The prognosis has as much to do with the nodal status as it does with the stage, such that when the stage is disregarded, there is an 80% survival rate for patients without lymphatic involvement, versus 20% if the nodes are involved. Most patients with stage IIB or III lesions are treated with external-beam radiation (total dose, 45–55 Gy), followed by intracavitary brachytherapy. Survival rates of 60% to 70% for stage IIB and 33% to 50% for stage III disease can be expected. Those patients with locally advanced disease at presentation (stage IVA) or locally recurrent cervical cancer after radiotherapy may be candidates for pelvic exenteration (surgical removal of the entire contents of the pelvis). Survival rates of 12% are quoted for stage IV disease. The overall cure rate for all stages is about 50% to 60%. Chemotherapy is used when radiation ports cannot encompass the extent of disease or when cancer recurs outside the pelvis. Cervical cancer is resistant to chemotherapy; the best single-agent treatment has been cisplatin, with response rates of about 38%. Combination therapy has been somewhat more successful, but median survival has not been improved, and toxicity is more severe. Recent studies, however, have shown marked improvement in survival with chemotherapy given concurrently with radiotherapy. Surgery, radiotherapy, and chemotherapy are discussed in greater detail in Chapters 98 through 100.

The recommended follow-up after therapy comprises history, physical examination, and vaginal cytologic studies at 4-month intervals for 2 years, then every 6 months for 3 years, and then annually. Chest x-ray studies and intravenous pyelograms are obtained only in symptomatic patients. Recurrences appear within 2 years in 80% of the patients; half of these are asymptomatic. The classic triad of recurrence consists of pain, unilateral leg edema, and ureteral obstruction. It is often difficult on clinical grounds to distinguish recurrence from radiation-induced changes. A tissue biopsy specimen should be obtained, and this may require surgical exploration if needle techniques are unsuccessful. Unfortunately, most recurrences are amenable to palliation only. Pain relief, using neurosurgical procedures where necessary, is an important aspect of therapy.

Occasionally the patient with cervical cancer is pregnant, and management depends on the extent of the tumor and the duration of the pregnancy. Before 24 weeks' gestation, the pregnancy may be disregarded and treatment with external-beam irradiation commenced. Abortion generally follows in 4 to 5 weeks, allowing internal therapy to be performed; if not, hysterotomy can be performed. In some pregnancies of more than 24 weeks' duration, fetal viability may be awaited, followed by cesarean delivery and the initiation of therapy. Surgical treatment may be chosen in place of irradiation, as in the nonpregnant woman.

Reviews
1. National Institutes of Health consensus development conference statement on cervical cancer. *Gynecol Oncol* 1997;66:351.
   A panel of experts provides a responsible assessment of current screening, prevention, and treatment approaches.
2. Burghardt E, Ostor A, Fox H. The new FIGO definition of cervical cancer stage 1A: a critique. *Gynecol Oncol* 1997;65:1.
   The staging of most cancers is periodically revised to incorporate new knowledge; this editorial critiques the 1994 modifications.
3. Ostor A, Rome R, Quinn M. Microinvasive adenocarcinoma of the cervix: a clinicopathologic study of 77 women. *Obstet Gynecol* 1997;89:88.
   Adenocarcinoma and squamous carcinoma of the cervix appear to share a similar prognosis and should probably be managed in the same way.

Epidemiology
4. Benedet JL, Anderson GH, Matisic JP. A comprehensive program for cervical cancer detection and management. *J Obstet Gynecol* 1992;166:1254.
   Comprehensive cytology and colposcopy programs reduce the incidence and mortality of cervical cancer, as well as the rates of in situ disease.
5. Bosch FX, et al. International biological study on cervical cancer (IBSCC) study group. *J Natl Cancer Inst* 1995;87:796.
   The prevalence of human papillomavirus in cervical cancer is discussed in terms of the worldwide perspective.
6. Larsen NS. Invasive cervical cancer rising in young white females. *J Natl Cancer Inst* 1994;86:6.

An upward trend in both incidence and mortality among younger women has been observed despite intensive screening efforts.

7. Fisher G, Harlow SD, Schottenfeld D. Cumulative risk of second primary cancers in women with index primary cancers of uterine cervix and incidence of lower anogenital tract cancers, Michigan, 1985–1992. *Gynecol Oncol* 1997; 64:213.
An increased incidence of vulvar, vaginal, and oral cancers suggests a shared etiology, probably human papillomavirus. An increase in smoking-related cancers, such as of the lung and bladder, also has been observed.

Diagnostic Evaluation

8. Maiman M, et al. Cervical cancer as an AIDS-defining illness. *Obstet Gynecol* 1997;89:76.
In this study, cervical cancer was the most common AIDS-related malignancy in women (55% of cases), followed by lymphoma (29%) and Kaposi's sarcoma (16%).
9. Fujiwara H, et al. Adenocarcinoma of the cervix: expression and clinical significance of estrogen and progesterone receptors. *Cancer* 1997;79:505.
Receptor status did not correlate with stage or survival.
10. Chou CY, et al. Accuracy of three-dimensional ultrasonography in volume estimation of cervical carcinoma. *Gynecol Oncol* 1997;66:89.
The authors describe an improvement over two-dimensional ultrasonography in estimating tumor volume.
11. Feigen M, Crocker EF, Read J. The value of lymphoscintigraphy, lymphangiography and computed tomography scanning in the preoperative assessment of lymph nodes involved by pelvic malignant conditions. *Surg Gynecol Obstet* 1987; 165:107.
Neither computed tomography, magnetic resonance imaging, nor lymphangiography demonstrate optimal sensitivity for lymph node metastases.
12. Chu K-K, et al. Laparoscopic surgical staging in cervical cancer–preliminary experience among Chinese. *Gynecol Oncol* 1997;64:49.
The authors suggest that laparoscopic pelvic and paraaortic lymphadenectomy was efficient and feasible for pretreatment evaluation.

Treatment

13. Lee Y-N, et al. Radical hysterectomy with pelvic lymph node dissection for treatment of cervical cancer: a clinical review of 954 cases. *Gynecol Oncol* 1989;32:135.
The authors suggest that radical hysterectomy is the treatment of choice in younger women with early invasive cancers because ovarian and vaginal function are preserved.
14. Massi G, Savino L, Susini T. Schauta-Amreich vaginal hysterectomy and Wertheim-Meigs abdominal hysterectomy in the treatment of cervical cancer: a retrospective analysis. *Am J Obstet Gynecol* 1993;168:928.
The extended vaginal hysterectomy (Schauta) yielded a high cure rate for stages IB and IIA cases, and may be indicated in the presence of obesity or elevated surgical risk.
15. Miller BE, et al. Carcinoma of the cervical stump. *Gynecol Oncol* 1984;18:100.
The survival rates were the same as those in patients with an intact uterus.
16. Hopkins MP, Morley GW. The prognosis and management of cervical cancer associated with pregnancy. *Obstet Gynecol* 1992;80:9.
The prognosis was not altered by pregnancy or the trimester at diagnosis.
17. Russell AH. Contemporary radiation treatment planning for patients with cancer of the uterine cervix. *Semin Oncol* 1994;21:30.
If the clinical staging is incorrect, such that tumor is actually present outside radiation fields, standard radiotherapy will be unsuccessful.
18. Choi DH, Huh SH, Nam KH. Radiation therapy results for patients undergoing inappropriate surgery in the presence of invasive cervical carcinoma. *Gynecol Oncol* 1997;65:506.
In patients who have undergone cut-through hysterectomy, possible treatments include radiation therapy and secondary radical surgery, with expectation of cure rates in the 75% range.

19. Malfetano JH, et al. Extended field radiation and cisplatin for stage IIB and IIIB cervical carcinoma. *Gynecol Oncol* 1997;67:203.
    The authors discuss prophylactic paraaortic node radiation and cisplatin as a radiation sensitizer, with an associated 75% survival rate.
20. Rose PG et al. Concurrent cisplatin-based radiotherapy and chemotherapy for locally advanced cervical cancer. *N Engl J Med* 1999;340:1144.
    Paclitaxel has moderate activity in squamous cell cancer of the cervix with a 17% response rate. The primary and dose-limiting toxicity is neutropenia.
21. Eddy GL. Neoadjuvant chemotherapy with vincristine and cisplatin followed by radical hysterectomy and pelvic lymphadenectomy for FIGO stage IB bulky cervical cancer: a Gynecologic Oncology Group pilot study. *Gynecol Oncol* 1995; 57:412.
    The author discusses the increased risk of failure for patients with a large volume of primary tumor, bilateral parametrial disease, nodal metastases, and poor performance status.

Recurrent Disease
22. Larson DM, et al. Diagnosis of recurrent cervical carcinoma after radical hysterectomy. *Obstet Gynecol* 1988;71:6.
    Ninety percent of patients who suffer recurrent carcinoma after radical hysterectomy do so within 2 years of surgery and must be monitored during this critical period.
23. Ito H, et al. Radiotherapy for centrally recurrent cervical cancer of the vaginal stump following hysterectomy. *Gynecol Oncol* 1997;67:154.
    Patients with local failure had a significantly higher incidence of metastases.
24. Al-Saleh E, et al. Cisplatin/etoposide chemotherapy for recurrent or primarily advanced cervical carcinoma. *Gynecol Oncol* 1997;64:468.
    The response rate was 39%, with a response duration of 5 to 36 months.

---

93. ENDOMETRIAL HYPERPLASIA

Michel E. Rivlin

Prolonged stimulation by either endogenous or exogenous estrogen, in the absence of progesterone, leads to endometrial hyperplasia in some premenopausal or postmenopausal women. Possible mechanisms include an abnormal estrogen metabolism, reduced levels of sex hormone-binding globulin, leading to a greater concentration of circulating steroid, and increased sensitivity of the endometrium. It is unclear why only some women respond in this manner. Hyperplasia may be defined as an abnormal increase in the amount of proliferative endometrium that exhibits varying degrees of architectural and cytologic atypia. Three distinct forms have been described: simple, complex, and atypical. Simple hyperplasias (cystic hyperplasia) are the most common. These conditions are characterized by the formation of dilated glands lined with cuboidal or tall columnar epithelium, producing the typical Swiss cheese appearance. The malignant potential is less than 1% in such patients, and most cases regress spontaneously. The complex hyperplasias (adenomatous hyperplasia and moderate adenomatous hyperplasia) are so named because of the complex architectural pattern involved, in which the glands become numerous and crowd the intervening stroma. The malignant potential of this entity is estimated at 1% to 4%. Atypical hyperplasias (severe adenomatous hyperplasia, adenomatous hyperplasia with atypia, and carcinoma in situ) are characterized by the existence of more glands, such that they are almost back to back; there is also cellular atypia (the cells display increased proliferation, enlarged vesicular nuclei, prominent nucleoli, and altered staining characteristics) and no separating stroma. An estimated 23% of these cases progress to cancer at a mean of 4 years. Adenocarcinoma is distinguished from atypical hyperplasia by the invasion of tumor cells into the stroma.

The risk factors for endometrial hyperplasia and endometrial cancer appear to be the same. There is overwhelming evidence that the unopposed effects of estrogen can bring about progression from normal proliferative endometrium through hyperplasia to malignant endometrium. The incidence of endometrial hyperplasia and malignancy is increased from two- to ten-fold in women treated with exogenous estrogens. The risk is related to both the dose and duration of exposure and diminishes with cessation of estrogen use. Anovulation may result from primary ovarian dysfunction, as it does in the setting of functioning ovarian tumors (e.g., granulosa cell tumor), or from disturbances in the neuroendocrine regulation of ovarian function, such as polycystic ovarian syndrome, with a consequent increased risk of hyperplasia and carcinoma. Other risk factors include nulliparity, early age of menarche, and late age at menopause. Obesity, hypertension, and diabetes are commonly associated with estrogen excess, and this is probably related to the conversion of adrenal androstenedione to estrone in adipose tissue. Progesterone-progestins oppose the mitogenic and proliferative stimuli of estrogen by suppressing deoxyribonucleic acid synthesis and the actions of the nuclear estradiol receptor. They also accelerate the conversion of estradiol to estrone by means of enzyme induction and stimulate inactivation of estrogen through the process of sulfurylation. The risk of hyperplasia and carcinoma in patients treated with exogenous estrogens for the alleviation of menopausal symptoms or as replacement therapy, such as for gonadal dysgenesis, can therefore be neutralized by the addition of progestin, given in a dosage and duration appropriate to those of the estrogen replacement therapy.

The sporadic bleeding that typically precedes menopause can make it difficult to know whether a full patient workup is necessary. Yet, because older women are at high risk for hyperplasia, any bleeding cannot be ignored. The most common definition of postmenopausal bleeding (PMB) is that which occurs more than 12 months after the last normal period. Hormonal correlates of the menopause include a level of follicle-stimulating hormone greater than 40 mU/ml, estradiol less than 25 pg/ml, and progesterone less than 0.5 ng/ml. No matter how minimal or remote the PMB occurs from the time of examination, it should always be investigated because endometrial cancer has been associated with all types of bleeding patterns. The causes of PMB include gynecologic malignancies in 10% to 20% of cases. The most common finding is endometrial atrophy, discovered in 60% to 80% of cases; vaginal atrophy may be the cause in about 15% of the cases. Hyperplasia causes 5% to 10% of the cases of PMB, and endometrial polyps 2% to 12%. The exogenous estrogens responsible for causing PMB vary with the population studied. Therefore, detailed questioning is vital to elicit information on the past or current use of estrogen medication. Gastrointestinal or urinary bleeding may be confused with vaginal bleeding and should be kept in mind.

The standard investigation of perimenopausal and postmenopausal bleeding includes a history directed at eliciting relevant risk factors, the bleeding pattern, and exogenous sources of estrogen. In the pelvic examination, obvious lesions and pelvic masses are sought and uterine size is evaluated. Pelvic ultrasonography is most helpful in identifying pelvic masses and in the measurement of endometrial thickness. Postmenopausal women with measurements under 5 mm are unlikely to have significant endometrial lesions. Sonography after installation of fluid into the cavity (saline sonohysterography) is effective in demonstrating intrauterine masses such as endometrial polyps. Special studies include cervical cytology, biopsy of any visible lesions, urinalysis, the stool guaiac test, hematocrit, and, in most instances, endometrial sampling. Papanicolaou (Pap) smear is positive in only 50% of the patients with invasive endometrial lesions, and although the results of endometrial cytology are reliable, they are insufficient for establishing a diagnosis in more than a third of the cases. The two usual methods for obtaining a histologic sample are (1) fractional dilatation and curettage (D&C), in which first the endocervix and then the endometrium are curetted, and (2) the endometrial aspiration biopsy. The former is usually a hospital-based procedure and therefore an expensive one; it carries about a 10%

false-negative rate. The latter procedure is inexpensive and can be performed in the physician's office, although it often is uncomfortable for the patient. It provides results similar to those yielded by D&C. Office sampling is appropriate as a first-step evaluation but may prove inadequate in older patients with cervical stenosis or in women with fibroids or an enlarged or irregular uterus. D&C is probably indicated in these patients. If hyperplasia is found, D&C should be performed to rule out the existence of adjacent foci of invasive disease. If atrophic endometrium is found, the patient should be closely monitored for the recurrence of bleeding.

In about half of the women with atrophic endometrium, no tissue is obtained; such patients may require a D&C or hysteroscopy, although some clinicians would await bleeding recurrence. Hysteroscopy is an important aid in the evaluation of abnormal bleeding and can be performed as an ambulatory procedure with a paracervical block. Failure rates of less than 5% have been achieved for this procedure, and failure is due to unsatisfactory visualization of the endometrial cavity. Recurrent bleeding requires further evaluation with D&C, hysteroscopy, and pelvic ultrasonography, as indicated in the individual patient, to rule out extrauterine malignancy. Younger patients with endometrial hyperplasia who desire children may be treated with ovulation induction. If attempts at ovulation induction fail and the hyperplasia persists, progesterone therapy followed by further attempts at ovulation induction should be tried. If atypical hyperplasia is present, hysterectomy is generally advisable. Management in older patients, the morbidly obese, or other patients with major surgical risk factors can consist of a progestational agent such as medroxyprogesterone acetate. Careful monitoring with endometrial biopsies is essential.

Endometrial cancer is the most common reproductive cancer in the United States and the fourth most common cancer in women. Three fourths of cases are diagnosed in postmenopausal women at an average age of 61 years. The incidence of endometrial carcinoma in women on combined estrogen-progestin regimens is not only reduced compared with the incidence in those on unopposed estrogen replacement, but it is also below that observed in untreated women. Some clinicians therefore recommend the performance of a progesterone challenge test in postmenopausal women. If withdrawal bleeding occurs, they recommend a monthly dosage with progestin to eliminate an unopposed estrogen action. If the progestin challenge yields negative results, the existence of endometrial atrophy and the absence of estrogen stimulation is presumed and the progestin therapy is discontinued.

In general, there may be two different types of endometrial cancer: one arising from endometrial hyperplasia and associated with hyperestrogenism, either endogenous or exogenous, and another (40%–50%) arising from an inert or atrophic endometrium and associated with compromised immune function secondary to aging. Of the two, the hormonally influenced group of endometrial cancers appears to be the less aggressive and to have a better prognosis.

Reviews
1. Burke TW, et al. Endometrial hyperplasias and endometrial cancer. *Obstet Gynecol Clin North Am* 1996;23:411.
   The risks of progression were described as follows: simple hyperplasia, 1%; complex hyperplasia, 3%; simple with atypia, 8%; and complex with atypia, 29%.
2. Skov BG, et al. Comparison of the reproducibility of the WHO classifications of 1975 and 1994 of endometrial hyperplasia. *Int J Gynecol Pathol* 1997;16:33.
   Squamous metaplasia or acanthosis (replacement of glandular cells by squamous cells) may be present. This change is found in normal endometrium but is more common (9.8%) in hyperplastic endometrium. This metaplastic squamous epithelium is capable of undergoing the same dysplastic and invasive changes as cervical, vaginal, or vulvar squamous epithelium.

Etiology
3. Woodruff JD, Pickar JH. Incidence of endometrial hyperplasia in postmenopausal women taking conjugated estrogens (Premarin) with medroxyprogesterone acetate or conjugated estrogens alone. *Am J Obstet Gynecol* 1994;170:1213.

After 3 years, women who were postmenopausal on no therapy had a 1.7% hyperplasia rate; those on estrogen and progesterone had a 0.5% to 2.9% rate; and those on estrogen only had a 20% to 62% rate.

4. McDonald TW, Malkasian GD, Gaffey TA. Endometrial cancer associated with feminizing ovarian tumor and polycystic ovarian disease. *Obstet Gynecol* 1977; 49:654.
   Endometrial cancer associated with a coexistent endogenous estrogen stimulus is usually low grade, low stage, and superficial, with a good prognosis.
5. Coulam CB, Annegers JF, Kranz JS. Chronic anovulation syndrome and associated neoplasia. *Obstet Gynecol* 1983;61:403.
   Women who do not ovulate are at increased risk for breast cancer, endometrial cancer, and pituitary adenoma.
6. Vitoratos N, et al. The role of androgens in the late-premenopausal woman with adenomatous hyperplasia of the endometrium. *Int J Gynecol Obstet* 1990;34:157.
   An increased availability of the precursor hormone androstenedione or an increased capacity for the extraglandular conversion of androstenedione to estrone occurs in older, obese women, the same population at high risk for endometrial neoplasia.
7. Cohen I, et al. Estrogen and progesterone receptor expression in postmenopausal Tamoxifen-exposed endometrial pathologies. *Gynecol Oncol* 1997;67:8.
   In the low estrogen environment of menopause, Tamoxifen acts as an estrogen agonist, rather than antagonist, inducing estrogen and progesterone receptors in the endometrium.
8. Cohen I, et al. Time-dependent effect of tamoxifen therapy on endometrial pathology in asymptomatic postmenopausal breast cancer patients. *Int J Gynecol Pathol* 1996;15:152.
   Of 164 women, 20% had an endometrial pathology, 11% had simple hyperplasia, 4% had polyps, 3% had complex hyperplasia, and 2% had cancer.

Pathology
9. Terakawa N, et al. The behavior of endometrial hyperplasia: a prospective study. Endometrial Hyperplasia Study Group. *J Obstet Gynaecol Res* 1997;23:223.
   The authors followed 51 patients with no therapy for 6 months. Most cases disappeared spontaneously, except for complex atypical cases, in which 80% persisted.
10. Kaku T, et al. Endometrial carcinoma associated with hyperplasia. *Gynecol Oncol* 1996;60:22.
    Of 115 carcinomas, 36% were associated with hyperplasia. The survival rate was 96% in those with hyperplasia compared to 73% in those without hyperplasia.
11. Van Bogaert LJ. Clinicopathologic findings in endometrial polyps. *Obstet Gynecol* 1988;71:771.
    Endometrial polyps may be the site of various types of hyperplasia and also may contain foci of carcinoma or accompany carcinoma elsewhere in the endometrium.
12. Michael H, et al. DNA ploidy, cell cycle kinetics, and low versus high grade atypia in endometrial hyperplasias. *Am J Clin Pathol* 1996;106:22.
    All hyperplasias and moderately differentiated cancers were diploid, and most poorly differentiated cancers were aneuploid. Neither S phase nor proliferative fractions could predict which hyperplasias were associated with cancer.

Diagnosis
13. Pickar JH, Archer DF. Is bleeding a predictor of endometrial hyperplasia in postmenopausal women receiving hormone replacement therapy? *Am J Obstet Gynecol* 1997;177:1178.
    Irregular bleeding was indicative of hyperplasia in women receiving unopposed estrogen but was not in women receiving concomitant progestins.
14. Haller H, et al. Transvaginal sonography and hysteroscopy in women with postmenopausal bleeding. *Int J Gynaecol Obstet* 1996;54:155.
    Hysteroscopy is particularly effective in the diagnosis of endometrial atrophy, polyps, and submucus fibroids.

15. Kufahl J, et al. Transvaginal ultrasound, endometrial cytology sampled by Gynoscann and histology obtained by Uterine Explora Curette compared to the histology of the uterine specimen. A prospective study in pre- and postmenopausal women undergoing elective hysterectomy. *Acta Obstet Gynecol Scand* 1997;76:790.

Of 181 women, ultrasonographic evaluation (cutoff limit of 4 mm endometrial thickness) missed one cancer and two hyperplasias, cytology missed two cancers and nine hyperplasias, and histology missed one cancer and two hyperplasias.

16. Goldstein SR. Saline infusion sonohysterography. *Clin Obstet Gynecol* 1996;39:248.

Filling the endometrial cavity with saline outlines any lesion projecting into the cavity, and this is particularly helpful in identifying submucosal fibroids and endometrial polyps.

17. Malinova M, Pehivanov B. Transvaginal sonography and progesterone challenge for identifying endometrial pathology in postmenopausal women. *Int J Gynaecol Obstet* 1996;52:49.

Withdrawal bleeding following progesterone administration in postmenopausal women indicates significant estrogen levels and therefore an increased risk of endometrial hyperplasia or neoplasia.

18. Ishii Y, Fujii M. Criteria for differential diagnosis of complex hyperplasia or beyond in endometrial cytology. *Acta Cytol* 1997;41:1095.

If endometrial cells are seen on Pap smears in postmenopausal women or if atypical endometrial cells are seen on Pap smears in premenopausal women, endometrial biopsy is indicated.

Management

19. Randall TC, Kurman RJ. Progestin treatment of atypical hyperplasia and well-differentiated carcinoma of the endometrium in women under age 40. *Obstet Gynecol* 1997;90:434.

Prolonged treatment, multiple endometrial biopsies, and careful monitoring are essential. Successful pregnancy can occur.

20. Kistner RW. Treatment of hyperplasia and carcinoma in situ of the endometrium. *Clin Obstet Gynecol* 1982;25:63.

In the postmenopausal patient, hysterectomy is indicated when any degree of endometrial hyperplasia is detected. In patients with major surgical risk factors, progestin therapy should be maintained for at least a year.

21. Persson I, et al. Risk of endometrial cancer after treatment with estrogens alone or in conjunction with progestogens: results of a prospective study. *Br Med J* 1989;298:147.

Estrogens alone are associated with a two- to threefold increase in the risk of neoplasia; the addition of progestins either removes this increased risk or delays its onset. Continuing follow-up is essential.

22. Effects of hormone replacement therapy on endometrial histology in postmenopausal women. The Postmenopausal Estrogen/Progestin Interventions (PEPI) Trial. The Writing Group for the PEPI Trial. *JAMA* 1996;275:370.

Endometrial hyperplasia caused by estrogen replacement therapy was reversed by progestin in 34 of 36 women.

23. Cerin A, Heldaas K, Moeller B. Adverse endometrial effects of long-cycle estrogen and progestogen replacement therapy. The Scandinavian Long Cycle Study Group. *N Engl J Med* 1996;334:668.

Hormone replacement therapy with progestin prescribed every third month was associated with 6.2% endometrial abnormalities after 3 years as compared with 0.8% with monthly progestin administration.

24. Agorastos T, et al. Treatment of endometrial hyperplasias with gonadotropin-releasing hormone agonists: pathological, clinical, morphometric, and DNA-cytometric data. *Gynecol Oncol* 1997;65:102.

Gonadotroph-releasing hormone agonists are an effective alternative to progesterone, as too are androgens (danazol).

25. Jick SS, Walker AM, Jick H. Oral contraceptives and endometrial cancer. *Obstet Gynecol* 1993;82:931.

Compared with never-users, women who had used oral contraceptives were 50% less likely to develop endometrial cancer.

94. ENDOMETRIAL CARCINOMA

Michel E. Rivlin

Endometrial carcinoma is the most common female pelvic malignancy in the United States. It is estimated that 37,400 women will develop this cancer and that 6,400 deaths will result from the disease in 1999. Carcinoma of the uterine corpus appears to be hormonally dependent, and epidemiologic factors are known. In obese women, androstenedione is converted to estrone in fatty tissue, and the resulting unopposed action of estrogen leads to a several-fold increase in the risk of endometrial cancer. Most estrogen-related cancers are well differentiated and superficially invasive, with an excellent prognosis. However, there is no room for complacency concerning endometrial cancer because the overall survival rate is lower in these women than in those with other early-stage gynecologic malignancies. The peak incidence occurs in those 58 to 60 years of age; only 10% of the cases arise in women under 50 years of age. Nulliparity, obesity, hypertension, and diabetes are frequently associated findings. Early menarche and late menopause are also risk factors.

The malignant epithelial tumors of the endometrium are usually classified using the World Health Organization (WHO) or International Federation of Obstetricians and Gynecologists (FIGO) systems. The two most common subtypes—endometrioid adenocarcinoma and adenocarcinoma with squamous metaplasia (previously referred to as adenoacanthoma)—have the best prognosis and constitute approximately 80% of the cases. Other subtypes, including papillary adenocarcinoma with squamous differentiation (previously adenosquamous carcinoma) and clear cell carcinoma, are associated with a much less favorable outcome. The tumors are graded according to the amount of non–gland-forming tumor. Grades 1, 2, and 3 indicate solid growth patterns in 5%, 6% to 50%, and more than 50% of the tumor, respectively. The less differentiated the tumor, the higher the incidence of deep myometrial penetration and of lymph node metastasis, and thus the worse the prognosis. The gross appearance is usually that of a friable tumor mass with areas of necrosis and hemorrhage. The tumor invades the myometrium and cervix. Lymphatic spread is to the pelvic nodes and then to the aortic nodes, although rarely direct spread to the aortic nodes may occur. Vaginal metastases are found in about 10% of the cases; hematogenous spread (to the lungs) occurs with advanced disease.

Abnormal bleeding occurs in about 80% of the cases. About 20% of the patients with postmenopausal bleeding have underlying cancer, and this increases to 50% to 60% after age 80. About 10% of the patients complain of uterine cramping and pain. If the uterine contents become infected, a pyometra develops, and signs of sepsis may supervene. The findings from physical examination are usually noncontributory unless the disease is advanced.

The revised system for staging endometrial cancer (FIGO, 1988) is based on the findings obtained at surgical exploration. Stage IA tumors are limited to the endometrium; stage IB tumors invade less than half the myometrium. Stage IC tumors invade more than half the myometrium. Stage IIA represents endocervical glandular involvement, stage IIB indicates cervical stromal invasion. In stage IIIA, tumor invades the serosa, or adnexa, or both, and peritoneal cytologic findings that are positive also place the patient in this stage. Stage IIIB represents vaginal metastases, and stage IIIC represents metastases to the pelvic or paraaortic lymph nodes, or both. In stage IVA tumors there is invasion of the bladder or bowel, and in stage IVB there are distant metastases, including intraabdominal or inguinal nodes, or both. In those patients (usually about 10% of the cases) who do not undergo surgical exploration because of medical contraindications to operation, the older FIGO (1979) clinical staging system is used.

Screening and initial diagnosis can be accomplished by either cytologic or histologic sampling (Papanicolaou smears are negative in 50% of cases); however, fractional dilatation and curettage (D&C; endocervix sampled before the endometrium) is the most reliable method. Sonography, sonohysterography, and hysteroscopy also have proved to be useful diagnostic adjuncts in skilled hands. The search for metastases includes chest x-ray studies and intravenous pyelography. Computed tomography or magnetic resonance imaging are rarely indicated. Clinical staging correlates poorly with surgical staging and may be incorrect in as many as 50% of women. Surgical evaluation includes removal of the uterus, tubes, and ovaries, sampling of the pelvic and paraaortic nodes, and cytologic examination of the washings from the pelvic cavity. Histopathologic evaluation of the depth of the myometrial invasion, the presence or absence of occult cervical or lymph node metastasis, the presence or absence of hormone receptors, and tumor grading complete the assessment for high-risk disease.

There appear to be two pathogenetic types of endometrial carcinoma. Type 1 is associated with obesity and estrogen excess, either exogenous or endogenous. The tumor is usually grade 1 or 2, depth of invasion is superficial, and nodal metastasis is infrequent. The stage is generally low, and the prognosis is excellent. Type 2 is not associated with obesity or estrogen; the tumor is often grade 3, with deep invasion; nodal metastasis is frequent; the stage high; and the prognosis poor. Individual cases may therefore be classified as low risk if they are stage 1, grade 1 or 2, nonserous and non–clear cell, with invasion of less than the inner third of the myometrium. They are intermediate risk if they are grade 3 or involve invasion of the middle third or deep third of the myometrium. And they are high risk if they are stage II or higher or serous or clear cell carcinoma.

Approximately 75% of cases are clinically stage I when diagnosed. Management of these women is primarily surgical, and often includes adjuvant radiotherapy in selected cases. Stage I grade 1 adenocarcinomas with less than one-third myometrial invasion and negative cytology are generally managed by extrafascial hysterectomy and adnexectomy. Features indicating a high likelihood of lymph node metastasis include grade 3 lesions, deep myometrial penetration, histologic cervical involvement, and a nonendometrioid histologic appearance. In these patients, selective pelvic and aortic node dissection is indicated. If the nodes contain cancer, postoperative pelvic and possibly also periaortic radiation therapy (45–50 Gy) is administered. This tailoring of therapy to the individual patient obviates the need for radiation treatment in the low-risk patient while providing the best available therapy for high-risk patients. Stage II carcinoma is diagnosed only if the histopathology indicates cervical stromal invasion, not only on an endocervical curettage containing floating fragments of adenocarcinoma. Treatment is the same as that for cervical cancer, with a choice between radical radiotherapy, radical surgery, and combinations of surgery and radiotherapy. Patients with stage III disease are not predictably cured of their disease. Following surgical staging, whole-pelvis radiotherapy (45–50 Gy) and paraaortic radiotherapy, if paraaortic nodes are positive, may be therapeutic choices. Stage IV disease may be treated with pelvic and abdominal radiotherapy or with progestins or chemotherapy. The overall response rate associated with progestin therapy has been reported to be 33% for patients with well-differentiated lesions and 10% for those with poorly differentiated lesions. Lesions with a high steroid receptor content respond more favorably than do those with a low receptor content. Cytotoxic chemotherapy is often used when hormonal therapy is ineffective. The combination of doxorubicin, cisplatin, and carboplatin yielded response rates of 15% or more, and paclitaxel has provided up to 35% response rates. Combining hormonal and cytotoxic chemotherapy does not appear to improve response. Five-year survival rates are 80% for patients in stage I, 70% in stage II, 30% in stage III, and 9% in stage IV.

Review
1. Rose PG. Endometrial carcinoma. *N Engl J Med* 1996;335:640.
   The estimated risk ratio for endometrial cancer is 3 for women 20 to 50 pounds overweight, and 10 for women more than 50 pounds overweight.
2. Boronow RC. Surgical staging of endometrial cancer: evolution, evaluation, and responsible challenge—a personal perspective. *Gynecol Oncol* 1997;66:179.
   Women with grade 1 lesions confined to the endometrium have a zero incidence of nodal metastasis; by contrast, those with grade 3 lesions and deep myometrial invasion have incidences of 34% pelvic and 23% paraaortic nodal metastases.

Diagnosis
  3. Langer RD, et al. Transvaginal ultrasonography compared with endometrial biopsy for the detection of endometrial disease. *N Engl J Med* 1997;337:1792.
     The anteroposterior two-layer thickness measured in the sagittal plane near the fundus generally does not exceed 4 or 5 mm in normal postmenopausal women.
  4. Bonilla-Musoles F, et al. Three-dimensional hysterosonography for the study of endometrial tumors: comparison with conventional transvaginal sonography, hysterosalpingography, and hysteroscopy. *Gynecol Oncol* 1997;65:245.
     Three-dimensional sonohysterography improved the determination of myometrial and cervical invasion.
  5. Hricak H, et al. MR imaging evaluation of endometrial carcinoma: results of an NCI cooperative study. *Radiology* 1991;179:829.
     Magnetic resonance imaging was better than sonography for the evaluation of myometrial invasion but is probably not sufficiently accurate to justify the cost.

Treatment
  6. Orr JW Jr, Holimon JL, Orr PF. Stage I corpus cancer: is teletherapy necessary? *Am J Obstet Gynecol* 1997;176:777.
     Extensive surgical staging including lymphadenectomy safely identified women who did not require adjunctive teletherapy without compromising their risk of survival.
  7. Rubin SC, et al. Management of endometrial adenocarcinoma with cervical involvement. *Gynecol Oncol* 1992;45:294.
     The preferred treatment of stage II disease has not been established. Some researchers advocate primary radical hysterectomy and others primary radiotherapy. Currently, an approach combining external and internal irradiation with surgery has yielded good results.
  8. Bloss JD, et al. Use of vaginal hysterectomy for the management of stage I endometrial cancer in the medically compromised patient. *Gynecol Oncol* 1991;40:74.
     The usual reasons for using the vaginal approach are obesity and coexistent medical problems. Careful case selection is the key to good results.
  9. Kim YB, et al. Progestin alone as primary treatment of endometrial carcinoma in premenopausal women: report of seven cases and review of the literature. *Cancer* 1997;79:320.
     Of the cases reviewed, 10 of 21 responded, and three had children after therapy.
 10. Price FV, et al. A trial of outpatient paclitaxel and carboplatin for advanced, recurrent, and histologic high-risk endometrial carcinoma: preliminary report. *Semin Oncol* 1997;24[Suppl 15):15–78.
     Systemic chemotherapy is used both as a salvage strategy and as adjuvant therapy in situations where the combination of surgery and radiation usually fail to provide a cure.
 11. Sood AK, et al. Value of preoperative CA 125 level in the management of uterine cancer and prediction of clinical outcome. *Obstet Gynecol* 1997;90:441.
     Levels less than 20 U/ml indicated a very low risk of extrauterine disease, and levels over 65 U/ml carried a 6.5-fold higher risk of extrauterine disease. Levels should be measured in all patients with endometrial cancer.
 12. Shumsky AG, et al. Risk-specific follow-up for endometrial carcinoma patients. *Gynecol Oncol* 1997;65:379.
     Recurrences occur within 3 years in 82% of patients who develop a recurrence, and 61% of these are symptomatic. The authors suggest that close follow-up should be reserved for symptomatic cases and those at high risk of recurrence.
 13. Chapman JA, et al. Estrogen replacement in surgical stage I and II endometrial cancer survivors. *Am J Obstet Gynecol* 1996;175:1195.
     There was no difference in recurrence or survival between patients given estrogen replacement and those from whom estrogen was withheld.

Pathology and Prognosis
 14. Yokoyama Y, et al. Indispensability of pelvic and paraaortic lymphadenectomy in endometrial cancers. *Gynecol Oncol* 1997;64:411.

Nodal metastases were found in all stages. Therefore, nodal sampling is necessary in order to select suitable postoperative therapy and to perform accurate FIGO staging in all patients except those with stage 1A grade 1 disease, those unfit for surgery, and those with stage IV cancer.

15. Descamps P, et al. Predictors of distant recurrence in clinical stage I or II endometrial carcinoma treated by combination surgical and radiation therapy. *Gynecol Oncol* 1997;64:54.

The most common sites for recurrence were peritoneal (28%), bone (28%), and lung (21%). Lymph node involvement was the strongest predictor for recurrence.

16. Milosevic MF, Dembo AJ, Thomas GM. The clinical significance of malignant peritoneal cytology in stage I endometrial carcinoma. *Int J Gynecol Cancer* 1992;2:225.

Malignant cytology is usually associated with other adverse prognostic factors that dominate the clinical course of the disease. Routine adjuvant treatment for this finding alone is therefore probably not justified.

17. Aalders JG, Abeler V, Kolstad P. Stage IV endometrial carcinoma: a clinical and histological study of 83 patients. *Gynecol Oncol* 1984;17:75.

The sites of extrapelvic extension of stage IV disease, in descending order of frequency, were the lungs (36%), multiple sites (23%), lymph nodes (13%), and bladder (13%).

18. Matthews RP, et al. Papillary serous and clear cell type lead to poor prognosis of endometrial carcinoma in black women. *Gynecol Oncol* 1997;65:206.

Patients are more likely to be black, to have advanced stage, and to have poor survival compared with women with endometrioid adenocarcinoma.

---

95. UTERINE SARCOMA

Michel E. Rivlin

Uterine sarcomas are a diverse group of malignancies that arise from connective tissue (mesenchymal) elements of the uterus. The most common are those that arise purely from the myometrium (leiomyosarcomas) or endometrial stroma (endometrial stromal sarcomas) and those with an epithelial component (malignant mixed müllerian, mesenchymal, or mesodermal tumors and adenosarcomas). Uterine sarcomas are rare and have a wide range of histologic appearance. They are classified into categories according to their histogenetic findings. Uterine sarcomas are described as pure if they contain only one cell type and as mixed if they contain more than one cell type. If the tissue elements are native to the uterus—for instance, smooth muscle—the tumor is termed *homologous*. If the tissue elements are not native to the uterus—for instance, striated muscle, cartilage, or bone—the tumor is termed *heterologous*. Uterine sarcomas constitute up to 4% of all uterine malignancies.

Abnormal uterine bleeding is the most common symptom (80%) of uterine sarcoma; abdominal pain or discomfort occurs in about 15% to 50% of patients; and about 10% are aware of an abdominal mass. Approximately 30% of patients complain of gastrointestinal or genitourinary symptoms. There may be a history of previous pelvic irradiation in as many as 10% of patients. Uterine sarcomas are classified using the International Federation of Obstetricians and Gynecologists (FIGO) staging system for uterine cancer: stage I, tumor confined to the corpus; stage II, tumor involving the cervix; stage III, tumor extending outside the uterus but confined to the pelvis; and stage IV, tumor extending beyond the pelvis or distant metastases. Leiomyosarcomas occur in younger age groups, with a median age of about 50 years; mixed mesodermal sarcomas afflict older patients, usually in the sixth and seventh decades of life; and endometrial stromal sarcomas typically arise in patients between the ages of 30 and

75 years, with a mean age of onset of 45 years. Mixed mesodermal sarcomas represent 60% of the cases; leiomyosarcomas, 30%; and other sarcomas, 10%.
Diagnostic workup is similar to that for endometrial cancer, although biopsy may miss deep-seated tumors. The main treatment modality is surgical and consists of total abdominal hysterectomy combined with bilateral salpingo-oophorectomy. Extended staging with washings for cytologic analysis and pelvic and paraaortic lymph node sampling is appropriate. Surgery alone carries a high risk of local recurrence and distant metastasis. Adjuvant radiation therapy enhances the pelvic control rate by sterilizing the primary tumor but has little influence on the final outcome. Adjuvant chemotherapy reduces the incidence of metastasis but effects no difference in survival.

Leiomyosarcoma arises from the myometrial smooth muscle and originates from a fibroid in approximately 5% to 10% of cases. The mitosis count (mitotic index) is helpful in distinguishing sarcoma from cellular smooth muscle tumors and is also a guide to prognosis because there is an inverse relationship between the mitotic index and the prognosis. When there are more than 10 mitoses per 10 high-power fields (hpf), the tumor is malignant; if there are less than five mitoses, the tumor is benign; and when there are five to nine mitoses, the tumor is malignant if cellular atypia is also present. Extension beyond the uterus is evidence of malignancy regardless of the mitosis count or pleomorphism. Spread occurs by means of local extension, vascular invasion, and peritoneal implantation. Distant metastases affect the lungs, kidneys, liver, brain, and bone. After surgery, neither radiotherapy nor chemotherapy has proved to be of added value in the management of this disease; however, adjuvant therapy is recommended if the tumor was not confined to the uterus or if the mitosis count is greater than 10 per 10 hpf. Other unusual smooth muscle tumors of the uterus include intravenous leiomyomatosis, in which fibrous extensions into vessels occur, sometimes involving the iliac veins, vena cava, and right heart. Most patients are premenopausal, and hormonal manipulation may be helpful in management. Because of the benign histology and slow growth of these tumors, repeated local excision is helpful. Benign metastasizing leiomyoma produces pulmonary metastases, which also appear to be hormonally influenced because they progress more rapidly in premenopausal than in postmenopausal women. Leiomyomatosis peritonealis disseminata features multiple peritoneal tumors. Chiefly found in blacks, it is often associated with pregnancy and usually regresses when the hormonal stimulus is removed.

Stromal sarcoma, arising from undifferentiated endometrial stromal cells, is the rarest of the three major uterine sarcomas. The diagnosis can be made based on the D&C findings in 75% of the patients. There are three distinct variants, based on the morphology, mitosis counts, and biologic behavior. The stromal nodule, with a mitosis count under five, is considered benign; endolymphatic stromal myosis is a low-grade infiltrating sarcoma that is also referred to as stromal endometriosis or stromatosis. This tumor is characterized by infiltrating margins, myometrial invasion, and a mitosis count of less than 10 per 10 hpf. Extension into lymphatic and venous channels is common. The tumor is associated with slow progression and late recurrences, with long-term survival the rule because repeated local excision can often control the disease. Endometrial stromal sarcomas are high-grade malignancies with mitosis counts above 10 per 10 hpf. Pelvic irradiation improves local control and is warranted even when the disease is confined to the uterus. The prognosis in these patients is poor.

Mixed mesodermal sarcomas characteristically occur in postmenopausal women, with the exception of embryonal rhabdomyosarcoma of the cervix or vagina (sarcoma botryoides), which afflicts infants and children. A significant number of patients may have a history of pelvic irradiation for the treatment of benign or malignant conditions. Microscopically, either the carcinoma or the sarcoma may be the major component. The carcinoma is usually endometrial and grade 2 or 3. The entire group exhibits a malignant endometrial stroma, usually in the form of an undifferentiated spindle cell or fusiform sarcoma. Mitosis counts are not useful in predicting outcome in this instance. It is not clear whether the heterologous mixed tumors have a worse prognosis than those composed entirely of native tissues. Metastases are usually composed of malignant glands, but sarcomatous elements also may be found. Because the tumor is endometrial in origin, diagnosis is made based on D&C findings in up to 75% of the cases. In most instances, the uterus is filled with fungating, hemorrhagic, necrotic tumor, and, in up to a third, lymphatic spread has taken place by the time of diagnosis. The standard therapy is surgical, followed by whole-pelvis radiotherapy; combination chemotherapy is given for the control of recurrence or metastases, with response rates as low as 10%. The prognosis depends on the extent of the tumor, with minimal survival likely if extrauterine spread has taken place. The exception is sarcoma botryoides, in which combination therapy consisting of surgery, irradiation, and chemotherapy has considerably improved the outlook and may be associated with a good prognosis.

The overall 3-year survival rate for women with uterine sarcomas is 20% to 50%. The survival rate in patients with stage I disease is better (50%–60%). Once a tumor extends to the cervix or outside the uterus, the survival rate decreases to about 10% to 15%; thus, the disease extent at diagnosis is the most important prognostic factor.

Review
1. Levenback CF, et al. Uterine sarcoma. *Obstet Gynecol Clin North Am* 1996;23:457.
   Sarcomas are rare tumors with unpredictable prognoses. Treatment is similar to that for endometrial cancers.
2. Nordal RR, Thoresen SO. Uterine sarcomas in Norway 1956–1992: incidence, survival and mortality. *Eur J Cancer* 1997;33:907.
   No change in 5-year survival was seen after the introduction of chemotherapy in management of the disease.

Classification
3. Ober WB, Tovell HMM. Mesenchymal sarcomas of the uterus. *Am J Obstet Gynecol* 1959;77:246.
   It is often difficult histologically to distinguish benign from malignant mesenchymal neoplasms.
4. Kempson RL, Bari W. Uterine sarcomas. Classification, diagnosis and prognosis. *Hum Pathol* 1970;1:331.
   This describes a modification of Ober's classification that is histogenetically correct and clinically applicable.

Pure Sarcomas
5. Leibsohn S, et al. Leiomyosarcoma in a series of hysterectomies performed for presumed uterine leiomyomas. *Am J Obstet Gynecol* 1990;162:968.
   The incidence of leiomyosarcoma in fibroids is estimated at 0.13% to 0.29%. Conservative therapy of fibroids can delay the diagnosis of leiomyosarcoma.
6. Soumakis S, et al. Quantitative pathology in uterine smooth muscle tumors: the case for the standard histologic classification criteria. *Eur J Gynaecol Oncol* 1997;18:203.
   Volume-corrected mitotic index and nuclear roundness coefficient were the two most significant prognostic factors.
7. Nordal RR, et al. The prognostic significance of surgery, tumor size, malignancy grade, menopausal status, and DNA ploidy in endometrial stromal sarcoma. *Gynecol Oncol* 1996;62:254.
   Free resection margins, malignancy grade, tumor diameter, and menopausal status are important prognostic factors.
8. Hall KL, et al. Analysis of Ki-ras, p53, and MDM2 genes in uterine leiomyomas and leiomyosarcomas. *Gynecol Oncol* 1997;65:330.
   Relatively few studies have addressed the molecular biology of uterine sarcomas. General genomic markers, specific genetic alterations, and markers of proliferation and differentiation may be helpful in management and prognosis.
9. Gadducci A, et al. Uterine leiomyosarcoma: analysis of treatment failures and survival. *Gynecol Oncol* 1996;62:25.
   Only early-stage disease is curable; therapy of advanced or recurrent disease is palliative.

Mixed Sarcomas

10. Marth C, et al. Parity as an independent prognostic factor in malignant mixed mesodermal tumors of the endometrium. *Gynecol Oncol* 1997;64:121.
    Outcome was better with increasing parity. Extent of tumor and depth of myometrial invasion were the most important prognostic factors.
11. Schwartz SM, et al. Exogenous sex hormone use, correlates of endogenous hormone levels, and the incidence of histologic types of sarcoma of the uterus. *Cancer* 1996;77:717.
    There may be a role for unopposed estrogen in the etiology of uterine sarcoma paralleling studies of endometrial carcinoma. For example, müllerian adenosarcoma has been associated with tamoxifen therapy.
12. Mark RJ, et al. Postirradiation sarcoma of the gynecologic tract. A report of 13 cases and a discussion of the risk of radiation-induced gynecologic malignancies. *Am J Clin Oncol* 1996;19:59.
    Postirradiation sarcoma occurred at a median interval of 17 years from therapy. The absolute risk is under 1%, and the prognosis is poor.
13. Nola M, et al. Prognostic parameters for survival of patients with malignant mesenchymal tumors of the uterus. *Cancer* 1996;78:2543.
    The most powerful prognostic indicator for stromal sarcomas was the DNA index; for leiomyosarcomas, clinical stage; and for mixed tumors, depth of myometrial invasion.
14. Arrastia CD, et al. Uterine carcinosarcomas: incidence and trends in management and survival. *Gynecol Oncol* 1997;65:158.
    Incidence in black women was twice that in white women. Adjunctive therapy shifted from radiation to cisplatin-based chemotherapy after 1980.
15. Balat O, et al. Sarcoma botryoides of the uterine endocervix: long-term results of conservative surgery. *Eur J Gynaecol Oncol* 1996;17:335.
    The botryoid type is a variant of embryonal rhabdomyosarcoma with a grapelike appearance. Excision with chemotherapy may be sufficient treatment for localized disease.
16. George E, et al. Malignant mixed müllerian tumor versus high-grade endometrial carcinoma and aggressive variants of endometrial carcinoma: a comparative analysis of survival. *Int J Gynecol Pathol* 1995;14:39.
    Mixed sarcomas are clinically more aggressive than endometrial carcinomas.
17. Kurjak A, et al. Uterine sarcoma: a report of 10 cases studied by transvaginal color and pulsed Doppler sonography. *Ultrasound Obstet Gynecol* 1997;9:101.
    All sarcomas studied had abnormal tumoral blood vessels with a mean resistance index of less than 0.40. Sonography may be useful in assessing the preoperative differential diagnosis.
18. Smith T, Moy L, Runowicz C. Müllerian mixed tumors: CT characteristics with clinical and pathologic observations. *Am J Roentgenol* 1997;169:531.
    Computed tomographic scanning was useful in defining the extent of disease, identifying metastases, and assessing therapeutic efficacy.
19. Barbazza R, et al. Role of fine-needle aspiration cytology in the preoperative evaluation of smooth muscle tumors. *Diagn Cytopathol* 1997;16:326.
    Fine-needle aspiration cytology may be helpful in distinguishing frankly benign from overtly malignant forms of smooth muscle tumors.

Treatment

20. Hoffman W, et al. Radiotherapy in the treatment of uterine sarcomas. A retrospective analysis of 54 cases. *Gynecol Obstet Invest* 1996;42:49.
    Adjuvant radiotherapy increased the rate of disease-free survival, especially if poor prognostic factors were present.
21. Chi DS, et al. The role of whole-pelvic irradiation in the treatment of early-stage uterine carcinosarcoma. *Gynecol Oncol* 1997;65:493.
    Whole-pelvic irradiation did not improve survival rates, but a trend toward improved pelvic control was observed.
22. Currie J, et al. Combination chemotherapy with hydroxyurea, decarbazine and etoposide in the treatment of uterine leiomyosarcoma. *Gynecol Oncol* 1996;61:27.
    These agents have moderate activity and moderate toxicity.

23. Resnik E, et al. A phase II study of etoposide, cisplatin, and doxorubicin chemotherapy in mixed müllerian tumors of the uterus. *Gynecol Oncol* 1995;56:370. *These agents are highly active in early-stage disease, moderately active in advanced.*

24. Sutton G, et al. Ifosfamide treatment of recurrent or metastatic endometrial stromal sarcomas previously unexposed to chemotherapy. *Obstet Gynecol* 1996;87:747. *Ifosfamide proved active in these patients.*

25. Wade K, et al. Uterine sarcoma: steroid receptors and response to hormonal therapy. *Gynecol Oncol* 1990;39:364. *The tumors are estrogen receptor positive in 48% and progesterone receptor positive in 30%; neither the receptor nor the use of adjuvant hormonal therapy affected survival.*

---

96. BENIGN OVARIAN NEOPLASMS

Michel E. Rivlin

Non-neoplastic functional ovarian cysts are the most common adnexal masses encountered in the reproductive years. Their significance lies in the fact that they must be differentiated from more serious ovarian or tubal lesions. Follicular and corpus luteum cysts are rarely larger than 6 cm in diameter, and they are unilateral and freely mobile. There may be associated menstrual abnormalities. Uncommonly, hemorrhage, torsion, or rupture of a cyst may constitute an acute abdomen. Observation, or a short course of oral contraceptive pills, is usually followed by disappearance of the cysts, which are dependent on gonadotropin stimulation. Theca lutein cysts are usually large and bilateral. They result from high levels of human chorionic gonadotropin (hCG), commonly stemming from trophoblastic disease. They also may appear after the use of ovulation-inducing agents such as clomiphene. Involution occurs once the hormonal stimulus is removed.

Most ovarian neoplasms (70%) are derived from the coelomic germinal surface epithelium. This epithelium is of paramesonephric (müllerian) origin, so these tumors contain epithelium similar to that lining adult müllerian structures (e.g., endocervix, endometrium, endosalpinx) and are named mucinous, endometrioid, or serous neoplasms, respectively. Serous cystadenomas account for 25% of benign ovarian tumors. In general, these neoplasms arise in the reproductive years. They may occur as unilateral, unilocular cysts, termed simple cystomas, but serous cystadenomas are usually multilocular and may have papillary excrescences; 20% may be bilateral. The papillary cystadenoma is the most likely to undergo malignant change. Symptoms depend on the size of the tumor and whether accidents, such as rupture or torsion, occur. They are treated by conservative surgical treatment in younger women and by removal of the uterus and adnexa in older women.

Mucinous cystadenomas account for 15% of benign ovarian tumors. Malignant change occurs in about 5%. They are multilocular tumors containing a thick mucinous substance secreted by the columnar epithelium lining the cyst. They are usually unilateral (bilateral in 10%) and can become very large. Papillary excrescences may develop and increase the malignant potential. The clinical picture and management of the mucinous cystadenomas are similar to those for serous tumors.

The remaining benign epithelial tumors are uncommon. Endometrioid and mesonephroid (clear cell) cysts are included in this category and are extremely rare. The Brenner tumor, composed of nests of epithelial cells in a fibrous stroma, accounts for 1% of ovarian tumors. Usually found in postmenopausal women, the malignant potential is low. The tumor also may occur in conjunction with mucinous or dermoid cysts. Management usually consists of removal of the uterus and adnexa because of the patient's age.

About 20% of primary ovarian neoplasms are derived from germ cells. The mature cystic teratoma (dermoid), the most common tumor of young women, is second only to the serous tumor in frequency in all age groups. The tumor may contain tissues derived from all three germ layers, although ectodermal elements (particularly sebaceous fluid and hair) usually predominate. In 15%, functional or nonfunctional thyroid tissue may be present. The tumor is mobile and may lie anterior to the uterus. Malignant change is rare. Symptoms are uncommon unless a complication (usually torsion) occurs. Dermoids display a characteristic sonographic pattern of sharply defined fluid levels, dense echoes, and cystic areas. The approach to management is generally conservative surgical treatment consisting of ovarian cystectomy and careful examination of the opposite ovary, because 15% are bilateral. In older patients, the uterus and adnexa should be removed.

Approximately 5% of primary ovarian neoplasms are derived from sexually undifferentiated mesenchymal tissue. The fibroma, a connective tissue tumor composed of fibroblasts and collagen, is relatively common and accounts for 20% of solid ovarian tumors. The tumors vary greatly in size and are bilateral in 10% of patients. Generally symptomless, or exerting pressure effects if large, about 75% have a degree of ascites, whereas 3% exhibit Meigs syndrome (hydrothorax with ascites). The average age at diagnosis is 48 years; the usual approach to therapy is hysterectomy with removal of the adnexa, although malignant change is rare and oophorectomy is sufficient in the younger patient. Other supporting tissue tumors, such as myxoma, lipoma, and hemangioma, are occasionally seen, but all are rare.

An additional 5% of ovarian tumors are derived from specialized gonadal stroma (sexually differentiated mesenchymal tissue). These are "functioning" tumors capable of producing either estrogen (granulosa-theca cell), androgen (Sertoli-Leydig cell), or both (gynandroblastoma). The majority of these tumors are potentially malignant, however, and therefore are not regarded as benign.

Generally, most ovarian neoplasms are clinically silent, except for pressure symptoms such as urinary frequency, constipation, and pelvic heaviness. Very large tumors cause abdominal swelling and discomfort and might be confused with pregnancy. Pain may be felt, owing to stretching of the ovarian capsule or to torsion, rupture, or intracystic hemorrhage. If the tumors are functional, menstrual abnormalities may occur.

On physical examination, most of the ovarian tumors will be found lying behind the uterus or they will have ascended into the abdomen, although dermoids may be anteriorly placed. Benign tumors tend to be unilateral, cystic, movable, and symmetrical; there is no ascites. By contrast, malignant growths are usually bilateral, solid, fixed, and nodular, and there is ascites. Diagnostic evaluation should include sonography, and in some circumstances chest and abdominal x-ray examination, as well as an intravenous pyelogram. Further investigations depend on the individual case and may include bowel x-ray studies and laparoscopy. Estimation of the CA 125 levels, which are elevated in many cases of serous ovarian cancers, may be helpful, although many benign conditions exhibit this elevation as well. Alternative imaging techniques, including computed tomography and magnetic resonance imaging, are also being used more frequently in the assessment of pelvic masses. Color Doppler sonographic studies for vascular resistance may be helpful because resistance is lowest in malignant tumors. The differential diagnosis of adnexal masses includes benign ovarian tumors, functional ovarian cysts, ovarian malignancies, paraovarian cysts (benign lesions in the broad ligament), endometriosis, acute and chronic inflammatory masses, ectopic gestation, pedunculated fibroids, congenital uterine anomalies, and gastrointestinal masses. Careful history, physical examination, and relevant ancillary investigations are essential to ensure adequate management.

Women between the ages of 15 and 45 years with clinically benign ovarian cysts less than 6 cm in diameter may be observed on a monthly basis for a short period of time, but premenarchal and postmenopausal females are at high risk for malignancy, and early diagnosis is thus essential. Cysts greater than 10 cm in diameter are probably neoplastic and require immediate evaluation and probable excision. Almost all solid ovarian tumors are neoplastic (with the exception of the rare luteoma of pregnancy) and mandate aggressive evaluation and therapy. If a cyst persists or enlarges during a period of observation, one should proceed with evaluation and probably surgical excision. If the cyst persists but gets smaller, the patient may be observed through a second cycle. Cyst aspiration for diagnosis/management is problematic because of the danger of leakage from a malignant tumor.

When laparotomy is indicated, it is performed as soon as diagnostic procedures are completed. If malignancy is a possibility, bowel preparation should precede operation and facilities for definitive staging surgery of ovarian cancer should be reserved. Features of benign disease include a unilateral, freely mobile, smooth cyst with no ascitic fluid, and smooth peritoneal surfaces. If there is any doubt, frozen sections should be obtained. In older patients, total abdominal hysterectomy with bilateral salpingo-oophorectomy is the treatment of choice, even in patients with benign neoplasms. In younger patients with benign disease, conservative surgical treatment is the rule. Ovarian cystectomy or unilateral salpingo-oophorectomy, performed with great care to determine whether there is disease in the remaining ovary, is the usual procedure. Because the lesions are benign, the prognosis is excellent.

If the diagnostic investigation reveals findings that are overwhelmingly in favor of benign disease, many clinicians currently approach the surgery of adnexal disease, including ovarian masses, laparoscopically. Because of the risk of mismanagement of a malignant growth, however, it should be used only in a highly select group of women and should be performed only by clinicians with special expertise in its application.

Functional Cysts
1. Expectant management of functional ovarian cysts: an alternative to hormonal therapy. *Int J Gynaecol Obstet* 1994;47:257.
   Nearly all functional cysts disappear without treatment. Oral contraceptives may hasten the time of resolution.
2. Lanes SF, et al. Oral contraceptive type and functional ovarian cysts. *Am J Obstet Gynecol* 1992;166:956.
   The protective effect of oral contraceptives against functional ovarian cysts reported previously for high-dose monophasic pills may be attenuated with newer pills of lower hormonal potency.
3. Gerber B, et al. Simple ovarian cysts in premenopausal patients. *Int J Gynaecol Obstet* 1997;57:4.
   Neither ultrasonography nor cyst fluid cytology nor clinical findings provided a reliable diagnosis. If simple cysts persist for 2 cycles or 8 weeks, they should be removed by laparoscopy and not by aspiration.
4. Ishihara K, Nemoto Y. Sonographic appearance of hemorrhagic ovarian cyst with acute abdomen by transvaginal scan. *Nippon Ika Daigaku Zasshi* 1997;64:411.
   Hemorrhage into functional cysts is more frequent in a younger age group (10–20 years old) and in the luteal phase. Laparotomy is seldom necessary, and conservative follow-up with clinical and sonographic monitoring is advised.
5. Oelsner G, et al. Long-term follow-up of the twisted ischemic adnexa managed by detorsion. *Fertil Steril* 1993;60:976.
   Detorsion at laparotomy or laparoscopy may obviate the need for adnexectomy, the generally accepted treatment.
6. Kobayashi H, et al. Changes in size of the functional cyst on ultrasonography during early pregnancy. *Am J Perinatol* 1997;14:1.
   Cysts larger than 10 cm in diameter should be removed in the second trimester. Urgent laparotomy is indicated if torsion, rupture, or obstructed labor occurs. Cysts between 5 and 10 cm can be managed conservatively, if they are simple, but they should be removed if they contain septae or nodules or are solid.
7. Foulk RA, et al. Hyperreactio luteinalis differentiated from severe ovarian hyperstimulation syndrome in a spontaneously conceived pregnancy. *Am J Obstet Gynecol* 1997;176:1300.
   Benign ovarian cysts that can cause virilization in pregnancy include theca lutein cysts and luteoma of pregnancy, and management is conservative because they regress after delivery.

Neoplasms Derived from Coelomic Epithelium
8. Parazzini F, et al. Risk factors for seromucinous benign ovarian cysts in northern Italy. *J Epidemiol Commun Health* 1997;51:449.
    Menstrual irregularity and infertility were risk factors for benign ovarian cysts in this study.
9. Woodruff JD, Novak ER. Papillary serous tumors of the ovary. *Am J Obstet Gynecol* 1954;67:1112.
    One fourth of papillary serous cystadenomas contain microscopic calcospherites (psammoma bodies), which may show up on x-ray.
10. Chaitin BA, Gershenson DM, Evans HL. Mucinous tumors of the ovary. A clinicopathologic study of 70 cases. *Cancer* 1985;55:1958.
    Mucinous tumors are frequently associated with other cystomas, particularly serous and Brenner tumors, as well as teratomas. Malignancy occurs in 5% to 10% of primarily benign mucinous cysts.
11. Kahn MA, Demopoulos RI. Mucinous ovarian tumors with pseudomyxoma peritonei: a clinicopathological study. *Int J Gynecol Pathol* 1992;11:15.
    Rupture of a mucinous tumor can lead to diffuse intraperitoneal spread, a syndrome called pseudomyxoma peritonei.
12. Yoonessi M, Abell MR. Brenner tumors of the ovary. *Obstet Gynecol* 1979;54:90.
    Three in 24 cases were malignant in this study.

Neoplasms Derived from Germ Cells
13. Caspi B, et al. The growth pattern of ovarian dermoid cysts: a prospective study in premenopausal women. *Fertil Steril* 1997;68:501.
    Teeth are present in nearly 50% of benign cystic teratomas and can be visualized on x-ray. Within the cyst wall, a nodule, Rokitansky's protruberance, may be noted.
14. Lack EE, Young RH, Scully RC. Pathology of ovarian neoplasms in childhood and adolescence. *Pathol Annu* 1992;27:281.
    Although rare, these ovarian tumors can be malignant; the most common are germ cell tumors. Surgical treatment, if indicated, should be conservative (cystectomy or unilateral oophorectomy) whenever feasible.
15. Kawai M, et al. Seven tumor markers in benign and malignant germ cell tumors of the ovary. *Gynecol Oncol* 1992;45:248.
    These tumor markers include alpha-fetoprotein in yolk sac tumor and immature teratoma, lactate dehydrogenase in dysgerminoma, CA 19-9 in teratomatous growths and CA 125 in all tumor types except mature cystic teratoma.
16. Kempers RD, et al. Struma ovarii—ascitic, hyperthyroid, and asymptomatic syndromes. *Ann Intern Med* 1970;72:883.
    The term struma ovarii is used when thyroid is the predominant tissue in a dermoid.

Neoplasms Derived from Nonspecific Mesenchyme
17. Aboud E. A review of granulosa cell tumours and thecomas of the ovary. *Arch Gynecol Obstet* 1997;259:161.
    Thecomas are regarded as benign and granulosa cells as likely to recur years after an apparent cure. Both tumors may produce estrogen and may be associated with endometrial hyperplasia or carcinoma.
18. Outwater EK, et al. Ovarian fibromas and cystadenofibromas: MRI features of the fibrous component. *J Magn Reson Imaging* 1997;7:465.
    The ovarian fibroma is not easily distinguishable from the thecoma clinically or histologically.
19. Meigs JV. Fibroma of the ovary with ascites and hydrothorax—Meigs' syndrome. *Am J Obstet Gynecol* 1954;67:962.
    This change occurs in less than 5% of fibromas.

Diagnosis
20. Lim FK, et al. Pre and intraoperative diagnosis of ovarian tumours: how accurate are we? *Aust N Z J Obstet Gynaecol* 1997;37:223.

Statistically, the likeliest diagnosis for an ovarian mass in women over age 50 would be cancer, endometriosis in women 30 to 49, and dermoid in women under age 30.

21. Levine CD, et al. Benign extraovarian mimics of ovarian cancer. Distinction with imaging studies. *Clin Imaging* 1997;21:350.
   A wide spectrum of benign extraovarian pathology may closely resemble ovarian cancer. Magnetic resonance imaging or computed tomography may be helpful in the presence of indeterminate sonographic findings.
22. Reles A, et al. Transvaginal color Doppler sonography and conventional sonography in the preoperative assessment of adnexal masses. *J Clin Ultrasound* 1997;25:217.
   Color Doppler sonography can detect the low-resistance intratumoral blood vessels characteristic of malignant tumors and is therefore a useful adjunct to conventional sonography.

Management
23. Magrina JF, Cornella JL. Office management of ovarian cysts. *Mayo Clin Proc* 1997;72:653.
   If benign on clinical and sonographic examination and CA 125 levels are normal, ovarian cysts are almost always truly benign.
24. Gallup DG, Talledo E. Management of the adnexal mass in the 1990s. *South Med J* 1997;90:972.
   Laparoscopy for suspicious masses is only acceptable if immediate appropriate surgical staging is available for patients found to have cancer.
25. Trimbos JB, Hacker NF. The case against aspirating ovarian cysts. *Cancer* 1993;72:828.
   Aspirating ovarian cysts, except for oocyte retrieval, is potentially dangerous and frequently followed by cyst recurrence.
26. Yuen PM, et al. A randomized prospective study of laparoscopy and laparotomy in the management of benign ovarian masses. *Am J Obstet Gynecol* 1997;177:109.
   Operative laparoscopy should replace laparotomy in the management of benign ovarian masses.
27. Gotlieb WH, et al. Borderline tumors of the ovary: fertility treatment, conservative management, and pregnancy outcome. *Cancer* 1998;82:141.
   Conservative treatment is usually adequate, and fertility, pregnancy outcome, and chances of survival remain excellent.
28. Schmahmann S, Haller JA. Neonatal ovarian cysts: pathogenesis, diagnosis and management. *Pediatr Radiol* 1997;27:101.
   Sonography can reveal fetal or neonatal ovarian cysts. Conservative treatment is generally successful, but torsion and amputation may occur, so prophylactic aspiration may be indicated if they are large.
29. Ng PH, Hewson AD. The residual adnexa syndrome. *Aust N Z J Obstet Gynaecol* 1993;33:71.
   Ovaries and tubes left in site at the time of hysterectomy may become symptomatic and require removal.
30. Lafferty HW, et al. Ovarian remnant syndrome: experience at Jackson Memorial Hospital, University of Miami, 1985 through 1993. *Am J Obstet Gynecol* 1996;174:641.
   Remnants of ovary left behind at previous surgery may cause pain. Surgical removal is difficult, and ureters and great vessels are at risk for injury.

97. OVARIAN CARCINOMA

Michel E. Rivlin

Cancer of the ovary are the second most common gynecologic malignancy. In 1999, 25,200 new cases are expected in the United States, with 14,500 deaths. The mean age at onset is 62 years. Late menarche, early menopause, pregnancy, and oral contraception all appear to confer a protective effect by effecting ovulation suppression. Hereditary disorders, diet, environmental factors, viral infection, and irradiation have been implicated in the etiology.

Ovarian cancer is classified histologically into epithelial, gonadal stromal, and germ cell tumors. Of the malignant tumors, 40% to 45% are serous, 5% to 10% are mucinous, 15% to 20% are endometrioid, and 4% to 6% are clear cell. Epithelial adenocarcinomas are further differentiated into borderline and malignant types. Borderline growths display nuclear abnormalities and cellular stratification but lack stromal invasion. Gonadal stromal tumors (e.g., granulosa cell, Sertoli-Leydig cell) constitute 5% to 10% of ovarian cancer. Of the germ cell tumors, dysgerminoma (1%–2%), embryonal carcinoma (1%–2%), and immature teratoma (1%–2%) are the most common. Metastatic tumors (4%–8%) are generally derived from the bowel, endometrium, breast, or thyroid. Spread takes place over the surface of the peritoneum and the bowel and then extends to the upper abdomen. If there is nodal involvement, it usually affects the retroperitoneal nodes of the upper abdomen. Iliac nodes are involved about a fourth as often as in cervical cancer. Hematogenous spread is rarely seen clinically, but transdiaphragmatic dispersion is common.

Staging of ovarian cancer is based on the findings at laparotomy. In stage IA, growth is limited to one ovary; in stage IB, both ovaries are involved. Stage IC is either stage IA or IB, but tumor is also on the surface of the ovary, the capsule is ruptured, ascites is present, or the cytologic analysis of peritoneal washings yields positive findings. Stage II disease involves one or both ovaries and there is pelvic extension. Stage IIA involves extension or metastases to the uterus or tubes; stage IIB involves extension to other pelvic tissues; and stage IIC is stage IIA or B, plus there is ascites or positive washings, a ruptured capsule, or tumor on the ovarian surface. In stage III, tumor growth extends outside the pelvis, with peritoneal implants or positive retroperitoneal or inguinal nodes, or both. Superficial liver metastases are considered stage III, and this stage is further divided into IIIA through IIIC. Stage IV represents distant metastasis and includes pleural effusions with positive cytology and parenchymal liver metastasis.

The detection of a pelvic mass is often the first indication of an ovarian tumor, although many patients experience vague gastrointestinal symptoms for several months before the mass is discovered. Rarely, endocrine activity of the tumor may lead to menstrual abnormality. Although pelvic findings can be inconclusive, palpation of an irregular, nodular ("a handful of knuckles"), insensitive, bilateral mass in the pelvis strongly suggests the presence of an ovarian tumor. The disease is bilateral in 70% of cases of ovarian carcinomas, compared with 5% for benign lesions. Ascites and a right-sided pleural effusion are common findings in advanced disease. Imaging techniques such as computed tomography, magnetic resonance imaging, and sonography are more useful for monitoring the course of the disease than for making an early diagnosis.

Serum tumor markers are useful in the diagnosis and management of several types of ovarian tumors. CA 125 levels are elevated in more than 80% of patients with serous epithelial cancers but in only 1% of the normal population. Levels of this marker also may be elevated in association with endometriosis, pelvic inflammatory disease, fibroids, and other malignancies, however. Alpha-fetoprotein serum levels are elevated in endodermal sinus tumors and embryonal cell cancers. Levels of human chorionic gonadotropin are elevated in ovarian trophoblastic disease and may be elevated in embryonal cell carcinoma and dysgerminoma. The lactate dehydrogenase may be elevated in patients with dysgerminoma. CA 19-9 may be elevated in the setting of mucinous ovarian and gastrointestinal cancers. Carcinoembryonic antigen levels are sometimes elevated in association with ovarian cancer, but this finding is not specific for this cancer. None of the tumor markers are sensitive or specific enough to be considered for routine screening, but they are helpful in the differential diagnosis of pelvic masses and in the follow-up of treated cases.

Prime indications for exploratory laparotomy include a pelvic mass appearing after menopause; an adnexal mass at any age, progressively enlarging beyond 5 cm in diameter; adnexal masses 10 cm in diameter or larger; and masses that cannot be identified definitely as either fibroid or carcinoma. The preoperative workup should include an upper and lower bowel series, intravenous pyelography, and bowel preparation. This evaluation documents the extent of disease and helps determine whether the cancer is primary or metastatic. The goal of the primary surgical procedure is to remove the entire cancer or, if this is not feasible, to remove as much of the cancer as possible (debulk) without causing excessive morbidity or mortality. The early results of these major procedures have been improved by the liberal use of hyperalimentation, antibiotics, and critical care monitoring techniques. Conservative surgical treatment has no place in patients over 40 years of age with epithelial tumors, which account for 90% of ovarian cancers.

After an adequate midline incision has been made, cytologic evaluation of the pelvis, paracolic gutters, and subphrenic areas is conducted. Palpation and inspection of all peritoneal surfaces, including the liver, diaphragm, and pelvic and periaortic nodes, are followed by biopsy of suspicious areas. Total hysterectomy, bilateral salpingo-oophorectomy, omentectomy, and appendectomy should then be performed. In young, nulliparous patients with stage IA lesions whose gross and microscopic pathologic findings are favorable, unilateral adnexectomy is an option.

Chemotherapy should be administered to patients with stage II, III, or IV tumors. The effect of adjuvant chemotherapy is unclear but can improve the quality of life. Chemotherapy for stage I disease can be either single or multiagent and make use of drugs such as melphalan or cisplatin. The benefit of therapy for low-grade lesions must be weighed against the risk of its causing subsequent acute leukemia. Stage III and IV disease is generally treated with multiagent regimens that include cisplatin and paclitaxel. External radiotherapy has been phased out as an adjuvant measure in most centers, with the exception of its use in the treatment of germ-cell and gonadal stromal tumors, which are more responsive to this modality. However, in some hands, external radiotherapy has yielded good results and is still used. Another form of adjuvant therapy, the intraperitoneal instillation of radioactive phosphorus or platinum, also has been used with some success. After initial or adjunctive therapy in patients with no evidence of disease, some oncologists proceed to second-look surgery, an operation designed to evaluate the presence and extent of residual disease, if present. The techniques of this procedure are similar to those used for the original staging procedure. Chemotherapy may then be discontinued in patients with no evidence of disease, whereas those found to have disease may receive agents different from those previously administered. However, there are no hard data to prove that the second-look operation has led to improved long-term survival.

Problems to be palliated in patients with advanced ovarian cancer include ascites, pleural effusions, intestinal or urinary tract obstruction, and bowel fistula. Repeated paracentesis, nasogastric intestinal decompression, total parenteral nutrition, and conservative bypass operation all play roles in the management of these difficult situations.

The prognosis varies: approximately 70% of stage I, 50% of stage II, 15% of stage III, and less than 5% of stage IV patients survive 5 years. Sixty percent to 70% are either stage III or IV at the time of initial diagnosis, however, so there is only a 15% to 25% overall 5-year survival rate. The cause of death is usually related to diminished immunocompetence (resulting in severe sepsis) and malnutrition (associated with bowel obstruction).

Germ cell cancers are highly malignant and arise predominantly in the second or third decade of life. Characteristically unilateral (66%), the most common is the dysgerminoma, a tumor that is similar to the seminoma and arises from the primitive germ cell. Stage IA dysgerminomas can be treated by unilateral adnexectomy.

Recurrences occur in 10% to 20% of cases, but subsequent chemotherapy or radio-therapy is successful in controlling disease in 90%. Advanced disease is treated by hysterectomy with adnexectomy and postoperative chemotherapy or irradiation administered to the pelvic and paraaortic nodes. The embryonal carcinoma and immature teratoma arise from embryonal cells. Patients with these tumors are good candidates for conservative operation, followed by combination chemotherapy, to which they generally respond well. The endodermal sinus tumor and choriocarcinoma are derived from extraembryonic tissue. The former responds well to combination chemotherapy, and conservative operation is recommended because up to 75% of cases can be cured even while preserving fertility. Adjuvant chemotherapy is often recommended even for stage IA tumors.

Gonadal stromal malignancies include granulosa and Sertoli-Leydig cell cancers, which are usually unilateral with low-grade malignancy, and recurrence is typically confined to the pelvis. Late recurrences are not uncommon. Early disease in young patients may be treated conservatively.

The gonadoblastoma is composed of both germ cell and gonadal stromal cell tumors, in varying combinations. Most patients are intersexual, and 90% are chromatin negative. The malignant potential is determined by the type of germ cell tumor present. Generally, bilateral gonadectomy is indicated.

The lifetime risk of ovarian cancer in the general population is one in 70; in a woman with one first-degree relative with the disease, the risk is 5%; if the woman has two or more first-degree relatives with the disease, 7%. In this last group, there is a 3% risk of having an autosomal-dominant syndrome, placing them at an approximately 40% risk. The three known hereditary syndromes are familial site-specific ovarian cancer syndrome, breast-ovarian cancer syndrome, and Lynch syndrome II (hereditary nonpolyposis colorectal cancer.) Women who are carriers of the mutated genes BRCA1 and BRCA2 have an increased risk for ovarian cancer, and gene testing may soon play a diagnostic role in women with a positive family history. Although there are no current recommendations for routine screening, women at high risk may benefit from annual pelvic examination, testing of CA 125 level, and transvaginal ultrasonography with Doppler analysis of ovarian vessels. Preventive strategies include oral contraceptive use and prophylactic oophorectomy after completion of childbearing for women at particularly high risk for the disease.

Reviews
1. National Institutes of Health (NIH) Consensus Conference. Ovarian cancer. Screening, treatment, and follow-up. *JAMA* 1995;273:491.
   NIH consensus statements are prepared by a nonadvocate, nonfederal panel of experts. They do not represent a policy statement of the NIH or the federal government.
2. Gershenson DM, et al. Ovarian intraepithelial neoplasia and ovarian cancer. *Obstet Gynecol Clin North Am* 1996;23:475.
   The authors provide a description of the nature of the disease, epidemiology, evaluation and treatment, diagnosis, and possible prevention.

Etiology
3. Boyd J, Rubin SC. Hereditary ovarian cancer: molecular genetics and clinical implications. *Gynecol Oncol* 1997;64:196.
   Breast and ovarian cancer families are frequently linked to the BRCA1 and BRCA2 genes.
4. Tortolero-Luna G, Mitchell MF, Rhodes-Morris HE. Epidemiology and screening of ovarian cancer. *Obstet Gynecol Clin North Am* 1994;21:1.
   Data do not yet justify annual screening of CA 125 levels and/or pelvic ultrasonography in all women.
5. Heintz AP, Hacker NF, Lagasse LD. Epidemiology and etiology of ovarian cancer: a review. *Obstet Gynecol* 1985;66:127.
   Sex cord tumors are found in women with Peutz-Jeghers syndrome; ovarian fibromas in those with basal cell nevus syndrome; and dysgerminomas and gonadoblastomas in streak (XY) gonads with gonadal dysgenesis.

6. Loft A, Lidegaard O, Tabor A. Incidence of ovarian cancer after hysterectomy: a nationwide controlled follow up. *Br J Obstet Gynaecol* 1997;104:1296.
   The risk of ovarian cancer is lower among women who have undergone hysterectomy, but the protection decreases with time.

7. Eltabbakh GH, et al. Epidemiologic differences between women with extraovarian primary peritoneal carcinoma and women with epithelial ovarian cancer. *Obstet Gynecol* 1998;91:254.
   These diseases can occur after oophorectomy; there are few epidemiologic differences between the two conditions.

Diagnosis

8. Reles A, Wein U, Lichtenegger W. Transvaginal color Doppler sonography and conventional sonography in the preoperative assessment of adnexal masses. *J Clin Ultrasound* 1997;25:217.
   The probable nature of ovarian tumors is now diagnosed based on patient age, tumor size, tumor markers, and ultrasound pattern, as well as the observation of hemodynamic characteristics.

9. Buist MR, et al. Radioimmunotargeting in ovarian carcinoma patients with indium-111 labeled monoclonal antibody OV-TL 3 F(ab')2: pharmacokinetics, tissue distribution, and tumor imaging. *Int J Gynecol Cancer* 1992;2:23.
   Diagnostic accuracy of immunoscintigraphy was compared with ultrasound, CT, MRI, and physical examination. The method proved superior in locating abdominal tumor deposits.

10. Calaminus G, et al. Juvenile granulosa cell tumors of the ovary in children and adolescents: results from 33 patients registered in a prospective cooperative study. *Gynecol Oncol* 1997;65:447.
    Most patients with stromal tumors can be cured by surgery alone. In advanced stages or with recurrence, chemotherapy or irradiation is indicated.

11. Culine S, et al. Cisplatin-based chemotherapy in the management of germ cell tumors of the ovary: the Institut Gustave Roussy experience. *Gynecol Oncol* 1997; 64:160.
    Despite the exquisite radiosensitivity of dysgerminomas, chemotherapy is usually preferred to prevent infertility and because good results can be expected.

Management

12. Gershenson DM. Primary cytoreduction for advanced epithelial ovarian cancer. *Obstet Gynecol Clin North Am* 1994;21:121.
    Cytoreductive or debulking surgery is directed toward removal of as much tumor as possible.

13. Stier EA, et al. Laparatomy to complete staging of presumed early ovarian cancer. *Obstet Gynecol* 1996;87:737.
    Re-exploration after initial incomplete staging may be better delayed until completion of a course of chemotherapy.

14. Curtin JP, Shapiro F. Adjuvant therapy in gynecologic malignancies. Ovarian, cervical, and endometrial cancer. *Surg Oncol Clin North Am* 1997;6:813.
    The authors discuss the feasibility and effectiveness of adjuvant chemotherapy and radiation therapy in gynecologic cancers.

15. McGuire WP, et al. Cyclophosphamide and cisplatin compared with paclitaxel and cisplatin in patients with stage III and stage IV ovarian cancer. *N Engl J Med* 1996;334:1.
    The paclitaxel and cisplatin combination provided better therapeutic efficacy and resulted in longer survival.

16. Barakat RR, et al. Salvage intraperitoneal therapy of advanced epithelial ovarian cancer: impact of retroperitoneal nodal disease. *Eur J Gynecol Oncol* 1997;18:161.
    Intraperitoneal platinum therapy is not contraindicated, even if retroperitoneal nodal disease is present.

17. Clarke-Pearson DL, et al. Surgical management of intestinal obstruction in ovarian cancer. I. Clinical features, postoperative complications, and survival. *Gynecol Oncol* 1987;26:11.
    Of 49 patients, progressive cancer caused intestinal obstruction in 86%. The need for clearer preoperative selection criteria is emphasized.

Prognosis

18. Cmelak AJ, Kapp DS. Long-term survival with whole abdominopelvic irradiation in platinum-refractory persistent or recurrent ovarian cancer. *Gynecol Oncol* 1997;65:453.
    Radiotherapy may still have a role in the management of ovarian cancer.
19. Schwartz PE. Cytoreductive surgery for the management of stage IV ovarian cancer. *Gynecol Oncol* 1997;64:1.
    Neoadjuvant chemotherapy may be as effective as aggressive cytoreductive surgery in stage IV disease.
20. Buller RE, et al. CA 125 kinetics: a cost-effective clinical tool to evaluate clinical trial outcomes in the 1990s. *Am J Obstet Gynecol* 1996;174:1241.
    The CA 125 regression curve can dictate treatment response and planning.
21. Katsoulis M, et al. The prognostic significance of second-look laparotomy in advanced ovarian cancer. *Eur J Gynaecol Oncol* 1997;18:200.
    The amount of residual tumor after the second-look laparotomy was the most important prognostic parameter.
22. Bjorge T, et al. Prognosis of patients with ovarian cancer and borderline tumors diagnosed in Norway between 1954 and 1993. *Int J Cancer* 1998;75:663.
    Borderline tumors provided an excellent prognosis even with conservative therapy.
23. Buttine M, Nicklin JL, Crandon A. Low malignant potential ovarian tumors: a review of 175 consecutive cases. *Aust N Z J Obstet Gynaecol* 1997;37:100.
    The ovarian epithelial tumors arise from the coelomic epithelium. There are three categories: benign, low malignant potential (borderline), and malignant.
24. Watkin W, Silva EG, Gershenson DM. Mucinous carcinoma of the ovary. *Cancer* 1992;69:208.
    The clinical stage and stromal invasion are the most important variables. The prognosis in patients with stage I mucinous carcinomas is excellent.

---

98. SURGERY

Michel E. Rivlin

Three gynecologic procedures are used specifically for the management of pelvic malignancies: radical hysterectomy, pelvic exenteration, and staging laparotomy.

Radical hysterectomy (Wertheim) is generally reserved for patients with stage IB and perhaps early stage IIA cervical carcinoma who have no medical contraindications to surgery. Further indications for this procedure include certain endometrial stage II cancers, some vaginal cancers, and cervical cancer unresponsive to radiotherapy when surgery is technically feasible.

The results from surgery and radiotherapy for stage I cervical cancer are comparable. Irradiation offers the major advantage of being useful in most patients, regardless of their age or medical condition, and is the choice for large cancers. On the other hand, surgery allows the ovaries to be conserved, provides the diagnostic accuracy of surgical staging, and does not adversely affect vaginal function, which are important advantages, especially for the younger patient. In general, we are fortunate to have two good methods for treating cervical cancer.

At laparotomy, it is decided whether surgical treatment is feasible. If biopsy specimens and frozen sections of the paraaortic nodes reveal tumor changes, the procedure is terminated. However, opinion is divided as to whether the presence of positive pelvic nodes should be a reason for terminating the procedure or whether it should still be completed.

Wertheim's operation includes total abdominal hysterectomy and excision of the upper third to half of the vagina, along with the uterosacral and cardinal ligaments, and the paracervical and paravaginal tissues out to the pelvic sidewalls. Pelvic lymphadenectomy is nearly always combined with removal of the pelvic nodes to the aortic bifurcation. The nodes removed include the obturator, hypogastric, and external iliac groups. The adnexa are removed in older patients or in those patients who will also receive adjunctive radiotherapy.

The operative mortality rate is low (0.3%–1.7%), but urinary complications are not uncommon because a major portion of the endopelvic fascia is removed and the bladder and ureters are extensively dissected. Voiding dysfunction and loss of vesical sensation are the most common problems. Rarer, but major, urinary problems are the formation of vesicovaginal or ureterovaginal fistulas (0.7%–1.6%), which are especially common in patients who also have been treated with radiotherapy.

Another, not uncommon, surgical complication is the formation of lymphocysts (3%–24%). Fortunately, these generally regress, although some, especially if they are infected or produce pressure effects, may require drainage. Other complications are those found with any major surgical procedure, and all are more common in patients treated with radiotherapy. For this reason, most surgeons prefer to avoid irradiation preoperatively, using it postoperatively only if positive pelvic nodes are encountered.

Pelvic exenteration is seldom used as primary therapy. When it is performed, it is usually for recurrence after radiation therapy, generally of cervical cancer. For the procedure to be feasible, it is essential that the tumor be considered completely resectable. This decision is based on clinical and operative findings. In general, a swollen leg or sciatic nerve pain is indicative of inoperable disease. Metastasis to common iliac or aortic nodes or outside the pelvis also indicates disease that is too extensive for resection.

For those few patients with operable central recurrence, anterior or total exenterations are usually performed, depending on the site of disease. Posterior exenteration alone is seldom performed because urinary fistulas frequently form as complications.

Exenteration involves removal of the pelvic lymph nodes, the internal genitalia, and the vagina. Because the bladder and often the rectum are also removed, urinary and fecal diversions become necessary. These generally take the form of ilial or colon conduits in conjunction with the creation of a sigmoid colostomy. A neovagina also may be constructed, at the same time or at a later procedure.

Several operative techniques have been developed for contending with the resulting large defect in the pelvic floor and the open pelvic cavity, which otherwise predispose to pelvic hematoma, abscess, bowel obstruction, or even evisceration. The other major complications of exenteration involve problems with the urinary anastomoses, especially if irradiated tissues have been used.

The operative mortality rate is about 3% to 14%, and the overall survival rate is about 25% to 40%. Improvements in all aspects of therapy are yielding steadily better outcomes, however. In view of the formidable nature of exenteration, it should be reserved for only those patients who have the physical and psychologic resources to cope with the therapy.

Exploratory celiotomy for the purposes of surgical staging is generally accepted for ovarian cancer and is also becoming a fairly common procedure for endometrial carcinoma because the operation is generally the primary treatment for patients with these conditions. Ovarian cancer patients are also sometimes managed with a second surgical staging operation (second-look). The rationale for second-look surgery is based on the serious short- and long-term side effects of chemotherapy that can arise and on the impossibility of ruling out residual tumor using noninvasive methods in patients who clinically appear to be free of disease. Because advanced cervical cancer is usually treated by radiotherapy, a staging laparotomy may turn out to be unnecessary surgery and is therefore still regarded as investigative. Typical risk estimates for periaortic node involvement in the setting of cervical cancer are 6%, 20%, and 30% for stages I, II, and III, respectively.

The underlying rationale for surgical staging to better evaluate the extent of cervical disease is based on the finding that clinical staging is incorrect in more than a third of the patients who come to surgery. Surgical staging usually requires laparotomy, although some clinicians claim good results with laparoscopy.

The staging celiotomy is directed primarily at biopsy of the common iliac and aortic lymph nodes. In addition, the pelvic and abdominal cavities are inspected, and perirectal or perivesical biopsy specimens are obtained, if indicated. The pelvic surgery performed is limited, lest it compromise treatment of the primary tumor. Surgery delays definitive therapy for an average of about 8 days, and there is an operative mortality rate of about 1%.

If the common iliac or aortic nodes are positive (about 20% of patients), routine radiation fields cannot encompass the disease process, and failure of standard therapy is inevitable. Therefore, treatment should be modified to include the involved areas, if this is technically possible. To justify the surgical staging procedure, treatment modifications should be shown to increase survival. In practice, the major modification consists of extended-field radiation, generally about 4,500 cGy to the paraaortic area, in addition to standard pelvic irradiation. The additional therapy seems unsuitable as a routine prophylactic measure because there is a definite complication rate, related in particular to small bowel problems. These complications, however, have been much reduced through the use of an extraperitoneal approach to node sampling. However, this approach does not permit intraperitoneal disease and visceral metastases to be assessed. The surgical staging for cervical cancer is still considered investigational because there are as yet no data to support a resulting increase in survival in the patients who undergo it. (Patients with positive aortic nodes often also have uncontrolled pelvic disease or metastasis elsewhere, resulting in a uniformly poor prognosis.)

The development of nonsurgical lymph node sampling techniques may obviate the need for staging laparotomy. Fine-needle aspiration of suspicious lymph nodes under computed tomographic guidance can predict disease if findings are positive, but has a significant false-negative rate of 14%, with up to 10% of the specimens unsatisfactory. Patients with periaortic nodal involvement can be cured, with 5-year survival rates ranging from 10% to 40%. The better results are reported for patients with early clinical stage disease and microscopic nodal involvement. Before any form of surgical staging is performed, the ability of the patient to tolerate the increased risk of extended-field radiotherapy must first be evaluated.

Radical Hysterectomy
1. Webb MJ. Radical hysterectomy. *Baillieres Clin Obstet Gynaecol* 1997;11:149.
   The degree of radicality may be tailored to the size and extent of the cervical lesion. This review summarizes the five types of extended hysterectomy.
2. Helmkamp BF, et al. Radical hysterectomy: current management guidelines. *Am J Obstet Gynecol* 1997;177:372.
   Use of Maylard incisions, suprapubic foley catheters, discontinuation of drains, early oral feeding, and initiation of a critical care pathway have decreased the length of stay in hospital to 3 to 5 days.
3. Roy M, et al. Vaginal radical hysterectomy versus abdominal radical hysterectomy in the treatment of early-stage cervical cancer. *Gynecol Oncol* 1996;62:336.
   The radical vaginal hysterectomy (Schauta) provides results comparable with the abdominal procedure. Unlike most European and Asian countries, the operation is seldom performed in the United States.
4. Spirtos NM, et al. Laparoscopic radical hysterectomy (type III) with aortic and pelvic lymphadenectomy. *Am J Obstet Gynecol* 1996;174:1763.
   The procedure should be considered investigational and reserved for oncology surgeons trained in extensive laparoscopic procedures.
5. Gerdin E, Cnattingius S, Johnson P. Complications after radiotherapy and radical hysterectomy in early-stage cervical carcinoma. *Acta Obstet Gynecol Scand* 1995;74:554.

Urinary tract complications dominated after these therapies for cervical carcinoma, voidance difficulties and incontinence being most common.

6. Feeney DD, et al. The fate of the ovaries after radical hysterectomy and ovarian transposition. *Gynecol Oncol* 1995;56:3.

Lateral ovarian transposition preserves ovarian function in only 50% of patients receiving pelvic radiotherapy following radical hysterectomy.

7. Monk BJ, Montz FJ. Invasive cervical cancer complicating intrauterine pregnancy: treatment with radical hysterectomy. *Obstet Gynecol* 1992;80:199.

Immediate treatment, low morbidity, acceptable survival rates, and preservation of ovarian function were all advantages of this treatment.

Pelvic Exenteration

8. Dottino PR, et al. Pelvic exenteration in gynecologic oncology: experience at the Mount Sinai Center, 1975–1992. *Mt Sinai J Med* 1995;62:431.

Thirty percent to 40% of the vulvar cancers, 60% to 70% of the vaginal cancers, 40% to 60% of the cervical cancers, 30% of the endometrial cancers, and 70% to 80% of the ovarian cancers recur and need further treatment. Regardless of the tumor origin or cell type, exenteration should be considered because, with careful patient selection, a salvage rate of 30% to 40% may be achieved. By contrast, repeated irradiation and chemotherapy are rarely curative.

9. Vergote IB. Exenterative surgery. *Curr Opin Obstet Gynecol* 1997;9:25.

Progress includes the use of continent intestinal reservoirs (Kock, Indiana, and Moring pouch) instead of the ileal conduit (Bricker), use of myocutaneous flaps to cover perineal or vulvar defects, and possible new indications such as sidewall relapse with palliative or even curative intent.

10. Woodhouse CR, et al. Exenteration as palliation for patients with advanced pelvic malignancy. *Br J Urol* 1995;76:315.

In general, exenteration is not considered a suitable means of palliation.

11. Magrina JF, Stanhope CR, Weaver AL. Pelvic exenterations: supralevator, infralevator, and with vulvectomy. *Gynecol Oncol* 1997;64:130.

Morbidity and survival were influenced by the type of exenteration: type I (supralevator), type II (infralevator), or type III (with vulvectomy).

12. Hawighorst-Knapstein S, et al. Pelvic exenteration: effects of surgery on quality of life and body image—a prospective longitudinal study. *Gynecol Oncol* 1997; 66:495.

Organ reconstruction should be performed whenever possible to improve body image, sexual function, and quality of life.

13. Miller B. Intestinal fistulae formation following pelvic exenteration: a review of the University of Texas M. D. Anderson Cancer Center experience, 1957–1990. *Gynecol Oncol* 1995;56:207.

In cases with significant infection, treatment should be surgical. In stable cases, conservative management with hyperalimentation and bowel decompression should be considered.

14. Bladou F, et al. Incidence and management of major urinary complications after pelvic exenteration for gynecological malignancies. *J Surg Oncol* 1995;58:91.

Reoperation is required for most urinary fistulas, but ureteral obstructions can be managed with percutaneous nephrostomy and ureteral stent.

Staging Laparotomy

15. Sartin AD, Parham GP. Routine lymph node dissection in the treatment of early stage cancer: are we doing the right thing? *Gynecol Oncol* 1998;68:1.

The authors suggest that only clinically involved regional nodes should be removed. Routine resection of primary tumor with lymphatic pathways is frequently unnecessary, resulting in equal salvage rates and lessened complications.

16. Possover M, et al. Value of laparoscopic evaluation of paraaortic and pelvic lymph nodes for treatment of cervical cancer. *Am J Obstet Gynecol* 1998;178:807.

Combination of laparoscopic evaluation and frozen section identified all patients with involved nodes correctly, and in 15% the results altered the originally planned primary therapy.

17. Fanning J, Nanavati PJ, Hilgers RD. Surgical staging and high dose rate brachytherapy for endometrial cancer: limiting external radiotherapy to node-positive tumors. *Obstet Gynecol* 1996;87:1041.
Postoperative external radiotherapy was avoided in 38% of patients without compromising survival.

18. Corn BW, et al. National trends in the surgical staging of corpus cancer: a pattern-of-practice survey. *Obstet Gynecol* 1997;90:628.
Complete surgical staging is not performed by most physicians caring for women with corpus cancer.

19. Bidzinski M, Mettler L, Ziclinski J. Endoscopic lymphadenectomy and LAVH in the treatment of endometrial cancer. *Eur J Gynecol Oncol* 1998;19:32.
Is this therapy an alternative to laparotomy for stage I and II endometrial cancer patients?

20. Yodducci A, et al. Analysis of failures after negative second-look in patients with advanced ovarian cancer: an Italian multicenter study. *Gynecol Oncol* 1998; 68:150.
A higher recurrence rate was found after negative laparoscopic reassessment than after negative reassessment by laparotomy.

21. Bor-Am A, et al. A second thought on second-look laparotomy. *Acta Obstet Gynecol Scand* 1993;72:386.
A high proportion of complete responders will subsequently develop recurrent disease.

22. Kohler MF, et al. Computed tomography–guided fine needle aspiration of retroperitoneal lymph nodes in gynecologic oncology. *Obstet Gynecol* 1990;76:612.
A positive result is significant; negative findings do not rule out nodal involvement (false-negative rate, 14%).

---

99. RADIATION THERAPY

Michel E. Rivlin

Radiation therapy is widely used in the treatment of gynecologic cancer and may be used either as the only therapy or in combination with surgical procedures, chemotherapy, or immunotherapy. Treatment may make use of radioactive isotopes, such as cesium, which is placed locally in the uterine and/or vaginal cavities (brachytherapy), or it may be administered from an external source. External irradiation (teletherapy) is usually performed with the megavoltage machines that have replaced the earlier orthovoltage instruments. Frequently, brachytherapy and teletherapy are combined, the former delivering the major radiation dosage to the tumor and the latter directed toward the draining lymph nodes.

The radiation therapy dosage is calculated in grays, which are the units of absorbed dosage. The dose of radiation delivered to a tumor depends on the energy of the source, the size of the treatment field, and the depth of the tumor beneath the surface. Using computer techniques, the dosimetry can be accurately calculated so that not too much radiation is delivered to normal tissues, while cancericidal doses are administered to the tumor and lymph nodes. Isodose curves are constructed by connecting points that receive equivalent radiation doses. Normal tissues composed of cells that are rapidly dividing, such as the epithelial tissues of the urinary and intestinal tracts, are less able to tolerate radiation than are the more stable tissues, such as those of the vagina and cervix.

Tumors differ in their radiosensitivity, frequently sharing this property with that of the parent tissue. The sensitivity depends on the histology, clinical variety, tumor bed, and oxygen tension. An anoxic tumor is radioresistant because oxygen is required for radiation damage to tissue, and this is frequently seen in the setting of large or recurrent tumors with an inadequate blood supply.

Ionizing radiation induces damage in the DNA. Radiation acts on cells primarily in the mitosis phase, making rapidly proliferating cells the most radiosensitive, although normal tissue recovers more efficiently than does tumor tissue. A given dose of radiation kills a constant fraction of tumor cells. Large tumors consist of a heterogeneous cell population and have variable growth fractions and a higher proportion of cells in the G_o (resting) phase of the cycle than do small tumors.

Efforts to improve the local control of bulky hypoxic tumors have included combinations of radiotherapy and hyperbaric oxygen or hypoxic cell sensitizers such as hydroxyurea, cisplatin, 5-fluorouracil, and misonidazole, which mimic oxygen in their ability to sensitize hypoxic cells. (A true radiosensitizer should augment tumor cell kill without adversely affecting normal tissues.) Refinements in treatment consisting of combinations of surgery, immunotherapy, or chemotherapy in conjunction with irradiation and unconventional radiation techniques are ongoing in attempts to improve results in patients with advanced disease.

Tolerance to radiation depends on several factors, including the total dosage administered, the period of time over which the dosage is given, and the volume of tissue irradiated. Tolerance is better when the dosage is fractionated and spread over a longer time period and where smaller, rather than larger, areas are treated. These factors must be taken into consideration when preparing a radiotherapeutic treatment plan.

The intensity of radiation from a source varies inversely as the square of the distance from the source. For example, in terms of a cervical tumor, the dosage rate at 1 cm from the cesium source is nine times that at 3 cm from the source. In this way, the sensitive bladder and rectal tissues receive dosages well within their individual safety margins, whereas 15,000 cGy or more may be delivered to the tumor site. However, it must be emphasized that generalizations regarding tissue tolerance in relation to total dosage must be regarded as only approximations.

Radiation sources are placed in systems designed to fit in the uterine and vaginal cavities. These systems include the uterine applicator (called the tandem) and the vaginal applicator (called the colpostat), which may require that the patient be under general anesthesia. Vaginal packing and a keel keep the systems stable and in place. Dosimetry films are then taken to ascertain position and to calculate isodose curves for various areas in the pelvis. The actual radioactive sources are inserted once satisfactory application is confirmed. This technique, called afterloading, minimizes exposure of personnel to radioactivity. Generally, sources are left in situ for 48 to 72 hours, and insertions are performed 2 to 4 weeks apart. This method of treatment is referred to as low dose rate brachytherapy. In the treatment of cervical cancer, two applications are usually administered, and these are given before, during, or after a concomitant course of external therapy.

The introduction of high-intensity sources and computer-controlled remote afterloading units have led to the use of high dose rate therapy lasting minutes instead of days and obviating the need for inpatient therapy as well as pulse dose rate therapy, which employs intermittent pulses of radiation, achieving the same overall time and total dose as low dose rate treatment. However, these novel techniques may produce more complications, and long-term efficacy must still be proved.

Computerized dosimetry is used to balance the dosage from the external and internal sources. External therapy is generally delivered from megavoltage instruments in doses fractionated over several weeks. The radiation is delivered in measured areas called portal-of-entry fields. The shape and size of ports vary with the lesions to be treated. In treating the whole pelvis, these ports generally measure 15 to 18 × 15 to 18 cm. Radiosensitive tissues may be protected with lead screens during external-beam therapy. For instance, a 4-cm central shield that protects the bladder and rectum may be used during whole-pelvis irradiation. In treating cervical cancer, a customary regimen is 4 to 5 weeks of external therapy (180–200 cGy/day), followed by two brachytherapy applications of 48 hours each, with 2 weeks intervening. A dose of 80 to 90 cGy is delivered to point A (2 cm proximal to the cervical os and 2 cm lateral, corresponding to the approximate point where the uterine artery crosses over the ureter) and 50 to 60 cGy to point B (3 cm lateral to point A and corresponding to the pelvic nodes). Treatment takes a total time of 8 to 10 weeks.

Therapeutic levels of radiotherapy damage cell nuclei and cause an obliterative endarteritis. These effects on normal tissue result in complications that are closely related to the dosage. It is the complication rate, rather than the cure rate, that places limits on radiation dosage. Local applications tend to cause focal injuries, whereas external therapy produces a more uniformly irradiated field.

Orthovoltage machines have power in the 125,000 to 400,000 electron volt range, whereas megavoltage machines are in the 2 to 35 million electron volt range. The higher-energy machines cause little skin or systemic reactions because the penetration is much greater than that of the older orthovoltage type, which caused marked skin and subcutaneous tissue damage.

Early side effects of radiotherapy include cystitis and proctosigmoiditis, both of which usually respond to dietary or medical management. Bone marrow suppression and radiation sickness are rarely encountered. An important early but occasional complication is acute pelvic sepsis, which necessitates termination of therapy until the infection is cleared.

The late complications are much more difficult to treat and are related to the ischemic and necrotizing effects of excessive ionizing radiation. They may appear months or years after the completion of therapy. Large bowel complications involving the rectum and sigmoid may consist of hemorrhage, ulceration, fistulas, or stricture. Milder forms may respond to conservative measures, whereas the more severe forms require the creation of a diverting colostomy.

Small bowel problems arise particularly when previous surgical treatment has resulted in loops fixed by adhesions or when the small bowel remains relatively immobile, most commonly at the terminal ileum. Enteritis, subacute obstruction, hemorrhage, ulceration, and perforation can all occur. These complications are more common when irradiation has been extended to the upper abdomen. Management is difficult and may involve surgical measures consisting of resection or bypass procedures.

Urinary tract problems involving the bladder and ureters include cystitis, ulceration, hemorrhage, stenosis, and fistula formation. If conservative measures are unsuccessful, surgical diversion of the urinary stream may be necessary.

The vaginal response to radiation consists of epithelial atrophy, erosions, and adhesion formation. Later, there may be stenosis and even complete vaginal obliteration. These changes can be partially prevented by the use of hormones and dilators, and, most important, by the resumption of intercourse as soon as possible after therapy. The cervix also commonly becomes stenotic with, occasionally, retention of secretions in the uterine cavity, thus leading to a pyometra that requires drainage. The most serious of the local complications, although rare, is complete vault necrosis, often with associated urinary or fecal fistulas.

In the management of complications after radiotherapy, it is vital to keep in mind the impaired healing of irradiated tissue. Frequently, it is difficult to differentiate recurrence from radiation injury and to perform diagnostic procedures, especially biopsies. Great care must be taken to prevent perforation or fistula formation. If surgical intervention is necessary, the poor healing and infection-resistant properties of irradiated tissue must be allowed for in the therapeutic plan.

Complications associated with radiation therapy are uncommon and chiefly afflict patients who receive an increased dosage as a calculated risk in an attempt to cure advanced disease. The incidence of complications from standard regimens with early disease is low, and the cure rate is excellent when the disease is localized.

Treatment should be individualized and a management team made up of a gynecologic oncologist, a chemotherapist, and a radiotherapist should arrive at a treatment plan after accurate staging of the disease. This plan should be reviewed at periodic intervals for response to therapy and the occurrence of complications that might necessitate a change in management.

Radiotherapy is the major modality of treatment for cervical cancer. In patients with endometrial cancer, radiotherapy is commonly used in conjunction with surgical measures. Ovarian cancer is now more frequently managed by surgery and chemotherapy, with radiotherapy used only for particularly radiosensitive tumors such as the dysgerminoma. Vaginal cancer is commonly managed by radiotherapy, often in conjunction with surgery. Although recurrent cancer may be treated with radiation therapy, previous treatment often limits the dosage that can be used, so the therapy is only for palliative purposes, as in the prevention or treatment of hemorrhage or the relief of pain. Further details on irradiation of pelvic cancer can be found in Chapters 90–97 in this section.

General

1. Iliakis G. Cell cycle regulation in irradiated and nonirradiated cells. *Semin Oncol* 1997;24:602.
   Cells have the ability to sense DNA damage and to activate repair pathways that restore the integrity of the DNA.
2. Bloomer WD, Hellman S. Normal tissue responses to radiation therapy. *N Engl J Med* 1975;293:80.
   The therapeutic ratio is the ratio between the lethal tumor dose and tissue tolerance.
3. DesRosiers PM, et al. New techniques in the radiotherapeutic treatment of gynecological malignancies. *Curr Opin Obstet Gynecol* 1998;10:21.
   The authors review the role of radiation therapy, alone or in combination with surgery and/or chemotherapy, for gynecologic malignancies.
4. Stitt JA, Thomadsen BR. Innovations and advances in brachytherapy. *Semin Oncol* 1997;24:696.
   Optimization in brachytherapy entails calculating the source strengths or source dwell times to satisfy a set of dose criteria to achieve the best dose distribution for a brachytherapy implant.
5. Gunderson LL, et al. Intraoperative irradiation: current and future status. *Semin Oncol* 1997;24:715.
   The purpose of intraoperative therapy is to decrease normal tissue damage.
6. Portenoy RK. Practical aspects of pain control in the patient with cancer. *CA* 1988;38:327.
   Therapeutic approaches of value in the control of cancer-related pain include pharmacologic, anesthetic, neuroaugmentative, physiatric, neurosurgical, and psychologic measures.

Cervical Cancer

7. Sardi JE, et al. Long-term follow-up of the first randomized trial using neoadjuvant chemotherapy in stage Ib squamous carcinoma of the cervix: the final results. *Gynecol Oncol* 1997;67:61.
   There are three possible strategies for integrating chemotherapy with local treatment: primary chemotherapy prior to local treatment (neoadjuvant), postoperative in high-risk cases (adjuvant), and radiosensitizing, in which drugs and irradiation are given together, with the goal to enhance the efficacy of the irradiation.
8. Rotman M, et al. Prophylactic extended-field irradiation of para-aortic lymph nodes in stages IIB and bulky IB and IIA cervical carcinomas. Ten-year treatment results of RTOG 79-20. *JAMA* 1995;274:387.
   A clear survival benefit was demonstrated with radiation to the paraaortic lymph node chain.
9. Malfetano JH, et al. Extended field radiation and cisplatin for stage IIB and IIIB cervical carcinoma. *Gynecol Oncol* 1997;67:203.
   Weekly cisplatin with prophylactic paraaortic radiation yielded a 75% survival benefit with minimal morbidity.
10. Thomas G, et al. A randomized trial of standard versus partially hyperfractionated radiation with or without concurrent 5-fluorouracil in locally advanced cervical cancer. *Gynecol Oncol* 1998;69:137.
    Hyperfractionation is a modification of standard radiotherapy in which fraction dose or frequency are increased, in this study together with concurrent chemotherapy.

11. Morris M, et al. Pelvic radiation with concurrent chemotherapy compared with pelvic and para-aortic radiation for high-risk cervical cancer. *N Engl J Med* 1999;340:1137.

    The addition of concurrent chemotherapy as a radio-sensitizer has markedly increased survival rates, and is now the standard of care.

Endometrial Cancer

12. Eltabbakh GH, et al. Excellent long-term survival and absence of vaginal recurrences in 332 patients with low-risk stage I endometrial adenocarcinoma treated with hysterectomy and vaginal brachytherapy without formal staging lymph node sampling: report of a prospective trial. *Int J Radiat Oncol Biol Phys* 1997;38:373.

    In low-risk, early-stage disease, the role of adjuvant therapy and of lymph node sampling are controversial.

13. Greven KM, et al. Which prognostic factors influence the outcome of patients with surgically staged endometrial cancer treated with adjuvant radiation? *Int J Radiat Oncol Biol Phys* 1997;39:413.

    This article discusses external beam and vaginal endocavitary brachytherapy for patients with close surgical margins, cervical involvement, capillary space invasion, or unfavorable histology.

14. Fishman DA, et al. Radiation therapy as exclusive treatment for medically inoperable patients with stage I and II endometrioid carcinoma of the endometrium. *Gynecol Oncol* 1996;61:189.

    Death from recurrent disease was the main problem, and among those who did not die of intercurrent disease the survival rates were close to those of patients who had surgery.

15. Nag S, et al. Perineal template interstitial brachytherapy salvage for recurrent endometrial adenocarcinoma metastatic to the vagina. *Gynecol Oncol* 1997;66:16.

    This treatment is an effective alternative to radical or exenterative pelvic surgery even after previous irradiation.

16. Reisinger SA, et al. A phase I study of weekly cisplatin and whole abdominal radiation for the treatment of stage III and IV endometrial carcinoma. A gynecologic oncology group pilot study. *Gynecol Oncol* 1996;63:299.

    Chemoradiation for advanced disease is a feasible regimen with acceptable toxicity, and is possibly effective.

Vaginal and Vulvar Cancer

17. Chyle V, et al. Definitive radiotherapy for carcinoma of the vagina: outcome and prognostic factors. *Int J Radiat Oncol Biol Phys* 1996;35:891.

    In a series of 301 patients, management relied on external-beam radiation and brachytherapy, and survival was 60% at 5 years, 49% at 10 years.

18. Xiang-E W, et al. Treatment of late recurrent vaginal malignancy after initial radiotherapy for carcinoma of the cervix: an analysis of 73 cases. *Gynecol Oncol* 1998;69:125.

    Reirradiation is possible and valuable, but radiation complications are common.

19. Manavi M, et al. Does T1, NO-1 vulvar cancer treated by vulvectomy but not lymphadenectomy need inguinofemoral radiation? *Int J Radiat Oncol Biol Phys* 1997;38:749.

    No difference was observed in 5-year survival rates between groups who did or did not receive postoperative inguinofemoral radiotherapy.

20. Cunningham MJ, et al. Primary radiation, cisplatin, and 5-fluorouracil for advanced squamous carcinoma of the vulva. *Gynecol Oncol* 1997;66:285.

    The authors describe effective chemoradiation with acceptable morbidity, and surgery is not necessary if the response is complete.

Ovarian Cancer

21. Lanciano R, et al. Update on the role of radiotherapy in ovarian cancer. *Semin Oncol* 1998;25:361.

    This article includes an assessment of the possible role of intraperitoneal radiocolloid therapy (chromic phosphate, P32) as primary or salvage treatment.

22. Cmelak AJ, Kapp DS. Long-term survival with whole abdominopelvic irradiation in platinum-refractory persistent or recurrent ovarian cancer. *Gynecol Oncol* 1997;65:453.

The actuarial 5-year survival rate was 57%, with 10% experiencing serious complications such as obstructions and fistulas.

Complications

23. Eifel PJ, et al. Time course and incidence of late complications in patients treated with radiation therapy for FIGO stage 1B carcinoma of the cervix. *Int J Radiat Oncol Biol Phys* 1995;32:1289.

The actuarial risk of grade 3 or higher radiation complications (gastrointestinal and genitourinary combined) is 9.3% at 5 years, 11.1% at 10 years, and 14.1% at 20 years.

24. Montana GS, Fowler WC. Carcinoma of the cervix: analysis of bladder and rectal radiation dose and complications. *Int J Radiat Oncol Biol Phys* 1989;16:95.

The authors report that the point A dose in patients with complications for all stages was greater than that in patients without complications.

25. McGonigle KF, et al. Complications of pelvic radiation therapy for gynecologic malignancies in elderly women. *Int J Gynecol Cancer* 1996;6:149.

Older women tolerate radiotherapy less well than younger women. Chronic intestinal and / or urinary problems occurred in 63% of the women in this study by 3 years of follow-up.

26. Shahin MS, Puscheck E. Reproductive sequelae of cancer treatment. *Obstet Gynecol Clin North Am* 1998;25:423.

Premature ovarian failure and sterility occur in women exposed to 800 rad or more.

27. Parkin DE, Davis JA, Symonds RP. Urodynamic findings following radiotherapy for cervical carcinoma. *Br J Urol* 1988;61:213.

Up to one-half of the long-term survivors had complaints of frequency, urgency, and urge incontinence. Detrusor instability was found in nearly all symptomatic women.

28. Lee RA, Symmonds RE, Williams TJ. Current status of genitourinary fistula. *Obstet Gynecol* 1988;72:313.

Successful repair of fistulas following radiation damage requires carefully planned and timed procedures using nonirradiated tissue to close the defect.

29. Krebs HB, Goperud DR. Mechanical intestinal obstruction in patients with gynecologic disease: a review of 38 patients. *Am J Obstet Gynecol* 1987;157:577.

In this series, 17% of small bowel and 26% of colon obstructions were associated with radiation therapy–related strictures and adhesions.

30. Allen-Mersh TG, et al. The management of late radiation-induced rectal injury after treatment of carcinoma of the uterus. *Surg Gynecol Obstet* 1987;164:521.

Florid proctitis resolved within 2 years of onset in 33%, and surgical treatment was necessary in 39%. Cancer-induced symptoms tended to occur after a median of 8 months, compared with radiation-induced symptoms, which appeared at a median of 16 months.

31. Beemer W, Hopkins MP, Morley GW. Vaginal reconstruction in gynecologic oncology. *Obstet Gynecol* 1988;72:911.

Vaginal reconstruction is feasible when the vagina has been obliterated by irradiation or surgery.

32. Muram D, et al. Postradiation ureteral obstruction: a reappraisal. *Am J Obstet Gynecol* 1981;139:289.

Differentiating periureteral radiation fibrosis from recurrent carcinoma may require laparotomy in some cases.

33. Mayr NA, Wen BC, Saw CB. Radiation therapy during pregnancy. *Obstet Gynecol Clin North Am* 1998;25:301.

The optimal radiotherapeutic management and the optimal management of the pregnancy involve directly opposing demands.

100. CHEMOTHERAPY IN GYNECOLOGIC CANCER

Michel E. Rivlin

Chemotherapeutic agents affect rapidly dividing cells, such as tumor cells, but spare static cell populations. However, renewing cell populations are also characteristic of some normal cell types, and these too are commonly damaged during cytotoxic drug treatment. Therefore, the bone marrow, mucous membranes, and gastrointestinal tract are frequently injured during chemotherapy, whereas muscle cells and bone are spared. It is usually this toxicity that dictates the drug dosage and not the tumor response.

The kinetics of individual tumor cells are important factors because different drugs act at different phases of the cell cycle. The mitotic phase of the cycle is followed by a variable period (G1), during which protein and ribonucleic acid (RNA) are synthesized. The S phase follows, with new deoxyribonucleic acid (DNA) synthesis; after this comes the G2 period, which is relatively short and precedes mitosis. The variation in duration of G1 is central to the proliferative behavior of cell populations. A short G1 period indicates proliferative behavior; if the postmitotic period is very long, it is termed G0 and represents nonproliferative populations.

Most cytotoxic agents act by disrupting some aspect of DNA, RNA, or protein synthesis, and rapidly dividing cells are the most sensitive to these agents. Certain agents are cell cycle specific and proliferation dependent (e.g., hydroxyurea and methotrexate); others kill in all phases of the cell cycle and are not too dependent on the proliferative rate (e.g., alkylating agents). Some drugs may have a greater effect on a particular phase of the cell cycle; for instance, doxorubicin (Adriamycin) is most effective in the late S phase, whereas cells in mitosis seem most sensitive to agents that disrupt the mitotic apparatus, such as vinblastine, vincristine, and taxol.

Cytotoxic agents kill a constant fraction of cells, rather than a constant number. This first-order kinetic concept means that only large log kills (>99%) with repetitive therapies can be curative. Furthermore, treatment applied early results in more cures than it does when the tumor is large and clinically obvious. Unfortunately, most tumors have already undergone 30 doublings before they are detected, and then are no longer early. In addition, at later stages of growth, only a few doublings markedly enlarge the tumor. However, two other factors influence tumor growth: cell death and the growth fraction. In most tumors, only a fraction of the cells are proliferating, and cell losses may range from 70% to 95%. It is estimated that doubling times in human tumors take about 50 days, but the range for individual growths is broad.

The terms *complete remission* and *partial remission* are used to indicate the response to therapy. A complete remission consists of a clinical response plus the disappearance of all objective evidence of tumor. The mean survival is usually prolonged in this setting. Partial remission indicates a 50% or greater reduction in the size of measurable lesions, with some clinical response and no new lesions, but the overall mean survival is usually not improved. In planning clinical trials of new agents or drug combinations, phase I trials determine the dosage and toxicity, phase II trials assess antitumor activity, and phase III trials compare efficacy against that of established regimens. Tumors may be primarily resistant to drug therapy or may develop drug resistance after an initial response. Acquired resistance may be either specific or broadly based to multiple drugs (pleiotropic). The mechanisms of resistance vary and include spontaneous biochemical mutations or the selecting out of resistant cell lines in the original tumor, because most tumors are not composed of homogeneous clonally derived cells with similar features, but of different populations with differing characteristics.

The balance between tumor sensitivity and normal tissue injury may leave only a narrow safety margin. The most common toxicity affects the bone marrow. Effects generally arise 7 to 10 days after the initial therapy and persist for 3 to 10 days. The toxicity is graded from 0 to 4, and grade 3 or 4 generally requires a delay in further therapy, or a dose modification, or both. In general, treatment is delayed if the leukocyte count is less than 3,000/µl or if the platelet count is less than 100,000/µl. If leukopenia is accompanied by fever, immediate culture and the institution of broad-spectrum antibiotic therapy while awaiting culture results are indicated. These are continued until granulocyte recovery occurs. Similarly, a platelet count of under 20,000/µl requires platelet transfusion, whereas a count of under 50,000/µl requires platelets only if hemorrhage occurs. Newer approaches to the management of myelosuppression include bone marrow transplantation and the use of hematopoietic growth agents, such as granulocyte colony-stimulating factor. The growth factors, however, have little effect on platelet recovery.

Most agents cause nausea, vomiting, and anorexia. Diarrhea, oral mucositis, esophagitis, and gastroenteritis are also problems. To prevent gastrointestinal toxicities, pretreatment may be required, especially when using drugs with severe emetogenic side effects, such as cisplatin or cyclophosphamide. Useful medications include antihistamines, phenothiazines, steroids, sedation, and the 5-hydroxytryptamine antagonist ondansetron. Other common adverse effects include alopecia, skin toxicity, neurotoxicity, and genitourinary toxicity. Examples of serious adverse reactions include the leukemogenic effect of the alkylating agents, the irreversible cardiomyopathy seen with cumulative doses of Adriamycin, the renal failure and hearing loss associated with cisplatin, the pulmonary fibrosis and death with cumulative doses of bleomycin, and the hemorrhagic cystitis that can occur with cyclophosphamide. Moreover, severe skin necrosis with extravasation from the vein can occur when plant alkaloids and antitumor antimetabolites are used, so that special precautions are necessary for their safe administration.

In view of the inevitable minor and major toxicities associated with antineoplastic drugs, the decision to use them is obviously a complex one. Factors related to the patient, the tumor, the chosen regimen, and the available therapeutic facilities must be taken into account. The probability of achieving a useful response must be shared with the patient. In general, with the exception of gestational trophoblastic disease, drug combinations are necessary to prolong survival or cure in patients with most disseminated tumors. The principles governing the use of combination drug therapy include their intermittent use so as to maximize their effect while minimizing toxicity. The drugs must be active as single agents against the tumor and should possess different mechanisms of action so as to diminish drug resistance. They should also have different spectra of toxicity to enable full dosage, and there should be a biochemical basis for additive or synergistic effects.

Combination chemotherapy used from the outset is termed induction chemotherapy. Adjuvant chemotherapy is that given if the risk of recurrence after definitive initial therapy, usually surgery or irradiation, is high. Neoadjuvant (or primary) chemotherapy is that used to treat local disease difficult to manage with other therapeutic modalities. Salvage chemotherapy is intended for palliation rather than cure. Cytotoxic drugs are generally administered parenterally or orally but also may be inserted into body cavities, including intraperitoneally. The advantage of intracavitary treatment is that many agents are cleared more slowly from body cavities than those given systemically. The major application of this approach is in patients with minimal residual disease because of the limited penetration achieved by this route.

The cytotoxic agents used in patients with gynecologic cancer may be classified as alkylating agents, antimetabolites, antitumor antibiotics, plant-derived alkaloids, hormones and antihormones, and lastly, a miscellaneous group consisting of various agents that do not fit into any of the other classes.

The alkylating agents include melphalan (Alkeran), cyclophosphamide (Cytoxan), and chlorambucil (Leukeran). All three are effective agents in the treatment of ovarian cancer, whereas Cytoxan is also active for cervical cancer and uterine sarcoma. Chlorambucil is active for gestational trophoblastic neoplasia (GTN). Alkylating agents form an unstable alkyl group that has a radiomimetic effect, resulting in breaks and cross-linkages of DNA, and thus preventing cell division.

Antimetabolites are cycle-specific agents that substitute for normal metabolites. They act on an enzyme regulatory site, bind to inhibitors of vital enzymes, or occupy a catalytic site of vital enzymes, thus interrupting normal DNA or RNA synthesis, or both. Methotrexate, 5-fluorouracil (5-FU), and hydroxyurea are antimetabolites; the first two are used for GTN and ovarian cancers, whereas the third is used as a radiosensitizer in the treatment of cervical cancer. Antitumor antibiotics are natural isolates of soil fungi. They act by forming complexes with DNA, but there is a narrow therapeutic index. Those used in the practice of gynecology are dactinomycin (Actinomycin-D), bleomycin, and doxorubicin (Adriamycin). The first two are useful for ovarian germ cell tumors, whereas dactinomycin is also used for GTN. Adriamycin is useful for ovarian, endometrial, and sarcomatous lesions.

The Vinca plant alkaloids, derivatives of the periwinkle, arrest cells in metaphase by binding the microtubular protein used in the formation of the mitotic spindle. Etoposide (VP-16) is a topoisomerase inhibitor. Vincristine (Oncovin), vinblastin, and VP-16 are useful for germ cell tumors. Oncovin is also active against sarcomas.

The hormonal agents include progestational drugs such as medroxyprogesterone acetate (Depo-Provera) and megestrol acetate (Megace), which are used for endometrial cancer, or antiestrogenic drugs such as tamoxifen, which is possibly useful in endometrial cancer, or leuprolide (Lupron), which is used for ovarian and endometrial cancer.

Miscellaneous agents include cis-dichlorodiammineplatinum (cisplatin) and carboplatinum, which form the basis of most ovarian cancer regimens and are also active against cervical cancer. Ifosfamide is used for sarcoma and ovarian cancer. Hexamethylmelamine and paclitaxel (taxol) are active against ovarian epithelial cancer. Taxol is a mitotic spindle poison but has many and novel toxicities, including anaphylaxis, hypotension, and cardiac toxicity, besides the usual toxicities such as myelosuppression. Nevertheless, in combination with cisplatin or carboplatin, it appears to be the most effective chemotherapy for ovarian cancer.

The chemotherapy of GTN is detailed in Chapter 3; however, the most common use of chemotherapy in gynecologic cancer is as a supplement to surgery in the treatment of epithelial cancer of the ovaries. The treatment of choice for ovarian cancer is a cisplatin-based combination of drugs (taxol with cisplatin or carboplatin). Patients with minimal residual disease postoperatively respond better than do those with bulkier disease. For the treatment of early-stage ovarian cancer, the place of adjuvant chemotherapy is less clear-cut, but it is usually indicated when high-risk findings are present. In squamous cell cervical cancer, cisplatin and ifosfamide both show modest activity. In addition, cisplatin, hydroxyurea, and 5-FU have been used as radiosensitizing agents for cervical cancer. Concurrent chemotherapy has improved results in association with radiotherapy.

For the management of endometrial cancer, progestins, tamoxifen, and Lupron given as single agents may be helpful for advanced disease, especially for receptor-positive cases. In the setting of treatment failure or receptor-negative disease, platinum-based multiagent therapy is indicated (Adriamycin plus platinum). Uterine sarcomas may be treated with doxorubicin (leiomyosarcoma) or ifosfamide or cisplatin (mixed mesodermal). Adjuvant chemotherapy has not proved helpful. Stromal and germ cell ovarian neoplasms respond well to cisplatin-based combination chemotherapy (bleomycin, etoposide, platinum), often with complete response. Adjuvant therapy for early-stage disease is of value. The standard chemotherapy for the less common vulvar, vaginal, and tubal cancers is not well established.

Chemotherapeutic agents that might be used in practice by gynecologists include Alkeran, Cytoxan, methotrexate, and hydroxyurea. Only specialists should administer Adriamycin, Actinomycin-D, taxol, or combination therapy. Cisplatin, 5-FU, and carboplatin occupy an intermediate position, and their use depends on the experience and facilities available to the individual practitioner.

General
1. Perry MC. Toxicity of chemotherapy. *Semin Oncol* 1992;19:453.
   This article includes a section on fertility after chemotherapy.
2. Rolston KV. Infections in the neutropenic cancer patient. *Cancer Bull* 1992;
   44:226.
   The author provides a useful algorithm for management of febrile episodes in neutropenic patients.
3. Buekers TE, Lallas TA. Chemotherapy in pregnancy. *Obstet Gynecol Clin North Am* 1998;25:323.

The authors discuss the integral role of chemotherapy in the treatment of breast and ovarian cancer, leukemia, and lymphoma. Benefits of therapy outweigh the risks to the fetus in most situations.

Carcinoma of the Ovary

4. Brown JV, et al. Three-hour paclitaxel infusion and carboplatin is an effective outpatient treatment for stage III epithelial ovarian cancer. *Gynecol Oncol* 1998;68:166.

   Tumor response to initial paclitaxel/platinum treatment is predictive of future response to second-line agents.

5. Coukos G, Rubin SC. Chemotherapy resistance in ovarian cancer: new molecular perspectives. *Obstet Gynecol* 1998;91:783.

   Alterations in specific oncogenes and tumor suppression genes appear to be directly associated with the loss of chemosensitivity.

6. Schilder RJ, Shea TC. Multiple cycles of high-dose chemotherapy for ovarian cancer. *Semin Oncol* 1998;25:349.

   The collection and reinfusion of peripheral blood progenitor cells after chemotherapy accelerate hematopoietic recovery compared with colony-stimulating factors alone or with autologous bone marrow.

7. Recio FO, et al. Five-year survival after second-line cisplatin-based intraperitoneal chemotherapy for advanced ovarian cancer. *Gynecol Oncol* 1998;68:267.

   Intraperitoneal cisplatin-based chemotherapy offers a viable option as salvage treatment.

8. Abu-Rustum NR, Aghajanian C. Management of malignant germ cell tumors of the ovary. *Semin Oncol* 1998;25:1.

   Initial conservative surgery and staging followed by combination chemotherapy cures the majority of the patients.

Carcinoma of the Cervix

9. Keys HM, et al. Cisplatin, radiation, and adjuvant hysterectomy compared with radiation and adjuvant hysterectomy for bulky stage 1B cervical carcinoma. *N Engl J Med* 1999; 340:1154.

   Reported improvements in survival with concurrent chemotherapy have not been noted with neoadjuvant chemotherapy.

10. Iwasaka T, et al. Adjuvant chemotherapy after radical hysterectomy for cervical carcinoma: a comparison with effects of adjuvant radiotherapy. *Obstet Gynecol* 1998;91:977.

    Similar results were observed, but more pelvic recurrences were seen with chemotherapy and more extrapelvic recurrences were seen with radiotherapy, suggesting that a combination of the two modalities might prove advantageous.

11. Sardi JE, et al. Long-term follow-up of the first randomized trial using neoadjuvant chemotherapy in stage Ib squamous carcinoma of the cervix: the final results. *Gynecol Oncol* 1997;67:61.

    Neoadjuvant chemotherapy prior to radical surgery and adjunctive radiation provided superior results as compared with standard therapy.

Endometrial Cancer

12. Covens A, et al. A phase II study of leuprolide in advanced/recurrent endometrial cancer. *Gynecol Oncol* 1997;64:126.

    The authors reported no responders among 25 patients, although other researchers have reported up to 28% response rates.

13. Ball HG, et al. A phase II trial of paclitaxel in patients with advanced or recurrent adenocarcinoma of the endometrium: a Gynecologic Oncologic Group study. *Gynecol Oncol* 1996;62:278.

    Four of 30 patients experienced complete responses, whereas six exhibited partial responses.

14. Piver MS, et al. A prospective trial of progesterone therapy for malignant peritoneal cytology in patients with endometrial carcinoma. *Gynecol Oncol* 1992;47:373.

    None of the 45 women in this study with tumor confined to the uterus and positive peritoneal cytology, who received progesterone therapy, experienced recurrence of their cancer.

Vulvar Carcinoma / Uterine Sarcoma
15. Eifel PJ, et al. Prolonged continuous infusion cisplatin and 5-fluorouracil with radiation for locally advanced carcinoma of the vulva. *Gynecol Oncol* 1995;59:51. *Overall, 6 of 12 patients remained disease-free 17 to 30 months after therapy.*
16. Sutton G, Blessing JA, Malfetano JH. Ifosfamide and doxorubicin in the treatment of advanced leiomyosarcomas of the uterus: a Gynecologic Oncology Group study. *Gynecol Oncol* 1996;62:226. *The role of adjuvant chemotherapy is unclear. Active agents include ifosfamide, doxorubicin, and cisplatin.*

---

101. BENIGN BREAST DISORDERS

Galen V. Poole

At some time during their lives most women will have a problem with their breasts. They often seek the advice of their gynecologist, who must be familiar with the initial evaluation of breast problems. Fortunately, most breast disorders are benign, and many can be handled by limited intervention and reassurance. Other problems will require early referral for complete investigation and appropriate management.

The principle importance of benign breast lesions is the need to differentiate them from breast cancer. Both benign and malignant lesions of the breast can present as a mass, breast pain, nipple discharge, or a mammographic abnormality. These symptoms may occur in combination. Less frequent problems include skin changes (dimpling, retraction, edema) and nipple eczema.

The evaluation of a breast complaint should include history of prior breast problems; menstrual history (menarche and menopause, if appropriate); age and parity; history of breast-feeding; relation of pain to menses; use of exogenous hormones, including oral contraceptives; family history of breast cancer; and history of irradiation to the chest. The breasts should be examined at least annually by a physician, and monthly by the woman. Breast self-examination should be taught to all adult women and is preferably performed in the shower or bath, as well as in front of a mirror. The breasts should be examined in both sitting and standing positions with arms at the side, arms raised, and with the hands on the hips to flex the pectoralis muscles. The latter might demonstrate skin retraction if there is an underlying malignancy. The breasts should be palpated with the patient in the upright and supine positions. The axillae are best evaluated with arms at the side to relax the pectoral and latissimus muscles. The supra- and infraclavicular fossae also should be palpated for adenopathy. If there is nipple discharge, the breasts should be compressed radially toward the nipple to localize the offending duct(s). No attempt should be made to probe the duct prior to surgery. If the breast examination is equivocal, the woman should be reexamined in 2 to 6 weeks, at a different phase of her menstrual cycle.

Mammography should be recommended to women who are 40 years of age or older, even if the physical examination is unrevealing. Breast ultrasonography can be used to differentiate a solid mass from a cystic mass (as can needle aspiration), and may facilitate the localization of mammographically identified but nonpalpable mass lesions, but ultrasonography has no role as a screening study. The American Cancer Society recommends that women 40 to 49 years of age have a screening mammogram every other year, and annually after the age of 50 years. Modern film screen mammography with breast compression is safe, with a radiation dose of less than 1 rad. With skilled interpretation the sensitivity is excellent, although most abnormalities identified mammographically are benign. Because of breast glandular density, mammography is of little value in women under the age of 40 years, but sometimes is obtained to provide reassurance. A negative mammogram should never defer the evaluation of a palpable breast mass or abnormal density. If a mass is palpated in one breast, bilateral mammography should be performed to exclude contralateral as well as ipsilateral occult lesions. If a mass is identified on examination or on mammography, it may require tissue sampling. Palpable lesions and those that can be localized on ultrasonography can be assessed by fine-needle aspiration, although experienced cytopathologists are required for interpretation. Because cancer cells adhere poorly to one another, they are more easily aspirated than normal cells. Only individual cells can be evaluated; therefore, fine-needle aspiration provides no information regarding invasiveness. The sensitivity of fine-needle aspiration ranges from 75% to 95%, with a specificity of 90% to 99%. Aspiration of a cyst is both diagnostic and potentially curative. Any cyst that recurs after two or three aspirations should be excised. Fluid obtained by cyst aspiration is often sent for cytologic examination, but this is of low yield since the overwhelming majority of cysts are benign. A high potassium content in cyst fluid suggests that the cyst is of apocrine origin and may have a higher probability of recurrence.

A core needle biopsy can be performed on a palpable mass, and the tissue sample is more easily interpreted by a pathologist. Negative (benign) fine-needle aspiration and core needle biopsy results should be regarded as inadequate samples, and a repeat sample should be obtained, or one should proceed to an open surgical biopsy. Complete excision of a lesion is preferred, but for a very large and probably malignant lesion, an incisional biopsy is adequate prior to definitive surgical management.

If mammography demonstrates a lesion in both the craniocaudal and mediallateral or medial-lateral oblique views, but cannot be palpated, it can be followed with subsequent reexamination and ipsilateral mammography in 3 to 6 months if it appears to be benign. If the lesion is mammographically indeterminate or suspicious, it should be evaluated by either a wire-directed or stereotactic biopsy. The entire lesion can be removed by wire-directed biopsy, but a stereotactic biopsy results in a smaller incision and can be done in an office-based setting. Cysts and other masses can be localized by either ultrasonography or mammography. Microcalcifications and subtle architectural changes require mammographic localization.

Most women between menarche and menopause will have some degree of breast tenderness or pain, engorgement, and nodularity, which typically occurs between ovulation and menses. These symptoms often become more intense in the fourth decade of life and subside after menopause. If exogenous hormones are administered following menopause, the symptoms can recur and may become especially prominent. This pattern of symptoms has been attributed to fibrocystic disease or chronic cystic mastitis, but these terms are not appropriate because the problem is neither a disease nor necessarily associated with either cysts or inflammation. *Fibrocystic changes* are often noted on breast biopsies performed for other purposes. The breasts are exquisitely sensitive to hormone-induced stimulation during puberty, menstruation, pregnancy, and lactation. The cyclic proliferation and involution of the breast during the menstrual cycle may precipitate breast pain and tenderness. The pain may be mild to severe, unilateral or bilateral, and does not necessarily correlate with physical findings. Examination usually demonstrates nodularity and tenderness, which can be diffuse or localized, especially in the subareolar area and in the upper outer quadrant. The nodularity can be impressive, but this is only infrequently due to large cysts, and there is usually no dominant mass.

Women with breast pain are often said to have fibrocystic changes, but there are no specific pathologic findings typical of *mastalgia*. The pain can be either cyclic or constant and can be very disconcerting to the patient. Treatment can be frustrating and requires reassurance and understanding from the physician. A supportive brassiere may provide some relief, and nonsteroidal antiinflammatory medications are beneficial. Narcotics should be avoided. Avoidance of caffeine has been recommended, and this is reasonably simple but is only occasionally helpful. Changing or eliminating oral contraceptives, or reducing the dose of exogenous estrogens, is often of benefit. A number of medications have been evaluated for the treatment of mastalgia, but placebo-controlled trials have not always substantiated the effectiveness of these agents. Vitamin E (alpha tocopherol) and other antioxidants have been widely used, but clinical studies have not confirmed their value. Evening primrose oil has been used in Europe, but is not widely available in the United States, and its benefit is only marginally superior to placebo. Bromocriptine, a prolactin inhibitor, is often effective for cyclic pain but is not approved for this use in the United States. In young women, oral contraceptives may alleviate some of the pain and nodularity, but can also increase these symptoms if they cause excessive hormonal stimulation. Danazol at a dose of 100 to 400 mg per day is the most effective drug for cyclic mastalgia, but its androgenic side effects of hirsutism, acne, oily skin and hair, reduction in breast size, and menstrual irregularity are often intolerable for the patient. Tamoxifen, an antiestrogen used to prevent recurrences of breast carcinoma, has been found to improve mastalgia at a dose of 10 mg per day. Side effects are less frequent and less intense than with danazol, but it is not approved for the treatment of mastalgia in the United States. Subcutaneous mastectomy with implantation of a prosthetic breast has been advocated for the treatment of mastalgia, especially when it has not responded to typical interventions. This treatment does not always alleviate pain, nor does it always prevent the problem of primary concern to the patient because carcinomas can develop in residual breast tissue.

Fibroadenomas are the most common breast masses in adolescents and young children, but they can occur at any age. They are typically between 0.5 and 3 cm in size. They can become quite large (>5 cm), especially just after menarche or just before menopause. These giant fibroadenomas are benign, but can mimic carcinoma due to their rapid growth and should be completely excised. In young women, smaller fibroadenomas can be observed, but many women prefer excision to alleviate their concerns and to avoid repeated examinations. On palpation, fibroadenomas are firm, well delineated, and quite mobile. There are no characteristic mammographic features, but they are usually well delineated and solid. This can be confirmed via ultrasonography if necessary. In older women, fibroadenomas may undergo degeneration, or regress entirely. If calcified, they are very hard to palpation, and very dense on mammography. There may be a small increased risk of subsequent breast cancer in women who have had a fibroadenoma excised.

Sclerosing adenosis is a variant of fibrocystic change that can mimic breast cancer both clinically and histologically. It may present as a poorly delineated mass on palpation or as clustered microcalcifications on mammography. Microscopically it is characterized by interlobular fibrosis and ductal proliferation. The fibrosis can be intense, and the lobules may lose their orientation, making differentiation from carcinoma difficult on frozen section. The nuclei are regular, however, and mitoses should not be present. They are adequately treated by complete excision. There appears to be a slight increased risk for development of breast cancer in women who have had sclerosing adenosis on biopsy.

Radial sclerosing lesions (radial scars) are typically small (<2 cm), stellate, irregular, and hard lesions that look and feel like carcinomas. They even mimic cancer on mammography. They are probably an intense form of fibrocystic change, with which they are often associated histologically. Simple excision is appropriate treatment, although women found to have these lesions may have a slightly increased risk for breast cancer.

Epithelial hyperplasia is often identified as an incidental finding on breast biopsies. This is defined as an increased number of cell layers lining the breast ducts. It can be mild (three to four cell layers), moderate (five or more layers), or florid, in which the ducts are packed with cells. If the cells lose their regularity, the term *atypical ductal hyperplasia* is used to describe this condition. This may be a precursor for ductal carcinoma in situ. Although florid epithelial hyperplasia is associated with a slight increased risk for breast cancer, atypical ductal hyperplasia is associated with a four- to fivefold increased frequency of invasive breast cancer compared with women without this finding. *Atypical lobular hyperplasia* is associated with a similar increase in the risk of development of breast cancer.

Injury to the breast may cause an area of *fat necrosis,* another sclerosing lesion that can be confused with breast cancer. Only about half the women with fat necrosis can recall a specific injury leading to this lesion. Fibrosis caused by the necrosis may result in the development of a poorly demarcated mass, sometimes with skin retraction.

Mammography also may demonstrate features worrisome for malignancy. Excision is both diagnostic and therapeutic.

Mammary duct ectasia (plasma cell mastitis) is an uncommon disorder that may cause either clear or thick nipple discharge, as well as periareolar abscesses. It is not an infectious disorder primarily, but secondary infections may require incision and drainage. Histologically, the mammary ducts are dilated, with inspissated secretions, periductal inflammation, and sometimes marked fibrosis. If subareolar abscesses recur, or periareolar fistulas develop, the involved subareolar area should be excised.

Mastitis and *breast abscesses* may occur in lactating women, but they are actually seen in fewer than 1% of breast-feeding women. The most common pathogen is *Staphylococcus aureus*, which tends to invade and destroy the milk-filled breast, causing abscesses and intense inflammation. An early infection presenting as simple cellulitis may respond to antibiotics alone. Needle aspiration of an abscess can be diagnostic, but definitive management must include open surgical drainage. A biopsy of the abscess wall should be obtained. Nursing need not be stopped, but can be painful on the affected side. Mechanical emptying of the affected breast can be performed until resolution of inflammation. If a woman chooses to stop breast-feeding, lactation can be suppressed if necessary. Any inflammatory changes in the breast of a woman beyond childbearing age should be considered inflammatory carcinoma. Evaluation should always include biopsy of the involved skin and breast.

Another lesion seen in lactating or recently lactating women is a *galactocele*. This is a cyst filled with milk, and although they are usually associated with lactation, they occasionally are seen in women near the menopause. They probably develop from obstruction of a breast duct, and typically present as a painless mass. Aspiration is diagnostic and is the only necessary treatment. Galactoceles only occasionally recur and can be excised if they fail to resolve on repeated aspiration.

Thrombosis of the thoracoepigastric (lateral thoracic) vein can cause a linear, cordlike mass in the breast, usually in the lower lateral aspect. This is known as *Mondor's disease*. Skin retraction may be present and can be accentuated by stretching the breast or raising the arms. The etiology is usually obscure, but it can follow minor breast injury or a breast biopsy. It can be mistaken for carcinoma, but careful physical examination and mammography will confirm the diagnosis. It is a self-limited condition that should be treated with reassurance, nonsteroidal antiinflammatory medications, and warm soaks if the lesion is tender.

Although bloody nipple discharge is a worrisome event, the most common cause is a benign *intraductal papilloma*. These 2- to 10-mm (rarely larger) lesions are usually solitary and develop within 1 to 3 cm of the nipple. They more commonly cause clear discharge than bloody drainage and cannot be palpated unless they are large. If the responsible duct can be identified, ductography may demonstrate the papilloma, but this is not necessary for management. Mammography should be obtained to exclude an occult breast carcinoma. At surgery the affected duct should be identified with a probe and excised by subareolar dissection. Multiple papillomas *(diffuse papillomatosis)* are uncommon. They usually cause serous nipple discharge, and the entire ductal system must be removed (with nipple-areolar preservation) to prevent recurrence. Unlike individual papillomas, diffuse papillomatosis seems to be associated with an increased risk of breast carcinoma.

Nipple invasion or creasing occurs occasionally and should be noted to avoid confusion with nipple retraction due to breast cancer. Nipple irritation may occur during breast-feeding, or from activities such as running, with abrasion of the nipple by clothing. Sebaceous cysts and other benign cysts may arise near the nipple or areola. Eczema of the nipple can occur but is usually bilateral and limited to the nipple and areola. Any rash involving the nipple should be suspected of representing Paget's disease (see Chapter 102) and must be examined via biopsy.

During lactation some women will become aware of tender swelling within one and rarely both axillae. This may be due to engorgement of the axillary tail of the breast, but might be caused by ectopic breast tissue that does not communicate with the rest of the breast. It may be quite tender, requiring suppression of lactation. This axillary breast tissue may require surgical excision to prevent recurrence in subsequent pregnancies.

Many women have undergone cosmetic breast enlargement or breast reconstruction following mastectomy. Anecdotal evidence has suggested that silicone gel prostheses might be responsible for the eventual development of rheumatoid arthritis, scleroderma, and other connective tissue diseases. Careful epidemiologic studies have failed to substantiate any link between breast implants and connective tissue diseases. Many women who have undergone breast augmentation have other risk factors that might increase their likelihood of developing connective tissue disorders.

General
1. Bland KI, Copeland EM III, eds. *The breast: comprehensive management of benign and malignant diseases,* 2nd ed. Philadelphia: WB Saunders, 1998.
   This is an excellent current textbook covering the entire spectrum of breast development, disorders, and treatment.
2. Kopans DB. *Breast imaging,* 2nd ed. Philadelphia: Lippincott-Raven, 1998.
   The author provides a thorough review of every aspect of diagnostic imaging of the breast, with high-quality illustrations.
3. Rosen PP. *Rosen's breast pathology.* Philadelphia: Lippincott-Raven, 1997.
   This is a superb reference on breast pathology, with numerous illustrations of histologic and cytologic specimens.
4. Tavassoli FA. *Pathology of the breast.* New York: Elsevier, 1992.
   This is a classic and still current reference on breast pathology.
5. Cady B, et al. Evaluation of common breast problems: guidance for primary care providers. *Cancer J Clin* 1998;48:49.
   This is a succinct review of common breast problems and their clinical evaluation.

Breast Imaging
6. Dershaw DD, et al. A comparison of screening mammography results from programs for women of different socioeconomic status. *Cancer* 1998;82:1692.
   Mammographic screening was effective for women of all socioeconomic status (SES), but more affluent women with cancer were more likely to have minimal cancers than were women of lower SES.
7. Frisell J, et al. Follow-up after 11 years update of mortality results in the Stockholm mammographic screening trial. *Breast Cancer Res Treat* 1997;45:263.
   Age at which benefit of screening could be confirmed was 50 years or greater, but methodologic weaknesses reduced the ability to assess the results in younger women.
8. Kopans DB. Updated results of the trials of screening mammography. *Surg Oncol Clin North Am* 1997;6:233.
   Screening mammography for women 40 to 49 years of age may reduce breast cancer mortality.
9. Wolverton DE, Sickles EA. Clinical outcome of doubtful mammographic finding. *Am J Roentgenol* 1996;167:1041.
   Only 1 ductal carcinoma in situ (DCIS) was identified among 543 probably benign mammographic abnormalities followed for a mean of 30 months.
10. Lidbrink E, et al. Neglected aspects of false positive findings of mammography in breast cancer screening: analysis of false positive cases from the Stockholm trial. *BMJ* 1996;312:1227.
    False-positive mammogram findings can consume time and resources, resulting in high costs and significant emotional distress for the women being evaluated.
11. Williams MB, et al. Future directions in imaging of breast diseases. *Radiology* 1998;206:297.
    This is a review of newer technologies and promising developments in early breast cancer detection and evaluation.

Tissue Sampling
12. The uniform approach to breast fine-needle aspiration biopsy. NIH Consensus Development Conference. *Am J Surg* 1997;174:371.
    This is a thorough review of the indications for techniques and cytologic evaluation of breast FNA.

13. Logan-Young W, et al. The cost-effectiveness of fine-needle aspiration cytology and 14-gauge core needle biopsy compared with open surgical biopsy in the diagnosis of breast carcinoma. *Cancer* 1998;82:1867.
When appropriate, less-invasive diagnostic procedures can result in substantial cost savings compared with open surgical biopsy.
14. Acheson MB, et al. Histologic correlation of image-guided core biopsy with excisional biopsy of nonpalpable breast lesions. *Arch Surg* 1997;132:815.
Stereotactic needle biopsy of the breast is accurate, with one missed carcinoma in 552 patients, 163 of whom had abnormal findings. The finding of atypical ductal hyperplasia requires subsequent excisional biopsy.

Mastalgia and Benign Lesions
15. Steinbrunn BS, Zera RT, Rodriguez JL. Mastalgia. Tailoring treatment to type of breast pain. *Postgrad Med* 1997;102:183.
A practical approach to the etiology and management of breast pain, with a review of currently used medications.
16. Euhus DM, Uyehara C. Influence of parenteral progesterones on the prevalence and severity of mastalgia in premenopausal women: a multi-institutional cross-sectional study. *J Am Coll Surg* 1997;184:596.
Medroxyprogesterone acetate was found to substantially reduce the frequency and severity of cyclic mastalgia.
17. Bruzzi P, et al. Cohort study of association of risk of breast cancer with cyst type in women with gross cystic disease of the breast. *BMJ* 1997;314:925.
Women with cysts having fluid with a potassium:sodium ratio of more than 1.5:1 seem to have a higher risk of breast cancer than those with ratios of less than 1.5:1.
18. Marshall LM, et al. Risk of breast cancer associated with atypical hyperplasia of lobular and ductal types. *Cancer Epidemiol Biomarkers Prev* 1997;6:297.
Both lesions are associated with increased risks for breast cancer. Atypical lobular hyperplasia has a very high risk for premenopausal breast cancer, and a substantial risk for postmenopausal breast cancer. The association between atypical ductal hyperplasia and cancer is weaker and does not vary with menopausal status.
19. Dixon JM, et al. Assessment of the acceptability of conservative management of fibroadenoma of the breast. *Br J Surg* 1996;83:2645.
Of 202 women under age 40 with 219 fibroadenomas, 18 were initially excised (all were benign), 13 increased in size over 2 years and were excised (all were again benign), 19 decreased in size, 42 resolved, and 89 showed no change in size.
20. Dixon JM, et al. Periductal mastitis and duct ectasia: different conditions with different aetiologies. *Br J Surg* 1996;83:820.
Periductal mastitis affected younger women, 90% of whom were cigarette smokers. Duct ectasia was more common in older women whose incidence of smoking was not different from age-matched controls.
21. O'Hara RJ, Dexter SP, Fox JN. Conservative management of infective mastitis and breast abscesses after ultrasonographic assessment. *Br J Surg* 1996;83:1413.
Ultrasonography was used to differentiate nonsuppurative inflammation from abscess. The former was treated with antibiotics (one formed an abscess and one was found to have inflammatory cancer). Twenty-two of 30 abscesses were treated by aspiration; three required subsequent incision and drainage.

Breast Implants
22. Park AJ, et al. Silicone gel-filled breast implants and connective tissue diseases. *Plast Reconstructive Surg* 1998;101:261.
A total of 317 patients with silicone gel implants were compared with matched controls. There was one patient with rheumatoid arthritis in each group; no other connective tissue disorders were identified, and there were no increases in antinuclear antibody or Rh factor.
23. Nyren O, Vin L, Josefsson S, et al. Risk of connective tissue disease and related disorders among women with breast implants: a nation-wide retrospective cohort study in Sweden. *BMJ* 1998;316:417.

A total of 7,742 women with cosmetic breast implants was compared with 3,353 women who had undergone breast reduction. There was a slight reduction in the risk for rheumatoid arthritis, systemic lupus erythematosus, scleroderma, dermatomyositis, and related disorders in the implant group compared with the breast reduction group.

24. Cook LS, et al. Characteristics of women with and without breast augmentation. *JAMA* 1997;277:1612.

Women who had breast augmentation procedures were more likely to use ethanol, were younger at their first pregnancy and had a greater likelihood of terminated pregnancies, were more likely to use oral contraceptives and hair dyes, and had a greater lifetime number of sexual partners. They were less likely to be obese. These differences may account for some of the perceived health problems in women who have had breast implants.

---

102. MALIGNANT BREAST DISEASE

Galen V. Poole

Breast cancer is the most common cancer in women in the United States. It is estimated that in 1999 about 180,000 women in the United States will be newly diagnosed with breast cancer, and it will cause nearly 44,000 deaths. About 30% of all new cancers in women are carcinomas of the breast, and breast cancer is responsible for 16% of cancer deaths. Considered by itself, breast cancer is the sixth leading cause of death for women in the United States. The age-adjusted death rate from breast cancer for U.S. women from 1992 to 1995 was 21 per 100,000. The death rate from breast cancer tends to be higher in western Europe, and lower in Asia and less-developed countries in the West. In the United States, the death rate from breast cancer has been nearly static since at least 1930. In comparison, lung cancer has increased greatly in incidence and is now the leading cause of cancer death for women in the United States.

The significance of age as a risk factor for breast cancer can be appreciated by the recognition that a 35-year-old woman has a 2.5% chance of developing breast cancer within 20 years. In comparison, a 55-year-old woman has a 5% chance of developing breast cancer by age 75. The annual incidence of breast cancer is less than 60 per 100,000 below age 40, but increases to about 100 per 100,000 by age 50, and is nearly 200 per 100,000 at age 70 years.

One of the chief risk factors for cancer of the breast is female gender; fewer than 1% of all breast cancers develop in men. The role of estrogens in the pathogenesis of breast cancer should be obvious. Longer exposure to uninterrupted menstrual cycles is seen in women who experience early menarche, late menopause, nulliparity, or delay in childbirth after age 30. All these are associated with a higher risk of breast cancer. Women who undergo bilateral oophorectomy before age 35 and do not take estrogen replacement have a two-thirds reduction in breast cancer risk. Exogenous estrogens nullify this benefit. Estrogens promote differentiation and proliferation of mammary epithelium, and they can also regulate neoplastic growth. Although it would not be accurate to say that estrogens cause breast cancer, they clearly function as tumor promoters. Estrogens probably function in concert with a variety of growth factors to control ductal epithelial growth, and to promote the development of breast cancer. Some of these growth factors include transforming growth factors alpha and beta, insulin-like growth factor, and platelet-derived growth factor. Despite the acknowledged role of endogenous estrogens on breast cancer development, exogenous estrogens should not be denied to women who have undergone oophorectomy, nor to postmenopausal women. The benefits outweigh the risks, with the possible exception of women who have a strong family history of breast carcinoma.

It has long been recognized that women with a first-degree relative with breast cancer have about a twofold increased probability of developing breast cancer compared with the normal population. Two first-degree relatives with breast cancer increase the risk by four- to sixfold. It should not be surprising that genetics plays a role in breast cancer development. Within the past decade, it has been discovered that an abnormality in the *BRCA-1* gene increases susceptibility to breast and ovarian carcinoma. This gene has been localized to the long arm of chromosome 17 and is transmitted by autosomal-dominant inheritance. Over half the women who inherit this gene—from mother or father—will develop breast cancer by 50 years of age, and the lifetime risk of breast cancer is over 80%. Male carriers of the gene are not at increased risk for breast cancer, probably due to the absence of estrogen exposure. A second gene, *BRCA-2*, has been mapped to chromosome 13. It confers a high risk for early onset of breast cancer but has little or no association with the development of ovarian cancer. However, it may be associated with male breast cancer. In reality, only about 5% of breast cancers are known to be associated with breast cancer susceptibility genes. Because breast cancer is common, it is not unexpected that about 20% of women with breast cancer have a relative who has had breast cancer. Most women who develop breast carcinoma do not have any recognizable genetic susceptibility or familial tendency to do so.

A well-recognized risk for the development of breast cancer is a prior history of breast cancer. The lifetime risk of metachronous breast cancer is about 10%. Obviously, the woman must survive the first cancer. For this reason, good prognosis cancers seem to have a greater risk of metachronous recurrence. Prior to the onset of breast conservation therapy for breast cancer, the risk was confined to the remaining breast. With more widespread use of lumpectomy and irradiation for primary treatment of breast cancer, the recurrence can be identified in either breast. The dose of radiation used to treat breast cancer is not likely to be carcinogenic. However, ionizing radiation to the chest was used to treat thymic enlargement, and is still used for treatment of Hodgkin's disease. Prior exposure to such radiation is clearly associated with an increased risk for developing breast cancer, and women treated with chest irradiation must be followed closely with annual examinations and mammography.

Environmental factors seem to play a role in the susceptibility to breast cancer. Japanese women have a relatively low risk of developing breast cancer, but their female children who are raised in the United States have an incidence of breast cancer that approaches that of native-born American women. Much of this increase in risk may be due to dietary factors. Diets high in fats seem to increase breast cancer risk, and obesity (high caloric intake) is clearly associated with a higher probability of developing breast cancer. Alcohol consumption, even in moderate amounts, also may increase breast cancer risk. There is no known association with smoking or with prior breast augmentation surgery.

Most breast cancers are discovered by the woman or by her physician on routine examination. Screening mammography identifies an increasing number of cancers, many of which are small and relatively early in development. Large-scale breast cancer detection projects have shown that rigorous screening can increase the proportion of women with localized breast cancer from about 50% to 80%, with a dramatic increase in the percentage of breast cancers less than 1 cm in maximum diameter. This should translate into mortality reduction with more widespread use of mammography, but data are not currently available to confirm this speculation.

If a suspicious nodule or lesion is detected on physical examination or mammography, a biopsy or tissue sampling procedure such as fine-needle aspiration or stereotactic biopsy should be performed. If the diagnosis of carcinoma is confirmed, counseling and planning can be pursued. Definitive treatment can be scheduled within the next 2 to 3 weeks. Only occasionally nowadays do women choose to undergo a biopsy followed by immediate mastectomy.

Breast cancers are either noninvasive or invasive (infiltrating). Noninvasive cancers can occur from either ductal or lobular epithelium. *Ductal carcinoma in situ* (DCIS) was previously referred to as intraductal carcinoma. Prior to screening mammography, most women with DCIS had a palpable mass. Currently, the vast majority of DCIS lesions are identified as clustered microcalcifications, or occasionally a mass, on mammography. About half of all mammographically identified breast cancers are DCIS. On sectioning, necrotic cancer cells may extrude from the ducts, which are packed with neoplastic cells. The cells are confined to the lumina of the ducts and do not invade the basement membranes. Fewer than 1% of patients with DCIS will have lymph node metastases. This probably occurs due to failure to identify an area of microinvasive cancer in the pathologic specimen. Either simple mastectomy (without axillary node dissection) or lumpectomy with negative histologic margins plus breast irradiation adequately treats DCIS. Radiation therapy must be included with lumpectomy because the risk of local recurrence is very high with lumpectomy alone. Long-term follow-up is mandatory because the lifetime risk of recurrence is 1% to 2% per year.

The second type of noninvasive breast cancer is *lobular carcinoma in situ* (LCIS). Unlike DCIS, LCIS usually has no clinical or radiographic evidence of its presence. It is virtually never palpable, and usually is not associated with microcalcifications. It is typically discovered incidentally within the biopsy specimen of a coexistent, radiographically detected benign lesion. LCIS is bilateral in 30% to 50% of cases. Histologically, neoplastic cells are identified in the acini and terminal ductules of the breast lobules. There is no invasion of the basement membrane. LCIS is a marker for the eventual development of invasive (ductal or lobular) breast cancer. At least one third of women with LCIS will develop invasive carcinoma, and that cancer can develop in either or both breasts. If LCIS is identified on biopsy, one of two courses of treatment can be selected: (1) observational management consists of monthly self-examinations, twice annual physical examinations, and annual mammography with lifelong follow-up; or (2) bilateral simple mastectomy, which might be most appropriate for a woman with a positive family history of breast cancer, or one who is overly anxious about observation and long-term follow-up. Immediate breast reconstruction can be performed to reduce the psychological impact of mastectomy.

The most common invasive breast cancer is *infiltrating ductal carcinoma,* which accounts for about 75% of all breast cancers. Grossly, these tumors are hard, poorly delineated masses that may infiltrate deeply into normal breast tissue. Mammographically, they tend to present as stellate masses that may contain calcifications. These cause the lesion to feel gritty when cut with a scalpel. Histologically, the malignant ductal cells are dispersed within a fibrous stroma, which can be quite intense. This stromal reaction led to the older term *scirrhous carcinoma.*

Invasive lobular carcinoma constitutes 6% to 8% of breast cancers. This cancer also presents as a firm, poorly demarcated mass, and the mammographic features are similar to those of infiltrating ductal carcinoma. Histologically this tumor is characterized by small round cells that infiltrate the stroma in a linear array known as Indian file fashion. A less common form of ductal carcinoma (2%–4% of breast cancers) is *medullary cancer.* These soft tumors can be very bulky. Microscopically they are composed of sheets of large anaplastic cells surrounded by a prominent lymphocytic infiltrate. Despite its aggressive histologic appearance, medullary carcinoma has a somewhat better prognosis than infiltrating ductal carcinoma. *Mucinous (colloid) carcinoma* is even less common (about 2%), and on physical examination this tumor also tends to be deceptively soft and well circumscribed. Histologically, the well-differentiated epithelial cells are surrounded by mucin, giving the appearance of islands within lakes. This variant also has a better prognosis than infiltrating ductal carcinoma. *Tubular carcinomas* (less than 2%) tend to be small firm tumors with a lower probability of nodal metastasis. Their microscopic appearance is characterized by tubular structures that are lined with a single layer of well-differentiated tumor cells that infiltrate the surrounding stroma. *Paget's disease* may be misdiagnosed as eczema of the nipple. It presents as a crusting, weeping erosion of the nipple that may burn or itch. A biopsy of the nipple can be diagnostic and demonstrates the characteristic Paget's cells: large clear cells with a large nucleus and prominent nucleoli. It is essentially always associated with intraductal carcinoma, which may be palpable in about half the women with this variant of breast cancer. Paget's disease is treated like any other breast carcinoma, and the prognosis depends on the stage of the underlying cancer.

Mesenchymal tumors of the breast are rare, and some of these arise as a complication of prior breast cancer treatment. *Cystosarcoma phylloides* was described more than 150 years ago, and despite the *sarcoma* term in its name and the occasional finding of marked cellular atypia and infiltration, most of these tumors have a benign behavior. For this reason many pathologists prefer the term *phylloides tumor*. They arise from lobular elements of the breast, and present as a firm mass that can be quite large. They rarely cause skin retraction or edema, and axillary node metastases essentially never occur. They are adequately treated by wide local excision without nodal dissection. Mastectomy should be reserved for large tumors in a small breast or for recurrent tumors following local excision. True sarcomas can arise from any of the stromal elements of the breast, but these are rare and are adequately treated by wide local excision. Sarcomas of the chest wall may arise within the radiation field following mastectomy and irradiation. The interval between treatment and development of carcinoma averages 10 years and may mimic a chest wall recurrence of the primary breast cancer. Treatment may require extensive chest wall resection and reconstruction. Lymphedema of the arm may occur following extensive axillary lymph node dissection, especially if radiotherapy was delivered to the axilla. *Lymphangiosarcomas* may occur in these chronically swollen extremities. These tumors present as multiple purplish nodules and may involve the entire arm and shoulder. They metastasize quickly and have a very poor prognosis.

As for most cancers, the American Joint Committee on Cancer staging of breast carcinoma is based on three variables: (1) tumor size or extension; (2) regional lymph node involvement; and (3) metastases. For each variable, the suffix X means that particular characteristic cannot be assessed. The suffix 0 means that the feature is not present. If the tumor is in situ, this is labeled as Tis. T1 lesions are subcategorized as 1a if the tumor is equal to or less than 0.5 cm in maximum dimension; 1b if more than 0.5 cm but not more than 1.0 cm; and 1c if more than 1 cm but not more than 2 cm. T2 tumors are greater than 2 cm but not more than 5 cm, and T3 tumors are greater than 5 cm. T4 lesions can be of any size and must meet one of the following criteria: 4a tumors extend to the chest wall; 4b tumors are characterized by edema (*peau d'orange*), skin retraction, or satellite skin lesions; 4c includes features of both 4a and 4b; and 4d is reserved for the variant known as inflammatory breast cancer. These tumors are characterized by diffuse breast edema, tenderness, and warmth. There may not be a palpable mass. This cancer is occasionally confused with an infectious process, but prompt biopsy of the involved skin and any associated mass will confirm the diagnosis. The dermis is invaded by malignant cells, which may fill the dermal lymphatics.

Ipsilateral lymph node involvement is denoted by N. Regional lymph nodes may not be involved (N0). If moveable, enlarged ipsilateral axillary nodes are present, this is considered N1. Fixed ipsilateral axillary nodes are characterized as N2. If ipsilateral internal mammary nodes are involved by metastatic disease, this is designated as N3. Distant metastases (including ipsilateral supraclavicular nodes) are either not present (M0) or present (M1).

Staging of breast cancer is determined by the TNM classification. Stage 0 is any in situ carcinoma. Stage I includes T1 lesions without lymph node involvement or distant metastases (T1/N0/M0). Stage II is subdivided into IIA (T1/N1/M0 or T2/N0/M0) and IIB (T2/N1/M0 or T3/N0/M0). Stage IIIA is characterized by any tumor smaller than T4 with fixed axillary nodes and no distant metastases (T1–3/N2/M0) or any T3 lesion with moveable nodes and no distant metastases (T3/N1/M0). Stage IIIB includes all T4 lesions without distant metastases plus all breast cancers with internal mammary node involvement (N3) and no distant metastases. Stage IV is defined as any breast cancer with distant metastases, regardless of size or nodal status. Staging can be based on either clinical or pathologic information. Accurate staging may require adjunctive laboratory studies and diagnostic imaging. All patients diagnosed with invasive breast cancer should have liver function tests and a chest radiograph. If transaminases or alkaline phosphatase levels are elevated, a CT scan of the abdomen and a bone scan should be obtained. For DCIS or LCIS, no diagnostic studies are necessary since metastases do not occur.

The prognosis of breast cancer is determined primarily by the stage of the cancer. Women with stage I cancers have a 5-year survival rate of 90% and a 10-year survival rate of about 80%. Stage II carcinomas are associated with a 5-year survival rate of 75%; the 10-year survival rate is only 50%. The 5-year survival rate of women with stage III breast cancer is about 50%, and only 30% will survive for 10 years. Prognosis for stage IV breast cancer is poor: 15% survival at 5 years, and less than 5% at 10 years. In addition to stage at presentation, the prognosis for women with breast cancer is influenced by a number of additional factors. Histologic grading is important because the less well-differentiated the cancer, the worse the prognosis. Outcome is also adversely affected by angiolymphatic invasion. At any stage, black women have worse outcomes than white women. The presence of hormone receptors in the nuclear material of cancer cells is associated with a more favorable prognosis. Estrogen and progesterone receptors can be identified and quantified as binding capacity in femtomoles (10^{-15} moles) of labeled steroid bound per milligram of protein. Levels less than 3 femtomoles are negative, and levels between 3 and 10 femtomoles are intermediate. Levels greater than 10 femtomoles are considered positive. Newer qualitative hormone receptor assays based on immunohistochemical analysis or enzyme-linked immunoassays can be performed on archival material or on samples that are too small for quantitative analysis. Postmenopausal women (over 55 years) are more likely to have positive assays for estrogen receptors (ERs) than are premenstrual women. There is no similar association between age and the presence of progesterone receptors (PRs). Women who have positive assays for both ERs and PRs have an 80% response rate to hormonal therapy. If only ERs are present, the response rate is about 35%, compared with a 45% response rate if only PRs are present. If both receptors are absent, the response to hormonal manipulation is only 5% to 10%.

Flow cytometry can be used to evaluate the DNA content of cells in a tumor. Diploid cells are those in which the DNA content is similar to nonmalignant reference cells. If the DNA content is altered, the cells are said to be aneuploid. Prognosis is worse with aneuploid cells, which are characteristic of undifferentiated tumors with greater nuclear atypia. Less well-differentiated tumors also are less likely to express hormone receptors. Tumors with a greater percentage of cells in the S and G_2 phases than reference tissue are said to have a greater proliferative activity. This also can be assessed by the incorporation of tritiated thymidine by tumor cells in vitro. Tumors with increased proliferative activity also are more likely to be ER negative and poorly differentiated. They tend to be associated with a worse prognosis than tumors with low proliferative activity. Other markers of poor prognosis include increased secretion of the protease cathepsin D, increased levels of the cytosolic p53 protein, and amplification of the *HER-2/neu* oncogene. These may not be independent predictors because they often are correlated with other histologic and biochemical features that are associated with a worse prognosis.

The management of breast cancer has undergone a number of changes in the past two decades, and newer developments in our understanding of the roles of genetics and nuclear abnormalities in breast cancer promise exciting changes for the future. It is now recognized that the treatment of breast cancer requires a multimodal approach, with treatment directed toward locoregional control, as well as interventions to obtain systemic control of cancer. Surgical excision and radiotherapy, either alone or in combination, are capable of providing control of the cancer within the breast and the regional lymph nodes. Chemotherapy and hormonal therapy are intended to address systemic control.

Surgical procedures for the treatment of breast cancer include wide local excision (often referred to as lumpectomy), simple (total) mastectomy, modified radical mastectomy, and radical mastectomy. *Wide local excision* implies that a circumferential margin of normal breast tissue is removed with excision of a malignant breast tumor, but this may prove difficult, especially for a large (>5 cm) lesion, or for a smaller mass within a small breast. Wide local excision for carcinoma of the breast should always be supplemented by radiation therapy; otherwise, the local recurrence rate will be excessive. *Simple mastectomy* involves removal of the entire breast, including the nipple-areola complex. A node dissection is not included. If the axillary lymph nodes are removed in continuity with the breast, this is referred to as a *modified radical mas-*

tectomy. The axillary lymph node dissection (ALND) is not truly therapeutic because it does not alter survival. However, node dissection is necessary to stage the tumor pathologically. *Radical mastectomy* includes removal of the pectoralis major and minor muscles, and traditionally was performed with an extensive ALND. Radical mastectomy is infrequently performed nowadays because it results in a substantial cosmetic deformity and does not improve outcome compared with less-ablative procedures. Reconstructive surgery is also more difficult following radical mastectomy.

Radiation therapy for local control should always be added to wide local excision of a breast carcinoma. The entire breast is treated with a dose of 4,500 to 5,000 cGy in 180- to 200-cGy fractions, 5 days per week for 5 weeks. A booster dose of 1,500 to 1,800 cGy often is provided to the primary site of the tumor. Lumpectomy and radiotherapy cannot be used to treat breast cancer if there are multiple tumors within the breast, if negative lumpectomy margins cannot be identified, if there is an extensive intraductal component in association with a primary cancer, if the chest wall has been previously irradiated, or if the patient is pregnant.

Radiotherapy can be delivered after mastectomy if the patient is felt to be at risk for locoregional failure. Circumstances in which this might be necessary would include women with multiple positive axillary nodes and those with large primary tumors or other situations in which the margin of resection was very narrow. Although radiation to the chest and axilla clearly reduces the risk of local failure, it does not improve survival.

Systemic control of breast cancer is approached by hormonal manipulation and by the use of cytotoxic chemotherapy. Although oophorectomy, ovarian irradiation, adrenalectomy, and even hypophysectomy were used in the past to reduce estrogen levels, the same effect can be more simply achieved by the use of antiestrogens such as tamoxifen. Hormonal manipulation is of greatest value if the breast cancer is both ER- and PR-positive, but positivity for only one hormone receptor is preferable to both being negative. Continuation of tamoxifen for 5 years after initial treatment of breast cancer confers a survival benefit, but longer periods of administration do not provide additional value.

Cytotoxic chemotherapy can be used for the systemic treatment of breast cancer. Women with cancers less than 1 cm in diameter and negative lymph nodes usually are not candidates for chemotherapy. Women whose breast cancers are larger than 1 cm, are ER and PR negative, and have no involvement of the axillary nodes may benefit from chemotherapy. Regardless of tumor size, all women who have metastases to the axillary lymph nodes should receive chemotherapy, with the exception of postmenopausal women with good prognosis tumors (ER positive). Postmenopausal women with ER-positive tumors and axillary node involvement are usually treated with tamoxifen alone because the addition of cytotoxic chemotherapy confers no appreciable survival benefit.

The standard chemotherapy protocol for breast carcinoma is a combination of cyclophosphamide, methotrexate, and 5-fluorouracil (CMF). Other agents may be used, principally vincristine, which is often added to CMF. Doxorubicin (Adriamycin) may be used in combination with cyclophosphamide and 5-FU (CAF). This combination of agents is typically used for advanced, recurrent, or metastatic breast cancer. The benefit of chemotherapy is more clearly seen when the disease-free survival is evaluated, and is less pronounced when overall survival is assessed. The benefit of cytotoxic chemotherapy is most apparent in premenopausal, node-positive women.

Noninvasive breast cancer is treated by local measures only: either simple mastectomy, or wide local excision and breast irradiation. No ALND or systemic therapy is necessary. Early localized breast cancer is treated by either modified radical mastectomy, or wide local excision with axillary node dissection and breast irradiation. An alternative to formal axillary dissection is removal of a sentinel axillary lymph node identified by uptake of a vital dye and/or a radioactive label. There are not yet sufficient data to support the widespread use of this approach. Tamoxifen should be given to all women with ER-positive tumors larger than 1 cm if axillary lymph nodes are negative, and to postmenopausal women with positive axillary nodes if the tumor is ER positive. Systemic chemotherapy should be recommended to all women with breast cancers larger than 1 cm regardless of nodal status, except postmenopausal women with ER-positive tumors. Locally advanced breast cancer (stages IIIa and IIIb) is treated by multimodal therapy. These tumors are often too large for wide local excision and irradiation. The typical sequence is a modified radical mastectomy followed by systemic chemotherapy. Chest wall irradiation may be added to improve local control. Inflammatory breast cancer is managed by an aggressive combination of induction chemotherapy followed by mastectomy and regional radiation. Some oncologists prefer aggressive chemotherapy with tumoricidal irradiation, and reserve mastectomy only if gross residual disease persists. This approach to inflammatory carcinoma has altered the prognosis substantially. Five-year survival has improved from less than 5% to greater than 50%.

Breast cancer that is metastatic at diagnosis cannot be cured. Nonetheless, it can be controlled, and many women with bone or soft tissue metastases can survive for many years. Management includes a combination of hormonal manipulation and chemotherapy, with the occasional use of radiotherapy for either local control or treatment of painful metastases. Mastectomy should be reserved for those cases in which the primary tumor is large and may interfere with chemotherapy, or if the tumor is fungating through the skin and causes significant wound management problems.

Some patients with metastatic disease may be treated by giving lethal doses of chemotherapy, with subsequent reinfusion of previously harvested autologous bone marrow. This approach requires substantial support due to its complexity and toxicity. The duration of response is often disappointing, and it is not clear that cures can be achieved.

A promising recent development for treatment of advanced breast cancer is the administration of an antibody to an oncogene that signals cancer cells to continue their uncontrolled multiplication. Whether this approach proves to have wide applicability, and whether new antibodies to other cell-signaling agents can be devised and shown to have therapeutic benefit, remains to be seen.

Breast cancer is extremely uncommon during pregnancy and lactation, with an occurrence of one in every 3,000 to 4,000 pregnancies. The engorgement, tenderness, and nodularity of the breast during pregnancy renders physical examination difficult and greatly reduces the sensitivity of mammography. The diagnosis of breast cancer during pregnancy therefore is often delayed, and when discovered these tumors tend to be large with axillary lymph node metastases. These factors adversely affect prognosis, but for any given stage the outcome for breast cancer during pregnancy is similar to that in nonpregnant women with equivalent carcinomas. If mastectomy is selected for treatment of breast cancer during pregnancy, this can be performed with careful anesthetic monitoring of mother and fetus. If breast conservation is chosen, or if chemotherapy must be administered, the pregnancy should be terminated due to the obvious toxicity of radiation and cytotoxic agents.

General
1. Bland KI, Copeland EM III, eds. *The breast: comprehensive management of benign and malignant diseases,* 2nd ed. Philadelphia: WB Saunders, 1998.
    This is a modern, authoritative text on diseases of the breast.
2. Rosen PP. *Rosen's breast pathology.* Philadelphia: Lippincott-Raven, 1997.
    This is a well-illustrated, well-written text on breast pathology.
3. Landis SH, et al. Cancer statistics, 1998. *Cancer J Clin* 1998;48:6.
    The authors present an annual overview of cancer statistics, with a wealth of useful information.

In Situ Breast Cancer
4. Winchester DP, Strom EA. Standards for diagnosis and management of ductal carcinoma in situ (DCIS) of the breast. *Cancer J Clin* 1998;48:108.
    The authors present a complete review of standards for diagnosis and treatment of ductal carcinoma in situ.
5. Ernster VL, et al. Incidence of and treatment for ductal carcinoma in situ of the breast. *JAMA* 1996;275:913.
    Because of the widespread adoption of screening mammography, the incidence of ductal carcinoma in situ has increased greatly since 1983.

6. Silverstein MJ, et al. Outcome after invasive local recurrence in patients with ductal carcinoma in situ of the breast. *J Clin Oncol* 1998;16:1367.
   About 10% of 707 women with DCIS had recurrences, which were invasive in 35 (5%). The 8-year probability of breast cancer mortality after breast preservation was about 2%.

Early / Operable Breast Cancer

7. Winchester DP, Cox JD. Standards for diagnosis and management of invasive breast cancer. *Cancer J Clin* 1998;48:83.
   The authors present a consensus statement for breast cancer.
8. Forrest AP, et al. Randomized controlled trial of conservation therapy for breast cancer: 6-year analysis of the Scottish trial. *Lancet* 1996;348:708.
   After local excision of breast cancer, breast irradiation reduced local relapses from 24.5% to 5.8%.
9. Fisher B, et al. Tamoxifen and chemotherapy for node-negative, estrogen receptor-positive breast cancer. *J Natl Cancer Inst* 1997;89:1673.
   Chemotherapy reduces the risk of treatment failure regardless of tumor size, hormone receptor status, or age.
10. Connolly JL, et al. Predictors of breast recurrence after conservative surgery and radiation therapy for invasive breast cancer. *Mod Pathol* 1998;11:134.
    The authors emphasize the importance of adequate excision with negative margins to reduce local recurrence.
11. Dees EC, et al. Does information from axillary dissection change treatment in clinically node-negative patients with breast cancer? An algorithm for assessment of impact of axillary dissection. *Ann Surg* 1997;226:279.
    Twenty-seven percent of clinically node-negative women had pathologically positive nodes. Eight percent of T1a tumors and 10% of T1b tumors had positive nodes. However, women over 60 years of age who were clinically node-negative rarely had their treatment changed by the findings of axillary dissection.
12. White RE, et al. Therapeutic options and results for the management of minimally invasive carcinoma of the breast; influence of axillary dissection for the treatment of T1a and T1b lesions. *J Am Coll Surg* 1996;183:575.
    Node positivity was present in 9.8% of T1a and 19.4% of T1b lesions. Omission of axillary dissection in these patients was associated with significant reductions in overall, disease-free, and breast cancer–specific survival.
13. Guenther JM, Kirgan DM, Giuliano AE. Feasibility of breast-conserving therapy for younger women with breast cancer. *Arch Surg* 1996;131:632.
    Despite attempts to perform breast-conserving therapy in women under 35 years of age with breast cancer, mastectomy was required in 56% either initially (34%) or eventually (22%) due to multifocal tumors, large tumors, or local recurrence. Only 21% of women over 35 years of age required mastectomy for local control.
14. Borgstein PJ, et al. Sentinel lymph node biopsy in breast cancer: guidelines and pitfalls of lymphoscintigraphy and gamma probe detection. *J Am Coll Surg* 1998;186:275.
    The failure rate was higher in patients who had a previous excisional biopsy (36%) than in those with a palpable tumor in place (4%). Overall success in the biopsy of a sentinel node was 94%. Only one of 60 patients (1.7%) with a negative sentinel node had positive nodes on axillary dissection.

Advanced Breast Cancer

15. Eltahir A, et al. Treatment of large and locally advanced breast cancers using neoadjuvant chemotherapy. *Am J Surg* 1998;175:127.
    Multimodality therapy resulted in a 48% 5-year survival rate, which was higher in those with a complete response. No patient without response survived 5 years.
16. Glinski B, et al. Multimodality treatment of noninflammatory stage IIIb breast cancer. *J Surg Oncol* 1997;66:179.
    A regimen of preoperative chemotherapy, mastectomy, postoperative radiotherapy and chemotherapy resulted in a 33% 5-year disease-free survival rate.

17. Ayash LJ, et al. High-dose multimodality therapy with autologous stem-cell support for stage IIIb breast carcinoma. *J Clin Oncol* 1998;16:1000.
    This aggressive regimen resulted in a 64% disease-free survival rate at 30 months. Women with a complete response (15%) had a 100% 30-month disease-free survival rate.
18. Brooks HL, et al. Inflammatory breast carcinoma: a community hospital experience. *J Am Coll Surg* 1998;186:622.
    Most patients presented with stage IV disease, all of whom died, with a mean survival of about 1 year. Mean survival was 45 months for the five survivors, all of whom were stage IIId.
19. Lannin DR, et al. Influence of socioeconomic and cultural factors on racial differences in late-stage presentation of breast cancer. *JAMA* 1998;279:1801.
    Black women were much more likely to present with advanced breast cancer. Socioeconomic factors alone did not explain the effect of race on breast cancer stage. Most of the effect was due to cultural beliefs.

Genetics of Breast Cancer
20. Green MH. Genetics of breast cancer. *Mayo Clin Proc* 1997;72:54.
    This is an excellent review on familial breast cancer and the associated genetic abnormalities.
21. Newman B, et al. Frequency of breast cancer attributable to *BRCA1* in a population-based series of American women. *JAMA* 1998;279:915.
    Only 2.6% of women with breast cancer had BRCA1 mutations. White women with a family history of ovarian cancer, or at least four relatives with either breast or ovarian cancer, had mutations of BRCA1 ranging from 13% to 33%.

Breast Cancer Prevention
22. Mezzett M, et al. Population attributable risk for breast cancer: diet, nutrition, and physical exercise. *J Natl Cancer Inst* 1998;90:389.
    The risk of breast cancer was increased in women who had an ethanol intake of more than 20 g/day, low beta-carotene intake, low vitamin E intake, and low levels of physical activity. Obesity increased breast cancer risk for postmenopausal women.
23. Powles TJ. Status of antiestrogen breast cancer prevention trials. *Oncology (Huntingt)* 1998;12[Suppl]:28.
    Several prospective, double-blind trials are being conducted to evaluate the use of tamoxifen to prevent breast cancer. Although some adverse effects have occurred, the long-term benefits will likely outweigh the risks.

Miscellaneous
24. Goss PE, Sierra S. Current perspectives on radiation-induced breast cancer. *J Clin Oncol* 1998;16:338.
    This is a current review of breast cancer due to environmental, occupational, or therapeutic exposure to radiation. The authors discuss links with genetic causation and propose plausible prevention strategies.
25. Rajan PB, Cranor ML, Rosen PP. Cystosarcoma phyllodes in adolescent girls and young women: a study of 45 patients. *Am J Surg Pathol* 1998;22:64.
    Recurrence was more likely if tumor borders were infiltrative and surgical margins were positive. Metastases were rare (one patient).
26. Kuerer HM, et al. Breast carcinoma associated with pregnancy and lactation. *Surg Oncol* 1997;6:93.
    The incidence of breast cancer occurring during pregnancy is increasing, possibly because many women are delaying pregnancy until their late thirties and early forties.
27. Surbone A, Petrek JA. Childbearing issues in breast cancer survivors. *Cancer* 1997;79:1271.
    Although no prospective studies exist, survival does not seem to be decreased by subsequent pregnancy. Many premenopausal women with breast cancer have been rendered amenorrheic by chemotherapy, obviating subsequent pregnancies.

SUBJECT INDEX

A

Abdominal pregnancy, 11
Abnormal glandular
cells of uncertain
significance
(AGCUS), 426
Abnormal squamous
cells of uncertain
significance
(ASCUS), 426
Abortion, 5–10
complications, 6–7, 10
defined, 5
diagnosis, 5, 8
elective, 5–6
etiology, 5, 7–8
incidence, 5
induced, 6
infection and, 7
mortality rate, 6
recurrent, 5
septic, 7
spontaneous, 5
surgical, 6
symptoms, 7
therapeutic, 5–6
treatment, 6–7, 8–9
Abruptio placentae, 21–25
characteristics, 21
classification, 22
complications, 23, 25
definition, 21
diagnosis, 22, 24
DIC and, 22–23
etiology, 22
hemorrhage in, 22
incidence, 21
perinatal mortality and,
21
symptoms, 22
treatment, 23, 24
Abscess, breast, 471
Abuse
domestic battering,
379–380
physical, during preg-
nancy, 128
sexual
of children, 379, 381
of the elderly, 380
incidence, 379
Acetaminophen
during pregnancy, 126
Acquired immunodefi-
ciency syndrome
(AIDS)

adolescents and, 360
classification, 297
described, 297–298
diagnosis, 299, 301
drug abuse and, 298
effect on nervous
system, 298
epidemiology, 301
etiology, 297, 298
histologic studies, 298
HIV infection and,
298–299
incidence, 297, 298, 301
during pregnancy,
58–59
counseling, 59
HIV transmission, 59
incidence, 58
pneumonia and, 67
prophylaxis, 59
treatment, 59
prevalence, 300
prevention, 301–302
progression of, 299
protective role of
condoms, 333
symptoms, 298–299
testing for, 299
therapy, 301–302
transmission, 297
Actinomyces
pelvic abscess and, 315
Actinomycin-D
(Dactinomycin)
chemotherapeutic
agent in gyneco-
logic cancer, 466
treatment for gesta-
tional tropho-
blastic disease, 15
Acupuncture
for labor and delivery,
158
Acute puerperal inversion
postpartum hemor-
rhage and, 191
Acute urethral syndrome,
290
Acyclovir
for herpes simplex
virus infection, 48
for varicella, 49
Adenomyosis, 258
Adenosis, sclerosing, 470
Adolescents. See also
Puberty

contraceptive use, 87,
360–361
dysfunctional uterine
bleeding in,
400–401
human papillomavirus
and, 294
pregnancy in, 85–91
adolescent fathers, 87
complications, 86,
90–91
diagnosis, 89
etiology, 87, 88
health care for, 86–87
incidence, 85
long-term conse-
quences of, 86
nutritional de-
mands, 86
obstetric complica-
tions, 86
prevention, 87
psychological prob-
lems, 85–86
social complications,
85
treatment, 86, 89–90
sexual behavior of,
359–363
characterization, 359
contraception and,
361–362
education, 360, 363
experimentation,
359, 360
incidence, 360
physician's role in,
360
psychological equi-
librium and, 359
substance abuse and,
360
Adriamycin
(Doxorubicin)
chemotherapeutic
agent in gyneco-
logic cancer, 465,
466
Adult respiratory
distress syndrome
(ARDS)
during pregnancy, 69,
70–71
symptoms, 69
therapy, 69
treatment, 69

AFP. *See* Serum alpha-
fetoprotein
screening
AGCUS. *See* Abnormal
glandular cells
of uncertain
significance
Age
adolescents. *See*
Adolescents
benign ovarian neo-
plasms and, 446
breast cancer and, 474
carcinoma of the endo-
metrium and, 438
carcinoma of the vulva
and, 422
children. *See* Children
elderly. *See* Elderly
maternal, advanced,
91–94
contraception for, 91,
92
counseling for, 92
diabetes in, 92
fetal risks and, 92
grand multipara,
92–93, 94
hypertension in, 92
incidence, 91
medical diseases and,
92
mortality due to, 92
sterilization for, 92
menopause and, 406
sexuality and,
363–364, 365
AIDS. *See* Acquired
immunodeficiency
syndrome
Albuterol
for asthma, 66
Aldara (Imiquimod)
for condyloma
acuminatum, 57
Aldomet (Methyldopa)
for hypertension dur-
ing pregnancy, 30
Alendronate
(Biphosphonates)
for osteoporosis, 407
Alkeran (Melphalan)
chemotherapeutic
agent in gyneco-
logic cancer, 465,
466
Allen-Master syndrome,
253
ALND. *See* Axillary lymph
node dissection
Alpha 1 antitrypsin
deficiency

DNA genetic screening
and, 218
Amenorrhea, 385–388
anovulation and, 353
conditions leading to,
385–386
definition, 385
diagnosis, 385, 386
differential diagnosis,
385
etiology, 385
evaluation, 385–386
primary, 385
secondary, 385
Aminoglycosides
for pelvic abscess, 315
Amphotericin B
for pneumonia, 67
Aminoglycosides
for urinary tract infec-
tion in pregnancy,
53
Amniocentesis, 222
for antepartum diag-
nosis of fetal
anomalies, 212
genetic screening and,
218–219
Amoxicillin
for *Chlamydia* infection,
290
Ampicillin, 7
for premature ruptured
membranes, 118
for urinary tract infec-
tion in pregnancy,
53
Amytal (Sodium
amobarbital)
for eclampsia, 40
Analgesia
for labor and delivery,
157–160
cesarean section, 158
complications,
157–158, 160
evaluation, 157
obesity and, 157
parenteral, 157, 159
patient controlled,
158
psychologic, 160
regional, 157–158,
159
risk assessment, 157
selection, 157
Androgens
anovulation and,
352–353
insensitivity, 412–415
ambiguous genitalia
and, 413

diagnosis, 413–414
etiology, 412
genetic disorders and,
412–413
incomplete form of
resistance, 413
presentation, 413
pseudohermaphro-
dism, 413
therapy, 414
sexuality and, 364
Androgen insensitivity
syndrome, 413
Anemia
during pregnancy,
108–113
complications, 110,
112–113
congenital, 108
diagnosis, 108–109,
111
etiology, 108, 111
follow-up, 110
iron deficiency and,
109
laboratory evaluation,
108–109
toxins and, 109
treatment, 110,
111–112
Anesthesia
in breech presentation,
145
and heparin, for deep
vein thrombosis,
201
for labor and delivery,
157–160
cesarean section, 158
complications,
157–158, 160
evaluation, 157
obesity and, 157
parenteral, 157, 159
patient controlled,
158
psychologic, 160
regional, 157–159,
159
risk assessment, 157
selection, 157
laparoscopy and, 265,
267
mortality rate
during pregnancy,
68–69
with surgical
abortions, 6
in pediatric patients,
260, 262
during pregnancy, 127
Anorgasmy, 368
dyspareunia and, 374

Anovulation, 351–356
androgen and, 352–353
central neuroendocrine
failure and, 353
chronic, 354
clomiphene nitrate for,
354
described, 351
endometrial hyper-
plasia and, 434
estrogen and, 352
gonadotropins and, 352
gonadotropin therapy
for, 354
hormones and, 352
polycystic ovarian
syndrome and,
352–353, 355
premenstrual syndrome
and, 403
prolactin and, 353
surgical ablation for,
354
treatment, 353–354,
355–356
Antibiotics
antitumor, 465
prophylactic, for pla-
centa previa, 19
treatment for urinary
tract infection in
pregnancy, 53
Anticardiolipin anti-
bodies, 5
Antihypertensive agents
sexuality and, 364
Antimetabolites
chemotherapeutic
agent in gyneco-
logic cancer,
465–466
Antiphospholipid anti-
body syndrome
abortion and, 5
Antipsychotic drugs
sexuality and, 364
Antitumor antibiotics
chemotherapeutic
agent in gyneco-
logic cancer, 465,
466
Aortic regurgitation
during pregnancy, 72
Aortic stenosis
during pregnancy, 72
Apgar score, 177
ARDS. See Adult respira-
tory distress syn-
drome
Arias-Stella reaction, 12
ART. See Assisted repro-
ductive technology

Arteriosclerosis
menopause and,
409–410
ASB. See Asymptomatic
bacteriuria
ASCUS. See Abnormal
squamous cells of
uncertain signifi-
cance
ASD. See Atrial septal
defect
Asherman's syndrome
(intrauterine
synechiae), 5, 191
Asphyxia, fetal, 175–179
acid-base evaluation,
177–178
amniotic fluid and,
176–177, 178
described, 175–176
heart rate, 176
management, 176
outcome, 177, 178–179
Assisted reproductive
technology (ART),
350
Asthma
during pregnancy,
65–66, 69–70
beta agonist med-
ications, 66
diagnosis, 65
etiology, 65
peak expiratory flow
rate (PEFR), 65
pulmonary function
testing, 65
treatment, 66
Asymptomatic bacteri-
uria (ASB), during
pregnancy, 51
Atrial septal defect (ASD)
during pregnancy, 72
Atrophic vaginitis,
303–305
Atypical ductal hyper-
plasia, 470
Atypical lobular hyper-
plasia, 470
Autosomal dominant
traits
genetic screening and,
215
Autosomal recessive traits
genetic screening and,
215
Autosome 5, 16
Axillary lymph node
dissection (ALND),
479
Azithromycin
for chancroid, 58

for Chlamydia infection,
290
for gonorrhea, 278
AZT (Zidovudine)
for HIV, 49–50, 59
Aztaareonam
for urinary tract
infection in
pregnancy, 53

B
Bacterial vaginosis, 304
Bacteroides fragilis
following abortion, 7
pelvic abscess and, 315
Becker's muscular
dystrophy
DNA genetic screening
and, 218
Beclomethasone
for asthma, 66
Benign breast disorders,
468–474
Benign ovarian neo-
plasms, 445–449
Beta-agonist drugs
during pregnancy, 66
for preterm labor, 114
Beta blockers
for hyperthyroidism, 79
sexuality and, 364
Betamethasone
for delivery of small
infants, 180
Bichloracetic acid
for human papillo-
mavirus, 295
Biphosphonates
(Alendronate)
for osteoporosis, 407
Bleeding. See
Hemorrhage
Bleomycin
chemotherapeutic
agent in gyneco-
logic cancer, 466
Blood dyscrasia
postpartum hemor-
rhage and, 189
BMD. See Bone mineral
density
Bone mineral density
(BMD)
menopause and, 407
Bonnevie-Ullrich
syndrome, 410
BPP. See Fetal bio-
physical profile
Breast disease
benign, 468–474
abscess, 471
atypical ductal hyper-
plasia, 470

Breast disease (contd.)
  atypical lobular
    hyperplasia, 470
  diagnosis, 468
  diet and, 469
  differentiation from
    malignant, 468
  diffuse papillo-
    matosis, 471
  epithelial hyper-
    plasia, 470
  evaluation of com-
    plaint, 468
  examination, 469
  family history and,
    468
  fat necrosis, 470
  fibroadenomas, 470
  fibrocystic changes,
    469
  galactoceles, 471
  imaging, 472
  implants, 473–474
  infection, 471
  injury, 470
  intraductal papil-
    loma, 471
  mammary duct ecta-
    sia (plasma cell
    mastitis), 471
  mammography and,
    468–469
  mastalgia and,
    469–470, 473
  mastitis, 471
  Mondor's disease, 471
  needle biopsy and,
    469, 472–473
  nipple invasion, 471
  pain and, 469
  radial sclerosing
    lesions (radial
    scars), 470
  sclerosing adenosis,
    470
  Staphylococcus
    aureus, 471
  swelling, 471
  tissue sampling,
    469, 472–473
  malignant, 473–482
    age as risk factor, 474
    axillary lymph node
      dissection
      (ALND), 479
    chemotherapy, 478
      cytotoxic, 479
      standard protocol,
        479
    classification, 477
    cytosarcoma phyl-
      lodes, 477

  diagnosis, 475
  diet and, 475
  ductal carcinoma in
    situ (DCIS),
    475–476
  environment and, 475
  estrogen and, 474
  etiology, 475
  family history and,
    475
  flow cytometry, 478
  genetics, 482
  hormonal therapy,
    478
  incidence, 474
  infiltrating ductal,
    476
  lobular carcinoma in
    situ (LCIS), 476
  lymph nodes and, 477
  lymphangiosarcomas,
    477
  mammography,
    475–476
  management, 478
  mastectomy, 478–479
    modified radical,
      478–479
    radical, 479
    simple, 478
  medullary, 476
  mesenchymal tumors,
    477
  metastases, 480
  mucinous (colloid),
    476
  Paget's disease, 476
  pathogenesis, 474
  phyllodes tumor, 477
    during pregnancy,
      480
  prevention, 482
  prognosis, 476, 478
  radiation therapy
    for, 476, 479
  radiotherapy for, 479
  risk factors for, 474
  scirrhosis carcinoma,
    476
  staging, 477
  surgical procedures,
    478
  survival rates, 478
  symptoms, 475
  systemic control, 479
  treatment, 477, 479
  tubular, 476
Breast engorgement, 186
  infection and, 196
Breast-feeding. See also
  Lactation
  cardiac medications
    and, 72

  engorgement, 186
  in HIV-infected
    patients, 50, 59
  let-down reflex and, 186
  nipple soreness and, 186
Breast implants,
  473–474
Breech presentation,
  143–146. See also
  Delivery; Labor
  anesthesia for, 145
  cesarean delivery for,
    143–144
  characterization, 143
  definition, 143
  diagnosis, 143
  etiology, 143
  incidence, 143
  management, 144
  predisposition, 143
  procedures for, 146
  risk factors, 143
  symptoms, 143
Brenner tumor, 445–446
Bromocriptine mesylate
  (Parlodel)
  to suppress lactation,
    187
Bupivacaine
  for labor and delivery,
    157

C
CAH. See Congenital
  adrenal hyper-
  plasia
Calcitonin
  for osteoporisis, 407
Calcium channel blockers
  for hypertension during
    pregnancy, 30–31
  for preterm labor, 115
Calcium replacement
  therapy
  menopause and, 407
Calymmatobacterium
  granulomatis, 58
Cancer. See also Oncology,
  gynecologic
  endometrial, 438–441
  endometrial hyper-
    plasia, 433–437
  hepatocellular, 48
  hormonal contra-
    ception and, 326
  human papilloma virus,
    carcinogenic poten-
    tial of, 293–294
  oral contraceptives and,
    326
  ovarian, 450–454

recurrent, and radiation therapy, 461
uterine, 441–445
Candida albicans, 303–304
Capreomycin
for genital tuberculosis, 320
Carbon dioxide laser vaporization
for vulval intraepithelial neoplasia, 420
Carboplatinum chemotherapeutic agent in gynecologic cancer, 466
Carcinoma in situ (CIS), 426, 429
Cardiac lesions, congenital, 72
Cardiomyopathy during pregnancy, 73
Cardiovascular disease during pregnancy, 71–74
breast feeding, cardiac medications and, 72
classification, 72
counseling, 74
fetal surveillance, 73
management, 73
maternal mortality, 71, 72
sterilization for, 73
Cardiovascular system physiologic changes during pregnancy, 71
Cefix
for gonorrhea, 56
Cefixime
for gonorrhea, 278
Cefotetan
for gonorrhea, 278
for pelvic inflammatory disease, 312
for puerperal infections, 195
Cefoxitin
for pelvic inflammatory disease, 312
for puerperal infections, 195
Ceftizoxime
for gonorrhea, 278
Ceftriaxone
for chancroid, 58
for gonorrhea, 56, 278
for syphilis, 282
Celioscopy, 265
Celiotomy, exploratory, 455–456

Cephalexin
for urinary tract infection in pregnancy, 53
Cephalopelvic disproportion (CPD), 171–175
categories, 171
cesarean section due to, 172
complications, 175
definition, 171
diagnosis, 171, 173–174
etiology, 171, 173
fetal risks, 172
incidence, 171
management, 172, 173–175
maternal risks associated with, 172
Cephalosporin
for pneumonia, 67
for puerperal infections, 196
for toxic shock syndrome, 308
for urinary tract infection in pregnancy, 53
Cervical cap, 333, 334
Cervical intraepithelial neoplasia (CIN), 425–429
cervical dysplasia and, 426
cytologic study of, 426
diagnosis, 426, 428
epidemiology, 427
epithelial abnormalities and, 425–426
etiology, 426, 427–428
human papillomavirus and, 426
treatment, 426, 428–429
Cervical pregnancy, 11
Cervix
carcinoma of, 429–433
age and, 429
bleeding and, 430
chemotherapy for, 431
diagnosis, 429, 432
epidemiology, 431–432
follow-up, 431
grading, 429
incidence, 429
in pregnancy, 431
pretreatment clinical evaluation, 429–430

prognosis, 430
radiation therapy for, 430–431, 460–461, 461–462
recurrence, 431, 433
risk factors for, 429
staging of, 430
survival rates, 431
symptoms, 430
treatment, 430–431, 432–433
incompetent, 5
Cesarean section
for abnormal presentations, 147, 148
anesthesia and analgesia for, 158, 164
for breech presentation, 143–144
due to cephalopelvic disproportion, 172
complications, 165, 167–168
definition, 163
diagnosis, 166–167
elective, 164
etiology, 166
extraperitoneal, 164
history of, 163–164
hysterectomy with, 164
incidence, 163–165
incisions used in, 164
indications, 164
for large infants, 180, 181
mortality rates in, 165
placenta previa and, 18, 19
prophylactic antibiotic use, 165
risk factors, maternal, 163–164, 165
treatment, 167
vaginal births after, 165
wound infection and, 195
Chancroid
during pregnancy, 58
Chemical contraceptives, 335
spermicides and, 333, 335
teratogenicity, 335
Chemotherapy
for breast cancer, 478
cytotoxic, 479
standard protocol, 479
for gestational trophoblastic disease, 14, 15

Chemotherapy (*contd.*)
  in gynecologic cancer,
    463–468
  adjuvant, 465
  adverse effects, 465
  antitumor antibiotics,
    465
  cervical, 467
  combination, 465
  cytotoxic agents and,
    464
  endometrial, 467
  neoadjuvant, 465
  ovarian, 467
  remission and, 464
  side effects, 465
  specific agents,
    465–466
  uterine, 468
  vulvar, 468
  for ovarian cancer, 451,
    467
Children
  gynecologic disorders
    in, 260–264
  incest and, 379
  sexual abuse of, 379,
    381
Chlamydia infection,
    289–292
  diagnosis, 290, 291
  genitourinary, 289
  incidence, 289, 290
  pelvic inflammatory
    disease and, 311
  prevalence, 289, 291
  symptoms, 290,
    291–292
  transmission, 289
  treatment, 290–291,
    292
Chlamydia psittaci, 289
Chlamydia trachomatis,
    58, 289, 290
Chlorambucil (Leukeran)
  chemotherapeutic
    agent in gyneco-
    logic cancer, 465
  for gestational tropho-
    blastic neoplasia,
    465
Chloramphenicol
  for pelvic inflammatory
    disease, 312
Chlorotrianisene (TACE)
  to suppress lactation,
    187
Choriocarcinoma
  gestational tropho-
    blastic disease
    and, 13, 15
Chorionic villus sam-
    pling (CVS), 223

for antepartum diagno-
    sis of fetal anom-
    alies, 212
  genetic screening and,
    218
Chromosomal abnorm-
    alities
  abortion and, 5
  genetic screening and,
    215
  gonadal dysgenesis
    and, 410
Chronic granulomatous
    disease
  DNA genetic screening
    and, 218
CIN. *See* Cervical intra-
    epithelial neoplasia
Ciprofloxacin
  for genital tuber-
    culosis, 320
Ciprofloxin
  for chancroid, 58
Circadian rhythm
  prolactin and, 388
Cirrhosis, 48
CIS. *See* Carcinoma in
    situ
Cis-dichlorodiammine-
    platinum
    (Cisplatin)
  chemotherapeutic
    agent in gyneco-
    logic cancer, 466
Cisplatin (Cis-dichlorodi-
    ammineplatinum)
  chemotherapeutic
    agent in gyneco-
    logic cancer, 466
Clindamycin, 7
  for *Chlamydia* infection,
    290
  for pelvic abscess, 315
  for pelvic inflammatory
    disease, 312
  for puerperal infections,
    195
  for vaginitis, 304
Clomiphene citrate
  for infertility, 349
Clomiphene citrate
  for anovulation, 354
Clostridia
  pelvic abscess and, 315
Clotrimazole
  for *Trichomonas
    vaginalis*, 56
CMV. *See*
    Cytomegalovirus
Coitarche, 360
Collagen vascular disease
  essential hypertension
    and, 29

Colpopexy, sacral, 243
Colpotomy
  for sterilization, 337
Computerized dosimetry
  in radiation therapy,
    459–460
Condom, 333
  female (vaginal pouch),
    333
  latex allergy to, 333
  protective role in sexu-
    ally transmitted
    diseases, 333
Condyloma acuminatum
    (venereal warts)
  during pregnancy,
    56–57
  treatment, 57
Congenital adrenal hyper-
    plasia (CAH)
  DNA genetic screening
    and, 218
  hirsutism and, 395,
    397–398
Congenital anomalies,
    261, 263
Conjunctivitis
  Chlamydia infection
    and, 290
Contraception
  adolescent use of, 87,
    361–362
  for advanced-age
    women, 91, 92
  barrier methods,
    333–336
    beneficial effects, 336
    cervical cap, 333, 334
    condom, 333
      latex allergy to, 333
      protective role in
      sexually trans-
      mitted diseases,
      333
    contraceptive
      sponge, 333
    diaphragm, 333–334
      contraindications,
      334
      effectiveness, 334
      side effects, 334
    effectiveness of, 333
    female condom (vagi-
      nal pouch), 333
    product information,
      335–336
    side effects, 333,
      333–335
    spermicides, 333
    chemical methods, 335
    spermicides and,
      333, 335
    teratogenicity, 335

diabetes mellitus and, 76
hormonal, 325–329
  benefits, 329
  cancer and, 326
  complications, 325–326
  contraindications, 326
  hypertension and, 325–326
  metabolic changes and, 327–328
  "morning-after" pill, 327
  pregnancy following, 327
  progestin only, 327
  protocol regimen, 326–327
  side effects of, 325, 328–329
intrauterine devices, 330–332
during lactation, 186
oral, 6
pelvic inflammatory disease and, 311
postcoital, 6
pregnancy failure rates, 325
sterilization, 336–340
Contraceptive sponge, 333
Contraction stress test (CST), 224
Convulsions
during eclampsia, 39–40
Cordocentesis, 223
  for antepartum diagnosis of fetal anomalies, 212
  genetic screening and, 219
Corticosteroids
  for delivery of small infants, 179–180
  for lichen sclerosis, 419
  for squamous cell hyperplasia, 419
CPD. See Cephalopelvic disproportion
Craniopharyngiomas, 388–389
Cromolyn sodium
  for asthma, 66
Cryopreservation, 350
CST. See Contraction stress test
Culdocentesis
  in ectopic pregnancy, 12
Cushing's syndrome
  hirsutism and, 395, 397–398

CVS. See Chorionic villus sampling
Cyclophosphamide (Cytoxan)
  chemotherapeutic agent in gynecologic cancer, 465
  treatment for gestational trophoblastic disease, 15
Cystadenomas, 445
Cystic fibrosis
  DNA genetic screening and, 218
  during pregnancy, 68, 70
Cystitis
  during pregnancy, 51–52
Cystocele, 241
Cystometrogram, 248
Cystoscopy, 247
Cystourethrocele, 241
Cysts
  benign ovarian neoplasms, 445–446
Cytomegalovirus (CMV)
  AIDS and, 297
  fetal effects of, 49
  during pregnancy, 49
  protective role of condoms, 333
Cytosarcoma phylloides, 477
Cystoscopy
  for evaluation of carcinoma of the cervix, 429–430
Cytoxan (Cyclophosphamide)
  chemotherapeutic agent in gynecologic cancer, 465–466
  treatment for gestational trophoblastic disease, 15

D
Dactinomycin (Actinomycin-D)
  chemotherapeutic agent in gynecologic cancer, 466
  treatment for gestational trophoblastic disease, 15
Danazol (Danocrine)
  for endometriosis, 257
Danocrine (Danazol)
  for endometriosis, 257
DCIS. See Ductal carcinoma in situ

Deep vein thrombosis (DVT), during pregnancy, 199–204
  complications, 202, 204
  described, 199
  diagnosis, 199–200, 203
  etiology, 199–200, 202–203
  incidence, 199
  mortality rates, 199
  risk factors, 201
  symptoms, 200
  treatment, 200–201, 203–204
Dehydroepiandrosterone sulfate (DHEAS)
  precocious puberty and, 392
Deladumone OB (Estradiol valerate)
  to suppress lactation, 187
Delivery. See also Breech presentation; Labor
  analgesia and anesthesia for, 157–160
  cesarean section. See Cesarean section
  eclampsia and, 40–41
  forceps extraction, 158, 160–163
  of large infants (macrosomia), 181–182
    cesarean section for, 180, 181
    risk factors, 181
    weight, 181–182
  of small infants, 179–181, 182
    cesarean section for, 180
    infection in, 180
    management, 180
    risk factors, 179–180
    vaginal delivery, 180
    weight, 181–182
  vacuum extraction, 161–162
  vaginal, spontaneous, 171
Demerol (Meperidine)
  for labor and delivery, 157
  during pregnancy, 126
Depo-Provera (Medroxyprogesterone acetate)
  chemotherapeutic agent in gynecologic cancer, 466

Depo-Provera (Medroxy-progesterone acetate) (contd.)
for dysfunctional uterine bleeding, 400
Depression
postpartum, 203–208
Dermoids, 446
Desogestrel
as hormonal contraceptive, 327
Dexamethasone
for delivery of small infants, 180
DGI. See Disseminated gonococcal infection
DHES. See Dehydroepiandrosterone sulfate
Diabetes mellitus
abortion and, 5
contraception and, 76
during pregnancy, 73–78
classification, 75
complications, 77–78
detection, 75, 76
essential hypertension and, 29
fetal surveillance, 76
management, 75, 76–77
monitoring during labor, 75
in the postpartum period, 75
preexisting, 75
sexuality and, 365
Diaphragm, 333–334
contraindications, 334
effectiveness, 334
side effects, 334
Diazepam (Valium)
contraindication for eclampsia, 40
Diet
breast cancer and, 475
benign breast disease and, 469
and premenstrual syndrome, 403
Diffuse papillomatosis, 471
Dilantin (Phenytoin sodium)
contraindication for eclampsia, 40
Dilation and curettage
endometrial hyperplasia and, 434
for termination of pregnancy, 6

Discriminatory zone, 12
Disseminated gonococcal infection (DGI), 278
Disseminated intravascular coagulopathy (DIC)
abruptio placentae and, 22–23
DNA
probes
for antepartum diagnosis of fetal anomalies, 212
genetic screening and, 218–219
radiation therapy damage and, 459
Donavania granulomatis, 58
Doppler velocimetry
fetal well-being and, 225, 226
Dosimetry
computerized in radiation therapy, 459–460
Down syndrome
genetic screening and, 216
Doxorubicin (Adriamycin)
chemotherapeutic agent in gynecologic cancer, 466
Doxycycline
for Chlamydia infection, 290
for gonorrhea, 278
for pelvic inflammatory disease, 312
for syphilis, 282
Drug abuse
AIDS and, 298
Dual-energy x-ray absorptiometry (DXA)
menopause and, 407
DUB. See Dysfunctional uterine bleeding
Duchenne muscular dystrophy
DNA genetic screening and, 218
Ductal carcinoma in situ (DCIS), 475–476
DVT. See Deep vein thrombosis
DXA. See Dual-energy x-ray absorptiometry
Dysfunctional uterine bleeding (DUB), 399–402

in adolescents, 400–401
complications, 401
conditions associated with, 400
definition, 399
etiology, 400
management, 401–402
menstruation cycle described, 399–400, 401
in perimenopausal women, 400
treatment, 400, 401
Dysmenorrhea, 253–255
definition, 251
diagnosis, 251
incidence, 251
PMS and, 251–252
primary, 251, 252
secondary, 251
symptoms, 251
treatment, 252
uterine fibroids and, 237
Dyspareunia, 373–377. See also Vaginismus
anorgasmy and, 374
definition, 374
diagnosis, 375–376
etiology, 375
incidence, 374
pain and, 375
symptoms, 374
treatment, 376
Dystocia, 168–171

E
Echocardiography
for antepartum diagnosis of fetal anomalies, 212
Eclampsia, 39–43. See also Hypertension, pregnancy-induced
complications, 39, 43
convulsions during, 39–40
definition, 39
delivery and, 40–41
diagnosis, 39, 42–43
etiology, 39, 42
hemorrhage and, 41
incidence, 39
mortality, 39
perinatal mortality, 39
postpartum, 39, 41
recurrence rate, 41
risk factors, 39
symptoms, 39, 41
treatment, 39–40
E. coli, 53

Ectopic pregnancy (EP),
   10–13
   causes, 11
   definition, 10
   diagnosis, 11
   incidence, 10–11
   IUDs and, 11
   mortality rate, 10
   PID and, 11
   risk factors, 11
   sonography and, 12
   symptoms, 11
   treatment
      nonsurgical, 12
      surgical, 12
Edema
   in pregnancy-induced
      hypertension, 34
Eisenmenger syndrome
   during pregnancy, 72
Elderly
   abuse of, 380
Embolectomy, 201–202
Embryoscopy
   for antepartum diagno-
      sis of fetal anom-
      alies, 212
Endocrine disorders
   amenorrhea, 385–388
   androgen insensitivity,
      412–415
   anovulation, 351–352
   dysfunctional uterine
      bleeding, 399–402
   gonadal dysgenesis,
      410–412
   hirsutism, 393–399
   hyperprolactinemia,
      388–390
   menopause, 406–410
   premenstrual syn-
      drome, 402–406
   puberty, precocious,
      391–394
   sexuality and, 365
Endometrial hyper-
      plasia, 433–437
   bleeding and, 433–435
   diagnosis, 433–435
   dilation and curettage
      for, 434
   diseases associated
      with, 434
   estrogen and, 434
   evaluation, 433–435
   incidence, 434
   management, 435
   menopause and, 434
   risk factors for, 434
   types, 433–434
Endometriosis, 256–260
   definition, 256

diagnosis, 256, 257, 259
etiology, 256, 258–259
incidence, 256
infertility and, 256,
   258, 349
laparoscopy and, 257
management, 257,
   259–260
pain and, 257
prognosis, 258
recurrence of, 257
symptoms, 256–257,
   259
treatment, 257
Endometrium
   carcinoma of, 438–441
      abnormal bleeding
         and, 438
      age as factor, 438
      associated diseases
         with, 438
      classification of, 438
      diagnosis, 438–439,
         440
      estrogen-related, 438
      histopathologic eval-
         uation, 439
      incidence, 438
      metastases, 438
      prognosis, 440–441
      progression, 439
      radiation therapy
         and, 462
      screening, 438–439
      staging, 438
      symptoms, 438–439
      treatment, 439, 440
Endomyometritis,
      193–195
   complications, 195
   risk factors, 194
   symptoms, 194
   treatment, 195
Endopelvic fascia, 242
Enoxacin
   for gonorrhea, 278
Enterobacter species, 53
Enterobius vermicularis,
   261
Enterocele, 241
Enterococcus, 195
EP. See Ectopic pregnancy
Epididymitis, 290
Epidural analgesia
   for cesarean section,
      164
   for labor and delivery,
      157
Episiotomy
   infection and, 195
Epithelial hyperplasia,
      470

Erythromycin
   for chancroid, 58
   for Chlamydia infection,
      290
   for gonorrhea, 278
   for pneumonia, 67
   for syphilis, 57
Escherichia coli
   following abortion, 7
   pelvic abscess and, 315
   postpartum, 194, 196
   during pregnancy, 66
Essential hypertension,
      in pregnancy,
      29–33
   complications, 31, 33
   counseling, preconcep-
      tion, 30
   diagnosis, 29, 32
   diuretics for, 30
   etiology, 29, 31–32
   evaluation, 30
   fetal surveillance in, 31
   incidence, 29
   management, 30
   perinatal mortality and,
      29
   pheochromocytoma,
      mortality rate
      and, 30
   PID and, 29
   risk factors of, 29
   small for gestational
      age (SGA) infants
      due to, 29
   symptoms, 29
   treatment, 30–31, 32–33
   versus pregnancy-
      induced hyper-
      tension (PIH), 29
Estradiol
   androgen insensitivity
      syndrome and, 413
Estradiol valerate
   (Deladumone OB)
   to suppress lactation,
      187
Estrogen
   adverse effects, 408
   anovulation and, 352
   breast cancer and, 474
   deprivation, long-term
      effects, 407
   for dysfunctional uter-
      ine bleeding, 401
   endometrial carcinoma
      and, 438
   endometrial hyper-
      plasia and, 434
   menopause and,
      407–408
   and premenstrual
      syndrome, 404

Estrogen (*contd.*)
  replacement therapy,
    407–408
  prolapse and, 243
Ethambutol
  for genital tuber-
    culosis, 320
  for tuberculosis, 68
Ethinyl estradiol
  as oral contraceptive,
    6, 325, 327
Ethynodial diacetate
  as hormonal contra-
    ceptive, 327
Etoposide (VP-16)
  chemotherapeutic
    agent in gyneco-
    logic cancer, 466
  treatment for gesta-
    tional tropho-
    blastic disease, 15
Exenteration, pelvic, 455,
    457
Exploratory celiotomy,
    455–456

F
Familial hyper-
    cholesterolemia
  DNA genetic screening
    and, 218
Fat necrosis, 470
Female condom (vaginal
    pouch), 333
Fetal anomalies
  antepartum diagnosis
    of, 211–214
  amniocentesis, 212
  chorionic villus
    sampling, 212
  cordocentesis, 212
  DNA probes, 212
  echocardiography in,
    212
  embryoscopy, 212
  fetal organ biopsy,
    212
  incidence, 211
  neural tube defect,
    211, 217–218
  genetic screening
    and, 217
  polymerase chain
    reaction (PCR),
    212
  prevention, 211
  prognosis, 214
  serum alpha-
    fetoprotein
    screening, 211
  sonographic screening
    for, 211

  techniques, 212,
    213–214
  therapy, 214
Fetal biophysical profile
    (BPP), 223–225
Fetal demise, 122–126
  antepartum, manage-
    ment of, 122–124
  coagulation studies in,
    123
  complications, 126
  detection of, 122
  diagnosis, 122, 125
  etiology, 123–125
  incidence, 122
  psychological reaction
    to, 123–124
  symptoms, 122
  treatment, 123, 125–126
Fetal distress, 175–179
  acid-base evaluation,
    177–178
  amniotic fluid and,
    176–177, 178
  described, 175–176
  heart rate, 176
  management, 176
  outcome, 177, 178–179
Fetal well-being, ante-
    partum assess-
    ment of, 223–226
  contraction stress test,
    224
  Doppler velocimetry,
    225, 226
  fetal biophysical profile,
    223–225
  maternal awareness of
    fetal activity, 224
  nonstress test, 224,
    225–226
  perinatal mortality rate,
    223
Fetus
  abnormal presentations
    of, 146–149
  breech presentation,
    143–146
  brow presentation,
    147, 148–149
  cesarean section for,
    147, 148
  compound presenta-
    tion, 148, 149
  diagnosis, 143
  etiology, 143
  face presentation,
    147, 148–149
  incidence, 147
  lie of, 146, 147, 148
  management, 147
  occipitoposterior
    position, 148, 149

  prolonged labor and,
    147
  risk factors, 147
  lung maturity, labora-
    tory tests for,
    226–231
  accuracy, 227
  lamellar body density
    test, 228–229
  L/S ratio, 227–228
  Lumadex Foam
    Stability Index,
    228
  phosphatidylglycerol,
    228
  sequential protocol
    for, 229
  strategies for, 229
  surfactant foam test,
    228
  Tdx FLM test, 229
  normal heart rate, 176
  organ biopsy, for ante-
    partum diagnosis
    of fetal anomalies,
    212
Fibroadenomas, 470
Fibrocystic changes, 469
Fibroids
  uterine, 237–241
  complications, 239
  described, 237
  diagnosis, 238, 240
  etiology, 237, 239–240
  features, 237
  management, 238,
    240–241
  outcome, 239
  pregnancy and, 238
  subserous, 237
  submucous, 237, 238
  symptoms, 237
  treatment, 238–239
Fibromas, 446
Fifth disease (human
    parvovirus B19),
    51
  diagnosis, 50
  infection rate, 50
  during pregnancy, 50
  symptoms, 50
FISH. *See* Fluorescence in
    situ hybridization
Fitz-Hugh-Curtis
    syndrome (peri-
    hepatitis), 278
5–Fluorouracil (5–FU)
  chemotherapeutic
    agent in gyneco-
    logic cancer, 466
  for human papillo-
    mavirus, 295

Flagyl (Metronidazole)
for pelvic abscess, 315
for pelvic inflamma-
tory disease, 312
for *Trichomonas
vaginalis*, 56
for vaginitis, 303, 304
FLM *See* Fetus, lung
maturity
Flow cytometry, 478
Fluorescence in situ hy-
bridization (FISH)
genetic screening and,
219
Folic acid
deficiency of, during
pregnancy, 109
genetic screening and,
217
Follicle-stimulating
hormone (FSH)
androgen insensitivity
syndrome and, 413
Forceps, types of, 158
Forceps extraction, 158,
160–163. *See also*
Vacuum extraction
categories of, 160
complications, 163
controversy regarding,
161
incidence, 161
indications, 160, 161,
162–163
prerequisites for, 161
Fragile X mental retarda-
tion, DNA genetic
screening and, 218
FSH. *See* Follicle-
stimulating
hormone

G
Galactoceles, 471
Galactorrhea
anovulation and, 353
Gamete intrafallopian
transfer (GIFT),
347
Gardnerella vaginalis, 53
Genetic counseling,
213–223
age as factor, 216
associations with
abnormal MSAFP
testing, 217
basic principles of,
213–215
breast cancer and, 482
diagnosis, 221
DNA analysis avail-
ability, 218

family history and, 216
indications for, 216
invasive testing, 218
methods, 216–219
objectives, 215
overview of disorders,
215–216
screening procedures
and, 215
sickle cell disease and,
110
Genetic disorders
androgen insensitivity
and, 412–413
Genital herpes. *See*
Herpes simplex
virus infection
Genital prolapse, 241
Genital tuberculosis.
See Tuberculosis,
genital
Genitalia, ambiguous, 413
Gentamycin, 7
for pelvic inflamma-
tory disease, 312
for premature ruptured
membranes, 118
for puerperal infections,
196
Gestational trophoblastic
disease (GTD),
13–18
chemotherapy for, 14,
15
choriocarcinoma in, 13,
15
complications, 15, 16–17
diagnosis, 13, 14, 16
etiology, 16
incidence, 13
management, 14, 15
metastatic, 13–15
molar pregnancy and,
13–14
nonmetastatic, 14
prognosis, 15, 17–18
radiotherapy, 15
remission, 14, 15
surgical treatment, 15
symptoms, 14
treatment, 14, 17
vaginal bleeding and,
14, 15
Gestational trophoblastic
tumors (GTTs), 13
Gestodene
as hormonal contra-
ceptive, 327
GIFT. *See* Gamete intra-
fallopian transfer
Glucocorticoids, anti-
inflammatory
for asthma, 66

Glucose-6–phosphate
deficiency
DNA genetic screening
and, 218
GnRH. *See* Gonadotropin-
releasing hormone
Goiter
during pregnancy,
78–79
Gonadal dysgenesis,
410–412
Bonnevie-Ullrich
syndrome, 410
chromosome abnor-
malities in, 410
definition, 410
diagnosis, 411
features, 410
forms of, 410–411
mosaicism and, 411
pregnancy and, 411
synthetic growth
hormone and, 411
treatment, 410
Gonadectomy, 414
Gonadotropin-releasing
hormone (GnRH)
for anovulation, 352,
354
for endometriosis,
257–258
hirsutism and, 396
for uterine fibroids, 239
Gonorrhea
complications, 279
described, 277
diagnosis, 278, 280
epidemiology, 279
incidence, 277
during pregnancy, 56,
278, 279
diagnosis, 56
incidence, 56
symptoms, 56
treatment, 56
follow-up, 278–279
rape and, 379
risk factors for, 277
symptoms, 277–278
transmission, 277, 278
treatment, 278,
280–281
Gonozyme test, 278
Grand multipara, 92–93,
94
definition, 92
mortality, 92
multiple gestation in,
93
uterine rupture in, 93
Granuloma inguinale
during pregnancy, 58

Granulomatous disease,
   chronic
   DNA genetic screening
   and, 218
Graves' disease
   during pregnancy, 79,
   80
GTD. See Gestational
   trophoblastic
   disease
GTTs. See Gestational
   trophoblastic
   tumors
Gynecology
   dysmenorrhea, 237,
      251–252, 253–255
   endometriosis, 256–260
   hysterectomy, 270–274
   hysteroscopy, 266–267,
      269
   laparoscopy, 263–266,
      267–269
   pediatric, 260–264
   pelvic pain, 252–254,
      255–256
   prolapse, 241–246
   stress incontinence,
      246–251
   uterine fibroids,
      237–241

H
Haemophilus ducreyi, 58
hCG. See Human chori-
   onic gonadotropin
HDN. See Hemolytic
   disease of the
   newborn
HELLP syndrome
   anemias during preg-
      nancy and, 109
   hypertension and,
      35–36
Hemoglobinopathies
   during pregnancy,
      108–113
Hemolytic disease
   anemias during preg-
      nancy, 109
   of the newborn (HDN),
      101
Hemophilia
   DNA genetic screening
      and, 218
Hemophilus influenzae,
      66, 67
Hemorrhage
   abortion and, 6–7
   abruptio placentae
      and, 21–25
   eclampsia and, 41
   ectopic pregnancy and,
      10–13

endometrial carcinoma
   and, 438
endometrial hyper-
   plasia and,
   433–435
gestational tropho-
   blastic disease
   and, 13–18
hysterectomy, post-
   operative bleeding
   and, 271
laparoscopy and, 266
placenta previa and,
   18–21
postpartum, 189–194
uterine, 441
Heparin
   for deep vein thrombo-
      sis, 200–201
   for puerperal infections,
      195
Hepatitis, acute viral, 50
   during pregnancy, 47
   symptoms, 47
   types, 47
Hepatitis B, 50
   during pregnancy, 47
   neonatal prophylaxis,
      47
   perinatal transmission,
      47
   protective role of
      condoms, 333
   transmission of, 47
Hepatitis C, 50
   diagnosis, 48
   during pregnancy,
      47–48
   risk factors, 47–48
   symptoms, 48
Herpes simplex virus
   infection (genital
   herpes), 50
   characteristics, 285,
      288
   diagnosis, 286, 288
   differential diagnosis,
      286
   etiology, 286
   incidence, 285
   neonatal infection, risk
      of, 48
   during pregnancy, 58,
      287
   prevention, 287
   protective role of
      condoms, 333
   psychological disability
      due to, 287
   recurrence of, 48, 285,
      286
   symptoms, 48, 285

transmission, 285, 287
   treatment, 48, 286–287,
      288–289
Herpes zoster (shingles),
      48
Hexamethylmelamine
   chemotherapeutic
      agent in gyneco-
      logic cancer, 466
Hirsutism, 393–399
   androgen secretion
      and, 393–395,
      396–397, 399
   classification, 395
   congenital, 397–398
   definition, 394
   evaluation, 393–395
   polycystic ovarian
      disease and, 398
   symptoms, 393–395
   treatment, 396,
      398–399
HIV. See Human immuno-
   deficiency virus
   infection
HMD. See Hyaline
   membrane disease
hMG See Human
   menopausal
   gonadotropin
Homosexuality, 368
Hormones
   chemotherapeutic
      agent in gyneco-
      logic cancer, 466
   during postpartum
      period, 205
Hormone therapy
   breast cancer and, 478
   to suppress lactation,
      187
HPV. See Human papil-
   loma virus
HSV. See Herpes simplex
   virus infection
Human chorionic gona-
   dotropin (hCG)
   benign ovarian neo-
      plasms and, 445
   and ectopic pregnancy,
      12
   in gestational tropho-
      blastic disease, 13
Human immunodeficiency
   virus infection
   (HIV), 51
   birth rate and, 49
   etiology, 49
   during pregnancy, 49
   protective role of
      condoms, 333
   syphilis and, 281

transmission, 49
treatment, 49
Human menopausal go-
    nadotropin (hMG)
    for infertility, 349
Human papilloma virus
    (HPV), 292–297
    carcinogenic potential
        of, 293–294
    cervical intraepithelial
        neoplasia and, 426
    classification, 293
    described, 294
    latent period, 294
    outcome, 293
    during pregnancy,
        56–57, 295, 296
    prevalence, 293
    recurrence, 294
    spectrum of disease,
        292–293
    symptoms, 293, 294
    treatment, 293–295,
        296–297
Human parvovirus B19
    (fifth disease, ery-
    thema infection),
    51
    diagnosis, 50
    infection rate, 50
    during pregnancy, 50
    symptoms, 50
Huntington's chorea
    DNA genetic screening
        and, 218
Hyaline membrane
    disease (HMD)
    cesarean section and,
        164
Hydramnios, 95–96,
    149–153
    chromosomal abnor-
        malities associ-
        ated with, 150
    complications, 150, 153
    definition, 149
    diagnosis, 150, 152
    etiology, 150, 152
    incidence, 150
    medical therapy, 150
    in multiple gestations,
        151
    treatment, 150, 153
Hydralazine
    for eclampsia, 40
    for pregnancy-induced
        hypertension, 35,
        36
Hydrocortisone
    for asthma, 66
    for thyroid disease
        during pregnancy,
        79

Hydronephrosis
    etiology, 52
    during pregnancy, 52
Hydroxyurea
    chemotherapeutic
        agent in gyneco-
        logic cancer, 466
Hyperbilirubinemia, 101
Hypercholesterolemia,
    familial
    DNA genetic screening
        and, 218
Hyperemesis gravidarum,
    130–134
    complications, 130, 134
    definition, 130
    diagnosis, 131, 133
    drug therapy for, 131
    etiology, 131, 133
    history, 131
    incidence, 131
    management, 132
    parenteral nutrition
        for, 131
    prognosis, 131
    symptoms, 131
    treatment, 131, 133–134
    versus morning sick-
        ness, 130–131
Hypernatremia
    abortion and, 6
Hyperplasia
    atypical ductal hyper-
        plasia, 470
    atypical lobular hyper-
        plasia, 470
    congenital adrenal,
        DNA genetic
        screening and, 218
    endometrial, 433–437
    epithelial, 470
    squamous cell, 419
Hyperprolactinemia,
    388–390
    described, 388
    etiology, 388
    evaluation, 389
    prolactin physiology,
        388, 389–390
    sexuality and, 364
    symptoms, 389
    treatment, 389, 390
Hypertension
    essential. See Essential
        hypertension, in
        pregnancy
    hormonal contracep-
        tion and, 325–326
    pregnancy-induced
        (PIH), 33–38. See
        also Eclampsia
    development, 34

diagnosis, 34, 37
    etiology, 33–34, 36
    HELLP syndrome
        and, 35–36
    hospitalization for,
        33–35
    incidence, 34
    invasive hemo-
        dynamic moni-
        toring and, 36
    management, 33–35
    mild, 34
    physiology, 34
    preeclampsia, 34
    proteinuria in, 34
    severe, 34
    symptoms, 34, 35
    treatment, 35–36,
        37–38
Hyperthyroidism
    during pregnancy, 79
Hypertonic saline
    for abortion induce-
        ment, 6
Hypnosis
    for labor and delivery,
        158
Hypoglycemia
    and premenstrual syn-
        drome, 402–403
Hypothalamic disorders,
    387
Hypothyroidism
    neonatal, 80
    during pregnancy, 78
Hysterectomy
    abdominal approach,
        270
    benign ovarian neo-
        plasms and, 446
    complications, 271,
        273–274
    counseling for, 270
    definition, 270
    emotional and psycho-
        sexual sequelae,
        271
    in gestational tropho-
        blastic disease, 14
    incidence, 270, 271
    management, 272
    postoperative bleeding,
        271
    procedure, 270, 271
    prolapse and, 243
    prophylactic antibi-
        otics and, 271
    radical (Wertheim),
        453–455, 456–457
    for sterilization, 270
    vaginal approach, 270
    vaginal vault and, 271

Hysterosalpingogram, 5
Hysterosalpingography, 239
Hysteroscopy, 266–267, 269
  complications, 266
  contraindications, 266
  definition, 266
  endometrial hyperplasia and, 435
  procedure, 266–267
Hysterosonography, 5

I
ICSI. See Intracytoplasmic sperm injection
IDA. See Iron deficiency anemia
Idiopathic hypertrophic subaortic stenosis (IHSS)
  during pregnancy, 72
Ifosfamide
  chemotherapeutic agent in gynecologic cancer, 466
IHSS. See Idiopathic hypertrophic subaortic stenosis
Imiquimod (Aldara)
  for condyloma acuminatum, 57
Immunoglobulin HBIG, 47
Implants, breast, 473–474
Incest, 379
Incontinence. See Stress incontinence; Urinary incontinence
Indomethacin
  for hydramnios, 150
  for preterm labor, 113–115
Infection
  acquired immunodeficiency syndrome (AIDS), 297–302
  Chlamydia, 289–292
  genital herpes. See Herpes simplex virus infection
  genital tuberculosis, 318–322
  gonorrhea, 56, 277–281
  herpes simplex virus infection, 47–48, 50, 58, 285–289
  human papilloma virus, 292–297
  in pediatric patients, 261

pelvic abscess, 313–318
pelvic inflammatory disease, 310–314
  during pregnancy, 59–61
  intrauterine, 49
  sexually transmitted diseases, 55–61
  urinary tract, 51–55
  venereal diseases, 55–61
  viral, 47–51
  puerperal, 193–199
  breast engorgement, 196
  respiratory, 195–196
  urinary tract, 196
  wound, 195
  syphilis, 57–58, 281–284
  toxic shock syndrome, 306–310
  vaginitis, 303–306
Infertility
  adoption and, 347
  anovulatory, 351–356
  artificial insemination and, 347–348
  couple, evaluation of, 343–344
  ovulatory dysfunction, 343, 344
  semen testing, 343, 344
  testing, 343
  therapy and, 343–344
  definition, 343
  diagnosis, 348
  endometriosis and, 256, 258
  female-associated, 348–351
  assisted reproductive technology, 350
  counseling, 348
  cryopreservation, 350
  endometriosis-associated, 349
  etiology, 348
  incidence, 348
  oocyte donation, 350
  ovulatory dysfunction, 349
  postcoital test and, 349–350
  therapy, 349
  treatment, 349
  tuboperitoneal factors, 348–349
  incidence, 345
  male-associated, 345–348

anti-sperm antibodies and, 346
  causes, 345
  diagnosis, 347
  incidence, 345
  endocrinologic-associated factors, 346–347
  evaluation, 345
  Klinefelter's syndrome and, 346
  laboratory evaluation, 345
  neurologic factors affecting, 346
  physical examination, 345
  semen analysis, 345
  testosterone levels and, 345–346
  treatment, 348
  varicoceles and, 346
  vasectomy, reversible effects of, 346
Influenza pneumonia
  during pregnancy, 67
Inheritance, genetic
  screening for, 216
Injuries, pediatric, 262
Intercourse
  painful, 368
Intracytoplasmic sperm injection (ICSI), 347
Intraductal papilloma, 471
Intrauterine devices (IUDs), 330–332
  complications, 330–332
  contraindications, 330
  described, 330
  ectopic pregnancy and, 11
  expulsion, 330
  insertion techniques, 330
  laparoscopy and, 264
  pelvic inflammatory disease and, 311, 332
  pregnancy with, 331, 332
  risk factors and, 330–331
  use of, incidence, 330
  vaginitis and, 303
Intrauterine growth restriction (IUGR), 133–139
  definition, 134
  etiology, 135, 137
  growth and evaluation of infant, 135–136
  incidence, 135

obstetric management, 135
postpartum management, 136
prenatal diagnosis, 135, 137–138
symptoms, 135
treatment, 136, 138–139
Intrauterine insemination (IUI), 346
Intrauterine pregnancy (IUP), 11
Intrauterine synechiae (Asherman's syndrome), 5, 191
In vitro fertilization (IVF), 347
In vitro fertilization, with embryo transfer (IVF-ET), 350
Iron deficiency anemia (IDA) during pregnancy, 109
Isoniazid
for genital tuberculosis, 320
for tuberculosis, 68
IUDs. See Intrauterine devices
IUGR. See Intrauterine growth restriction
IUI. See Intrauterine insemination
IUP. See Intrauterine pregnancy
IVF. See In vitro fertilization
IVF-ET. See In vitro fertilization, with embryo transfer

J
Jarisch-Herxheimer reaction, 282

K
Kaposi's sarcoma
AIDS and, 297
Kernicterus, 101, 126
Kidney disease, adult-onset polycystic
DNA genetic screening and, 218
Klebsiella pneumoniae, 66
postpartum, 194
Klebsiella species, 53
Klinefelter's syndrome
infertility and, 346

L
Labetalol
for hypertension during pregnancy, 30

Labial adhesion, 261
Labor. See also Breech presentation; Delivery
analgesia and anesthesia for, 157–160
calcium channel blockers for, 115
cephalopelvic disproportion, 171–175
failure to progress in (dystocia), 168–171
cephalopelvic disproportion and, 168–169
cervical dilatation, arrest of, 168
etiology, 169–170
management, 169, 170
outcome, 170–171
fetal distress, 175–179
normal, 171
preterm, 113–117
complications, 114
diagnosis, 113
incidence, 113
management, 114
neonatal problems, 114, 115, 116–117
risk factors for, 113, 115–116
testing, 113–114
treatment, 113–115, 116
progression, 171
stages of, 168
Lactation, 185–189. See also Breast-feeding
breast engorgement and, 186, 196
complications, 188–189
composition of human milk, 185
contraception during, 186
drug ingestion during, 186–187
energy cost of, 186
etiology, 187
hormones affecting, 185
management, 185–186, 188
milk supply during, 186
nutritional status of mother during, 185–186
oxytocin release and, 185
process of, 185
prolactin and, 185
suppression of, 187

Lactobacilli, 53
Lactogenesis
hyperprolactinemia and, 388
Lamellar body density test, for lung maturity testing, 228–229
Laparatomy
in ectopic pregnancy, 12
indications for exploratory, 451
staging, 456, 457–458
Laparoscopy
anesthesia and, 265, 267
complications, 265–266, 268–269
contraindications, 265
definition, 264
diagnostic purpose, 264
in ectopic pregnancy, 12
endometriosis and, 257
hemorrhage and, 266
incidence, 265
indications for use, 264
mortality rate, 265
procedure, 265, 267
for sterilization, 337
LCIS. See Lobular carcinoma in situ
Leiomyomatosis peritonealis disseminata, 238
Leiomyosarcomas, 441–442
age as factor in, 441–442
benign metastasizing, 238
diagnosis, 442
incidence, 238
malignancy, 238
postmenopause, 238
treatment, 442
Lesch-Nyhan disease
DNA genetic screening and, 218
LETZ. See Loop excision of the transformation zone
Leukeran (Chlorambucil)
chemotherapeutic agent in gynecologic cancer, 465
for gestational trophoblastic neoplasia, 465
Levothyroxine
for hypothyroidism, 79
LH. See Luteinizing hormone
Lichen sclerosus, 261, 419

Lidocaine
for labor and delivery,
157, 158
Ligaments
cardinal, 242
Mackenrodt's, 242
transverse cervical, 242
Lithotripsy
contraindication during
pregnancy, 52
Lobular carcinoma in situ
(LCIS), 476
lymph nodes and, 477
lymphangiosarcomas,
477
Lomefloxacin
for gonorrhea, 278
Loop excision of the
transformation
zone (LETZ), 427
Lumadex Foam Stability
Index, for lung
maturity testing,
228
Lupron
chemotherapeutic
agent in gyneco-
logic cancer, 466
Luteal phase deficiency
abortion and, 5
Luteinizing hormone (LH)
androgen insensitivity
syndrome and, 413
dysfunctional uterine
bleeding and, 399
Lymph nodes
breast cancer and, 477
Lymphangiosarcomas,
477
Lymphogranuloma
venereum
during pregnancy, 58
Lymphoma, non-
Hodgkin's
AIDS and, 297

M
Mackenrodt's ligaments,
242
Macrosomia, 181–182
cesarean section for,
180, 181
risk factors, 181
weight, 181–182
Magnesium gluconate
for preterm labor, 114
Magnesium sulfate
for eclampsia, 39
for placenta previa, 19
for pregnancy-induced
hypertension, 35
for preterm labor, 114

Malignant melanoma
carcinoma of the vulva
and, 423
Mammary duct ectasia
(plasma cell
mastitis), 471
Mammography
benign breast disease
and, 468–469
breast cancer and,
475–476
Marfan's syndrome
during pregnancy,
72–73
Marshall (Bonney) test,
247
Mastalgia
benign breast disease
and, 469–470, 473
Mastectomy, 478–479
modified radical,
478–479
radical, 479
simple, 478
Mastitis
plasma cell, 471
Maternal serum alpha-
fetoprotein
(MSAFP)
genetic screening and,
215
Medroxyprogesterone
acetate (Depo-
Provera; MPA)
chemotherapeutic
agent in gyneco-
logic cancer, 466
for dysfunctional uter-
ine bleeding, 400
Megace (Megestrol
acetate)
chemotherapeutic
agent in gyneco-
logic cancer, 466
Megestrol acetate
(Megace)
chemotherapeutic
agent in gyneco-
logic cancer, 466
Meigs syndrome, 446
Melanoma, malignant
carcinoma of the vulva
and, 423
Melphalan (Alkeran)
chemotherapeutic
agent in gyneco-
logic cancer, 465
Men
condom, protective role
in sexually trans-
mitted diseases,
333

contraception and, 333
erectile dysfunction
(impotence),
371–372
diagnosis, 371, 373
drug therapy, 372
etiology, 371
evaluation, 371
hormonal factors,
372
management, 371
premature ejacula-
tion, 372, 374
psychologic therapy,
372
therapy, 371–372
treatment, 373–374
infertility and, 345–348
anti-sperm anti-
bodies and, 346
causes, 345
diagnosis, 347
incidence, 345
endocrinologic-
associated
factors, 346–347
evaluation, 345
Klinefelter's syn-
drome and, 346
laboratory evalua-
tion, 345
neurologic factors
affecting, 346
physical examination,
345
semen analysis, 345
testosterone levels
and, 345–346
treatment, 348
varicoceles and, 346
vasectomy, reversible
effects of, 346
sexual response,
370–372
Menopause, 406–410
age of, 406
arteriosclerosis,
409–410
calcium replacement
therapy, 407
definition, 406–407
endometrial hyper-
plasia and, 434
estrogen deprivation,
long-term effects,
407
estrogen replacement
therapy, 407–408
adverse effects, 408
osteoporosis and, 407,
409
perimenopause and,
408

symptoms, 407
therapy, 407–408
Menorrhagia
uterine fibroids and,
237
Menstruation. *See also*
Premenstrual
syndrome
dysfunctional uterine
bleeding and,
399–402
irregular, hirsutism
and, 396
normal cycle described,
399–400, 401
Mental retardation
Fragile X, DNA genetic
screening and, 218
Meperidine (Demerol)
for labor and delivery,
157
during pregnancy, 126
Mesenchymal tumors,
477
Mestranol
as hormonal contra-
ceptive, 327
Metaproterenol
for asthma, 66
Methotrexate
abortion and, 6
chemotherapeutic
agent in gyneco-
logic cancer, 466
ectopic pregnancy and,
12
treatment for gesta-
tional trophoblas-
tic disease, 15
Methoxyflurane
for labor and delivery,
158
Methyldopa (Aldomet)
for hypertension dur-
ing pregnancy, 30
Methylprednisolone
for asthma, 66
Metronidazole (Flagyl)
for pelvic abscess, 315
for pelvic inflamma-
tory disease, 312
for *Trichomonas
vaginalis*, 56
for vaginitis, 303, 304
Mezlocillin
for puerperal infections,
195
for urinary tract infec-
tion in pregnancy,
53
$MgSO_4$
for eclampsia, 40

Mifepristone (RU-486)
as oral contraceptive, 6
for uterine fibroids,
239
Minilaparotomy
for sterilization, 337
Miscarriage, 5–10
Misoprostol
abortion and, 6
Mitral regurgitation
during pregnancy, 72
Mitral stenosis
during pregnancy, 72
Mixed mesodermal
sarcoma, 442–443
Molimina, 402. *See also*
Premenstrual
syndrome
Molluscum contagiosum
during pregnancy, 58
Mondor's disease, 471
Monosomy X, 5
Morphine
during pregnancy, 126
Mosaicism
gonadal dysgenesis and,
410
Moxalactam
for puerperal infections,
195
MPA. *See* Medroxypro-
gesterone acetate
Mucopurulent cervicitis,
290
Müller-Hillis maneuver,
168, 172
Multifetal gestations,
95–100
complications, 96–97,
100
diagnosis, 96, 98–99
etiology, 95, 98
evaluation, 96
gestational age verifi-
cation in, 97
hypertension in, 95–96
incidence, 95
intrapartum manage-
ment, 97
management, 96–97,
99–100
morbidity in, 95
mortality rate in, 95
nonstress testing in, 97
perinatal mortality in,
96
selective pregnancy
reduction, 96
symptoms, 96
zygosity in, 95
Multiparity, sterilization
and, 336

Multivitamins
for hyperthyroidism, 79
Muscular dystrophy
Becker's, DNA genetic
screening and, 218
Duchenne, DNA genetic
screening and, 218
*Mycobacterium tubercu-
losis*, 67–68, 318
Mycoplasma hominis, 311
Myocardial infarction
during pregnancy, 73
Myotonic dystrophy,
DNA genetic
screening and, 218

N
Nafcillin
for toxic shock
syndrome, 30
Narcotics
for labor and delivery,
157–158
Necrosis, fat, 470
Neisseria gonorrhoeae,
261, 277, 310–311
Neonatal viability
defined, 5
Neurofibromatosis (NF),
DNA genetic
screening and, 218
Nerve stimulation, tran-
scutaneous
for labor and delivery,
158
Neural tube defect (NTD),
211
genetic screening and,
217–218
Neuroendocrine failure
and anovulation, 353
NF. *See* Neurofibro-
matosis
NGU. *See* Nongonococcal
urethritis
Nifedipine
for hypertension dur-
ing pregnancy, 31
for preterm labor, 115
Nitrofurantoin
contraindication dur-
ing pregnancy, 53
for urinary tract infec-
tion in pregnancy,
53
Nitrous oxide
for labor and delivery,
158
Nongonococcal urethritis
(NGU), 289
Nonstress test (NST),
224, 225–226

Norethindrone
as hormonal contra-
ceptive, 327
Norethindrone acetate
as hormonal contra-
ceptive, 327
Norethynodrel
as hormonal contra-
ceptive, 327
Norfloxacin
for gonorrhea, 278
Norgestimate
as hormonal contra-
ceptive, 327
Norgestrel
as hormonal contra-
ceptive, 327
Norrie's disease
DNA genetic screening
and, 218
NST. See Nonstress test
NTD. See Neural tube
defect
Nutrition
breast cancer and, 475
benign breast disease
and, 469
and lactation, status of
mother during,
185–186
and premenstrual
syndrome, 403

O

Obsessive-compulsive
disorder
postpartum period
and, 205
Ofloxacin
for Chlamydia infection,
290
for pelvic inflamma-
tory disease, 312
Oligohydramnios, 151
Oncology, gynecologic.
See also Cancer
benign breast disorders,
468–474
benign ovarian neo-
plasms, 445–449
carcinoma of the
cervix, 429–433
carcinoma of the vulva,
422–425
cervical intraepithelial
neoplasia,
425–429
chemotherapy. See
Chemotherapy
endometrial, 438–441
endometrial hyper-
plasia, 433–437

malignant breast
disease, 473–482
non-neoplastic and
intraepithelial
neoplastic vulval
conditions,
419–421
ovarian cancer, 450–454
radiation therapy,
458–464
surgery, 453–458
uterine sarcoma,
441–445
Oncovin (Vincristine)
chemotherapeutic
agent in gyneco-
logic cancer, 466
treatment for gesta-
tional trophoblas-
tic disease, 15
Oocyte donation, 350
Orgasm
male, 370–374
anatomy, 370
erectile dysfunction
(impotence),
371–372
diagnosis, 371, 373
drug therapy, 372
etiology, 371
evaluation, 371
hormonal factors,
372
management, 371
premature ejacu-
lation, 372, 374
psychologic ther-
apy, 372
therapy, 371–372
treatment,
373–374
Ornithine transcarba-
mylase deficiency
DNA genetic screening
and, 218
Osteoporosis
menopause and, 407,
409
Otitis media
Chlamydia infection
and, 290
Outflow tract disorders,
387
Ovary(ies)
benign neoplasms of,
445–449
age as factor, 446
Brenner tumor,
445–446
cysts, 445–446
dermoids, 446
diagnosis, 446,
448–449

differential diagnosis,
446
etiology, 445
features, 446
fibroma, 446
functional, 447
hysterectomy and,
446
incidence, 445
management, 449
mucinous cysta-
denomas, 445
physical exam-
ination of, 446
prognosis, 447
serous cysta-
denomas, 445
symptoms, 445
treatment, 447
cancer of, 450–454
advanced disease and,
452
chemotherapy for,
451
classification of, 450
complications, 451
detection, 450, 453
etiology, 452
incidence, 450
indications for
exploratory
laparotomy, 451
management,
453–454
metastatic tumors
and, 450
oral contraceptives
and, 326
preoperative
workup, 451
prognosis, 451, 454
radiation therapy
and, 451, 461,
462
recurrence, 452
risk factors for, 452
staging, 450
surgery and, 451
tumor markers and,
450–451
disorders of, 387
Ovulatory dysfunction,
349
Oxacillin
for toxic shock
syndrome, 308
Oxytocin (Pitocin)
for abruptio placentae,
23
for breech presentation,
144
for cephalopelvic dis-
proportion, 172

for fetal demise, 123
grand multipara and,
93
hypertension and, 31, 35
lactation and, 185
for nonbreech abnormal
presentations, 147
for postpartum hemor-
rhage, 190

P

Paclitaxel (Taxol)
chemotherapeutic
agent in gyneco-
logic cancer, 466
Paget's disease, 476
Pain
chronic pelvic, 255–256
ectopic pregnancy and,
11–12
Papanicolaou (Pap)
smear
cervical cap and, 334
Papilloma, intraductal,
471
Papillomatosis, diffuse,
471
Paraphilia, 368
Parlodel (Bromocriptine
mesylate)
to suppress lactation,
187
Parvovirus B19 (fifth
disease, erythema
infection), 51
diagnosis, 50
infection rate, 50
during pregnancy, 50
symptoms, 50
Patent ductus arteriosus
(PDA)
during pregnancy, 72
PCOS. See Polycystic
ovarian syndrome
PCP. See Pneumocystis
carinii pneumonia
PDA. See Patent ductus
arteriosus
Pearl index, 333
Pediatric gynecology,
260–264
anesthesia and, 260, 262
congenital anomalies,
261, 263
in early childhood, 260
examination, 260
infection, 261
injuries, 262
labial adhesion, 261
lichen sclerosus, 261
in the newborn, 260
in the premenarche
period, 260

in puberty, 260
symptoms, 261
treatment, 261
tumors, 262, 263–264
uterine anomalies, 261
vaginal anatomy, 261
vulvar pruritus, 261
vulvovaginitis, 261, 263
Pelvic abscess, 313–318
complications, 315
described, 313–315
differential diagnosis,
315, 317
etiology, 313–315, 317
mortality rate, 315
pregnancy following,
316
rupture of, 315, 318
surgical management,
316
symptoms, 315, 316
treatment, 315–316,
317–318
Pelvic congestion, pelvic
pain due to, 253
Pelvic exenteration, 455,
457
Pelvic inflammatory
disease (PID),
310–314
ambulatory care, 312
Chlamydia infection
and, 290
definition, 310
ectopic pregnancy and,
11, 310, 312
etiology, 311, 313
gonorrhea and,
310–311
hospitalization for, 312
incidence, 310
infertility due to, 312
management, 311
risk factors for,
310–311
symptoms, 311,
313–314
therapy, 311–312, 314
types, 311
Pelvic pain, chronic,
255–256
age as factor in, 253
definition, 252
diagnosis, 253
evaluation, 253
management, 254
nerves and, 253
psychologic evaluation,
253
symptoms, 253
therapy, 253
treatment, 253

Penicillin
for puerperal infections,
195
for syphilis, 57, 282
for urinary tract infec-
tion in pregnancy,
53
Peptococcus, 193–195, 315
Peptostreptococcus,
193–195, 315
Percutaneous umbilical
blood sampling.
See Cordocentesis
Perihepatitis (Fitz-
Hugh-Curtis
syndrome), 278
Perimenopause
dysfunctional uterine
bleeding and, 400
menopause and, 408
Peritoneoscopy, 265
Pessaries, vaginal, 243
Phenergan
(Promethazine)
for hyperemesis
gravidarum, 131
Phenobarbitol
for hyperemesis
gravidarum, 131
Phenylketonuria (PKU)
DNA genetic screening
and, 218
Phenytoin sodium
(Dilantin)
contraindication for
eclampsia, 40
Phylloides tumor, 477
PID. See Pelvic inflam-
matory disease
PIH. See Hypertension,
pregnancy-induced
Piperacillin
for urinary tract infec-
tion in pregnancy,
53
Pitocin (Oxytocin)
abortion and, 6
for abruptio placentae,
23
for breech presentation,
144
for cephalopelvic
disproportion, 172
for fetal demise, 123
grand multipara and,
93
hypertension and, 31,
35
lactation and, 185
for nonbreech abnor-
mal presentations,
147

Pitocin (Oxytocin) (*contd.*)
for postpartum hemor-
rhage, 190
for premature rup-
tured membranes,
119
Pituitary disorders, 387
PKU. *See*
Phenylketonuria
Placenta previa, 18–21
cesarean section and,
18, 19
classification, 18
complications, 19, 21
definition, 18
diagnosis, 18–19, 20
etiology, 18, 20
incidence, 18
management, 19
outcome, 19
recurrence rate, 18
risk factors for, 18
symptoms, 18–19
treatment, 19, 21
vaginal bleeding and,
19
Plasma cell mastitis
(mammary duct
ectasia), 471
Plummer's disease
during pregnancy, 79
PMDD. *See* Premen-
strual dysphoric
disorder
PMS. *See* Premenstrual
syndrome
Pneumocystis carini
pneumonia (PCP),
67, 297
Pneumonia
during pregnancy,
66–67, 70
diagnosis, 66–67
risk factors, 66
symptoms, 66
treatment, 67
Podophyllin
contraindication dur-
ing pregnancy, 57
for human papillo-
mavirus, 294
Polycystic kidney disease,
adult onset
DNA genetic screening
and, 218
Polycystic ovarian
syndrome (PCOS)
anovulation and,
352–353, 355
dysfunctional uterine
bleeding and, 400
Pomeroy method of
sterilization, 337

Porphyria
during pregnancy, 109
Postpartum hemorrhage
(PPD). *See* Post-
partum period,
hemorrhage in
Postpartum period
depression during,
203–208
counseling for, 206
effect on family, 206
incidence, 204
management,
205–206
psychosocial risk
factors, 205
psychotherapy for,
205–206
symptoms, 203–205
treatment, 205–206
eclampsia and, 39, 41
hemorrhage in, 189–194
complications, 191,
193–194
definition, 189
diagnosis, 189, 192
etiology, 189, 191–192
acute puerperal
inversion, 191
blood dyscrasia, 189
uterine atony, 189
uterine inversion,
189
incidence, 189
management,
189–190
risk factors, 189
treatment, 190,
192–193
vaginal and cervical
lacerations,
190–191
obsessive-compulsive
disorder and, 205
Poststerilization
syndrome, 338
Posttraumatic stress
disorder
rape and, 378
PPD. *See* Postpartum
period, depression
during
PPH. *See* Postpartum pe-
riod, hemorrhage in
Prednisone
for asthma, 66
Pregnancy
abdominal, 11
in adolescents, 85–91
advanced maternal age
in, 91–94
AIDS and, 58–59

anemias during,
108–113
anesthesia during, 127
aortic regurgitation and,
72
aortic stenosis and, 72
ARDS and, 69, 70–71
asthma during, 65–66,
69–70
breast cancer and, 480
carcinoma of the cervix
and, 431
calcium channel block-
ers during, 30–31
cardiomyopathy during,
73
cardiovascular disease
during, 71–74
cervical, 11
condyloma acuminatum
(venereal warts)
and, 56–57
cystic fibrosis and, 68,
70
cytomegalovirus during,
49
diabetes mellitus
during, 73–78
ectopic. *See* Ectopic
pregnancy
fetal demise, 122–126
genital herpes and, 58
goiter and, 78–79
gonadal dysgenesis and,
410
gonorrhea and, 56
hemoglobinopathies
during, 108–113
hepatitis and, 47–48
herpes and, 48
HIV transmission and,
49
hormonal contracep-
tion prior to, 327
HPV virus and, 56–57
hyperemesis gravi-
darum in, 130–134
hypertension during,
29–33
infection during. *See*
Infection
influenza during, 67
intrauterine, 11
intrauterine growth
restriction in,
133–139
iron deficiency anemia
during, 109
labor, preterm,
113–117
mitral regurgitation
during, 72

mitral stenosis during,
72
molar, 13–14
multifetal, 95–100
multiple reduction, 6
parvovirus and, 50
patent ductus arterio-
sus and, 72
pneumonia and, 66–67,
70
postterm, 105–108
cervical status, 105
diagnosis, 105
examination, 105
fetal surveillance in,
106
incidence, 105
labor induction in,
106
management,
105–106,
107–108
maternal risks, 105
nonstress testing in,
105
perinatal mortality,
105
premature ruptured
fetal membranes
in, 117–122
prolapse and, 242
pulmonary disease and,
65–71
pyuria and, 53
RH isoimmunization
and, 101–104
rubella during, 47
shunts and, 72
sickle cell disease and,
109
smoking and, 34
spherocytosis and, 109
surgery during,
126–130
syphilis and, 57–58
termination. See
Abortion
thyroid disease and,
78–82
trauma during, 126–130
tuberculosis and, 67–68,
70
urinary tract infection
during, 51–55
uterine fibroids and,
238
vaginitis during, 303
valvular heart disease
and, 72
varicella during,
48–49, 67
x-rays during, 127

Premarin
for dysfunctional uter-
ine bleeding, 401
Premature ruptured
fetal membranes
(PROM), 117–122
complications, 118–119,
121
diagnosis, 117–118, 120
etiology, 117, 119–120
evaluation, 117–118
fetal morbidity, 117
incidence, 117
labor induction and, 119
management, 118,
121–122
neonatal outcome, 118
preterm delivery, 117
risk factors for, 117
treatment, 118, 120
Premenstrual dysphoric
disorder (PMDD),
402
Premenstrual syndrome
(PMS), 402–406
anovulation and, 403
diagnosis, 402
dietary therapy, 403
disorders mimicking,
403
etiology, 402–403
pathogenesis, 403
pathophysiology, 403,
403–405
symptoms, 402
therapy, 403–404,
405–406
Proctitis, 290
Progestin
for dysfunctional uter-
ine bleeding, 401
as hormonal contra-
ceptive, 327
Progesterone
during pregnancy, 65
measurement, 5
Progestins
chemotherapeutic
agent in gyneco-
logic cancer, 466
Prolactin
for anovulation, 353
hyperprolactinemia
and, 388, 389–390
lactogenesis and, 388
Prolactinoma, 388
Prolapse, 241–246
complications, 242
diagnosis, 242–243,
243–245
etiology, 242, 244
genital, defined, 241,
244

medical therapy, 245
postoperative care, 242
pregnancy and, 242
stress urinary inconti-
nence, 242
surgical procedures,
242, 245–246
symptoms, 242
treatment, 242
PROM. See Premature
ruptured fetal
membranes
Promethazine
(Phenergan)
for hyperemesis
gravidarum, 131
Propranolol
for thyroid disease
during pregnancy,
79–80
Propylthiouracil (PTU)
for hyperthyroidism,
79
Prostaglandin $F_{2\alpha}$
abortion and, 6
postpartum hemor-
rhage and, 190
Prostaglandin E_1 (PGE$_1$),
6
Prostaglandin E_2 (PGE$_2$),
6
Prostatitis, 290
Proteus mirabilis, 53
Pseudohermaphrodism,
413
Pseudomonas
aeruginosa, 68
Psychoprophylaxis
for labor and delivery,
158
PTU. See
Propylthiouracil
Puberty. See also
Adolescents
precocious, 391–394
classification, 391
described, 391
diagnosis, 391–392
etiology, 391
incidence, 391
LHRH-dependent,
392
LHRH-independent,
392
premature adrenar-
che, 392
treatment, 392, 394
PUBS. See Cordocentesis
Puerperal infections,
193–199
complications, 198–199
diagnosis, 197

Puerperal infections,
(contd.)
etiology, 197
fever and, 194
risk factors and, 194
symptoms, 194
treatment, 197–198
Pulmonary disease
during pregnancy,
65–71
Pulmonary embolism,
201–202
Pyelonephritis, acute
during pregnancy, 52
symptoms, 52
Pyrazinamide
for genital tuber-
culosis, 320
for tuberculosis, 68
Pyrid
for tuberculosis, 68
Pyuria
during pregnancy, 53
functional residual
capacity (FRC),
65
pulmonary function
testing, 65

Q
Q-tip test, 247
Quinolones
contraindication dur-
ing pregnancy, 53
for gonorrhea, 278

R
Radial sclerosing lesions
(radial scars), 470
Radiation therapy,
458–464
for breast cancer, 476,
479
for cervical cancer,
430–431, 460–461,
461–462
complications, 460, 463
computerized dosime-
try in, 459–460
described, 458
DNA damage and, 459
dosage required, 458
for endometrial cancer,
462
intensity variation,459
management, 460
for ovarian cancer,
451, 461, 462
radiosensitivity to,
458–459
recurrent cancer and,
461
side effects, 460

small bowel problems
and, 460
tolerance to, 459
treatment time, 460
urinary tract problems
and, 460
for vaginal cancer, 461,
462
vaginal response to, 460
for vulvar cancer, 462
Radical hysterectomy
(Wertheim),
453–455, 456–457
Radiotherapy
for breast cancer, 479
Rape, 377–382
evaluation of victim,
378, 380
incidence, 378
posttraumatic stress
disorder and, 378
sexually transmitted
diseases and, 379
Rapid plasma reagin
(RPR) test
for syphilis, 282
Rathke's pouch, 388–389
RDS. See Respiratory
distress syndrome
Reciprocal translocation,
5
Rectocele, 241
Renal disease
essential hypertension
and, 29
Renal ultrasound imaging,
247
Respiratory distress syn-
drome (RDS), 227
Respiratory infection,
195–196
diagnosis, 195–196
risk factors for, 195
symptoms, 195
treatment, 196
Retinoblastoma, DNA
genetic screening
and, 218
Retropubic urethro-
cystopexy, 243
RH isoimmunization,
101–104
amniocentesis and, 102
complications, 101, 104
Coomb's test for, 101
diagnosis, 101, 103
etiology, 103
fetal monitoring, 102
incidence, 101
management, 102,
103–104
premature delivery
and, 102

prevalence, 101
prophylaxis, 104
Rifampin
for Chlamydia infection,
290
for genital tuberculosis,
320
for tuberculosis, 68
Ritrodrine
for preterm labor, 114
Robertsonian trans-
location, 5
RPR. See Rapid plasma
reagin
Rubella
during pregnancy, 47
immunity to, 211
vaccine, contraindica-
tion during preg-
nancy, 47

S
Sacral colpopexy, 243
Saddle block
for labor and delivery,
158
Salpingectomy
in ectopic pregnancy,
12
partial, sterilization
and, 337
Salpingitis isthmica
nodosa
Chlamydia infection
and, 290
and ectopic pregnancy,
11
Salpingostomy
in ectopic pregnancy, 12
Sarcoma
mixed mesodermal,
442–443
stromal, 442
uterine, 441–445
Scirrhosis carcinoma,
476
Sclerosing adenosis, 470
Septic pelvic throm-
bophlebitis, 195
diagnosis, 202
symptoms, 195
treatment, 195, 202
Serotinergic transmission
and premenstrual
syndrome, 403
Serotonin reuptake
inhibitors (SSRIs)
postpartum period
and, 206
Serum alpha-fetoprotein
screening (AFP),
211

Sex hormone-binding
    globulin (SHBG)
    hirsutism and, 395
Sexual abuse
    of children, 379, 381
    domestic battering
        and, 379–380
    of the elderly, 380
    incidence, 379
Sexual assault, 377. See
    also Rape
Sexual deviation, 378
Sexual dysfunction
    counseling and, 368
    female, 367
    following sterilization,
        338
    therapy, 368
    treatment, 368
Sexual offense, 379
Sexual response
    male, 370–372
    female, 367
Sexuality
    adolescent, 359–363
    aging process and,
        363–364, 365
    alterations and,
        363–365
    drugs and, 363–365,
        366
    dyspareunia, 373–377
    illness and, 365, 366
    rape and, 377–382
    sexual assault, 377
    treatment, 365
    vaginismus, 376, 377
Sexually transmitted dis-
    eases (STDs)
    acquired immunodefi-
        ciency syndrome
        (AIDS), 297–302
    Chlamydia infection,
        289–292
    genital tuberculosis,
        318–322
    gonorrhea, 56, 277–281
    herpes simplex virus
        infection (genital
        herpes), 50,
        285–289
    human papilloma
        virus, 292–297
    during pregnancy,
        55–61
    protective role of
        condoms, 333
    rape and, 379
    syphilis, 57–58,
        281–284
    vaginitis, 303–306
Sheehan's syndrome, 191,
    389

Shingles (Herpes zoster),
    48
Shunts
    during pregnancy, 72
Sickle cell disease (SCD)
    DNA genetic screening
        and, 218
    genetic counseling, 110
    during pregnancy, 109
Sigmoidoscopy
    for evaluation of carci-
        noma of the cervix,
        429–430
SIL. See Squamous intra-
    epithelial lesion
Small bowel
    radiation therapy,
        problems and, 460
Smoking, cigarette
    hypertension during
        pregnancy and, 34
Sodium amobarbital
    (Amytal)
    for eclampsia, 40
Sonography
    ectopic pregnancy and,
        12
Spectinomycin
    for gonorrhea, 278
Spherocytosis
    during pregnancy, 109
Squamocolumnar
    junction, 425
Squamous cell hyper-
    plasia, 419
Squamous intraepithelial
    lesion (SIL), 426
Squamous metaplasia,
    425
SSRIs. See Serotonin re-
    uptake inhibitors
Staging laparotomy, 456,
    457–458
Staphlococcus aureus
    breast engorgement
        and, 196
    breast infection and,
        471
    toxic shock syndrome
        and, 307
Staphylococcus sapro-
    phyticus, 53
STDs. See Sexually
    transmitted
    diseases
Sterilization, 336–340
    benefits, 339
    complications, 337,
        339–340
    counseling, 339
    definition, 336
    experimental methods,
        338, 339

failure rates, 337–338
    incidence, 336
    indications, 336
    interval, 337
    laparoscopy, 337
    long-term effects, 338
    during postpartum
        period, 337
    poststerilization
        syndrome, 338
    reversal of, 338
    safety, 338
    sexual dysfunction
        following, 338
    techniques, 336–337
Streptococcus pneumo-
    niae, 67
    pelvic abscess and, 315
    postpartum, 195
Streptomycin
    for genital tuber-
        culosis, 320
Stress incontinence,
    246–251
    definition, 246
    diagnosis, 247, 250
    examination, 247–248
    etiology, 246, 247
    surgical treatment, 249
    symptoms, 247
    testing, 247
        cystometrogram, 248
        cystoscopy, 247
        Marshall (Bonney),
            247
        Q-tip, 247
        renal ultrasound
            imaging, 247
        urethroscopy, 247
    therapy, 248, 250–251
    urethral pressure and,
        248
Stromal sarcoma, 442
SUI. See Urinary inconti-
    nence, stress
Sulfa-methoxazole-
    trimethoprim
    for Chlamydia infection,
        290
Sulfonamides
    during pregnancy, 126
Surfactant foam test, for
    lung maturity, 228
Surgery. See also
    Cesarean section;
    Hysterectomy
    in cancer treatment,
        453–458
    complications, 455
    exploratory celiotomy,
        455–456
    mortality rate, 455

Surgery (*contd.*)
  pelvic exenteration,
    455, 457
  radical hysterectomy
    (Wertheim),
    453–455,
    456–457
  risk factors for, 456
  staging laparotomy,
    456, 457–458
  during pregnancy,
    126–130
Syntocinon
  let-down reflex and, 186
Synthetic growth
  hormone, 411
Syphilis
  blood tests for, 282
  diagnosis, 281,
    283–284
  epidemiology, 283
  etiology, 281
  follow-up, 283
  incidence, 281
  incubation period, 281
  latent, 281
  during pregnancy,
    57–58, 282–283
  congenital, 57
  effect on fetus, 57
  incidence, 57
  perinatal, 284
  symptoms, 57
  testing, 57
  treatment, 57–58
  rape and, 379
  secondary, 281
  tertiary, 281
  transmission, 281
  treatment, 282, 283
Systemic lupus erythe-
  matosis
  abortion and, 5

T
TACE. *See*
  Chlorotrianisene
Tamoxifen
  chemotherapeutic
    agent in gyneco-
    logic cancer, 466
Tampons, toxic shock
  syndrome and, 308
Taxol (Paclitaxel)
  chemotherapeutic
    agent in gyneco-
    logic cancer, 466
Tay-Sachs disease
  DNA genetic screening
    and, 218
Tdx FLM test, for lung
  maturity, 229

Terbutaline
  for asthma, 66
  for preterm labor, 114
Testosterone enanthate
  to suppress lactation,
    187
Testosterone
  androgen insensitivity
    syndrome and, 413
  hirsutism and, 394
  infertility and,
    345–346
Tetanus toxoid
  during pregnancy,
    126–127
Tetracycline
  for *Chlamydia* infection,
    290
  contraindication during
    pregnancy, 53, 126
  for gonorrhea, 278
  for pelvic inflammatory
    disease, 312
Tetralogy of Fallot, 72
Thalassemia
  DNA genetic screening
    and, 218
  during pregnancy,
    109–110
Theophylline
  for asthma, 66
Thermography
  for deep vein thrombo-
    sis during preg-
    nancy, 200
Thiazides
  sexuality and, 364
Thyroid disease
  abortion and, 5
  during pregnancy,
    78–82
  characteristics, 78
  complications, 82
  diagnosis, 79, 81–82
  etiology, 78–79,
    80–81
  prognosis, 79
  symptoms, 79
  treatment, 79, 82
Thyroid-releasing hor-
  mone (TRH), 388
Thyroid-stimulating
  hormone (TSH), 5
  hyperprolactinemia
    and, 388–389
Thyrotoxicosis
  in the newborn, 80
Thyroxine
  for hypothyroidism, 79
Tissue sampling, breast,
    469, 472–473
TOA. *See* Tuboovarian
  abscess

Tocolysis
  contraindications to,
    114
Toxic shock syndrome
  (TSS), 306–310
  complications, 308
  definition, 307
  diagnosis, 307
  diaphragm and, 334
  etiology, 307, 309
  incidence, 307
  menstruation and,
    307–308, 309
  organ system involve-
    ment in, 308
  recurrence, 308
  symptoms, 307–308
  treatment, 308
Toxic streptococcal syn-
  drome, 309, 310
Toxoplasmosis
  AIDS and, 297
Transcutaneous nerve
  stimulation
  for labor and delivery,
    158
Transitional zone (TZ),
    425
Trauma, during preg-
  nancy, 126–130
  adnexal mass, 128
  appendicitis, 127
  drug treatment,
    126–127
  electric shock, 128
  fetal assessment,
    128–129
  gallbladder disease,
    127–128
  gunshot wound, 128
  incidence, 128
  laboratory evaluation,
    127
  laparatomy, 127, 128
  motor vehicle accidents,
    128
  physical abuse, 128
  small-bowel obstruction,
    128
  stabbing, 128
  thermal injury, 128
  Treponema pallidum, 57,
    281
TRH. *See* Thyroid-
  releasing hormone
Triamcinolone
  for asthma, 66
Trichloroacetic acid
  for human papillo-
    mavirus, 295
Trichomonas vaginalis,
    303

during pregnancy, 56
  prevalence, 56
  risk factors, 56
  symptoms, 56
  treatment, 56
Triploidy, 5
TSH. See Thyroid-
  stimulating
  hormone
TSS. See Toxic shock
  syndrome
Tubal ligation
  for sterilization, 11
Tuberculosis
  genital, 318–322
    age as factor in, 318
    AIDS and, 319
    diagnosis, 319–320,
      321
    family history of, 319
    incidence, 318–319
    infertility due to, 319,
      320
    patient workup, 320
    physical examination,
      319
    pregnancy and, 320
    surgical intervention,
      320
    therapy, 320,
      321–322
    treatment, 319, 320
  pelvic, 318
  during pregnancy,
    67–68, 70
Tuboovarian abscess
  (TOA), 315
Turner's syndrome, 410
  genetic screening and,
    216
21–hydroxylase deficiency
  DNA genetic screening
    and, 218
Twilight sleep
  for labor and delivery,
    158
Twins
  abnormal presenta-
    tions, 146
TZ. See Transitional zone

U
Ultrasound
  genetic counseling and,
    216–217, 221–222
Ureaplasma urealyticum,
  53, 311
Urethral syndrome (fre-
  quency-urgency
  syndrome), 51–52
Urethrocystopexy,
  retropubic, 243
Urethroscopy, 247

Urinary incontinence,
  stress
  prolapse and, 242
Urinary status
  during pregnancy, 52
Urinary tract infection
  (UTI)
  diaphram and, 334
  during pregnancy,
    51–55
    asymptomatic, 51
    complications,
      52–53, 55
    diagnosis, 52–53,
      53–55
    etiology, 52, 54
    prevention, 51, 53
    recurrence, 51
    symptomatic, 51–52
    treatment, 53, 55
  puerperal, 196
    diagnosis, 196
    symptoms, 196
    treatment, 196
    radiation therapy and,
      460
Uterine atony
  postpartum hemor-
    rhage and, 189
Uterine curettage
  in ectopic pregnancy,
    12
Uterine fibroids,
  237–241
Uterine inversion
  postpartum hemor-
    rhage and, 189
Uterus
  Couvelaire, 22
  malformation, 5
  sarcoma of, 441–445
    abnormal uterine
      bleeding and,
      441
    classification, 441,
      443
    described, 441
    diagnosis, 442
    incidence, 442
    metastases, 442
    postmenopause and,
      442
    survival rate, 443
    symptoms, 441
    therapy, 443
    treatment, 442,
      443–445
UTI. See Urinary tract
  infection

V
Vacuum extraction,
  161–162. See also
  Forceps extraction

advantages, 161–162
  contraindications, 162
  disadvantages, 162
  indications, 162
Vaginal cancer
  radiation therapy and,
    460, 461, 462
Vaginal hysterectomy
  prolapse and, 243
Vaginal pessaries, 243
Vaginal pouch (female
  condom), 333
Vaginismus, 376, 377.
  See also
  Dyspareunia
  described, 376
  etiology, 376
  symptoms, 376
  therapy, 377
Vaginitis, 303–306
  allergic and chemical,
    305
  Candida albicans,
    303–304
  diagnosis, 303, 305–306
  epidemiology, 305
  etiology, 303
  incidence, 304
  during pregnancy, 303
  symptoms, 303, 304
  transmission, 303
  treatment, 304, 306
Valium (Diazepam)
  contraindication for
    eclampsia, 40
Valvular heart disease
  during pregnancy, 72
Vancomycin
  for toxic shock syn-
    drome, 308
Varicella, during preg-
  nancy
  diagnosis, 49
  incidence, 48
  incubation period, 48
  neonatal mortality
    and, 49
  pneumonia, 67
  treatment, 49
  vaccination for, 49
Varivax
  contraindication dur-
    ing pregnancy, 49
Vascular disease
  sexuality and, 365
Vasectomy, reversible
  effects of, 346
VDRL. See Venereal
  Disease Research
  Laboratory test
Venereal diseases. See
  Sexually transmit-
  ted diseases

Venereal Disease Research Laboratory (VDRL) test, for syphilis, 282
Ventricular septal defect (VSD) during pregnancy, 72
VIN. See Vulval intraepithelial neoplasia
Vinblastin chemotherapeutic agent in gynecologic cancer, 466
Vinca plant alkaloids chemotherapeutic agent in gynecologic cancer, 466
Vincristine (Oncovin) chemotherapeutic agent in gynecologic cancer, 466 treatment for gestational trophoblastic disease, 15
Virilism, 393–399
Vitamin B complex for hyperemesis gravidarum, 131
Vitamin B₆ for hyperemesis gravidarum, 131
Vitamin C for hyperemesis gravidarum, 131
Vitamin E for breast feeding, 196
Von Willebrand's disease DNA genetic screening and, 218
VP-16 (Etoposide) chemotherapeutic agent in gynecologic cancer, 466

treatment for gestational trophoblastic disease, 15
VSD. See Ventricular septal defect
Vulva carcinoma of, 422–425 age and, 422 conditions associated with, 423 diagnosis, 422 differential diagnosis, 422 etiology, 424 malignant melanoma and, 423 metastasis and, 422 pathology, 424 preoperative workup, 422 prognosis, 423 radiation therapy and, 462 staging system for, 422 surgery for, 423 symptoms, 422 therapy, 423 treatment, 423, 423–425 vulvar intraepithelial neoplasia and, 422 non-neoplastic and intraepithelial neoplastic conditions, 419–421 classification of, 419–420 diagnosis, 419 dermatoses of, 419 symptoms, 419 treatment, 419, 420

Vulval intraepithelial neoplasia (VIN), 419–421 diagnosis, 419 recurrence, 420 symptoms, 419, 420 treatment, 419, 420
Vulvar pruritus, 261
Vulvar vestibulitis syndrome, 420, 421
Vulvodynia, 419
Vulvovaginitis, 261, 263

W
Warfarin for deep vein thrombosis, 201
Wertheim hysterectomy, 453–455, 456–457
Wound infections, 195 diagnosis, 195 morbidity and mortality, 195 symptoms, 195 treatment, 195

X
X-linked recessive traits genetic screening and, 216
X-rays during menopause, 407 during pregnancy, 127

Z
Zidovudine (AZT) for HIV, 49–50, 59
ZIFT. See Zygote intrafallopian transfer
Zygote intrafallopian transfer (ZIFT), 347, 350

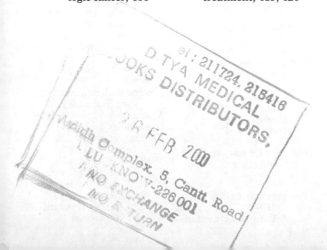